Novel Developments in Stem Cell Mobilization

Stefan Fruehauf • W. Jens Zeller • Gary Calandra
Editors

Novel Developments in Stem Cell Mobilization

Focus on CXCR4

Springer

Editors
Stefan Fruehauf
Center for Tumor Diagnostics and Therapy
Paracelsus Klinik
Osnabrueck, Germany
prof.stefan.fruehauf@pk-mx.de

W. Jens Zeller
German Cancer Research Center
Heidelberg, Germany
j.zeller@dkfz.de

Gary Calandra, MD, PhD
Private Consultant, Cresco, PA, USA
calandra@sunlink.net

ISBN 978-1-4614-1959-4 e-ISBN 978-1-4614-1960-0
DOI 10.1007/978-1-4614-1960-0
Springer New York Dordrecht Heidelberg London

Library of Congress Control Number: 2011945168

Printed on acid-free paper

Springer is part of Springer Science+Business Media (www.springer.com)

Preface

Systemic cancer treatment led to increasing survival rates and even cures in an impressive number of tumor types within the last five decades, especially in patients with high-growth-fraction tumors benefitted from this development.

Autologous transplantation of bone marrow or peripheral blood hematopoietic stem and progenitor cells (PB HSC/HPC) following high-dose chemotherapy allowed an up to sixfold increase in dose intensity and was a further milestone enabling cure or long-term disease control in lymphoma, myeloma, and solid tumors. Introduction of cytokines (e.g., G-CSF) in the 1980s significantly improved PB HSC/HPC collection for blood stem cell transplantation. Since then, no significant progress beyond chemotherapy-supported and cytokine-based HSC/HPC mobilization had been made.

In the early 1990s, AMD3100, now plerixafor—chemically a bicyclam—was originally developed as an anti-HIV drug; the chemokine receptor CXCR4 was identified as the target for plerixafor. In the late 1990s, CXCR4 was discovered as a crucial factor for HSC/HPC retention in the bone marrow. As with a considerable number of drugs, serendipity played a decisive role in elucidating the potency of plerixafor for HSC/HPC mobilization: in HIV-infected patients plerixafor induced an unexpected dose-dependent leukocytosis and in healthy volunteers it was found that these increased peripheral blood mononuclear cells were enriched by $CD34^+$ HSC/HPC. Subsequently, it became clear that the number of patients who can profit from PB HSC/HPC transplantation could be increased since older patients and poor mobilizers following standard mobilization strategies (G-CSF, chemotherapy) also showed increased numbers of circulating $CD34^+$ HSC/HPC after addition of plerixafor. This action and the synergism of plerixafor with G-CSF led to the clinical approval of plerixafor as a first in class compound for mobilization of HSC/HPC. The amount of HSC/HPC mobilization and the rapid kinetics compare favorably with classical mobilization protocols and are a quantum leap for hard-to-mobilize patients who now become eligible for potentially curative treatment.

Increased HSC/HPC mobilization by compounds interacting with their adhesion in bone marrow niches is a substantial step toward improvement of PB HSC/HPC transplantation, so that meanwhile, further compounds with potent mobilizing capacity were developed and are presently in clinical phase I and II trials.

An exciting new role for CXCR4 inhibitors emerged by the discovery that cells of different tumor types—leukemias and solid tumors—express CXCR4 as well and that SDF-1–CXCR4 interaction is involved in adhesion and movement of cancer cells. Although there are concerns regarding side effects to normal cells, it is a fascinating idea for oncologists that mobilization of tumor cells (e.g., by interruption of the SDF-1–CXCR4 axis) could someday eliminate the threat of minimal residual disease, since mobilization of MRD cells from protective niches to the blood might increase their chemotherapeutic sensitivity.

Last but not least, use of CXCR4 antagonists in tissue repair and in inflammatory diseases has led to exciting new approaches that will be reviewed in this book, too.

Finally, we would like to express our thanks to all contributors, who facilitated a timely publication of this book and we are greatly obliged to Springer for their competent support.

Osnabrueck, Germany — Stefan Fruehauf
Heidelberg, Germany — W. Jens Zeller
Cresco, PA, USA — Gary Calandra

Contents

Contributors

Anupriya Agarwal Division of Hematology and Medical Oncology, Oregon Health & Science University, Knight Cancer Institute, Portland, OR, USA

George Ansstas Division of Oncology, Siteman Cancer Center, Washington University School of Medicine, St. Louis, MO, USA

Linda J. Bendall Westmead Institute for Cancer Research, Westmead Millennium Institute, University of Sydney, Westmead, NSW, Australia

Kenneth Bradstock Westmead Institute for Cancer Research, Westmead Millennium Institute, University of Sydney, Westmead, NSW, Australia

Hal E. Broxmeyer Department of Microbiology and Immunology, Indiana University School of Medicine, Indianapolis, IN, USA

Jan A. Burger Department of Leukemia, Unit 428, The University of Texas M.D. Anderson Cancer Center, Houston, TX, USA

Eike C. Buss Department of Internal Medicine V, Heidelberg University Hospital, Heidelberg, Germany

Nelson J. Chao Division of Cellular Therapy/BMT, Duke University, Durham, NC, USA

Eric Chevalier Polyphor Ltd, Allschwil, Switzerland

Patricia A. Cronin Department of Academic Surgery, Cork University Hospital, Cork, Ireland

Alessandra D' Addio Hematology Unit, Azienda Istituti Ospitalieri, Cremona, Italy

David C. Dale University of Washington, Seattle, WA, USA

Michael Deininger Division of Hematology and Hematologic Malignancies, Huntsman Cancer Institute, University of Utah, Salt Lake City, UT, USA

Klaus Dembowsky Polyphor Ltd, Allschwil, Switzerland

John F. DiPersio Division of Oncology, Siteman Cancer Center, Washington University School of Medicine, St. Louis, MO, USA

Kenneth Douglas Clinical Apheresis Unit, Beatson West of Scotland Cancer Centre, Glasgow, UK

Cynthia E. Dunbar Molecular Hematopoiesis Section, Hematology Branch, National Heart, Lung and Blood Institute, National Institutes of Health, Bethesda, MD, USA

Linda Eissenberg Division of Oncology, Siteman Cancer Center, Washington University School of Medicine, St. Louis, MO, USA

Neal Flomenberg Thomas Jefferson University, Philadelphia, PA, USA

Maximilian M. Fresen Internal Medicine, University Clinic Köln, Köln, Germany

Stefan Fruehauf Center for Tumor Diagnostics and Therapy, Paracelsus Klinik, Osnabrück, Germany

Rainer Haas Department of Hematology, Oncology and Clinical Immunology, University Hospital Düsseldorf, Heinrich Heine University Düsseldorf, Düsseldorf, Germany

Jessie Hanrahan Genzyme Corporation, Cambridge, MA, USA

Nadia Harun Westmead Institute for Cancer Research, Westmead Millennium Institute, University of Sydney, Westmead, NSW, Australia

Anthony D. Ho Department of Internal Medicine V, Heidelberg University Hospital, Heidelberg, Germany

Frank J. Hsu Genzyme Corporation, Cambridge, MA, USA

Kai Hübel Internal Medicine, University Clinic Köln, Köln, Germany

Esa Jantunen Department of Medicine, Kuopio University Hospital and University of Eastern Finland/Clinical Medicine, Kuopio, Finland

Yubin Kang Division of Hematology-Oncology, Medical University of South Carolina, Charleston, SC, USA

Guido Kobbe Department of Hematology, Oncology and Clinical Immunology, University Hospital Düsseldorf, Heinrich Heine University Düsseldorf, Düsseldorf, Germany

Andre Larochelle Molecular Hematopoiesis Section, Hematology Branch, National Heart, Lung and Blood Institute, National Institutes of Health, Bethesda, MD, USA

Roberto M. Lemoli Department of Hematology and Oncological Sciences "L. & A. Seràgnoli", Istitute of Hematology, University of Bologna, Bologna, Italy

W. Conrad Liles University Health Network/University of Toronto, Toronto General Hospital, Toronto, ON, Canada

Christian Ludin Polyphor Ltd, Allschwil, Switzerland

Amy R. MacKenzie Thomas Jefferson University, Philadelphia, PA, USA

John M. McCarty Bone Marrow Transplant Program, Massey Cancer Center, VCU Medical Center, Richmond, VA, USA

Fazia Mir Division of Oncology, Siteman Cancer Center, Washington University School of Medicine, St. Louis, MO, USA

Arnon Nagler Chaim Sheba Medical Center, Tel-Hashomer, Israel

Sridhar Nimmagadda Russell H. Morgan Department of Radiology and Radiological Science, Johns Hopkins University, Baltimore, MD, USA

Tapio Nousiainen Department of Medicine, Kuopio University Hospital, Kuopio, Finland

Daniel Obrecht Polyphor Ltd, Allschwil, Switzerland

Thomas O'Hare Division of Hematology and Hematologic Malignancies, Huntsman Cancer Institute, University of Utah, Salt Lake City, UT, USA

Amnon Peled Hadassah Hebrew University Hospital, Goldyne Savad Institute of Gene Therapy, Jerusalem, Israel

Sara M. Rankin Leukocyte Biology Section, NHLI Division, Faculty of Medicine, Imperial College, London, UK

H. Paul Redmond Department of Academic Surgery, Cork University Hospital, Cork, Ireland

Michael P. Rettig Division of Oncology, Siteman Cancer Center, Washington University School of Medicine, St. Louis, MO, USA

Catherine H. Roberts Bone Marrow Transplant Program, Massey Cancer Center, VCU Medical Center, Richmond, VA, USA

Barbara Romagnoli Polyphor Ltd, Allschwil, Switzerland

Mette Marie Rosenkilde The Laboratory of Molecular Pharmacology, Department of Neuroscience and Pharmacology, University of Copenhagen, The Panum Institute, Copenhagen, Denmark

Mark Schroeder Division of Oncology, Siteman Cancer Center, Washington University School of Medicine, St. Louis, MO, USA

Anne Steen The Laboratory of Molecular Pharmacology, Department of Neuroscience and Pharmacology, University of Copenhagen, The Panum Institute, Copenhagen, Denmark

Guido Tricot Department of Medicine, Utah Blood and Marrow Transplant and Myeloma Program, University of Utah School of Medicine, Salt Lake City, UT, USA

Matias E. Valsecchi Thomas Jefferson University, Philadelphia, PA, USA

Lauren E. Woodard Russell H. Morgan Department of Radiology and Radiological Science, Johns Hopkins University, Baltimore, MD, USA

Johann Zimmermann Polyphor Ltd, Allschwil, Switzerland

Part I
Basic Science and Experimental Studies on Stem Cell Mobilization

Chapter 1
Preclinical Experience with AMD3100 for Mobilization of Hematopoietic Stem and Progenitor Cells

Hal E. Broxmeyer

Abstract The SDF-1/CXCL12–CXCR4 axis is involved in a number of functional activities of hematopoietic stem (HSC) and progenitor cells (HPC). This includes migration, chemotaxis, homing, and survival. AMD3100, also known as Plerixafor or Mozobil, is a small molecular weight Bicyclam known to specifically antagonize the binding of stromal cell-derived factor-1 (SDF-1)/CXCL12 to one of its receptors, CXCR4. This chapter reviews preclinical studies demonstrating the first proof-of-principle that AMD3100 is a potent and rapid mobilizer of HSC/HPC to the blood in mice and that AMD3100 synergizes with the main HSC/HPC-mobilizing agent, granulocyte-colony-stimulating factor (G-CSF) to greatly enhance G-CSF-induced mobilization of HSC/HPC. Preclinical studies, which led to clinical evaluation of AMD3100 were possible in part because of the nonspecies specificity of AMD3100 which allowed for mobilization studies first in mice, and subsequently in dogs and monkeys, including transplantation of the mobilized cells into conditioned animals of their own species. Preclinical studies in higher animals and the first, and subsequent human clinical studies with AMD3100 are described. Also, discussed are the use of AMD3100 with other mobilizing agents, such as GRO-β, and potential uses of AMD3100 to enhance engraftment of HSC, to treat inflammatory disorders involving SDF-1/CXCL12–CXCR4 interactions, and as a tool to dissect out cell and intracellular events mediated by SDF-1/CXCL12.

Keywords Stem cells • Progenitor cells • Mobilization • AMD3100 • G-CSF

H.E. Broxmeyer, PhD (✉)
Department of Microbiology and Immunology, Indiana University School of Medicine, 950 West Walnut Street, R2-302, Indianapolis, IN 46202-5181, USA
e-mail: hbroxmey@iupui.edu

S. Fruehauf et al. (eds.), *Novel Developments in Stem Cell Mobilization: Focus on CXCR4*, DOI 10.1007/978-1-4614-1960-0_1,

Introduction

Blood cell production (hematopoiesis) is regulated by a number of biologically active molecules termed cytokines [1]. Specific cytokines act alone, or in combination, to regulate the functional outcomes of hematopoietic stem (HSC) and progenitor (HPC) cells [2–4]. HSC self-renew (make more of themselves) and upon demand differentiate through intermediary lineage-restricted HPC to various blood cell lineages: erythroid, granulocyte, macrophage, lymphoid, and megakaryocyte/platelet [3, 4]. HSC and HPC are first found developmentally in the aorta-gonad-mesonephros (AGM) region and the yolk sack, next in fetal liver, and then in fetal bone marrow and spleen [3, 4]. At birth, placental and umbilical cord blood are rich sources of HSC and HPC [2–4]. Through childhood and adult life, the major source of HSC and HPC production is the bone marrow, with small numbers of these cells circulating in the blood. This low level of circulating HSC/HPC is considered to be physiologically relevant [5, 6]. Various agents and treatments have enhanced mobilization of HSC/HPC from bone marrow of children and adults into their circulating blood [7–10]. Increase in circulating levels of HSC and HPC is noted after blood cell rebound from cytotoxic effects of chemotherapy and/or irradiation used to treat patients with blood disorders or tumors, but can also be found after infusion of selected cytokines. The past and present "gold-standard" for HSC/HPC mobilization in humans is the cytokine, granulocyte-colony-stimulating factor (G-CSF), although other members of the cytokine/chemokine family of molecules have been used [9, 10]. Mechanisms mediating cytokine-induced mobilization of HSC/HPC are described elsewhere [9–16]. However, many patients cannot be adequately mobilized with G-CSF alone, highlighting the need to find other mobilizing agents that can act alone or with G-CSF more effectively in these hard to mobilize patients.

HSC/HPC transplants from bone marrow, mobilized peripheral blood, and cord blood have been used successfully in the clinic to treat a wide variety of malignant and nonmalignant disorders. What the major tissue source of HSC/HPC for clinical transplantation will be in the future remains to be determined, but mobilized peripheral blood has for years replaced bone marrow as the most often used source of transplantable HSC/HPC. For unknown reasons, not all patients respond well to the HSC/HPC mobilizing effects of G-CSF. "Poor"- or "non"-responders to G-CSF-induced mobilization include, but are not limited to, patients with anemia (e.g., Fanconi anemia) and lymphoma [7, 8]. Enhancing HSC/HPC mobilization in these "poor"- or "non"-G-CSF responders would clearly be of great clinical advantage. The value of mobilized cells not only resides in the quantity of HSC/HPC that can be obtained, but also reflects the quality of these cells. HSC and HPC compartments each include a hierarchy of cells at various stages of differentiation and activity. HSC can be found that have extensive competitive repopulating and self-renewal capacity or that have less of these capabilities. A mobilized blood product could contain a mixture of different quality HSC. There are assays that allow one to assay HSC and HPC through phenotypic and functional means [1–4]. Cells are defined phenotypically by the presence and absence of an array of cell surface proteins that are recognized by antibodies specific to these cell surface proteins [17]. Murine HSCs are much better phenotypically defined than human HSCs. Murine HSCs are found in the phenotypically defined populations that are Sca1$^+$ and lineage (Lin)$^-$ for mature blood cell types, and more defined cell types in this lineage are Sca1$^+$c-kit$^+$lin$^-$ and CD34$^{lo/-}$ Sca1$^+$c-kit$^+$lin$^-$ or via use of SLAM markers. Human HSCs are considered to reside in a CD34$^+$CD38$^-$ population. CD34$^+$CD38$^-$ human cell populations are not nearly as purified for HSC as are murine Sca1$^+$lin$^-$, Sca1$^+$c-kit$^+$lin$^-$, or CD34$^{lo/-}$Sca1$^+$c-kit$^+$lin$^-$ cells. This relates to both a lack of identified cell surface molecules that define human HSC, as many of those markers that rigorously define murine marrow HSC are of no use for human HSC from any tissue source, and the functional assays available to detect these populations. In the mouse system, HSC home to the bone marrow, take up residence in the marrow, and are nurtured to grow and engraft a lethally irradiated recipient for the life-time of the engrafted mouse. Human HSCs are less rigorously defined functionally. Assays for functional HSC deal with engraftment of sublethally irradiated mice with severe combined immunodeficiency (SCID), such as nonobese diabetic (NOD)/SCID mice [2, 4]. Here, human cells engraft the mouse bone marrow but cannot save the life of such mice given a lethal dose of irradiation. While the human assay for functional HSC is not perfect, it is the best we have at this time and there are second and third generation mice with NOD/SCID that have been used to assay engraftment of human HSCs [18]. Functional assays are extremely important to use, as phenotype does not always recapitulate function, especially when phenotyped cells have been subjected to in vitro culture maneuvers to expand or differentiate them or after stress in vivo. Without functional back-up assays, it is not clear what the phenotype tells us, other than that the cell is likely there. It is in the context of phenotypically and functionally- defined HSC, as well as HPC, that efforts have been made to identify alternative means to mobilize HSC and HPC, especially in patients who are not optimally responsive to the HSC/HPC mobilizing effects of G-CSF.

AMD3100 is a Bicyclam. It has the formation $C_{28}H_{54}N_8$, with a molecular mass of 502.782 g/mol and the structure 1,1′-[1,4-Phenylenebis(methylene)]bis[1,4,8,11-tetraazacyclotetradecane] as noted by Wikipedia. It is also called Plerixafor, with the trade name Mozobil. Herein, this mobilizing agent is referred to as AMD3100, as this name is used for the preclinical studies that I and others performed which led to the clinical testing of the agent. This chapter thus focuses on AMD3100, originally recognized as a specific antagonist of the binding of the chemokine stromal cell-derived factor (SDF)-1/CXCL12 to its 7-transmembrane spanning Gαi-linked chemokine receptor, CXCR4, in terms of its capacity to mobilize HSC/HPC from mice and humans by itself, and also to synergize with G-CSF to enhance G-CSF-induced mobilization of HSC and HPC.

SDF-1/CXCL12–CXCR4 Axis and AMD3100

SDF-1/CXCL12 is a potent chemotactic molecule that induces directed movement of cells expressing CXCR4 [1, 19–24]. This includes CXCR4-expressing HSC and HPC. The SDF-1/CXCL12–CXCR4 axis has been linked to in vivo homing and engrafting capacity of HSC/HPC. SDF-1/CXCL12 induces a number of intracellular signals through CXCR4, including activation of the MAP Kinase and AKT/PI3 Kinase pathways, which apparently mediate migratory and cell survival functions of HSC and HPC [25, 26], among other leukocyte cell types, and even tumor cells. The exact intracellular and extracellular mechanisms mediating SDF-1/CXCL12 migration of responsive cell types, including HSC and HPC have not been entirely elucidated, but knowledge of SDF-1/CXCL12–CXCR4 effects on migration and engraftment of HSC/HPC was crucial to the identification of AMD3100 as a potent HSC/HPC mobilizing agent. SDF-1/CXCL12 has a number of other very important and physiologically relevant activities. It acts as a survival enhancing factor for HSC/HPC [25–28], and is believed to function as a retention factor for these cells within the bone marrow [12, 20, 29], effects enhanced by the inhibition of CD26/Dipeptidylpeptidase IV, an enzyme that truncates and inactivates many activities of SDF-1/CXCL12, including the chemotactic activity of this chemokine [29, 30]. AMD3100 is a symmetric small molecular weight bicyclam that functions as an antagonist with great specificity for SDF-1/CXCL12–CXCR4 interactions [31–34]. CXCR4 is a major co-receptor for HIV infection [35, 36], and original clinical studies evaluated the efficacy of AMD3100 as an anti-HIV treatment modality.

For HIV, the drug was being dosed with continuous (24 h) daily infusion which was impractical. In addition, there was a potential issue of cardiac arrhythmia in two patients, plus an apparent lack of effect. For the clinical studies proposed and undertaken below, this amount of toxicity was not encountered, as we were able to demonstrate that the short time frame of administration of AMD3100 for manifestation of its mobilizing capacity for HSC and HPC did not have such side effects.

It was in the context of understanding the role of SDF-1/CXCL12 and CXCR4 in migration, homing, retention, nurturing, and engraftment of HSC/HPC, and the effectiveness of AMD3100 as an antagonist of SDF-1/CXCL12 binding to CXCR4 for both murine and human cells that the author and his laboratory, in collaboration with Dr. Gary Bridger, AnorMed Corporation (Langley, British Columbia), evaluated the first proof-of-principle that AMD3100 acted as a mobilizer of HPC and HSC in mice, and synergistically enhanced G-CSF-induced mobilization of murine HPC and HSC [37]. Dr. Bridger called me one evening after reading my review articles on chemokine molecules and their hematopoietic activities, including those of SDF-1/CXCL12. After some discussion about chemokines and hematopoiesis, Dr. Bridger asked me what I might do if I had access to a specific inhibitor of SDF-1/CXCL12 binding to CXCR4. I mentioned that I had been looking for such an agent that could be used with mouse cells and in mice, but in all my years of going to Gordon Conferences on chemotactic cytokines, and networking with those in the field, the only such reagents available were for use with human cells. However, I noted that if I had access to such a mouse active reagent, one of the first experiments I would do would be to test the hypothesis, that I long believed, that interfering with SDF-1/CXCL12–CXCR4 chemokine-receptor binding would allow for rapid mobilization of HSC/HPC from marrow to peripheral blood. Dr. Bridger assured me that AMD3100 would work on both human and mouse cells as an antagonist for SDF-1/CXCL12 binding to CXCR4, and within months I had enough AMD3100 to begin testing its capacity to mobilize HPC. The in vivo studies, assessing the mobilizing effects of AMD3100 on HPC release to peripheral blood of mice, based on the dosing range of AMD3100 suggested by Dr. Bridger demonstrated rapid mobilizing effects, within 15–30 min of subcutaneous administration of AMD3100 to the mice.

I am sometimes asked why, if we did the first proof-of-principle studies on mobilization of HSC/HPC in mice with AMD3100, that the clinical papers from Dr. Dale's group in collaboration with Dr. Gary Bridger and Dr. Gary Calandra (also of AnorMed) with me as co-author [38, 39] came out before the mouse studies [37]. The reason being that as fast as I relayed the experimental data to Dr. Bridger, Dr. Dale's group was translating the studies in human volunteers. It is difficult to publish mouse studies when the exact type studies are so quickly available in human clinical reports. This occurred not only for use of AMD3100 alone, but also for our first proof-of-principle studies in which a single dose of AMD3100 was used in mice to greatly enhance mobilization of HPC induced by administration of multiple additions over a number of days of G-CSF [37]. These results were also rapidly translated by Dr. Dale's group in human volunteers [40]. Thus, all the preclinical work that my group did in mice, with mobilizing HPC alone with AMD3100 or with AMD3100 plus G-CSF were published [37] after the clinical studies when we had enough information above and beyond the clinical studies [38–40] to warrant publication in a high impact journal. One key to getting our laboratory-based proof-of-principle study published [37] was the additional proof inherent in the paper that AMD3100, either alone or in combination with G-CSF in mice, and in man also greatly enhanced release into peripheral blood of long-term marrow competitive and noncompetitive HSCs with extensive self-renewal capacity. These donor cells in a mouse–mouse transplant assay could save the life of the mouse, and long-term repopulate the complete hematopoietic system of lethally irradiated mouse recipients. In a human donor cell, mouse recipient mouse chimera study known to detect human HSCs, the human cells engrafted the hematopoietic system of sublethally irradiated NOD/SCID mice [37]. At the time we reported these mouse and human HSC assays [37], cells mobilized in humans, by AMD3100 had not yet been shown to repopulate human recipients long-term. Our mouse data was published in abstract form [41], and given as a presentation at the American Society of Hematology meeting in the year 2001. While human $CD34^+$ cell mobilization studies were reported in 2003 and 2004 [38, 39], CD34 is a phenotypic, not functional, marker for HSC and HPC. HSCs are extremely rare in $CD34^+$ populations and CD34 does not distinguish long-term from short-term repopulating human HSC, or even if the cells within the $CD34^+$ cell population actually have HSC activity. The $CD34^+$ cell populations are more highly enriched for HPC, which at best only provide short-term engraftment. Not all $CD34^+$ cells are HPC, as CD34 is also a marker for endothelial and other cell types. Our report demonstrating the functional HSC content of mobilized human $CD34^+$ cells, done in collaboration with Drs. Christie Orschell, Edward Srour, and Artur Plett at the Indiana University School of Medicine [37], was subsequently verified by actual transplantation of AMD3100-mobilized $CD34^+$ cells into human recipients. Moreover, our studies predicted that AMD3100 would be especially useful in situations where G-CSF-induced mobilization was below par [37], in patients who were difficult to adequately mobilize by G-CSF alone. Hence our studies [37] provided the first proof that HSC, as well as HPC, were being extensively mobilized by AMD3100, and that AMD3100 greatly enhanced the HSC mobilizing activity of G-CSF-induced mobilization.

Other Rapid Mobilizers and Detailed Preclinical Results with AMD3100

Mobilization of HSC and HPC in mice and humans in response to G-CSF is not quick, and usually occurs over a protracted period of time in which G-CSF is given a few times a day for a number of days in order to maximize the numbers of HSC/HPC circulating in the blood for collection purposes [7, 8]. In contrast, chemokines such as macrophage inflammatory protein (MIP)-1α/BB10010 [42–44], interleukin (IL)-8 [45–47], MIP-2 [48], and GRO-β [9, 10, 16, 49, 50] rapidly mobilize HPC to peripheral blood in minutes to hours after injection into mice. Therefore, our first studies used s.c. injection of 5 mg/kg AMD3100 into mice and subsequent evaluation of effects beginning at 15 min through 24 h [37]. Mobilization of HPC to the blood in C57Bl/6 mice occurred as early as 15 min, and peaked at 1 h with maintenance of low but significantly enhanced mobilization seen between 2 and 24 h after a single injection of AMD3100. Using a 1-h time interval, we found a dose-dependent induction of HPC mobilization to the blood with a plateau maximum dosage seen for the most part with 2.5–10.0 mg/kg AMD3100. A single injection of AMD3100 once a day for 3 days yielded maximal mobilization of HPC within 1 h after each injection, demonstrating that within this time frame of AMD3100 injections, mice did not become tolerant to the HPC mobilizing effects of AMD3100. The shortest length of time between which AMD3100 can be administered with maintenance of maximal mobilizing activity was not been determined.

Since G-CSF-induced mobilization does not occur rapidly, but rather occurs over days of administration of G-CSF in mouse models and when administered to humans, but effects of AMD3100 are rapid, we chose to evaluate the combined effects of G-CSF and AMD3100 on mobilization of HPC in the context of administration of G-CSF to the mice twice a day for 2–4 days, followed within 12–24 h of the last dose of G-CSF by a single one time administration of AMD3100 [37]. These studies were performed in mice of three different genetic strain backgrounds. This was done because the effectiveness of G-CSF-induced mobilization in humans is known to vary greatly among different individuals [7, 8], effects not yet predictable due to an incomplete knowledge of the mechanisms involved in G-CSF mobilization, and because different mouse strains are known to differ in the degree to which G-CSF induces HPC mobilization in these mice [51–53]. C57Bl/6 and DBA/2 mice are respectively "poor" and "good" responders to the HPC mobilizing capacity of G-CSF, with C3H/HeJ mice considered "intermediate" responders. The reported differential responsiveness in these different strains of mice to G-CSF-induced mobilization was confirmed in our studies [37]. In contrast to G-CSF, there was no clear distinction in HPC mobilization responses of these different mouse strains to AMD3100. A single injection of AMD3100 to mice of these three different genetic strains given after that of 2–4 days G-CSF resulted in significant, and in many cases synergistic, enhancement in HPC mobilization compared to mice given only G-CSF or AMD3100. That AMD3100 significantly enhanced G-CSF-induced mobilization in C57Bl/6 mice, which are relatively "poor" responders to G-CSF-induced mobilization, suggested that AMD3100 given after G-CSF administration might also enhance mobilization of HPC in mouse models of genetic disease associated with "poor" response to G-CSF-induced mobilization [37]. For such a test model, we chose to evaluate mice in which the Fanconi Anemia Complement C group gene (Fancc) was deleted (Fancc –/– mice). Patients with Fanconi anemia respond very poorly to the mobilization effect of G-CSF [54], and there are similarities to this noted in the Fancc –/– mice [37]. In collaboration with Dr. D. Wade Clapp and his group at the Indiana University School of Medicine, we demonstrated an incredible HPC mobilizing response in Fancc –/– mice with combined treatment of these mice with G-CSF followed by AMD3100 [37]. In fact, the synergistic effects of G-CSF plus AMD3100 in Fancc –/– mice was greater than that seen in the litter-mate control wild-type (+/+) mice, even though G-CSF by itself was less effective in mobilizing HPC from Fancc –/–, compared to +/+ mice, and AMD3100 was about equally effective by itself in mobilizing HPC in Fancc –/– and +/+ mice. We believe that Fancc –/– or other Fanconi anemia complement group –/– mice may serve as a useful model to better understand the mechanisms involved in synergistic induction of HPC mobilization by combined treatment with G-CSF and AMD3100.

The above results with mobilization of mouse HPC, while setting the stage for the human clinical trials and their assessment of the effects of AMD3100 on mobilization of human $CD34^+$ cells and HPC, did not address the mobilizing capacity of AMD3100, alone or in combination with G-CSF, on HSC. The only true tests for functional HSC are in vivo engraftment tests, and in the mouse HSC situation, transplantation that saves the life of lethally irradiated mice [4]. A competitive mouse transplant setting was used to evaluate the competitive nature of the mobilized HSC in lethally irradiated primary mice. Secondary transplantation was done in which bone marrow cells from lethally irradiated primary mice that had engrafted with donor cells were transplanted into secondary lethally irradiated mice in order to determine the self-renewal capacity of the original donor cells. AMD3100 mobilized a competitive repopulating and self-renewing population of mouse HSC, and AMD3100 synergized with G-CSF to enhance mobilization of these HSCs [37]. HSCs were also mobilized from Fancc –/– mice by the combination of G-CSF plus AMD3100 [55].

The effects of AMD3100, alone and in combination with G-CSF, noted for mobilization of mouse HPC and HSC, were confirmed for mobilization of human HPC and HSC [37, 40]. Except for differences in timing and dosage effects between mouse and man, the overall effects in humans were similar to that in mice. In mice, mobilization of HPC and HSC occurred within an hour, while in man maximal mobilization occurred after 6–9 h, depending on AMD3100 dosage used, results likely reflecting different pharmacokinetics of AMD3100 in mouse and man.

Evaluation of mobilization of human NOD/SCID repopulating cells (SRC; considered to be equivalent or close to human HSC) [4] not only demonstrated enhanced mobilization of SRC from human donors when AMD3100 was used in combination with G-CSF, in comparison to that of only G-CSF or AMD3100, but also suggested that a single dose of AMD3100 alone might be more effective than 4–5 days of multiple injections of G-CSF for mobilization of human SRC [37]. Interestingly, human $CD34^+$ cells isolated from the blood after treatment of the donors with G-CSF plus AMD3100 expressed a phenotype characteristic of highly engrafting mouse HSC [37], suggesting that the combination of G-CSF and AMD3100 mobilizes a high-quality population of HSC.

Mobilization of Transplantable Hematopoietic Stem Cells in Dogs and Monkeys

AMD3100 was evaluated for its capacity to mobilize dog HSC for use in autologous and allogeneic canine transplantation models [56]. In the autologous model, neutrophil and platelet recovery in 920 cGy total body irradiated dogs occurred respectively at medians of 9 and 25 days. Dogs had normal marrow function at 1 year post-transplantation. Evaluation of long-term engraftment was in the setting of dog leukocyte antigen-identical littermate donor cell transplants into irradiated recipients. Recovery was similar to that of the autologous model. Blood-donor chimerism was 97–100% with a median follow-up of 53 weeks.

Study of the engrafting capability of AMD3100 mobilized monkey $CD34^+$ cells utilized Neo^R-containing retroviral vector-marked cells from rhesus macaques transplanted into myeloblated rhesus macques [57]. Neo^R gene-marked myeloid and lymphoid cells were detected up to 32 months after transplantation. In vivo marking was superior to that noted with G-CSF mobilized cells that were also transduced prior to transplantation. This, plus the fact that more AMD3100-mobilized cells of the CD34 phenotype were in G_1 phase of the cell cycle and expressed CXCR4 and the integrin VLA-4 [57], compared with that of G-CSF mobilized cells, was interpreted to suggest that there were fundamental differences in populations of $CD34^+$ cells mobilized by G-CSF vs. AMD3100.

Clinical Results with AMD3100

Immediately after our first proof-of-principle experiment was performed that demonstrated that AMD3100 acted as a single injection to rapidly mobilize granulocyte macrophage (CFU-GM), erythroid (BFU-E), and multipotential (CFU-GEMM; CFU-MIX) progenitors into the blood of mice (reported subsequently in [37]), a clinical study was started in ten healthy human volunteers, in which a single dose of AMD3100 was given s.c. at 80 μg/kg [38]. This induced rapid, generalized leukocytosis, an increase in circulating CD34$^+$ counts, and a concomitant increase in CFU-GM, BFU-E, and CFU-GEMM, the latter colony assessment of HPC being performed in the author's laboratory. The effects on CD34$^+$ cells and HPC peaked at 6–9 h postadministration of AMD3100. Effects of AMD3100 were dose-dependent at this time for both CD34$^+$ cells and HPC. As in mice [37], serial administration of AMD3100 resulted in consistent, reversible increases in peripheral blood CD34$^+$ cells and HPC in man [37, 38].

A recent review has provided a comprehensive analysis of the clinical effects of AMD3100 [58]. At first, rapid mobilization of CD34$^+$ cells was also induced by AMD3100 in patients with multiple myeloma and non-Hodgkin's lymphoma [59]. As we originally predicted [37], AMD3100 served as an especially relevant HSC/HPC mobilizing agent in patients in whom mobilization with G-CSF has been sub-par resulting in not nearly enough cells for transplant purposes. A number of clinical studies have now borne out this prediction in patients in whom G-CSF alone was not an optimal mobilizing agent [60–63]. Because certain tumor cells also express CXCR4 and may respond to mobilization by AMD3100, caution is required in the evaluation of the use for transplantation of cells mobilized by AMD3100 in patients with cancer; this has been discussed by others [64–67].

A pharmacokinetic–pharmacodynamic model was elucidated for mobilization of CD34$^+$ cells in humans by AMD3100, in which a two-compartment model was proposed with first-order absorption [68]. This model may be of use in evaluating relevant covariates and optimization of AMD3100 for use in various patient populations.

Clinical Results with the Combination of G-CSF and AMD3100

That AMD3100, by itself was a potent mobilizer of HPC and HSC in mice, and also synergized with G-CSF to enhance mobilization of HPC in mice [37], set the ground-work to begin evaluating effects of combination of G-CSF and AMD3100 on mobilization of HPC and HSC in man. The protocol for humans was similar to that for mice in that the donors received G-CSF for 4–5 days, and then a single injection of AMD3100 prior to collection of the blood cells at times after AMD3100 administration [40]. A single injection of AMD3100 after the full schedule of G-CSF administration resulted in significantly enhanced numbers of circulating HPC and SRC (=HPC). Peak of mobilization was 6–9 h after administration of AMD3100.

In a follow-up clinical study for mobilization of autologous CD34$^+$ cells and HPC, two objectives were met [69]. The first objective evaluated whether more CD34$^+$ cells and functionally defined HPC were mobilized per unit of blood volume of apheresis after administration of G-CSF plus AMD3100, compared to that of G-CSF alone. The second was to determine whether the combination of G-CSF plus AMD3100 required fewer apheresis procedures to reach a target level of at least 5×10^6 CD34$^+$ cells/kg bodyweight for transplantation and if patients mobilized with the combination of G-CSF plus AMD3100 had at least a 90% rate of success with autologous transplantation as defined by neutrophil engraftment by 21 days after transplantation of the mobilized autologous peripheral blood.

The suggestion that combination of G-CSF plus AMD3100 not only enhanced the quantity of mobilized HPC/HSC, but also the quality of these cells received support from a genomics study that analyzed expression of differentially expressed genes from $CD34^+$ cells mobilized from three patients each with either combination of G-CSF plus AMD3100, or with G-CSF only [70]. The differentially expressed genes were analyzed by Affymetrix GeneChip Human Genome U133 Plus 2.0 and a software package, Micro Array Solutions 1.3. Some selected genes were validated by quantitative real-time polymerase chain reaction. A pattern of 81 genes and 21 genes were respectively expressed at higher and lower levels in the G-CSF plus AMD3100, compared to AMD3100, group. Increased expression was noted in genes for antiapoptosis (survival), cell cycle, replication/DNA repair, cell motility, and oxygen transport. Decreased expression was seen in the proapoptosis gene group. It was concluded that $CD34^+$ cells mobilized with the combination of G-CSF and AMD3100 expressed significantly higher levels of genes that could potentially promote superior engraftment after myeloablative therapy, than $CD34^+$ cells mobilized with only G-CSF [70].

A full profile of different types of cells mobilized by the combinations of G-CSF plus AMD3100 compared with that of G-CSF alone has yet to be reported. In this context, it was demonstrated that either G-CSF or AMD3100 significantly stimulated angiogenesis in a mouse model of acute hind limb ischemia [71]. The kinetics of mobilization of angiogenic cells was different between the two mobilizing agents, with AMD3100 inducing more rapid revascularization. The combination of G-CSF and AMD3100 induced the earliest and most complete recovery in blood flow to the hind limb site of ischemia. It appeared that mobilized monocytes mediated angiogenesis through a paracrine mechanism [71].

Preclinical Models Evaluating Mobilization of HPC Using AMD3100 Plus Chemokines

Efforts to further enhance mobilization of HSC/HPC in humans are warranted, especially in the context of patients who do not respond well to the mobilizing effects of G-CSF alone.

Several members of the chemokine family, including MIP-1α/CCL3 [42–44], IL-8/CXCL8 [45–47], MIP-2 [48], and GRO-β/CXCL2 [9, 10, 16, 49, 50] mobilize HPC into the blood of mice. This mobilization is rapid and usually peaks within an hour or less of injection of the chemokine into mice. MIP-1α, which acts through the CCR1 chemokine receptor for mobilization of HPC [44], and AMD3100 each alone significantly enhanced mobilization of CFU-GM, BFU-E, and CFU-GEMM in C3H/HeJ mice by 2.3–5.1% within 1 h of injection (AMD3100 at 5 mg/kg s.c.; MIP-1α at 5 μg/mouse i.p.) [41, 72]. When administered simultaneously, the combination of AMD3100 plus MIP-1α resulted in 8.8–13.2-fold enhancement in circulating levels of HPC that was greater than additive compared to either reagent alone. The combination of G-CSF given twice a day at 2.5 μg/mouse/injection s.c. followed 16 h later by AMD3100 and/or MIP-1α resulted 1 h later in enhanced numbers of HPC/mL peripheral blood compared to that of G-CSF alone. The largest fold increase in circulating levels of HPC occurred with the combination of G-CSF, AMD3100, and MIP-1α. This combination, while mobilizing significantly greater numbers of HPC than that of AMD3100 plus MIP-1α, was only borderline significant or not statistically different from the numbers of HPC mobilized by the combination of G-CSF plus AMD3100.

GRO-β/CXCL2 or the truncated form of GRO-β, which both bind the CXCR2 receptor, also acts as a rapid mobilizer of HPC, as well as HSC [16, 49, 50]. This mobilization peaks at 15 min, and GRO-β significantly enhances G-CSF-induced mobilization of HPC/HSC. The combination of AMD3100 and GRO-β resulted in synergistic mobilization of CFU-GM as well as HSC with short- and long-term repopulating activity. The combination of AMD3100 plus GRO-β mobilized 2–4-fold more competitive repopulating units than that of G-CSF [73, 74]. The combination of G-CSF with AMD3100 plus GRO-β resulted in suprasynergistic mobilization of CFU-GM, an effect also noted in Fancc −/− mice [74–76], which respond poorly to the mobilizing effects of G-CSF alone.

The MIP-1α analogue BB10010 was not found to be a very active mobilizer of HPC in patients with breast cancer [43], and thus, may not be useful in humans for enhancing G-CSF and/or AMD3100 mobilization of HPC/HSC. GRO-β may be more useful in such combined reagent studies.

AMD3100 as a Tool to Enhance Engraftment of HSC

Efforts are ongoing to enhance efficacy of HSC transplantation for nonmyeloablative conditioning regimens, since myeloblative conditioning is associated with significant morbidity and mortality. It was reasoned that mobilizing HSC/HPC from environmental niches in the bone marrow, prior to transplantation of donor HSC, might open up "spaces" in the marrow for enhanced "take" of the infused donor cells. This possibility was considered based on the use of parabiotic mice [77]. After infusion of AMD3100 into one partner of a parabiotic pair of mice, HSC exited the marrow of the mouse, and engrafted in niches of the partner mouse. Treatment of regular mice (no parabiotic linking) with AMD3100, followed by donor cell infusion in otherwise nonconditioned mice resulted in over 4% donor cell engraftment. This engraftment was increased to about 9% when mice received weekly injections of AMD3100 for 3 consecutive weeks, each followed by transplantation of donor cells 2 h after injection of AMD3100. Interestingly, if a mouse strain was used in which AMD3100 was less effective as a mobilizing agent, the AMD3100 did not enhance donor cell engraftment beyond that seen with only the cells themselves (which was approximately 1% engraftment). Strategies such as this to enhance engraftment in non- or minimally ablated patients warrant further evaluation for reproducibility of results by other investigators; combination of reagents that enhance migration of HSC and HPC out of their bone marrow niches prior to infusion of donor HSC/HPC may be useful in this effort. Conditioning of recipients with HSC/HPC mobilizing agents (e.g., AMD3100, GRO-β, or MIP-1α) may be useful in combination with procedures that enhance the competitive homing capabilities of donor HSC/HPC. An example of enhancing HSC homing and engraftment is through inhibition of dipeptidylpeptidase IV activity of cell surface molecule CD26 [29, 30, 78]. Inhibition or deletion of CD26 results in enhanced homing and engraftment of a long-term bone marrow competitive repopulating cell with extensive self-renewal capacity. More recent studies have demonstrated that inhibition of CD26 on human cord blood $CD34^+$ cells enhances engraftment of these cells into sublethally irradiated NOD/SCID mice [79]. It would be of interest to see if preconditioning NOD/SCID mice with mobilizing agents such as AMD3100 with or without other rapid mobilizers, such as GRO-β, MIP-1α, or even IL-8, might further enhance the engrafting capability of CD26-inhibited human $CD34^+$ cells into NOD/SCID mice or mice with other forms of SCID, in the context of sublethal irradiation or no irradiation. In another context, selective enhancement of donor cell engraftment was demonstrated by AMD3100 in a mouse transplant model [80].

AMD3100 as a Tool to Evaluate SDF-1/CXCL12–CXCR4 Interactions

AMD3100 has been used to study the specificity of SDF-1/CXCL12 effects on migration/chemotaxis, and survival of HPC [28] and mouse embryonic stem cells [81], as well as intracellular effects mediating SDF-1/CXCL12 actions [26]. It has also been used to demonstrate that the inhibition of CD26 enhancement of homing of mouse bone marrow cells into lethally irradiated mice involved SDF-1/CXCL12–CXCR4 interactions [29].

Mechanisms of AMD3100-Induced Mobilization

A number of papers have implicated various interactions as being important in AMD3100-induced mobilization and enhancement of mobilization of HSC and HPC. This includes the complement system [82], and the activity of the proto-oncogene receptor molecule c-kit [83]. However, while it is clear that AMD3100 acts as a selective antagonist for binding of SDF-1/CXCL12 to CXCR4, and most studies automatically suggest that this may be the mechanism involved in mobilization, new information has come to light suggesting that at least in part, the mobilizing activity of AMD3100 for HSC and HPC may be mediated through AMD3100 effects on CXCR4-dependent SDF-1/CXCL12 release from bone marrow stromal cells [84]. This study demonstrated that AMD3100 in mice and nonhuman primates enhanced release of SDF-1/CXCL12 to the circulation, alone with HPC, that these effects were blocked by anti-CXCR4, anti-SDF-1/CXCL12, or beta2-adrenergic antagonism. Moreover, AMD3100 induced increased SDF-1/CXCL12 release from human bone marrow cell populations of osteoblasts and endothelial cells, both intricately involved in the bone marrow microenvironmental niche regulation of hematopoiesis.

Additional Roles for AMD3100

As a result of its specificity for antagonizing binding to and subsequent intracellular signaling of SDF-1/CXCL12 through CXCR4, AMD3100 could potentially serve to treat patients with clinical problems triggered by SDF-1/CXCL12–CXCR4 interactions. In this context, AMD3100 was found to be efficacious in down-regulating development of cockroach allergy-induced inflammation and airway hyperreactivity in a mouse model of asthma [85]. Treatment of allergic mice reduced airway hyperreactivity, peribronchial eosinophilia, as well as overall responses to inflammation. Moreover, there was a reduction in IL-4 and IL-5, and increases in IL-12 and interferon-γ levels in lungs of treated mice with this allergy-induced inflammation. AMD3100 also inhibited autoimmune joint inflammation in mice deficient for interferon-γ receptor [86]. The beneficial effect of AMD3100 in this model was apparent within the time frame of initiation of immunization and appearance of first symptoms. AMD3100 also reduced delayed-type hypersensitivity to autoantigen, collagen type II. It is believed that this effect was due to blocking migration of leukocytes into the joint [86].

Another interesting use of AMD3100 is as conjugate components of targeted nonviral gene delivery systems to CXCR4-expressing cells [87]. Polyplexes made with AMD3100-labeled polymers, enhanced gene transfer into CXCR4-expressing T-lymphocyte cell line, JURKAT. Effects were more apparent when nonspecific transfection pathways were decreased, and also when phorbol myristate acetate (PMA) was used. PMA triggered CXCR4 receptor endocytosis of AMD3100-labeled polyplexes to a greater extent than respective nonlabeled AMD3100.

The SDF-1/CXCL12–CXCR4 pathway is involved in the movement of cancer cells, with mediation through NF-κB [88] and p53 [89]. Potential consequences of cancer cell mobilization must be taken into careful account when AMD3100 is used to mobilize HSC/HPC from patients with leukemia or other cancers [60–65]. However, AMD3100 is also being considered for use in mobilizing cancer cells to the blood where they may be, once outside their protective niche within the body, more susceptible to kill by chemotherapeutic and/or other treatment modalities [90]. It remains to be seen in animal models whether or not, AMD3100 can be used to enhance the efficacy of tumor cell kill in such circumstances, without damaging normal cells, since normal HSC and HPC may also be more responsive to kill by these treatments when they are outside a "protective niche."

Concluding Remarks

AMD3100 has already demonstrated clinical efficacy in the context of mobilization of HSC and HPC, and may have other clinically relevant uses. One reason so much has been learned so quickly of the clinical activities of AMD3100, is that AMD3100 is not species specific. Thus, the same compound is capable of antagonizing SDF-1/CXCL12 binding to CXCR4 in mouse, canine, monkey, and human cells, thus greatly increasing the extent of preclinical studies that can be and have already been done.

Circadian rhythms influence circulating levels of HSC and HPC [91]. It will be of practical value to see how timing of AMD3100 administration in the context of HSC/HPC mobilization may further allow for optimization of enhanced mobilization of HSC/HPC.

Most recently, the human HSC has been more precisely defined as $Lin^-CD34^+CD38^-CD45RA^-Thy1^+Rho^{lo}CD49f^+$ such that a single such cell is capable of long-term multilineage engraftment in immune deficient mice [92]. Such information may be of future use in assessing mobilized peripheral blood HSC numbers and activity.

Acknowledgments The studies cited in references from the author's laboratory were supported in part by US Public Health Service RO1 Grants HL56416 and HL67384 from the US National Institutes of Health and Project 1 in PO1 HL053586 from National Heart Lung Blood Institute to HEB.

References

1. Shaheen M, Broxmeyer HE (2009) The humoral regulation of hematopoiesis. In: Hoffman R, Benz EJ Jr, Shattil SJ, Furie B, Silberstein LE, McGlave P, Heslop H, Anastasi J (eds) Hematology: basic principles and practice, 5th edn. Elsevier Churchill Livingston, Philadelphia, pp 253–275, Part III, Chapter 24
2. Broxmeyer HE, Smith FO (2009) Cord blood hematopoietic cell transplantation. In: Appelbaum FR, Forman SJ, Negrin RS, Blume KG (eds) Thomas' hematopoietic cell transplantation, 4th edn. Wiley-Blackwell, West Sussex, pp 559–576, Section 4, Chapter 39
3. Broxmeyer HE (2004) Proliferation, self-renewal, and survival characteristics of cord blood hematopoietic stem and progenitor cells. In: Broxmeyer HE (ed) Cord blood: biology, immunology, banking, and clinical transplantation. Amer. Assoc, Blood Banking, Bethesda, pp 1–21, Chapter 1
4. Broxmeyer HE, Srour E, Orschell C, Ingram DA, Cooper S, Plett PA, Mead LE, Yoder MC (2009) Cord blood hematopoietic stem and progenitor cells. In: Klimanskaya I, Lanza R (eds) Essentials of stem cell biology. Academic, Elsevier Science, San Diego, pp 151–156, Chapter 7
5. Wright DE, Wagers AJ, Gulati AP, Johnson FL, Weissman IL (2001) Physiological migration of hematopoietic stem and progenitor cells. Science 294:1933–1936. doi:10.1126/science.1064081
6. Abkowitz JL, Robinson AE, Kale S, Long MW, Chen J (2003) Mobilization of hematopoietic stem cells during homeostasis and after cytokine exposure. Blood 102:1249–1253. doi:10.1182/blood-2003-01-0318
7. Ng-Cashin J, Shen T (2004) Mobilization of autologous peripheral blood hematopoietic cells for support of high-dose cancer therapy. In: Blume KG, Forman SJ, Appelbaum FR (eds) Thomas' hematopoietic cell transplantation, 3rd edn. Blackwell Publishing, Ltd., Malden, pp 576–587
8. Schmitz N (2004) Peripheral blood hematopoietic cells for allogeneic transplantation. In: Blume KG, Forman SJ, Appelbaum FR (eds) Thomas' hematopoietic cell transplantation, 3rd edn. Blackwell Publishing, Ltd., Malden, pp 588–598

9. Pelus LM, Fukuda S (2008) Chemokine-mobilized adult stem cells; defining a better hematopoietic graft. Leukemia 22:466–473. doi:10.1038/sj.leu.2405021
10. Pelus LM (2008) Peripheral blood stem cell mobilization: new regimens, new cells, where do we stand. Curr Opin Hematol 15:285–292. doi:10.1097/MOH.0b013e328302f43a
11. Papayannopoulou T (2004) Current mechanistic scenarios in hematopoietic stem/progenitor cell mobilization. Blood 103:1580–1585. doi:10.1182/blood-2003-05-1595
12. Dar A, Kollet O, Lapidot T (2006) Mutual, reciprocal SDF-1/CXCR4 interactions between hematopoietic and bone marrow stromal cells regulate human stem cell migration and development in NOD/SCID chimeric mice. Exp Hematol 34:967–975. doi:10.1016/j.exphem. 2006.04.002
13. Cancelas JA, Jansen M, Williams DA (2006) The role of chemokine activation of Rac GTPases in hematopoietic stem cell marrow homing, retention, and peripheral mobilization. Exp Hematol 34:976–985. doi:10.1016/j.exphem.2006.03.016
14. Ratajczak MZ, Reca R, Wysoczynski M, Yan J, Ratajczak J (2006) Modulation of the SDF-1-CXCR4 axis by the third complement component (C3)—implications for trafficking of CXCR4+ stem cells. Exp Hematol 34:986–995. doi:10.1016/j.exphem.2006.03.015
15. Winkler IG, Levesque JP (2006) Mechanisms of hematopoietic stem cell mobilization: when innate immunity assails the cells that make blood and bone. Exp Hematol 34:996–1009. doi:10.1016/j.exphem.2006.04.005
16. Pelus LM, Fukuda S (2006) Peripheral blood stem cell mobilization: the CXCR2 ligand GRObeta rapidly mobilizes hematopoietic stem cells with enhanced engraftment properties. Exp Hematol 34:1010–1020. doi:10.1016/j.exphem.2006.04.004
17. Kondo M, Wagers AJ, Manz MG, Prohaska SS, Scherer DC, Beilhack GF, Shizuru JA, Weissman IL (2003) Biology of hematopoietic stem cells and progenitors: implications for clinical application. Annu Rev Immunol 21:759–806. doi:10.1146/annurev.immunol.21.120601.141007
18. Liu Y, Hangoc G, Campbell TB, Goodman M, Tao W, Pollok K, Srour EF, Broxmeyer HE (2008) Identification of parameters required for efficient lentiviral vector transduction and engraftment of human cord blood CD34(+) NOD/SCID-repopulating cells. Exp Hematol 36:947–956. doi:10.1016/j.exphem.2008.06.005
19. Aiuti A, Webb IJ, Bleul C, Springer T, Gutierrez-Ramos JC (1997) The chemokine SDF-1 is a chemoattractant for human CD34+ hematopoietic progenitor cells and provides a new mechanism to explain the mobilization of CD34+ progenitors to peripheral blood. J Exp Med 185:111–120. doi:10.1084/jem.185.1.111
20. Kim CH, Broxmeyer HE (1998) In vitro behavior of hematopoietic progenitor cells under the influence of chemoattractants: stromal cell-derived factor-1, steel factor, and the bone marrow environment. Blood 91:100–110
21. Jo DY, Rafii S, Hamada T, Moore MA (2000) Chemotaxis of primitive hematopoietic cells in response to stromal cell-derived factor-1. J Clin Invest 105:101–111. doi:10.1172/JCI7954
22. Wright DE, Bowman EP, Wagers AJ, Butcher EC, Weissman IL (2002) Hematopoietic stem cells are uniquely selective in their migratory response to chemokines. J Exp Med 195:1145–1154. doi:10.1084/jem.20011284 DOI:dx.doi.org
23. Peled A, Petit I, Kollet O, Magid M, Ponomaryov T, Byk T, Nagler A, Ben-Hur H, Many A, Shultz L, Lider O, Alon R, Zipori D, Lapidot T (1999) Dependence of human stem cell engraftment and repopulation of NOD/SCID mice on CXCR4. Science 283:845–848. doi:10.1126/science.283.5403.845 DOI:dx.doi.org
24. Lapidot T, Kollet O (2002) The essential roles of the chemokine SDF-1 and its receptor CXCR4 in human stem cell homing and repopulation of transplanted immune-deficient NOD/SCID and NOD/SCID/B2m(null) mice. Leukemia 16:1992–2003. doi:10.1038/sj.leu.2402684
25. Lee Y, Gotoh A, Kwon HJ, You M, Kohli L, Mantel C, Cooper S, Hangoc G, Miyazawa K, Ohyashiki K, Broxmeyer HE (2002) Enhancement of intracellular signaling associated with hematopoietic progenitor cell survival in response to SDF-1/CXCL12 in synergy with other cytokines. Blood 99:4307–4317. doi:10.1182/blood.V99.12.4307 DOI:dx.doi.org
26. Joo EK, Broxmeyer HE, Kwon HJ, Kang HB, Kim JS, Lim JS, Choe YK, Choe IS, Myung PK, Lee Y (2004) Enhancement of cell survival by stromal cell-derived factor-1/CXCL12 involves activation of CREB and induction of Mcl-1 and c-Fos in factor-dependent human cell line MO7e. Stem Cells Dev 13:563–570. doi:10.1089/1547328042417318

27. Broxmeyer HE, Kohli L, Kim CH, Lee Y, Mantel C, Cooper S, Hangoc G, Shaheen M, Li X, Clapp DW (2003) Stromal cell-derived factor-1/CXCL12 directly enhances survival/antiapoptosis of myeloid progenitor cells through CXCR4 and G(alpha)i proteins and enhances engraftment of competitive, repopulating stem cells. J Leukoc Biol 73:630–638. doi:10.1189/jlb.1002495 DOI:dx.doi.org
28. Broxmeyer HE, Cooper S, Kohli L, Hangoc G, Lee Y, Mantel C, Clapp DW, Kim CH (2003) Transgenic expression of stromal cell-derived factor-1/CXC chemokine ligand 12 enhances myeloid progenitor cell survival/antiapoptosis in vitro in response to growth factor withdrawal and enhances myelopoiesis in vivo. J Immunol 170:421–429
29. Christopherson KW, Hangoc G, Mantel CR, Broxmeyer HE (2004) Modulation of hematopoietic stem cell homing and engraftment by CD26. Science 305:1000–1003. doi:10.1126/science.1097071
30. Christopherson KW, Hangoc G, Broxmeyer HE (2002) Cell surface peptidase CD26/dipeptidylpeptidase IV regulates CXCL12/stromal cell-derived factor-1 alpha-mediated chemotaxis of human cord blood CD34+ progenitor cells. J Immunol 169:7000–7008
31. De Clercq E (2003) The bicyclam AMD3100 story. Nat Rev Drug Discov 2:581–587. doi:10.1038/nrd1134
32. Hatse S, Princen K, Bridger G, De CE, Schols D (2002) Chemokine receptor inhibition by AMD3100 is strictly confined to CXCR4. FEBS Lett 527:255–262. doi:10.1016/S0014-5793(02)03143-5 DOI:dx.doi.org
33. Rosenkilde MM, Gerlach LO, Jakobsen JS, Skerlj RT, Bridger GJ, Schwartz TW (2004) Molecular mechanism of AMD3100 antagonism in the CXCR4 receptor: transfer of binding site to the CXCR3 receptor. J Biol Chem 279:3033–3041. doi:10.1074/jbc.M309546200
34. Gerlach LO, Jakobsen JS, Jensen KP, Rosenkilde MR, Skerlj RT, Ryde U, Bridger GJ, Schwartz TW (2003) Metal ion enhanced binding of AMD3100 to Asp262 in the CXCR4 receptor. Biochemistry 42:710–717. doi:10.1021/bi0264770
35. Labrosse B, Brelot A, Heveker N, Sol N, Schols D, De CE, Alizon M (1998) Determinants for sensitivity of human immunodeficiency virus coreceptor CXCR4 to the bicyclam AMD3100. J Virol 72:6381–6388
36. Blanco J, Barretina J, Henson G, Bridger G, De CE, Clotet B, Este JA (2000) The CXCR4 antagonist AMD3100 efficiently inhibits cell-surface-expressed human immunodeficiency virus type 1 envelope-induced apoptosis. Antimicrob Agents Chemother 44:51–56. doi:10.1128/AAC.44.1.51-56.2000 DOI:dx.doi.org
37. Broxmeyer HE, Orschell CM, Clapp DW, Hangoc G, Cooper S, Plett PA, Liles WC, Li X, Graham-Evans B, Campbell TB, Calandra G, Bridger G, Dale DC, Srour EF (2005) Rapid mobilization of murine and human hematopoietic stem and progenitor cells with AMD3100, a CXCR4 antagonist. J Exp Med 201:1307–1318. doi:10.1084/jem.20041385
38. Liles WC, Broxmeyer HE, Rodger E, Wood B, Hubel K, Cooper S, Hangoc G, Bridger GJ, Henson GW, Calandra G, Dale DC (2003) Mobilization of hematopoietic progenitor cells in healthy volunteers by AMD3100, a CXCR4 antagonist. Blood 102:2728–2730. doi:10.1182/blood-2003-02-0663
39. Hubel K, Liles WC, Broxmeyer HE, Rodger E, Wood B, Cooper S, Hangoc G, Macfarland R, Bridger GJ, Henson GW, Calandra G, Dale DC (2004) Leukocytosis and Mobilization of CD34+ Hematopoietic Progenitor Cells by AMD3100, a CXCR4 Antagonist. Support Cancer Ther 1:165–172. doi:10.3816/SCT.2004.n.008
40. Liles WC, Rodger E, Broxmeyer HE, Dehner C, Badel K, Calandra G, Christensen J, Wood B, Price TH, Dale DC (2005) Augmented mobilization and collection of CD34+ hematopoietic cells from normal human volunteers stimulated with granulocyte-colony-stimulating factor by single-dose administration of AMD3100, a CXCR4 antagonist. Transfusion 45:295–300. doi:10.1111/j.1537-2995.2005.04222.x
41. Broxmeyer HE, Hangoc G, Cooper S, Bridger G (2001) Interference of the SDF-1/CXCR4 axis in mice with AMD3100 induces rapid high level mobilization of hematopoietic progenitor cells, and AMD3100 acts synergistically with G-CSF and MIP-1α to mobilize progenitors. Blood 98(Suppl 1):811a (abstract #3371)

42. Lord BI, Woolford LB, Wood LM, Czaplewski LG, McCourt M, Hunter MG, Edwards RM (1995) Mobilization of early hematopoietic progenitor cells with BB-10010: a genetically engineered variant of human macrophage inflammatory protein-1 alpha. Blood 85:3412–3415
43. Broxmeyer HE, Orazi A, Hague NL, Sledge GW Jr, Rasmussen H, Gordon MS (1998) Myeloid progenitor cell proliferation and mobilization effects of BB10010, a genetically engineered variant of human macrophage inflammatory protein-1alpha, in a phase I clinical trial in patients with relapsed/refractory breast cancer. Blood Cells Mol Dis 24:14–30. doi:10.1006/bcmd.1998.0167
44. Broxmeyer HE, Cooper S, Hangoc G, Gao JL, Murphy PM (1999) Dominant myelopoietic effector functions mediated by chemokine receptor CCR1. J Exp Med 189:1987–1992. doi:10.1084/jem.189.12.1987 DOI:dx.doi.org
45. Laterveer L, Lindley IJ, Hamilton MS, Willemze R, Fibbe WE (1995) Interleukin-8 induces rapid mobilization of hematopoietic stem cells with radioprotective capacity and long-term myelolymphoid repopulating ability. Blood 85:2269–2275
46. Fibbe WE, Pruijt JF, Velders GA, Opdenakker G, van KY, Figdor CG, Willemze R (1999) Biology of IL-8-induced stem cell mobilization. Ann N Y Acad Sci 872:71–82. doi:10.1111/j.1749-6632.1999.tb08454.x DOI:dx.doi.org
47. Laterveer L, Zijlmans JM, Lindley IJ, Hamilton MS, Willemze R, Fibbe WE (1996) Improved survival of lethally irradiated recipient mice transplanted with circulating progenitor cells mobilized by IL-8 after pretreatment with stem cell factor. Exp Hematol 24:1387–1393
48. Wang J, Mukaida N, Zhang Y, Ito T, Nakao S, Matsushima K (1997) Enhanced mobilization of hematopoietic progenitor cells by mouse MIP-2 and granulocyte colony-stimulating factor in mice. J Leukoc Biol 62:503–509
49. King AG, Horowitz D, Dillon SB, Levin R, Farese AM, MacVittie TJ, Pelus LM (2001) Rapid mobilization of murine hematopoietic stem cells with enhanced engraftment properties and evaluation of hematopoietic progenitor cell mobilization in rhesus monkeys by a single injection of SB-251353, a specific truncated form of the human CXC chemokine GRObeta. Blood 97:1534–1542. doi:10.1182/blood.V97.6.1534 DOI:dx.doi.org
50. Pelus LM, Bian H, King AG, Fukuda S (2004) Neutrophil-derived MMP-9 mediates synergistic mobilization of hematopoietic stem and progenitor cells by the combination of G-CSF and the chemokines GRObeta/CXCL2 and GRObetaT/CXCL2delta4. Blood 103:110–119. doi:10.1182/blood-2003-04-1115
51. Roberts AW, DeLuca E, Begley CG, Basser R, Grigg AP, Metcalf D (1995) Broad inter-individual variations in circulating progenitor cell numbers induced by granulocyte colony-stimulating factor therapy. Stem Cells 13:512–516. doi:10.1002/stem.5530130508
52. Roberts AW, Foote S, Alexander WS, Scott C, Robb L, Metcalf D (1997) Genetic influences determining progenitor cell mobilization and leukocytosis induced by granulocyte colony-stimulating factor. Blood 89:2736–2744
53. de Haan G, Ausema A, Wilkens M, Molineux G, Dontje B (2000) Efficient mobilization of haematopoietic progenitors after a single injection of pegylated recombinant human granulocyte colony-stimulating factor in mouse strains with distinct marrow-cell pool sizes. Br J Haematol 110:638–646. doi:10.1046/j.1365-2141.2000.02252.x DOI:dx.doi.org
54. Croop JM, Cooper R, Fernandez C, Graves V, Kreissman S, Hanenberg H, Smith FO, Williams DA (2001) Mobilization and collection of peripheral blood CD34+ cells from patients with Fanconi anemia. Blood 98:2917–2921. doi:10.1182/blood.V98.10.2917 DOI:dx.doi.org
55. Pulliam AC, Hobson MJ, Ciccone SL, Li Y, Chen S, Srour EF, Yang FC, Broxmeyer HE, Clapp DW (2008) AMD3100 synergizes with G-CSF to mobilize repopulating stem cells in Fanconi anemia knockout mice. Exp Hematol 36:1084–1090. doi:10.1016/j.exphem.2008.03.016
56. Burroughs L, Mielcarek M, Little MT, Bridger G, Macfarland R, Fricker S, Labrecque J, Sandmaier BM, Storb R (2005) Durable engraftment of AMD3100-mobilized autologous and allogeneic peripheral-blood mononuclear cells in a canine transplantation model. Blood 106:4002–4008. doi:10.1182/blood-2005-05-1937
57. Larochelle A, Krouse A, Metzger M, Orlic D, Donahue RE, Fricker S, Bridger G, Dunbar CE, Hematti P (2006) AMD3100 mobilizes hematopoietic stem cells with long-term repopulating capacity in nonhuman primates. Blood 107:3772–3778. doi:10.1182/blood-2005-09-3592

58. Pusic I, DiPersio JF (2010) Update on clinical experience with AMD3100, an SDF-1/CXCL12-CXCR4 inhibitor, in mobilization of hematopoietic stem and progenitor cells. Curr Opin Hematol 17:319–326. doi:10.1097/MOH.0b013e328338b7d5
59. Devine SM, Flomenberg N, Vesole DH, Liesveld J, Weisdorf D, Badel K, Calandra G, DiPersio JF (2004) Rapid mobilization of CD34+ cells following administration of the CXCR4 antagonist AMD3100 to patients with multiple myeloma and non-Hodgkin's lymphoma. J Clin Oncol 22:1095–1102. doi:10.1200/JCO.2004.07.131
60. Calandra G, McCarty J, McGuirk J, Tricot G, Crocker SA, Badel K, Grove B, Dye A, Bridger G (2008) AMD3100 plus G-CSF can successfully mobilize CD34+ cells from non-Hodgkin's lymphoma, Hodgkin's disease and multiple myeloma patients previously failing mobilization with chemotherapy and/or cytokine treatment: compassionate use data. Bone Marrow Transplant 41:331–338. doi:10.1038/sj.bmt.1705908
61. Giralt S, Stadtmauer EA, Harousseau JL, Palumbo A, Bensinger W, Comenzo RL, Kumar S, Munshi NC, Dispenzieri A, Kyle R, Merlini G, San MJ, Ludwig H, Hajek R, Jagannath S, Blade J, Lonial S, Dimopoulos MA, Einsele H, Barlogie B, Anderson KC, Gertz M, Attal M, Tosi P, Sonneveld P, Boccadoro M, Morgan G, Sezer O, Mateos MV, Cavo M, Joshua D, Turesson I, Chen W, Shimizu K, Powles R, Richardson PG, Niesvizky R, Rajkumar SV, Durie BG (2009) International myeloma working group (IMWG) consensus statement and guidelines regarding the current status of stem cell collection and high-dose therapy for multiple myeloma and the role of plerixafor (AMD 3100). Leukemia 23:1904–1912. doi:10.1038/leu.2009.127
62. Dugan MJ, Maziarz RT, Bensinger WI, Nademanee A, Liesveld J, Badel K, Dehner C, Gibney C, Bridger G, Calandra G (2010) Safety and preliminary efficacy of plerixafor (Mozobil) in combination with chemotherapy and G-CSF: an open-label, multicenter, exploratory trial in patients with multiple myeloma and non-Hodgkin's lymphoma undergoing stem cell mobilization. Bone Marrow Transplant 45:39–47. doi:10.1038/bmt.2009.119
63. Toledano H, Yahel A, Cohen IJ, Yaniv I, Stein J (2010) Successful mobilization, harvest and transplant of peripheral blood stem cells using AMD3100 and G-CSF following high dose craniospinal irradiation for medulloblastoma in a young child. Pediatr Blood Cancer 54: 613–615. doi:10.1002/pbc.22370
64. Grignani G, Perissinotto E, Cavalloni G, Carnevale SF, Aglietta M (2005) Clinical use of AMD3100 to mobilize CD34+ cells in patients affected by non-Hodgkin's lymphoma or multiple myeloma. J Clin Oncol 23:3871–3872. doi:10.1200/JCO.2005.55.250
65. Devine S, Gazitt Y, Calandra G (2005) Reply to Editor. J Clin Oncol 23:3872–3873
66. Tavor S, Eisenbach M, Jacob-Hirsch J, Golan T, Petit I, Benzion K, Kay S, Baron S, Amariglio N, Deutsch V, Naparstek E, Rechavi G (2008) The CXCR4 antagonist AMD3100 impairs survival of human AML cells and induces their differentiation. Leukemia 22:2151–5158. doi:10.1038/leu.2008.238
67. Fruehauf S, Ehninger G, Hubel K, Topaly J, Goldschmidt H, Ho AD, Muller S, Moos M, Badel K, Calandra G (2010) Mobilization of peripheral blood stem cells for autologous transplant in non-Hodgkin's lymphoma and multiple myeloma patients by plerixafor and G-CSF and detection of tumor cell mobilization by PCR in multiple myeloma patients. Bone Marrow Transplant 45:269–275. doi:10.1038/bmt.2009.142
68. Lack NA, Green B, Dale DC, Calandra GB, Lee H, MacFarland RT, Badel K, Liles WC, Bridger G (2005) A pharmacokinetic-pharmacodynamic model for the mobilization of CD34+ hematopoietic progenitor cells by AMD3100. Clin Pharmacol Ther 77:427–436. doi:10.1016/j.clpt.2004.12.268
69. Flomenberg N, Devine SM, DiPersio JF, Liesveld JL, McCarty JM, Rowley SD, Vesole DH, Badel K, Calandra G (2005) The use of AMD3100 plus G-CSF for autologous hematopoietic progenitor cell mobilization is superior to G-CSF alone. Blood 106:1867–1874. doi:10.1182/blood-2005-02-0468
70. Fruehauf S, Seeger T, Maier P, Li L, Weinhardt S, Laufs S, Wagner W, Eckstein V, Bridger G, Calandra G, Wenz F, Zeller WJ, Goldschmidt H, Ho AD (2006) The CXCR4 antagonist AMD3100 releases a subset of G-CSF-primed peripheral blood progenitor cells with specific gene expression characteristics. Exp Hematol 34:1052–1059. doi:10.1016/j.exphem.2006.06.003

71. Capoccia BJ, Shepherd RM, Link DC (2006) G-CSF and AMD3100 mobilize monocytes into the blood that stimulate angiogenesis in vivo through a paracrine mechanism. Blood 108:2438–2445. doi:10.1182/blood-2006-04-013755
72. Broxmeyer HE, Hangoc G, Cooper S, Campbell T, Ito S, Mantel C (2007) AMD3100 and CD26 modulate mobilization, engraftment, and survival of hematopoietic stem and progenitor cells mediated by the SDF-1/CXCL12-CXCR4 axis. Ann N Y Acad Sci 1106:1–19. doi:10.1196/annals.1392.013
73. Pelus LM, Fukuda S, Bridger G (2006) The CXCR4 antagonist AMD3100 and the CXCR2 agonist GROβ synergistically mobilize hematopoietic stem cells (HSC) with short and long term repopulating activity. Blood 108(suppl Part 1):105a (abstract #339)
74. Hoggatt J, Pelus LM (2010) Hematopoietic stem cell mobilization with agents other than G-CSF. In: Methods in molecular biology. Stem cell mobilization: methods and protocols. Humana Press (in press)
75. Pelus LM, Clapp DW, Bridger G (2006) Suprasynergistic peripheral blood stem cell mobilization in normal and Fanconi anemia knockout mice by the combination of G-CSF plus the CXCR4 antagonist AMD3100 and the CXCR2 agonist GROβ. Blood 108(suppl Part 1):909a (abstract #3185)
76. Pelus LM, Singh P (2008) The combination of AMD3100 plus GROβ rapidly mobilizes hematopoietic stem cells with enhanced homing, adhesion and survival properties. Blood (Abstract) 112:34, abstract 71
77. Chen J, Larochelle A, Fricker S, Bridger G, Dunbar CE, Abkowitz JL (2006) Mobilization as a preparative regimen for hematopoietic stem cell transplantation. Blood 107:3764–3771. doi:10.1182/blood-2005-09-3593
78. Broxmeyer HE, Christopherson KW II (2004) Stromal cell derived factor-1/CXCL12, CXCR4 and CD26 in the mobilization and homing of hematopoietic stem and progenitor cells. Curr Med Chem Anti-Inflamm Anti Allergy Agents 3:303–311, In special issue: Guest Editor: Kim CH (guest ed) Lymphocyte migration and chemokines
79. Campbell TB, Hangoc G, Liu Y, Pollok K, Broxmeyer HE (2007) Inhibition of CD26 in human cord blood CD34+ cells enhances their engraftment of nonobese diabetic/severe combined immunodeficiency mice. Stem Cells Dev 16:347–354. doi:10.1089/scd.2007.9995
80. Kang Y, Chen BJ, Deoliveira D, Mito J, Chao NJ (2010) Selective enhancement of donor hematopoietic cell engraftment by the CXCR4 antagonist AMD3100 in a mouse transplantation model. PLoS One 5:e11316
81. Guo Y, Hangoc G, Bian H, Pelus LM, Broxmeyer HE (2005) SDF-1/CXCL12 enhances survival and chemotaxis of murine embryonic stem cells and production of primitive and definitive hematopoietic progenitor cells. Stem Cells 23:1324–1332. doi:10.1634/stemcells.2005-0085
82. Lee HM, Wysoczynski M, Liu R, Shin DM, Kucia M, Botto M, Ratajczak J, Ratajczak MZ (2010) Mobilization studies in complement-deficient mice reveal that optimal AMD3100 mobilization of hematopoietic stem cells depends on complement cascade activation by AMD3100-stimulated granulocytes. Leukemia 24:573–582. doi:10.1038/leu.2009.271
83. Cheng M, Zhou J, Wu M, Boriboun C, Thorne T, Liu T, Xiang Z, Zeng Q, Tanaka T, Tang YL, Kishore R, Tomasson MH, Miller RJ, Losordo DW, Qin G (2010) CXCR4-mediated bone marrow progenitor cell maintenance and mobilization are modulated by c-kit activity. Circ Res 107:1083–1093. doi:10.1161/CIRCRESAHA.110.220970
84. Dar A, Schajnovitz A, Lapid K, Kalinkovich A, Itkin T, Ludin A, Kao W-M, Battista M, Tesio M, Kollet O, Netzer Cohen N, Margalit R, Buss EC, Baleux F, Oshi S, Fujii N, Larochelle A, Dunbar CE, Broxmeyer HE, Frenette PS, Lapidot T (2010) Rapid mobilization of hematopoietic progenitors by AMD3100 and catecholamine is mediated by CXCR4-dependent SDF-1 release from bone marrow stromal cells. Leukemia 25(8):1286–1296
85. Lukacs NW, Berlin A, Schols D, Skerlj RT, Bridger GJ (2002) AMD3100, a CxCR4 antagonist, attenuates allergic lung inflammation and airway hyperreactivity. Am J Pathol 160:1353–1360
86. Matthys P, Hatse S, Vermeire K, Wuyts A, Bridger G, Henson GW, De CE, Billiau A, Schols D (2001) AMD3100, a potent and specific antagonist of the stromal cell-derived factor-1 chemokine receptor CXCR4, inhibits autoimmune joint inflammation in IFN-gamma receptor-deficient mice. J Immunol 167:4686–4692

87. Le BB, Van CN, Daoudi JM, Di GC, Domb AJ, Vierling P (2004) AMD3100 conjugates as components of targeted nonviral gene delivery systems: synthesis and in vitro transfection efficiency of CXCR4-expressing cells. Bioconjug Chem 15:413–423. doi:10.1021/bc034220o
88. Helbig G, Christopherson KW, Bhat-Nakshatri P, Kumar S, Kishimoto H, Miller KD, Broxmeyer HE, Nakshatri H (2003) NF-kappaB promotes breast cancer cell migration and metastasis by inducing the expression of the chemokine receptor CXCR4. J Biol Chem 278:21631–21638. doi:10.1074/jbc.M300609200
89. Mehta SA, Christopherson KW, Bhat-Nakshatri P, Goulet RJ Jr, Broxmeyer HE, Kopelovich L, Nakshatri H (2007) Negative regulation of chemokine receptor CXCR4 by tumor suppressor p53 in breast cancer cells: implications of p53 mutation or isoform expression on breast cancer cell invasion. Oncogene 26:3329–3337. doi:10.1038/sj.onc.1210120
90. Andreeff M, Konoplev S, Wang RY, Zeng Z, McQueen T, Shi YX, Medeiros LJ, Estey E, McCarty JM, Elkins S, Champlin R, Calandra G, Bridger G, Konopleva M (2006) Massive mobilization of AML cells into circulation by disruption of leukemia/stroma cell interactions using CXCR4 antagonist AMD3100: First evidence in patients and potential for abolishing bone marrow microenvironment-mediated resistance. Blood 108(suppl Part 1):171a (abstract #568)
91. Mendez-Ferrer S, Chow A, Merad M, Frenette PS (2009) Circadian rhythms influence hematopoietic stem cells. Curr Opin Hematol 16:235–242. doi:10.1097/MOH.0b013e32832bd0f5
92. Notta F, Doulatov S, Laurent E, Peoppl A, Jurisica I, Dick JE (2011) Isolation of single human hematopoietic stem cells Capable of long-term multilineage engraftment. Science 333:218–221

Chapter 2
Molecular Pharmacology of CXCR4 Inhibition

Anne Steen and Mette Marie Rosenkilde

Abstract In recent years, the chemokine receptor CXCR4 has been shown to be implemented in the mobilization of progenitor cells from the bone marrow. This finding has prompted a search for CXCR4 antagonists acting as stem cell mobilizing agents. In accordance, it is important to look into the molecular pharmacology of well-known CXCR4 antagonists in order to augment the potency and affinity and to increase the specificity of future CXCR4-targeting compounds. In this chapter, binding modes of CXCR4 antagonists that have been shown to mobilize stem cells are discussed. In addition, comparisons between results obtained from structure–function studies and findings from newly released crystal structures are drawn.

The Activation of 7TM Rcceptors (G Protein-Coupled Receptors)

Chemokine receptors belong to the largest family of proteins in the human genome, namely the seven transmembrane spanning receptors (7TM receptors). Drugs targeting these receptors represent the majority of prescribed pharmaceuticals [1]. Therefore, it is expected that many more of these receptors are potential drug targets and numerous experiments have been performed in order to determine the exact activation mechanism.

A. Steen • M.M. Rosenkilde (✉)
The Laboratory of Molecular Pharmacology, Department of Neuroscience and Pharmacology, University of Copenhagen, The Panum Institute, Copenhagen DK-2200, Denmark
e-mail: annesteen@sund.ku.dk; rosenkilde@sund.ku.dk

S. Fruehauf et al. (eds.), *Novel Developments in Stem Cell Mobilization: Focus on CXCR4*, DOI 10.1007/978-1-4614-1960-0_2,

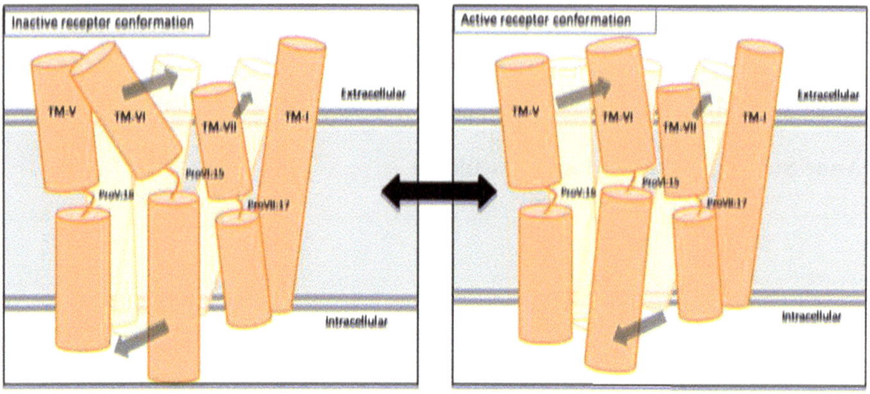

Fig. 2.1 Schematic drawing of the 7TM receptor activation mechanism as proposed by the Global Toggle Switch Model. TM-VI and TM-VII move around a weak point generated by the two highly conserved prolines in each helix. *Left panel*: The inactive receptor conformation. *Right panel*: The active conformation, in which the extracellular ends of TM-VI and TM-VII move toward each other, meanwhile the intracellular parts move away from one another, creating space for the binding of the signaling molecules. Redrawn from Schwartz et al. [2]

One theory of what occurs during the activation of 7TM receptors is the Global Toggle Switch Model described by Schwartz and coworkers [2–4]. Generally speaking, it is believed that all family A 7TM receptors are activated in much the same way, despite the fact that these receptors are activated by highly diverse ligands [5, 6]. Many of the studies that have been performed indicate that relatively large overall changes in the arrangement of the intracellular parts of the helices occur during receptor activation [7, 8]. This has led to the Global Toggle Switch Model, in which transmembrane domain VI (TM-VI) in particular performs a vertical "see-saw" movement, or a so-called toggle motion. This implies that the extracellular end of the helix tilts into the main ligand-binding pocket, meanwhile the intracellular end moves outward. In the assumed active state, an agonist binds and stabilizes this conformation. The extra space that is created on the intracellular side of the receptor allows for an associated molecule (e.g., the activated G protein or arrestin) to bind and elicit the signaling cascade (Fig. 2.1). However, due to the difficulty of crystallizing a stabilized active 7TM receptor, it has been difficult to provide proof of this theory. In fact, only recently rhodopsin (more specifically opsin, the ligand-free form of rhodopsin) was crystallized in what is presumed to be an active representation (despite the fact that the agonist, all-*trans* retinal, was lacking) [9, 10]. This crystal structure showed that compared to the dark inactive state of rhodopsin, the cytoplasmic half of TM-VI is tilted outward away from the helical bundle by 6–7 Å.

Furthermore, the crystallization indicated that TM-V is longer, very straight, and more inclined with a resulting shift of the cytoplasmic end by 2–3 Å toward TM-VI. Unlike the activation of rhodopsin by light, agonists are very inefficient in stabilizing an active state of the β_2 adrenergic receptor (β_2AR), making it difficult to secure the receptor in this conformation [11]. Moreover, even in complex with an agonist, the β_2AR crystallizes in an inactive conformation [12]. Experiments have shown that stabilization of the active state requires both binding of an agonist as well as the G protein [13]. In 2011, Kobilka and coworkers published the structure of a stabilized active conformation of the β_2 adrenergic receptor [11]. They employed a so-called nanobody that exhibits G protein-like behavior toward the β_2AR, preferentially binds to and stabilizes the active conformation, and furthermore, are more stable in detergent solutions the inherent G protein. Creating a complex of the β_2AR (coupled to a T4 lysosome which stabilizes the receptor [14]), the nanobody as well as a high-affinity agonist with favorable efficacy and a very slow off-rate made it possible to create a stabilized structure of an active β_2AR. When the β_2AR structure was superimposed with the opsin structure they were remarkably similar both in respect to the outward movement of the intracellular end of TM-VI as well as TM-V. Thus, these two active crystal structures provide further proof that overall conformational changes occur, including the toggle of TM-VI.

Molecular Pharmacology of CXCR4 Antagonists

Several CXCR4-targeting antagonists have been published since this chemokine receptor was discovered in 1996 (for recent review, see [15]). However, as the preponderance of these compounds are treated as anti-HIV compounds, only compounds which have been shown to act as stem cell mobilizing agents are included in the following sections.

The Cyclam Family

AMD3100 (Plerixafor/Mozobil™)

The cyclam-related compounds include the only CXCR4-targeting stem cell mobilizer that have reached the clinic (AMD3100 (Plerixafor, Mozobil™)). In general, these compounds are small-molecule antagonists of which AMD3100 is the prototype. It is composed of two 1,4,8,11-tetraazacyclotetradecane (cyclam) moieties linked together by a conformationally constraining aromatic linker (Fig. 2.2a). As the original indication of AMD3100 was anti-HIV therapy, the majority of published structure–function assays describe its potency in the inhibition of HIV-infection and not in the mobilization of stem cells.

Bicyclams are strongly basic at physiological pH due to the presence of four primary amines in each cyclam ring [16] and x-ray together with neutron diffraction structures have shown that the protonated cyclam ring has a tendency to form complexes with carboxylic acid groups by hydrogen bonds [17]. Accordingly, several studies have focused on the negatively charged domains facing the binding pocket of CXCR4.

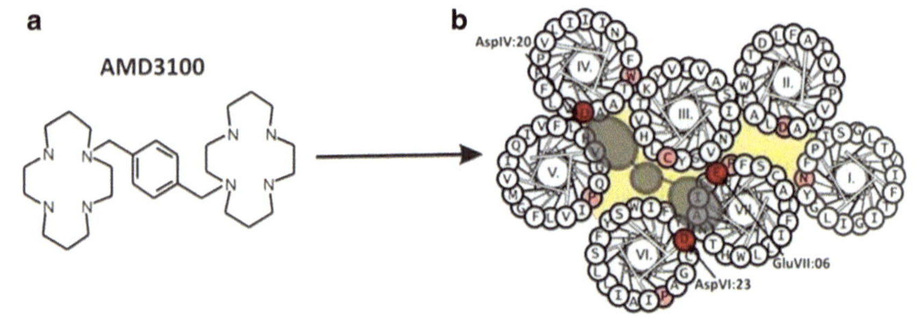

Fig. 2.2 (**a**) Chemical structure of the bicyclam AMD3100. (**b**) Schematic presentation of the proposed binding mode of AMD3100. Inserted is a helical wheel diagram of the chemokine receptor CXCR4. The *gray marking* shows the assumed position of the antagonist within the receptor and residues shown to be involved in the interaction are indicated in *red*. Conserved residues are colored *light red*

One of the first studies described a series of mutations in the extracellular loop 2 (ECL2) and TM-IV and the association with the degree of drug resistance [18]. In this study, it was found that mutating aspartates to neutral amino acids (asparagine, alanine, or glycine) in the examined domains of CXCR4 markedly increased the resistance to AMD3100 and thus are important for the interaction between the compound and the receptor. Specifically, they suggested that Asp^{181}, Asp^{182}, Asp^{187}, and Asp^{193} in ECL2 and Asp^{171} (IV:20) in TM-IV were involved in AMD3100 interaction (the numbers in parentheses indicate the Schwartz generic numbering system modified from Baldwin's system [19, 20]). Furthermore, they noticed that mutating phenylalanines in the same two regions of CXCR4 (Phe^{172} (IV:21) and Phe^{174} (IV:23) in TM-IV and Phe^{199} and Phe^{210} in ECL2) to nonaromatic amino acids also decreased the efficacy of AMD3100. It was speculated that the importance of the phenylalanines was due to interactions with the aromatic linker of AMD3100. The authors argued that the reasons for this could be both direct interaction of the residues with the compound or that altering an amino acid could change the overall configuration of the receptor and indirectly affect the interaction between AMD3100 and CXCR4.

In 2001, Gerlach et al. performed a comprehensive mutagenesis study of all aspartate residues facing the binding pocket of CXCR4 [21]. Furthermore, in a previous study it had been shown that the cyclam rings are able to chelate metal ions and in fact that transition metal ion chelated by the two macrocyclic rings of AMD3100 increase the affinity [22–24]. Based on this finding, Gerlach et al. also included metal ion-binding histidine residues facing the binding pocket. Testing all the mutants in competition binding, it was clear that especially two aspartate residues in the extracellular ends of TM-IV (Asp^{171}) and TM-VI (Asp^{262} (VI:23)) are involved in the binding of AMD3100. Testing a single cyclam unit or a monocyclam against the same mutations indicated that only Asp^{171}, and not Asp^{262}, was important for monocyclam-based compounds. Taken together, these findings led to a proposal of the interaction mode, in which AMD3100 spans the ligand-binding pocket and each cyclam ring binds to the two aspartate residues located at the extracellular ends of the transmembrane domains.

The authors speculated that because of the conformationally constraining aromatic linker, AMD3100 could simply prevent the receptor from changing into an—at that time unknown—active conformation. The decreased affinity of the compounds containing only one cyclam ring in the receptor where Asp^{171} had been mutated could represent the affinity to Asp^{262}. Alternatively, the single cyclam does bind to Asp^{262}, but this does not interfere with binding of the radioactive-labeled competing ligand (CXCL12/SDF-1α) and would not be detected.

Through mutational substitutions of 16 residues located in TM-III, -IV, -V, -VI, and -VII of CXCR4, it was shown that AMD3100 depends strongly on not only the two aspartate residues previously mentioned (Asp^{171} and Asp^{262}), but also a glutamate (Glu^{288} (VII:06)) in TM-VII [25]. When chelating zinc to AMD3100 it increased the dependency on Asp^{262} tenfold and a number of other residues on the inner face of TM-IV, -V, and -VI also appeared to be involved. The combination of these three acidic residues is unique to CXCR4, which is in agreement with the fact that AMD3100 is known to be highly selective for CXCR4 [26]. However, when aligning the chemokine receptors, it was discovered that two of the three residues (Asp^{171} and Asp^{262}) are present in the CXCR3 receptor, which otherwise is structurally rather distinct in the remaining binding pocket. On the other hand, a lysine is present in position 300 (LysVII:02), which possibly forms a neutralizing salt bridge with Asp^{278} (corresponding to Asp^{272} (VI:23) in CXCR4). To verify the assumed binding site of AMD3100, the construction of two mutations was necessary in CXCR3 (Ser^{304} (VII:06) to Glu and Lys^{300} to Ala (to interrupt the salt bridge)). Testing the mutant receptors in an inositol phosphate-signaling assay showed that AMD3100 was not able to inhibit activation induced by the endogenous chemokines on the CXCR3 wild-type receptor or on a receptor where only one of the mutations had been introduced. However, when combining the two mutations in CXCR3, and thereby reconstituting the tri-dentate acidic binding site in CXCR4, partial inhibition was seen when testing AMD3100 and the zinc-chelated form acted as a full antagonist. This finding supports the notion that these three acidic residues are essential and sufficient for AMD3100 binding. Previous studies have shown that the function of the linker is not based on its aromatic properties, but rather that it constrains the mobility and distance between the cyclam moieties [27, 28]. Based on this knowledge and the fact that the mutational analysis did not suggest that the side chains of any of the surrounding amino acids in proximity of the aromatic linker are involved in AMD3100-interaction, a binding mode of the compound was suggested: one cyclam ring interacts with the aspartate in TM-IV, while the other is sandwiched in between the aspartate in TM-VI and the glutamate in TM-VII. The linker then acts, as previously suggested, as a constraint, preventing TM-VI from moving inward and into the active conformation (Fig. 2.2b).

AMD3465 (A Monocyclam)

In the pursuit of orally bioavailable compounds, eradicating the cyclam moieties of AMD3100 is essential, because as mentioned before each cyclam ring has a

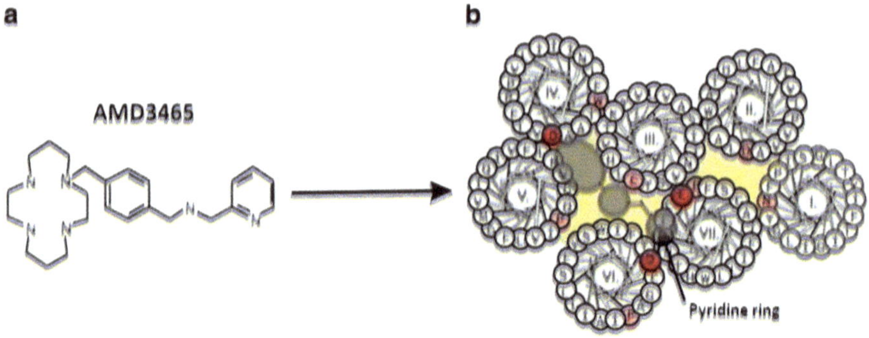

Fig. 2.3 (**a**) Chemical structure of the monocyclam AMD3465. (**b**) Schematic presentation of the proposed binding mode of the antagonist shown in a helical wheel diagram of CXCR4. The position of the compound is shown in *gray*, the pyridine ring of the molecule is indicated. Residues shown to be involved in the interaction are shown in *red*. In addition, His[281], placed at the extracellular end of TM-VII, is believed to be involved in the binding of the pyridine ring. Conserved residues are indicated in *light red*

positive charge of +2. As the original indication was as an antiviral therapeutic, a related compound with a higher oral bioavailability was sought after. However, as a stem cell mobilizing compound the lack of oral bioavailability does not pose any hindrances.

One such compound is AMD3465, the prototype monocyclam—constructed as a derivative of AMD3100 where one of the cyclam rings has been substituted by a pyridinemethylene moiety (Fig. 2.3a). In a publication from 2007, the complete binding mode of AMD3465 was described [29]. By mutational analysis it was shown that the monocyclam was dependent on the same three acidic residues as AMD3100 (Asp[171], Asp[262], and Glu[288]). Additionally, a number of mutational hits were discovered in the extracellular ends of TM-III, -V, -VI, and -VII, especially mutation of a histidine residue in the top of TM-VII (His[281] (VII:-02)) decreased the binding affinity >4,500-fold of AMD3465. By employing monocyclam compounds that varied in the "non-cyclam" and cyclam part, respectively, the authors were able to establish a very likely interaction mode between AMD3465 and CXCR4. As mentioned previously, Gerlach et al. [21] suggested that the cyclam ring in a monocyclam compound interacts with the aspartate in TM-IV. On the basis of this, it was expected that the pyridine moiety would bind to residues in the extracellular ends of TM-VI and -VII. Indeed, testing the compounds that varied in the "non-cyclam" part showed that they were not influenced by mutations made in the pocket surrounded by TM-III, -VI, and -VII but the mutational hits found for AMD3100 and AMD3465 in TM-IV and -V were still present. Moreover, these alternative monocyclam compounds displayed a much lower affinity than AMD3465 and this indicates that the pyridine interaction of AMD3465 with the residues in TM-VI and -VII—especially His[281]—is necessary for high-affinity

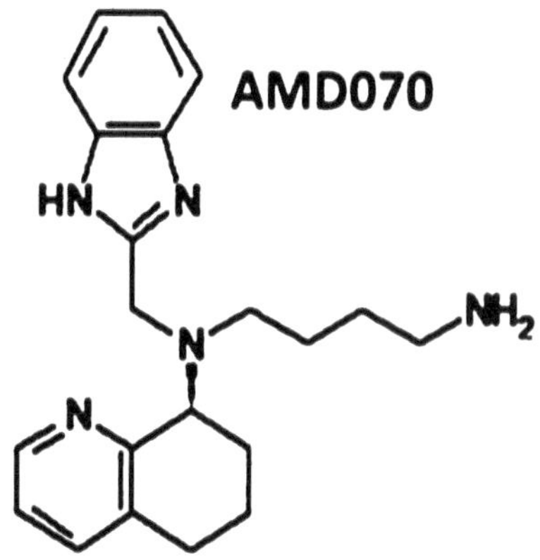

Fig. 2.4 Chemical structure of the noncyclam AMD070

binding to CXCR4. Accordingly, neither of the compounds varying in the cyclam part (by incorporation of a Cu^{2+} or a Ni^{2+}) of the molecule differed from AMD3465 in respect to affinity and was influenced by the same mutations as AMD3465. In conclusion, AMD3465 is believed to mimic the binding mode of AMD3100, with the cyclam ring interacting with Asp^{171} in TM-IV and neighboring residues in TM-III and -V, whereas the pyridine domain interacts with residues in the extracellular end of TM-VI and -VII, in particular His^{281}, which are not involved in AMD3100 binding (Fig. 2.3b).

AMD070 (A Noncyclam)

Because of the "remaining" cyclam moiety in AMD3465, the compound still needs to be administered by a parental route. The monocyclam could therefore be considered to constitute a medical intermediate compound—a step on the way to accomplish orally bioavailable compounds. Indeed, such a molecule has been developed, namely AMD070 (or AMD11070), in which the second cyclam ring has been replaced by a more drug-like chemical moiety (Fig. 2.4).

Not much work has been published on the molecular pharmacology of AMD070, but one publication has suggested that the compound overlaps with the binding sites that are shared between AMD3100 and AMD3465, i.e., Asp^{171}, Asp^{262}, and Glu^{288} [30]. In addition to the shared tri-acidic motif, the authors found that AMD070 also exhibited dependence on residues in the corner between TM-I, -II, -III, and -VII, namely Asp^{97} (II:23), Trp^{94} (II:20) (both in TM-II), and Tyr^{45} (I:07) (in TM-I). AMD070 has been tested in Phase II clinical trials as an anti-HIV agent, and has in general been well tolerated, but is currently on clinical hold due to histologic changes to the liver observed in long-term animal studies [31]. Additional preclinical safety assessments are pending.

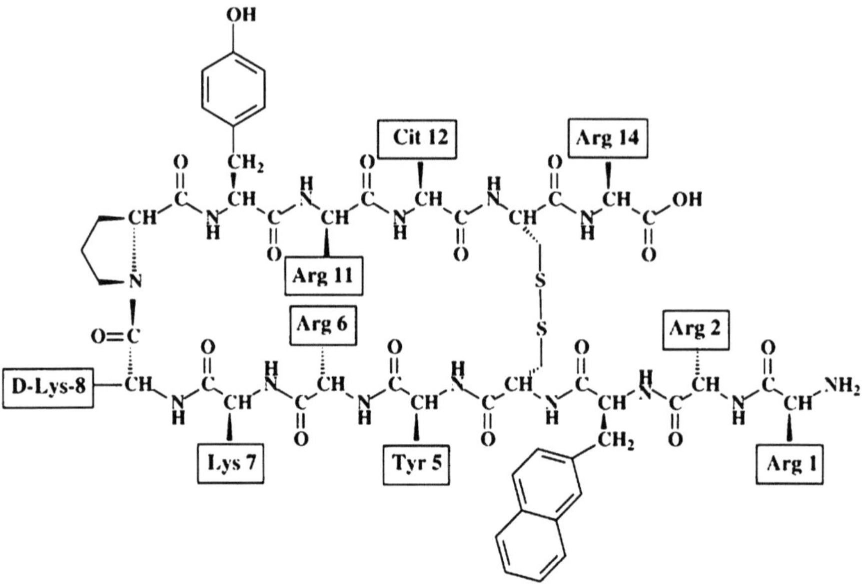

Fig. 2.5 Chemical structure of T140

Peptidic Compounds

T22, T140, and Derivatives

T22 is an 18-mer and a potent inhibitor of CXCR4 through an interaction with the N terminus and extracellular loop 1 and 2 [32–34]. However, the compound is highly basic and has poor oral bioavailability. Hence, smaller, more potent derivatives of T22, e.g., T140, have been constructed in which some of the basic amino acids have been replaced (Fig. 2.5). In a study from 2009, it was shown that administration of T140 to bone marrow-transplanted mice increases the production of progenitor and mature cells and exit to the periphery [35].

In 2003, a computational model of CXCR4 in a solvated lipid bilayer in complex with T140 was published [36]. The authors identified key residues by mutagenesis and used these as a basis for a plausible docking mode of T140. The computational model showed that the N terminal of T140 interacted with ECL2, while the C terminal was oriented inferiorly and interacted with residues in TM-IV as well as in ECL2 and ECL3. Four key residues of T140 had previously been identified as indispensable for CXCR4 antagonism, namely Arg^2, Nal^3, Tyr^5 (in the N terminus of T140), and Arg^{14} (in the C terminus) [37] and were predicted to act directly with CXCR4. In fact, the four key residues all had multiple interactions with residues in CXCR4, including amino acids in the N terminus, TM-IV, TM-V, ECL2, and ECL3, mainly in the extracellular regions. The modeling showed that Arg^{14} of T140 forms strong hydrogen bonds with Asp^{171} of CXCR4 (also seen to be important for binding of compounds belonging to the cyclam family). The authors also showed that mutation of Asp^{262} to alanine decreased the efficiency of T140. They speculated that this was due to a crucial role of ECL3 for the interactions with the C terminal of T140.

FC131 is a cyclic pentapeptide, derived from the critical residues of T140 for CXCR4 inhibition. In an extensive study from 2006, 11 derivatives of FC131, which were believed to share a common binding mode, were docked to a three-dimensional model of the transmembrane region of CXCR4 [38]. The authors had previously published a minimalistic 3D pharmacophore model for cyclopentapeptides suggesting the spatial arrangement of the domains required for CXCR4 binding [39], and the ligands were docked according to this model to further elucidate the atomic details of the CXCR4 interaction. By comparing the result of the ligand poses only two of the binding modes were common for all 11 compounds indicating likely binding modes.

The two proposed binding modes partly overlapped. However, the first binding mode indicates that the compounds mostly interact with residues in the "minor" ligand-binding pocket, i.e., the area that is defined by TM-I, -II, -III, and -VII, albeit part of the cyclopentapeptides might interact with hydrophobic residues in the "major" binding pocket (delimited by TM-III, -IV, -V, -VI, and -VII). On the other hand, the second proposal for a binding mode places the ligands in the CXCR4 "hotspot", in between TM-III, -V, -VI, and -VII. Interestingly, in both binding modes Arg^4 of the ligands forms a salt bridge with Glu^{288}, which also had been shown to be highly involved in the interaction between CXCR4 and the cyclam compounds [25]. However, in the computational modeling of the complex between CXCR4 and T140, the residue did not seem to interact with the compound [36].

The First Crystal Structure of a Chemokine Receptor: CXCR4

In 2010, the first crystal structure of a chemokine receptor, namely CXCR4, was published [40]. Stevens and coworkers described five independent inactive structures (three different constructs) of CXCR4 where either a small-molecule compound derived from isothiourea, IT1t, or a cyclic peptide, CVX15 was bound. In order to stabilize the receptor structure, they employed a T4 lysozyme fusion inserted between TM-V and -VI on the cytoplasmic side as well as additional thermostabilizing mutations. The authors describe the most distinctive differences between the structure of CXCR4 and other published crystal structures of 7TM receptors and indicate that homology models of CXCR4 based on these previously published structures might give a wrong impression of which residues are in the proximity and interacting with the ligands.

The ligand-binding pocket differs from other published structures of 7TM receptors in that it is larger, more open, and is located more proximal to the extracellular surface. The small-molecule antagonist, IT1t, occupies the part of the pocket that is delimited by side chains of TM-I, -II, -III, and -VII (the so-called "minor" binding pocket) and makes no contact with TM-IV, -V, and -VI. This is in stark contrast to ligands complexed to other 7TM receptor structures and is not consistent with the molecular pharmacology for other CXCR4 small-molecule antagonists predicted by mutational analysis, as discussed above. IT1t contains nitrogen molecules that could be protonated with a net positive charge. One of them forms a salt bridge with Asp^{97} in TM-II while another could make a polar interaction with a cysteine in ECL2 (residue 186). Both cyclohexane rings of IT1t fit into small pockets and form hydrophobic contacts with CXCR4. The imidazothiazole ring is connected to the rest of the molecule by a short flexible linker and appears to make a salt bridge to Glu^{288}.

The bulky 16-residue cyclic peptide compound, CVX15, fills most of the binding pocket volume. The peptide forms a β-hairpin loop and both the N terminal and C terminal of the compound are buried in the pocket. The first four amino acids in the N terminus of the peptide form hydrogen bonds to CXCR4 with backbone residues in ECL2. The first residue in the peptide, an arginine, makes polar interactions with Asp^{187} (in ECL2), while the second amino acid, also an arginine, interacts with Thr^{117} (III:09), Asp^{171}, and possibly His^{113} (III:05). An arginine in the C terminal of the peptide makes a salt bridge with Asp^{262} and a salt bridge is also observed between Asp^{193} in the top of TM-V and a lysine at position 7 in the peptide. Finally, a proline in the C terminal makes a water-mediated interaction with the Glu^{288}.

Concluding Remarks

Studying the molecular pharmacology of a compound is vital when optimizing the properties of the compound. Learning the exact binding mode and which residues the compound interacts with is crucial for the drug development process. The knowledge provides clues in the further pursuit of a more potent compound. Furthermore, increasing the specificity of the compound to its target will decrease the possibility of side effects. The experimental methods to obtain knowledge about the specific interactions between a compound and a corresponding receptor are plentiful, and the amount of publications of crystal structures has, since the first published crystal structure of rhodopsin in 2001, increased substantially and provides a unique insight into how ligands may bind and 7TM receptors are activated. However, the crystal structures are instant images of an inactive or an active receptor and not of the dynamic process that happens when a receptor is activated. This is why the functional receptor studies are also important and over the last two decades the functional studies have led to, in combination with crystal structures, a unifying mode of 7TM receptor activation, namely the Global Toggle Switch Model.

As can be deduced from the crystal structures of CXCR4 in complex with the small-molecule antagonist IT1t, the binding mode of the compound clearly stands out from what has been published previously. The interaction pattern between CXCR4 and IT1t differs from results obtained from mutational studies as well as homology models of CXCR4 based on crystal structures of other 7TM receptors. This shows that there is still a need for a more specific description of the molecular requirements for receptor activation and the detailed molecular interaction and binding modes of different ligands. The recently presented crystal structure of CXCR4 constitutes an important step toward further understanding of the molecular requirements for CXCR4 action.

Acknowledgments The authors are supported from The Danish Research Council for Independent Research | Medical Sciences, The NovoNordisk Foundation, The Lundbeck Foundation and the European Community's Sixth Framework program (INNOCHEM: LSHB-CT-2005-518167), the AP-Moller Foundation and the Aase and Einar Danielsen Foundation.

References

1. Klabunde T, Hessler G (2002) Drug design strategies for targeting G-protein-coupled receptors. Chembiochem 3(10):928–944. doi:10.1002/1439-7633(20021004)3:10<928::AID-CBIC928>3.0.CO;2-5
2. Schwartz TW, Frimurer TM, Holst B, Rosenkilde MM, Elling CE (2006) Molecular mechanism of 7TM receptor activation—a global toggle switch model. Annu Rev Pharmacol Toxicol 46:481–519. doi:10.1146/annurev.pharmtox.46.120604.141218
3. Nygaard R, Frimurer TM, Holst B, Rosenkilde MM, Schwartz TW (2009) Ligand binding and micro-switches in 7TM receptor structures. Trends Pharmacol Sci 30(5):249–259. doi:S0165-6147(09)00054-6 [pii] 10.1016/j.tips.2009.02.006
4. Benned-Jensen T, Rosenkilde MM (2009) The role of transmembrane segment II in 7TM receptor activation. Curr Mol Pharmacol 2(2):140–148
5. Schwartz TW, Rosenkilde MM (1996) Is there a "lock" for all agonist "keys" in 7TM receptors? Trends Pharmacol Sci 17(6):213–216. doi:0165614796100171 [pii]
6. Pierce KL, Premont RT, Lefkowitz RJ (2002) Seven-transmembrane receptors. Nat Rev Mol Cell Biol 3(9):639–650. doi:10.1038/nrm908 nrm908 [pii]
7. Hubbell WL, Altenbach C, Hubbell CM, Khorana HG (2003) Rhodopsin structure, dynamics, and activation: a perspective from crystallography, site-directed spin labeling, sulfhydryl reactivity, and disulfide cross-linking. Adv Protein Chem 63:243–290
8. Altenbach C, Kusnetzow AK, Ernst OP, Hofmann KP, Hubbell WL (2008) High-resolution distance mapping in rhodopsin reveals the pattern of helix movement due to activation. Proc Natl Acad Sci USA 105(21):7439–7444. doi:0802515105 [pii] 10.1073/pnas.0802515105
9. Scheerer P, Park JH, Hildebrand PW, Kim YJ, Krauss N, Choe HW, Hofmann KP, Ernst OP (2008) Crystal structure of opsin in its G-protein-interacting conformation. Nature 455(7212):497–502. doi:nature07330 [pii] 10.1038/nature07330
10. Park JH, Scheerer P, Hofmann KP, Choe HW, Ernst OP (2008) Crystal structure of the ligand-free G-protein-coupled receptor opsin. Nature 454(7201):183–187. doi:nature07063 [pii] 10.1038/nature07063
11. Rasmussen SG, Choi HJ, Fung JJ, Pardon E, Casarosa P, Chae PS, Devree BT, Rosenbaum DM, Thian FS, Kobilka TS, Schnapp A, Konetzki I, Sunahara RK, Gellman SH, Pautsch A, Steyaert J, Weis WI, Kobilka BK (2011) Structure of a nanobody-stabilized active state of the beta(2) adrenoceptor. Nature 469(7329):175–180. doi:nature09648 [pii] 10.1038/nature09648
12. Rosenbaum DM, Zhang C, Lyons JA, Holl R, Aragao D, Arlow DH, Rasmussen SG, Choi HJ, Devree BT, Sunahara RK, Chae PS, Gellman SH, Dror RO, Shaw DE, Weis WI, Caffrey M, Gmeiner P, Kobilka BK (2011) Structure and function of an irreversible agonist-beta(2) adrenoceptor complex. Nature 469(7329):236–240. doi:nature09665 [pii] 10.1038/nature09665
13. Yao XJ, Velez Ruiz G, Whorton MR, Rasmussen SG, DeVree BT, Deupi X, Sunahara RK, Kobilka B (2009) The effect of ligand efficacy on the formation and stability of a GPCR-G protein complex. Proc Natl Acad Sci USA 106(23):9501–9506. doi:0811437106 [pii] 10.1073/pnas.0811437106

14. Rosenbaum DM, Cherezov V, Hanson MA, Rasmussen SG, Thian FS, Kobilka TS, Choi HJ, Yao XJ, Weis WI, Stevens RC, Kobilka BK (2007) GPCR engineering yields high-resolution structural insights into beta2-adrenergic receptor function. Science 318(5854):1266–1273. doi:1150609 [pii] 10.1126/science.1150609
15. Steen A, Schwartz TW, Rosenkilde MM (2009) Targeting CXCR4 in HIV cell-entry inhibition. Mini Rev Med Chem 9:1605–1621. doi:MRMC Epub-055 [pii]
16. Izatt RM, Pawlak K, Bradshaw JS, Bruening RL (1991) Thermodynamic and kinetic data for macrocycle interactions with cations and anions. Chem Rev 91(8):1721–2085. doi:10.1021/cr00008a003
17. Adam KR, Antolovich M, Atkinson IM, Leong AJ, Lindoy LF, McCool BJ, Davis RL, Kennard CHL, Tasker PA (1994) On the nature of the host-guest interaction between cyclam and 4-tert-butylbenzoic acid-a system pre-assembled for metal complex formation. J Chem Soc Chem Commun 13:1539–1540
18. Labrosse B, Brelot A, Heveker N, Sol N, Schols D, De Clercq E, Alizon M (1998) Determinants for sensitivity of human immunodeficiency virus coreceptor CXCR4 to the bicyclam AMD3100. J Virol 72(8):6381–6388
19. Schwartz TW (1994) Locating ligand-binding sites in 7TM receptors by protein engineering. Curr Opin Biotechnol 5(4):434–444
20. Baldwin JM (1993) The probable arrangement of the helices in G protein-coupled receptors. EMBO J 12(4):1693–1703
21. Gerlach LO, Skerlj RT, Bridger GJ, Schwartz TW (2001) Molecular interactions of cyclam and bicyclam non-peptide antagonists with the CXCR4 chemokine receptor. J Biol Chem 276(17):14153–14160. doi:10.1074/jbc.M010429200 M010429200 [pii]
22. Troutner DE, Simon J, Ketring AR, Volkert W, Holmes RA (1980) Complexing of Tc-99m with cyclam: concise communication. J Nucl Med 21(5):443–448
23. Este JA, Cabrera C, De Clercq E, Struyf S, Van Damme J, Bridger G, Skerlj RT, Abrams MJ, Henson G, Gutierrez A, Clotet B, Schols D (1999) Activity of different bicyclam derivatives against human immunodeficiency virus depends on their interaction with the CXCR4 chemokine receptor. Mol Pharmacol 55(1):67–73
24. Gerlach LO, Jakobsen JS, Jensen KP, Rosenkilde MR, Skerlj RT, Ryde U, Bridger GJ, Schwartz TW (2003) Metal ion enhanced binding of AMD3100 to Asp262 in the CXCR4 receptor. Biochemistry 42(3):710–717. doi:10.1021/bi0264770
25. Rosenkilde MM, Gerlach LO, Jakobsen JS, Skerlj RT, Bridger GJ, Schwartz TW (2004) Molecular mechanism of AMD3100 antagonism in the CXCR4 receptor: transfer of binding site to the CXCR3 receptor. J Biol Chem 279(4):3033–3041. doi:10.1074/jbc.M309546200 M309546200 [pii]
26. Hatse S, Princen K, Bridger G, De Clercq E, Schols D (2002) Chemokine receptor inhibition by AMD3100 is strictly confined to CXCR4. FEBS Lett 527(1–3):255–262. doi:S0014579302031435 [pii]
27. Bridger GJ, Skerlj RT, Padmanabhan S, Martellucci SA, Henson GW, Abrams MJ, Joao HC, Witvrouw M, De Vreese K, Pauwels R, De Clercq E (1996) Synthesis and structure–activity relationships of phenylenebis(methylene)-linked bis-tetraazamacrocycles that inhibit human immunodeficiency virus replication. 2. Effect of heteroaromatic linkers on the activity of bicyclams. J Med Chem 39(1):109–119. doi:10.1021/jm950584t jm950584t [pii]
28. Joao HC, De Vreese K, Pauwels R, De Clercq E, Henson GW, Bridger GJ (1995) Quantitative structural activity relationship study of bis-tetraazacyclic compounds. A novel series of HIV-1 and HIV-2 inhibitors. J Med Chem 38(19):3865–3873
29. Rosenkilde MM, Gerlach LO, Hatse S, Skerlj RT, Schols D, Bridger GJ, Schwartz TW (2007) Molecular mechanism of action of monocyclam versus bicyclam non-peptide antagonists in the CXCR4 chemokine receptor. J Biol Chem 282(37):27354–27365. doi:M704739200 [pii] 10.1074/jbc.M704739200
30. Wong RS, Bodart V, Metz M, Labrecque J, Bridger G, Fricker SP (2008) Comparison of the potential multiple binding modes of bicyclam, monocylam, and noncyclam small-molecule CXC chemokine receptor 4 inhibitors. Mol Pharmacol 74(6):1485–1495. doi:mol.108.049775 [pii] 10.1124/mol.108.049775

31. Moyle G, DeJesus E, Boffito M, Wong RS, Gibney C, Badel K, MacFarland R, Calandra G, Bridger G, Becker S (2009) Proof of activity with AMD11070, an orally bioavailable inhibitor of CXCR4-tropic HIV type 1. Clin Infect Dis 48(6):798–805. doi:10.1086/597097 10.1086/597097 [pii]
32. Murakami T, Zhang TY, Koyanagi Y, Tanaka Y, Kim J, Suzuki Y, Minoguchi S, Tamamura H, Waki M, Matsumoto A, Fujii N, Shida H, Hoxie JA, Peiper SC, Yamamoto N (1999) Inhibitory mechanism of the CXCR4 antagonist T22 against human immunodeficiency virus type 1 infection. J Virol 73(9):7489–7496
33. Tamamura H, Imai M, Ishihara T, Masuda M, Funakoshi H, Oyake H, Murakami T, Arakaki R, Nakashima H, Otaka A, Ibuka T, Waki M, Matsumoto A, Yamamoto N, Fujii N (1998) Pharmacophore identification of a chemokine receptor (CXCR4) antagonist, T22 ([Tyr(5,12), Lys7]-polyphemusin II), which specifically blocks T cell-line-tropic HIV-1 infection. Bioorg Med Chem 6(7):1033–1041. doi:S0968-0896(98)00061-3 [pii]
34. Tamamura H, Murakami T, Masuda M, Otaka A, Takada W, Ibuka T, Nakashima H, Waki M, Matsumoto A, Yamamoto N et al (1994) Structure–activity relationships of an anti-HIV peptide, T22. Biochem Biophys Res Commun 205(3):1729–1735. doi:S0006291X84728683 [pii]
35. Abraham M, Beider K, Wald H, Weiss ID, Zipori D, Galun E, Nagler A, Eizenberg O, Peled A (2009) The CXCR4 antagonist 4F-benzoyl-TN14003 stimulates the recovery of the bone marrow after transplantation. Leukemia 23(8):1378–1388. doi:leu200956 [pii] 10.1038/leu.2009.56
36. Trent JO, Wang ZX, Murray JL, Shao W, Tamamura H, Fujii N, Peiper SC (2003) Lipid bilayer simulations of CXCR4 with inverse agonists and weak partial agonists. J Biol Chem 278(47):47136–47144. doi:10.1074/jbc.M307850200 M307850200 [pii]
37. Tamamura H, Omagari A, Oishi S, Kanamoto T, Yamamoto N, Peiper SC, Nakashima H, Otaka A, Fujii N (2000) Pharmacophore identification of a specific CXCR4 inhibitor, T140, leads to development of effective anti-HIV agents with very high selectivity indexes. Bioorg Med Chem Lett 10(23):2633–2637. doi:S0960-894X(00)00535-7 [pii]
38. Vabeno J, Nikiforovich GV, Marshall GR (2006) A minimalistic 3D pharmacophore model for cyclopentapeptide CXCR4 antagonists. Biopolymers 84(5):459–471. doi:10.1002/bip. 20508
39. Vabeno J, Nikiforovich GV, Marshall GR (2006) Insight into the binding mode for cyclopentapeptide antagonists of the CXCR4 receptor. Chem Biol Drug Des 67(5):346–354. doi:JPP387 [pii] 10.1111/j.1747-0285.2006.00387.x
40. Wu B, Chien EY, Mol CD, Fenalti G, Liu W, Katritch V, Abagyan R, Brooun A, Wells P, Bi FC, Hamel DJ, Kuhn P, Handel TM, Cherezov V, Stevens RC (2010) Structures of the CXCR4 chemokine GPCR with small-molecule and cyclic peptide antagonists. Science 330(6007):1066–1071. doi:science.1194396 [pii] 10.1126/science.1194396

Chapter 3
Combination Strategies for Stem Cell Mobilization Targeting CXCR4 and S1P Receptors

Nadia Harun, Kenneth Bradstock, and Linda J. Bendall

Clinical Application of Stem Cell Mobilization

Hematopoietic stem cell (HSC) transplantation (HSCT) is now increasingly used to treat a wide range of hematological malignancies as well as certain nonmalignant diseases such as bone marrow failure and immunodeficiency syndromes, metabolic disorders, and autoimmune diseases [1]. In addition, HSC have been investigated for the treatment of ischemic heart disease and stroke, with some encouraging results [2, 3]. The use of mobilized peripheral blood HSC has now largely overtaken that of HSC collected from pelvic bone marrow due to two significant advantages of the former over the latter. Firstly, the collection of mobilized HSC is less invasive, requiring only venous access and leukapheresis, as opposed to the need for general anesthesia and a surgical procedure with a bone marrow harvest. Secondly, there is a higher yield of hematopoietic stem and progenitor cells (as measured by $CD34^+$ cell counts) with mobilized peripheral blood collections than with bone marrow harvests. As a consequence, there is a significant reduction in the duration of both severe neutropenia as well as thrombocytopenia after peripheral blood stem cell transplantation (PBSCT) compared to bone marrow transplantation, with corresponding reductions in toxicity and incidence of serious complications [4]. Peripheral blood stem cells (PBSC) are now used almost exclusively in autologous HSCT, and also in the majority of collections from normal donors for allogeneic HSCT.

Despite these clinical improvements with the widespread adoption of mobilized HSC, significant problems remain [1]. For collection from normal donors, the mobilization procedure involves the parenteral administration of granulocyte-colony-stimulating factor (G-CSF), a potent "stress" cytokine, over a 4-day period. Although this regimen has proven to be relatively safe, the majority of donors develop transient

N. Harun • K. Bradstock • L.J. Bendall (✉)
Westmead Institute for Cancer Research, Westmead Millennium Institute, University of Sydney, Westmead, NSW 2145, Australia
e-mail: linda.bendall@sydney.edu.au

S. Fruehauf et al. (eds.), *Novel Developments in Stem Cell Mobilization: Focus on CXCR4*, DOI 10.1007/978-1-4614-1960-0_3,

but significant side effects, including moderate to severe bone pain (>80%) and headaches (50%), fatigue (50%), often disruptive of normal activities [5]. In addition, G-CSF is associated with rare potentially life-threatening adverse events in PBSC donors, the most serious of which is splenic rupture [6, 7]. Other potentially life threatening adverse events described in PBSC donors include sickle cell crises in donors with hemoglobinopathies, unstable angina, myocardial infarction, stroke, capillary leak syndrome, and IgA neuropathy [5, 8]. Approximately, one-third of normal donors do not mobilize well enough to collect sufficient numbers of $CD34^+$ cells with one apheresis procedure, and are required to have additional doses of G-CSF and a further apheresis. Older donors, often with significant medical co-morbidities, are being increasingly used, and there are concerns about the risks to their health from undergoing the mobilization regimen [9]. Clinical trials investigating this are currently underway. In addition, there are concerns about the long-term side effects of G-CSF particularly in healthy donors, as safety data are still incomplete [5, 10]. Certain recent innovations in allogeneic HSCT, in particular, the use of extensively T cell-depleted transplants from haplo-identical donors, require collection of very high numbers of $CD34^+$ cells. This is only achievable in a minority of normal donors with a single apheresis. In autologous PBSCT, now mainly used for delivery of high-dose chemotherapy for treatment of multiple myeloma and lymphoma, the collection of autologous HSC is usually carried out by the administration of G-CSF following myelosuppressive chemotherapy, such as high-dose cyclophosphamide [11]. However, a proportion of cases, in particular those heavily pretreated with chemotherapy, fail to mobilize adequate numbers to safely undergo transplantation. In multiple myeloma patients who have an incomplete response to a first autograft, there may have been insufficient HSC to carry out a second procedure to produce a complete response. Thus, despite the clinical success of PBSCT, HSC mobilization procedures that are better tolerated by normal donors, and reliably result in adequate yields of stem and progenitor cells for transplantation are needed. In order to improve HSC mobilization techniques further consideration of the mechanisms of stem cell trafficking is required.

Current Understanding of Stem Cell Trafficking

HSC and hematopoietic progenitor cells (HPC) normally reside in the bone marrow where their growth and maturation are tightly regulated by a combination of contact and cytokine-mediated signals provided by the bone marrow microenvironment [12, 13]. HSC are believed to localize to one of two proposed hematopoietic stem cell niches: one juxtaposed to the endosteum and the other to the bone marrow vasculature [14]. Exactly what controls the localization of HSC in the niche is not completely understood but a number of factors and their receptors have suspected or known roles including transmembrane stem cell factor (SCF)/c-kit [15], osteopontin [16], VCAM-1/VLA-4 [17, 18], N-cadherin [19], annexin II [20], and the calcium sensing receptor (CaR) [21]. However, the primary factor responsible for the retention of HSC in the bone marrow is the chemokine CXCL12, which is present at high concentration on osteoblasts and bone marrow endothelial cells [22]. The importance of CXCL12 in retaining HSC within the niche under physiological conditions is evident from the poor retention of *CXCR4*$^{-/-}$ HSC, with large numbers circulating in the blood [23]. Fluctuations in CXCL12 levels in the bone marrow have been shown to be responsible for the circadian rhythm underlying the basal HSC numbers in the peripheral blood, with peripheral blood HSC numbers peaking when CXCL12 levels in the bone marrow are low [24]. Furthermore, pharmacological disruption of CXCL12 binding to its receptor, CXCR4, by specific peptide or small-molecule antagonists, results in the rapid and substantial mobilization of HSC into the blood [25]. Together these data define CXCL12 as the primary factor responsible for retaining HSC within the bone marrow [23, 25, 26]. HSC and HPC can be mobilized from the marrow into the blood in experimental models by a large number of agents, including those that disrupt VLA-4 binding to VCAM-1 [17], the cytokines G-CSF, granulocyte-macrophage colony-stimulating factor (GM-CSF), interleukin (IL)-7, IL-3, IL-12, SCF [27], and flt-3 ligand, chemokines such as IL-8, Mip-1α, Groβ [28], or CXCL12, parathyroid hormone [29] and the chemotherapeutic agents cyclophosphamide (Cy) and paclitaxel [22]. However, only a few have been investigated clinically. The mechanisms involved are not fully understood, but the disruption of CXCL12/CXCR4 interactions is a recurring theme (Fig. 3.1). Indeed, the most common clinically utilized agent, G-CSF, and the chemotherapeutic agent cyclophosphamide, result in proteolytic degradation of both CXCL12 and its receptor CXCR4 [30]. In addition, proteases released by the expanded neutrophil population in the bone marrow during G-CSF-induced mobilization also cleave adhesion molecules including VCAM-1, the ligand of the integrin VLA-4, and c-kit, the receptor of membrane-bound SCF [15, 18].

CXCR4 Antagonists as Mobilizing Agents

Bicyclams were initially identified incidentally as an impurity in commercially available cyclam preparations being screened for anti-HIV activity. Exploration of modifications of the original compound indentified AMD3100 as the most potent and this compound was selected for development as an anti-HIV drug specific for T-lymphotropic X4 strains of the virus [31]. The target of AMD3100 was identified as CXCR4. During phase I clinical trials in normal volunteers, AMD3100 induced an unexpected dose-dependent increase in the total white cell count [32]. It was subsequently noted that these peripheral blood mononuclear cells (PBMC) were enriched for CD34^{+} hematopoietic stem and progenitor cells [33]. AMD3100 also proved to act synergistically with G-CSF, prompting its entry into the clinic where it is primarily used in combination with G-CSF under the name Plerixafor [34]. This agent produces rapid mobilization following a single administration with relatively few side effects. AMD3100 has been successfully used to mobilize normal allogenic donors with all recipients achieving adequate engraftment, although this required more than one round of mobilization in a significant proportion of the donors [35].

Although AMD3100 is the only CXCR4 antagonist currently approved for HSC mobilization, a number of alternative agents are in development for HSC mobilization. Among the more advanced of these is POL6326, a 16-amino acid cyclic peptide based on the polyphemusin II peptide which was originally derived from the American horseshoe crab (*Limulus polyphemus*) [36]. In mice and monkeys a single injection of POL6326 gives an 11–12-fold increase in circulating progenitor cells with a peak at 2–4 h after injection, and in a phase I study of 74 healthy volunteers, POL6326 was well tolerated and effectively mobilized $CD34^+$ stem cells. In an interim report on a phase II clinical trial of HSC mobilization in patients with multiple myeloma 600–1,200 μg/kg of POL6326 was infused over 1–2 h on 4 consecutive days, 3 weeks after the last injection of induction treatment [37]. HSC were collected with consecutive leukaphereses 30 min after the end of infusion and sufficient ($\geq 2 \times 10^6$/kg) $CD34^+$ cells were collected in 66% of 16 patients with the majority of patients requiring two leukaphereses. All patients successfully engrafted between 10 and 19 days after receiving cells. This suggests that POL6326 may be used as a single agent in the future.

BKT140 is another polyphemusin II-derived peptide antagonist of CXCR4 otherwise known as 4F-benzoyl-TN14003. It has also demonstrated potent mobilizing capacity in preclinical studies and is also in phase I/II trials for mobilization of multiple myeloma patients. An interim report on this study was presented at the 2010 American Society of Hematology (ASH) scientific meeting [38]. In this study, BKT140 (30–900 μg/kg) was administered on day 10 of the mobilization protocol, which consisted of high-dose cyclophosphamide (2 g/m^2) and daily G-CSF (5 μg/kg) commencing on day 5. Like POL6326, BKT140 was well tolerated, however, the $t_{1/2}$ was extremely short (0.7 h) as compared to POL6326, where the $t_{1/2}$ was 6–8 h. A significant dose-dependent increase in the white cell count and $CD34^+$ cells above the baseline was achieved with G-CSF/Cy, with a peak within 8 h of injection. BKT140 reduced the number of leukaphereses from 2.25 to 1 at the highest dose. Patients receiving the collected HSC engrafted rapidly, with a median time to neutrophil recovery being 11 days.

Finally, the CXCR4 antagonist TG-0054, the structure of which has not been published, has completed phase I testing in normal volunteers with results presented at the ASH meeting in 2009 [39]. In this study, the maximum tolerated dose was not reached in healthy volunteers with 4.40 mg/kg having maximal efficacy with 29.2 ± 12.9 $CD34^+$ cells/μL of blood being obtained. Minor adverse events included abdominal pain (11%), diarrhea (8%), dizziness (5%), nausea (5%), and diaphoresis (5%), which can be described as minor compared to the side effect profile of G-CSF. The $t_{1/2}$ was approximately 2.5–5 h with peak mobilization occurring between 4 and 6 h. TG-0054 is now in phase II/III clinical trials for the mobilization of HSC in patients with multiple myeloma, non-Hodgkin's lymphoma, and Hodgkin's lymphoma.

In addition to CXCR4 antagonists, a CXCL12 inhibitor, NOX-A12 is also in clinical trial for HSC mobilization. NOX-A12 is an L-enantiomeric RNA oligonucleotide or Spiegelmer that inhibits the activity of CXCL12 with a half-maximal inhibitory concentration (IC_{50}) of 300 pmol/L. NOX-A12 was covalently linked to 40-kDa branched polyethylene glycol on the 5′-terminus for in vivo use [40].

The first human studies of NOX-A12 have been completed and it is currently in phase I clinical trial in healthy volunteers, both alone and in combination with G-CSF. However, no data is available regarding the safety or efficacy of this compound and the current testing regimen seems cumbersome with the agent being administered by IV infusion (2 or 4 mg/kg) over 15 min, daily for 5 days.

A number of additional CXCR4 antagonists are in clinical trial for other indications including AMD070 for HIV, MDX-1338/BMS-936564, a CXCR4 antibody, for AML, and MSX-122: the latter was trialed in advanced cancer, however, this study was suspended. Whether these or derivatives of these agents will be useful in HSC mobilization is not known. Clearly, the future of HSC mobilization lies with compounds such as AMD3100 that specifically target HSC retention factors within the bone marrow. However, at this stage these are not sufficiently effective to be routinely used as single agents.

Sphingosine-1-Phosphate

Sphingosine-1-phosphate (S1P) is a bioactive zwitterionic lyso-phospholipid acting both as a ligand for the G protein-coupled receptors $S1P_{1-5}$ [41, 42] and as a second messenger [43]. Although the effects of S1P on cell trafficking are thought to be mediated by binding to surface receptors, altered intracellular S1P concentrations can shunt sphingolipid metabolites away from the ceramide system to enhance cell survival, and enhance growth via effects on sphingosine kinase. Sphingosine is generated from the metabolism of plasma-membrane sphingolipids such as sphingomyelin and is subsequently phosphorylated by one of two sphingosine kinases (SphK) SphK1 or SphK2 to produce S1P [41]. S1P is maintained at nanomolar concentrations in most tissues, including secondary lymphoid organs [44], due to high levels of the S1P degrading enzyme S1P lyase [45]. In contrast to tissues, S1P levels are much higher in the blood, reaching the low micromolar range. Production of S1P by red blood cells and platelets, as well as contributions from lymph where S1P levels can be in the hundred-nanomolar range, are thought to be responsible for maintaining this level [46].

As an extracellular factor, S1P mediates its effects through S1P receptors. There are five separate receptors with varying signaling mechanisms that provide diverse responses to S1P in different conditions. While $S1P_1$, $S1P_2$, and $S1P_3$ are widely expressed, $S1P_4$ and $S1P_5$ are limited to the immune and nervous system [47–49]. Within the hematopoietic system, $S1P_1$ is the predominant receptor and is expressed on most lymphocyte subsets, while $S1P_3$ and $S1P_2$ are expressed on dendritic cells and macrophages, and $S1P_4$ on some B cell subtypes and during late development stages of T cells [50]. $S1P_1$ and $S1P_3$ are also expressed by endothelial cells and so have the potential to modulate hematopoietic cell trafficking by altering endothelial function [51, 52]. S1P receptors are not expressed in a fixed state, but undergo constant recycling and re-expression [53]. $S1P_1$ expression is dramatically increased as T cells mature from $CD4^+CD8^+$ thymocytes to immature and then mature $CD4^+$ or $CD8^+$ T cells [54]. Although all S1P receptors are coupled to G proteins, individual receptors associate with specific G proteins. $S1P_1$ exclusively associates with the G_i protein [55], while $S1P_2$ and $S1P_3$ are promiscuous associating with G_i, G_q, and $G_{12/13}$ proteins [56]. $S1P_4$ and $S1P_5$ can signal through both G_i and $G_{12/13}$ proteins [48, 57]. The varying G protein associations may at least partially explain the different responses elicited by activation of individual S1P receptors such as the opposing effects of the binding of S1P to $S1P_2$ as compared to $S1P_1$ [58].

Activation of S1P receptors induces a variety of cellular processes, including cell migration, angiogenesis, vascular maturation, heart development, and neurite retraction [59]. The interaction of S1P with its primary receptor, $S1P_1$, results in decreased apoptosis, improved cell survival as well as increased proliferation and motility [59]. S1P is also involved in physiological processes such as lymphoid egress from secondary lymphoid organs and bone marrow, inflammation and the stimulation of vascular maturation and permeability [41, 60] and its role in hematopoietic cell trafficking is discussed later in this chapter.

S1P in Lymphocyte Trafficking

The function of S1P in lymphocyte egress from secondary lymph nodes is well characterized. The identification of S1P as the factor promoting the egress of lymphoid cells from peripheral lymph nodes arose from studies of the mechanism of action of the immunosuppressant drug, FTY720. FTY720 is rapidly phosphorylated in vivo and in in vitro cultures, and in this form it acts as an agonist for $S1P_1$, $S1P_3$, $S1P_4$, and $S1P_5$ [61]. However, extended exposure of cells to FTY720 down-regulates S1P receptors including $S1P_1$ [62]. Systemically administered FTY720 results in significant lymphopenia due to the retention of lymphocytes in lymph nodes [62, 63]. Confirmation that this phenotype was due to loss of $S1P_1$ function came from studies on $S1P_1$ deficient mice. Deletion of $S1P_1$ results in embryonic lethality but, by using lethally irradiated wild-type animals reconstituted with fetal liver cells from $S1P_1$ gene knockout (KO) animals, it was demonstrated that loss of $S1P_1$ in hematopoietic cells resulted in the same phenotype as that observed in FTY720-treated mice [54]. The role of the S1P gradient between the lymphoid tissues (low S1P levels) and the blood (high S1P levels) in the egress of lymphocytes from secondary lymphoid organs into the peripheral circulation was demonstrated using inhibitors of the S1P degrading enzyme, sphingosine lyase. Treatment of animals with 2-acetyl-4-tetrahydroxybutylimidazole (THI) or 4′ deoxypyridoxine (DOP), to block sphingosine lyase function and eliminate the S1P gradient, resulted in lymphopenia due to the retention of lymphocytes in lymph nodes and thymus [46]. These investigations have highlighted the role of S1P as a factor facilitating the egress of lymphoid cells out of the secondary lymphoid organs back into the peripheral blood [46, 54].

Although the S1P/$S1P_1$ axis provides a chemokine gradient facilitating lymphocyte egress from secondary lymphoid organs, there is also evidence of endothelial cell involvement. $S1P_1$ is abundantly expressed in human endothelial cells [64] and S1P has been shown to strengthen endothelial barrier integrity in vitro by activating signaling events that promote adherens junction assembly [65, 66]. Activation of $S1P_1$ on endothelial cells using $S1P_1$ agonists such as SEW2871 can inhibit transendothelial migration of T cells into lymphatic sinuses [67]. This suggests that the egress of lymphocytes from secondary lymphoid organs may be more complex. Although a role for endothelial regulated lymphocyte egress has not been shown under physiological conditions, it is possible that the addition of a S1P agonist could have similar effects on lymphocyte retention as suppression of $S1P_1$ expression.

S1P in Stem Cell Trafficking

The role of S1P in HSC trafficking has been a relatively recent concept and as yet is not fully understood. However, primitive human $CD34^+CD38^-$ cells and murine HSC and HPC were shown to express S1P receptors by RT-PCR. Furthermore, functional activity of these receptors on hematopoietic progenitors has been demonstrated using in vitro chemotaxis assays where S1P acted as the chemokine [68–70]. S1P produces a bell-shaped migratory response in HPC with high concentrations being inhibitory [71]. The ability of HPC to undergo chemoattractant in response to S1P suggests that a difference in the concentration of S1P between the peripheral blood and bone marrow microenvironment may provide a gradient, similar to that involved in lymphocyte egress from lymph nodes, driving a small number of HSC into the circulation under steady-state conditions. This hypothesis is supported by the decline in circulating HPC in the blood of mice following administration of FTY720. Furthermore, circulating hematopoietic stem/progenitor cells (HSPC) can traffic to peripheral nonlymphoid tissues, and S1P mediates the egress of HSPC from these tissues into the lymphatic system [72]. These HSPC then return to the blood stream and eventually the bone marrow. These data show that HSPC can respond to S1P in a manner similar to that of mature lymphoid cells.

In the absence of $S1P_1$, both B and T cells accumulate in the bone marrow. This accumulation does not appear to be due to increased short-term homing, but rather increased long-term retention, suggesting a role for $S1P_1$ in the migration of these cells into the peripheral blood. This is analogous to the retention observed in lymph nodes [73]. Consistent with this, mature T cells, including antigen-specific T_H cells are sequestered in the bone marrow of mice 3 h after intravenous administration of FTY720, the selective $S1P_1$ agonist SEW2871, or 24 h after oral administration of the S1P lyase inhibitor, THI [74]. This shows that the exit of lymphoid cells from the bone marrow is mediated by S1P in a manner similar to that observed for their exit from lymph nodes. In contrast to lymphoid tissue, bone marrow lacks a lymphatic system, so egress from the bone marrow must occur via the bloodstream. More recently, it has been shown that S1P and $S1P_1$ are required for the egress of B cell progenitors from the bone marrow, with the number of immature-B cells in the bone marrow increasing, while those in the blood decreasing, in both S1P- and $S1P_1$-conditionally deficient mice. Moreover, evidence from bromodeoxyuridine incorporation experiments suggested that immature-B cells were retained in the

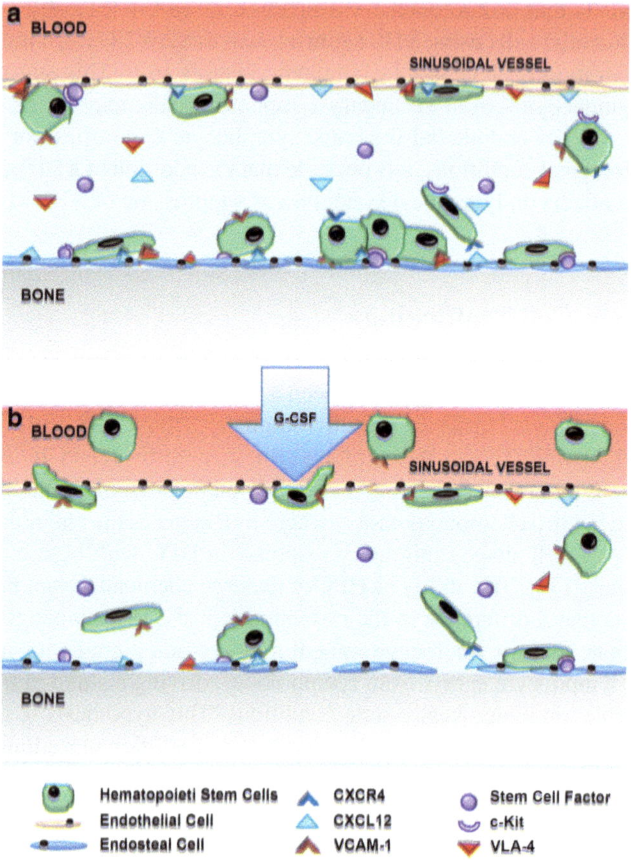

Fig. 3.1 (**a**) During steady-state conditions, HSC are retained in the bone marrow niche by adhesive and retentive interactions with endosteal cells and endothelial cells lining the bone marrow compartment. These axes include CXCL12/CXCR4, VCAM-1/VLA-4, and SCF/c-Kit. (**b**) Administration of G-CSF results in the cleavage of CXCR4, CXCL12, VCAM, and c-Kit, attenuating the retentive forces. Therefore, HSC are able to migrate across the vascular endothelium into the circulation

bone marrow for extended periods in mice where the S1P/S1P$_1$ axis was disrupted. Although the development of these cells appeared to be unaffected, there was an increase in the number of immature B cells undergoing apoptosis in the bone marrow [75, 76].

S1P was also recently identified as the major chemoattractant for HPC in the plasma. Following administration of G-CSF to mice, S1P levels increased as a result of activation of the complement cascade and lysis of S1P-containing red blood cells [71]. Decreased SphK1 mRNA and increased sphingosine phosphatase 1 mRNA levels in the bone marrow of G-CSF-treated mice may also contribute to the increased S1P concentrations [77]. However, Harun et al. observed a decrease from baseline S1P concentrations in human plasma collected following G-CSF administration for the mobilization of normal stem cell donors and patients undergoing autologous

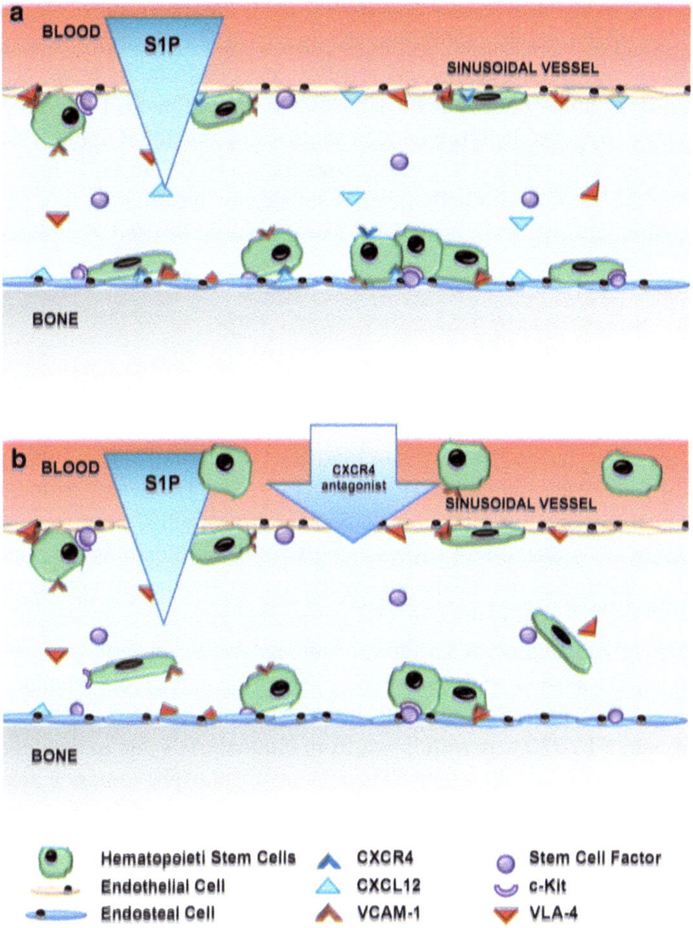

Fig. 3.2 (**a**) HSC are retained in the bone marrow by the retentive strength of CXCL12 binding to CXCR4, despite the presence of a S1P gradient attracting HSC toward the blood. (**b**) Upon blockage of the CXCR4 receptor with CXCR4 antagonists, HSC migrate toward the S1P gradient in the blood

HSCT [78]. Overall, changes in S1P concentrations in the bone marrow and blood and their effect on HSC mobilization remain to be clarified. Similar to the finding for B-cell progenitors, a significant reduction in the mobilization of HPC in response to AMD3100 was observed in DOP-treated mice [71, 78], however, the role of S1P and $S1P_1$ in G-CSF-mediated mobilization is less clear with conflicting data being reported [77, 78]. More recently, Ratajczak et al. suggested that bone marrow ceramide-1-phosphate (C1P) also acts as a bone marrow retention factor for HPC with levels increasing subsequent to cell damage induced by myeloablative therapy [79]. Together this suggests that under steady-state conditions, CXCL12 mediates the attraction and retention of HSC in the bone marrow but in the absence of CXCL12, a situation that occurs during mobilization, chemotactic activity of S1P can act unopposed, facilitating the egress of HSC from the bone marrow to the blood (Fig. 3.2).

Although activation of $S1P_1$ on endothelial cells has been shown to strengthen endothelial barrier integrity, inhibiting the egress of T cells from secondary lymphoid organs, this is unlikely to apply to egress of cells from the bone marrow. The endothelial layer lining bone marrow sinusoids is discontinuous [80], as opposed to the tight barrier imposed by lymph node endothelium, making it unlikely that effects on endothelium are involved in the mobilization of HPC and HSC from the bone marrow into the peripheral blood. Taken together, this information raises the possibility that stimulation of $S1P_1$ using $S1P_1$ agonists could be used to mobilize HSC.

S1P Receptor Agonists

The best-studied S1P receptor agonist is FTY720. As mentioned earlier, FTY720 requires phosphorylation before it can bind S1P receptors [81], but then activates four of the five S1P receptors, $S1P_1$ and $S1P_{3-5}$ [61]. However, receptor binding induces the internalization and degradation of the receptor, ultimately inhibiting S1P signaling. This dual effect makes using FTY720 difficult, as the outcome can be agonistic or antagonistic depending on the timing and the dose of the drug used. However, FTY720 is one of the few S1P agonists to be tested in clinical trials. It has been extensively examined as an immunosuppressive agent with the predominant side effect being transient bradycardia [82]. The cardiac effects are mediated through the actions of FTY720 on $S1P_3$, with the effect being lost in $S1P_3$ deficient mice [83]. However, FTY720 was withdrawn from clinical trials due to the development of macular degeneration in patients. The reasons for this phenomenon are not clear since FTY720 has been shown to have anti-angiogenic activity in cancers [84], although S1P itself has pro-angiogenic effects [85]. FTY720 also has a number of other effects, including activation of the TGFβ/Smad pathway, the sphingosine transporter ABCB1, the leukotriene C4 transporter Abcc1, and inhibition of cannabinoid receptor CB1 [86–89].

The only other S1P receptor agonist tested in the clinic is RG3477/ACT-128800 from Actelion. This more specific $S1P_1$ inhibitor is in a phase II clinical trial for relapsing multiple sclerosis. It was also used in a phase II trial of psoriasis, however, there is no information regarding this compound in the literature and Roche has recently withdrawn their support for this agent.

SEW2871 is highly specific for the $S1P_1$ receptor with an ED_{50} of 13 nM [90]. Although SEW2871 also induces receptor internalization, this is followed by recycling to the cell surface rather than the degradation seen with FTY720. Therefore, SEW2871 is not thought to down-regulate receptor expression [67], but this feature of SEW2871 and other $S1P_1$ agonists remains controversial. However, SEW2871 also induces lymphopenia 5–6 h after injection into mice [83]. This is thought to be the result of $S1P_1$-induced contraction of tight junctions in lymphatic endothelium, thereby impeding the transit and egress of lymphocytes [67]. Considering the lack of lymphatics in the bone marrow, and lack of endothelial tight junctions in bone marrow sinusoids, this phenomenon would be unlikely to impede HSC egress from the bone marrow. Interestingly, SEW2871 has been reported to down-regulate

VCAM-1 expression on endothelial cells over relatively short time frames [91]. Whether SEW2871 could have the same effect on bone marrow stromal and niche cells is not known, but if this were to occur this could contribute to the mobilizing effects of this agent since VCAM-1 is an important retention factor for HSC in the bone marrow [18]. However, SEW 2871 has not been tested in humans and there is limited preclinical data available.

A relatively new immunosuppressant, KRP-203, also has considerable selectivity for $S1P_1$ despite structural similarity with FTY720 [83], and like FTY720 it is the phosphorylated form of KRP-203 that is active. Whether SEW2871 or KRP-203-phosphate promote macular degeneration awaits further investigations, although neither compound is in clinical development.

Can $S1P_1$ Agonists Enhance HSC Mobilization?

If the S1P gradient between the blood and bone marrow provides a force attracting HSC into the peripheral blood, it may be possible to manipulate this axis to enhance HSC mobilization. Although there is some evidence to suggest that S1P acting via $S1P_1$ in the steady state does play a role in HSC trafficking [72], the effect appears to be small and it is difficult to imagine that addition of a $S1P_1$ receptor agonist would induce mobilization if used in isolation. Combining such an agent with current mobilization protocols to improve mobilization is a more realistic proposal. There are conflicting reports regarding the role of S1P in G-CSF-induced HSPC mobilization, with Golan et al. reporting an inhibitory effect of FTY720 [77], while others have not observed any effect of FTY720 [72, 78]. In contrast S1P appears to play a clearer role in mobilization induced by CXCR4 antagonists, such as AMD3100, with multiple mechanisms of disrupting the $S1P/S1P_1$ axis, including the S1P lyase inhibitor DOP [71], FTY720 and SK1 gene deletion [78], impeding mobilization. To date the only study looking at the effects of $S1P_1$ agonists suggests that such agents may improve mobilization using CXCR4 antagonists but not G-CSF-mediated mobilization [78]. The reason for this discrepancy is not entirely clear but G-CSF-mediated mobilization of HSC is undoubtedly more complex than that of CXCR4 antagonists, with not only CXCL12/CXCR4 being disrupted but also a myriad of other factors including VLA-4/VCAM1 and c-kit/SCF. The development of more suitable agents is needed in order to take $S1P_1$ agonists into the clinic. Stimulation of $S1P_1$ using FTY720 has problems due to its opposing effects, and the only clinically suitable agent, ACT-128800, although in trial for other indications, is not a candidate as a stem cell mobilizing agent at this stage.

Effects on the HPC Graft

The mechanism of mobilization used is likely to alter the proportion of various leukocyte subsets contributing to the graft, with the potential to impact on graft vs. host disease (GVHD) and graft vs. malignancy effects. Grafts collected following mobilization with AMD3100 or G-CSF have similar numbers of T cells, however, the makeup of the T cell subsets differs significantly. G-CSF results in a skewing toward T cells with a T_H2 phenotype. G-CSF also increases Tr1 regulatory T cells through IL-10 production. Tr1 cells do not express significant FoxP3 or CD25 but they produce IL-10 and TGF-β and have a similar regulatory function as the better known T_{regs} [92]. G-CSF also expands regulatory antigen presenting cells within the donor, which generate classical $CD4^+CD25^+$ IL-10-producing T_{regs} in the recipient, further inhibiting the inflammatory phase of GVHD [93]. Together this potentially explains the lack of increased GVHD despite larger number of T cells infused in a G-CSF primed PBSCT as compared to bone marrow transplantation [94, 95]. In contrast to G-CSF, AMD3100 does not appear to produce the same T_H2 effects, suggesting that increased GVHD may result [96]. However, the only study where the outcome of patients receiving grafts mobilized with AMD3100 alone was examined, reported a GVHD incidence of 35%. This is consistent with rates in recipients of G-CSF-primed grafts, despite a doubling in the number of $CD3^+$ and $CD4^+$ cells infused [35].

Considering the effects of manipulating the S1P/S1P_1 axis on lymphocyte trafficking, it likely that the addition of a S1P_1 agonist to AMD3100 will alter the immunological makeup of the graft. Intravenous administration of a S1P_1 agonist would be expected to result in increased numbers of lymphoid cells in the peripheral blood due to the anticipated increase in lymphocyte egress from secondary lymphoid organs. However, Wei et al. demonstrated that S1P_1 agonists retained lymphocytes in the medullary cords of lymph nodes [67]. This failure of lymphocytes to re-enter the lymphatic system would be expected to ultimately reduce peripheral blood lymphocyte numbers. Therefore, it is possible that addition of a S1P_1 agonist may reduce the number of lymphocytes in the graft.

S1P_1 was shown to inhibit T_{reg}-mediated peripheral maintenance and suppressive activity resulting in reduced tolerance and increased adaptive immune responses in knockout and over expression mouse models [97]. Although, much of this effect resulted from a reduction in the development and maturation of T_{reg} cells in these mice, there was evidence of cell intrinsic inhibition of T_{reg} function as a result of S1P_1 over expression. Furthermore, S1P_1 has also been shown to increase the differentiation of pro-inflammatory T_H1 cells [98]. These experiments have been conducted using 2–5-day exposures to S1P_1 agonists and whether a single administration of an S1P_1 agonists is likely to influence the activity of T cell subsets such as T_{reg} or T_H1 remains to be determined. However, the addition of a S1P_1 agonist has the potential to increase the pro-inflammatory nature of the graft and increase the risk of GVHD.

Summary

PBSC have become an essential part of therapy for an increasing number of conditions. Although mostly successful, protocols for HSC mobilization remain imperfect, with the principal mobilization agent, G-CSF, being relatively nonspecific in its action. Over the last two decades our understanding of the HSC niche and in particular factors that influence HSC trafficking has rapidly grown, providing opportunities for more rational strategies to be developed. AMD3100, the agent at the forefront of this targeted approach, stands at the beginning of a new era in HSC mobilization. While blocking CXCL12/CXCR4 interactions in isolation is not sufficient to replace G-CSF, it permits us to envision a quicker, less toxic method, particularly for normal PBSC donors who should not be exposed to any significant risks to their own health. In this chapter, we have focused on the role of the CXCL4/CXCR12 and S1P/S1P$_1$ axes in HSC trafficking. There is evidence emerging to suggest that manipulation of the S1P/S1P$_1$ axis can further enhance HSC mobilization, particularly that mediated by CXCR4 antagonists. However, this evidence is still preliminary and further studies need to be undertaken to determine the plausibility of this approach. Many questions remain unanswered. To what extent can S1P$_1$ agonists improve HSC mobilization and in combination with which agents? Could S1P$_1$ agonists reduce the need for G-CSF in some settings? What agents could be used clinically and will their side effects be acceptable? Finally, what effect will the use of such agents have of the nature of the graft produced and what consequences may this have for the recipient? Manipulation of the S1P/S1P$_1$ axis is only one potential strategy to improve HSC mobilization procedures, but one worthy of consideration. Whether agents targeting this or other HSC/niche interactions enter the clinic remains to be seen but inevitably more specific agents will be implemented and change the face of HSC mobilization in the future.

References

1. Jansen J, Hanks S, Thompson J, Dugan M, Akard L (2005) Transplantation of hematopoietic stem cells from the peripheral blood. J Cell Mol Med 9:37–50
2. Schächinger V, Erbs S, Elsässer A et al (2006) Improved clinical outcome after intracoronary administration of bone-marrow-derived progenitor cells in acute myocardial infarction: final 1-year results of the REPAIR-AMI trial. Eur Heart J 27:2775–2783
3. Sprigg N, Bath P, Zhao L et al (2006) Granulocyte-colony-stimulating factor mobilizes bone marrow stem cells in patients with subacute ischemic stroke: the Stem cell Trial of recovery EnhanceMent after Stroke (STEMS) pilot randomized, controlled trial (ISRCTN 16784092). Stroke 37:2979–2983
4. Schmitz N, Beksac M, Hasenclever D et al (2002) Transplantation of mobilized peripheral blood cells to HLA-identical siblings with standard-risk leukemia. Blood 100:761–767
5. D'Souza A, Jaiyesimi I, Trainor L, Venuturumili P (2008) Granulocyte colony-stimulating factor administration: adverse events. Transfus Med Rev 22:280–290
6. Tigue CC, McKoy JM, Evens AM, Trifilio SM, Tallman MS, Bennett CL (2007) Granulocyte-colony stimulating factor administration to healthy individuals and persons with chronic neutropenia or cancer: an overview of safety considerations from the Research on Adverse Drug Events and Reports project. Bone Marrow Transplant 40:185–192
7. Anderlini P (2009) Effects and safety of granulocyte colony-stimulating factor in healthy volunteers. Curr Opin Hematol 16:35–40
8. Funakoshi Y, Nazneen A, Nakashima Y et al (2010) Possible involvement of G-CSF in IgA nephropathy developing in an allogeneic peripheral blood SCT donor. Bone Marrow Transplant 45:1477–1478

9. Lysak D, Koristek Z, Gasova Z, Skoumalova I, Jindra P (2011) Efficacy and safety of peripheral blood stem cell collection in elderly donors; does age interfere? J Clin Apher 26:9–16
10. Gutierrez-Delgado F, Bensinger W (2001) Safety of granulocyte colony-stimulating factor in normal donors. Curr Opin Hematol 8:155–160
11. To L, Haylock D, Simmons P, Juttner C (1997) The biology and clinical uses of blood stem cells. Blood 89:2233–2258
12. Metcalf D (1993) Hematopoietic regulators: redundancy or subtlety. Blood 82:3515–3523
13. Whetton A, Dexter T (1993) Influence of growth factors and substrates on differentiation of haemopoietic stem cells. Curr Opin Cell Biol 5:1044–1049
14. Raaijmakers M, Scadden D (2008) Evolving concepts on the microenvironmental niche for hematopoietic stem cells. Curr Opin Hematol 15:301–306
15. Levesque J, Hendy J, Winkler I, Takamatsu Y, Simmons P (2003) Granulocyte colony-stimulating factor induces the release in the bone marrow of proteases that cleave c-KIT receptor (CD117) from the surface of hematopoietic progenitor cells. Exp Hematol 31:109–117
16. Nilsson SK, Johnston HM, Whitty GA et al (2005) Osteopontin, a key component of the hematopoietic stem cell niche and regulator of primitive hematopoietic progenitor cells. Blood 106:1232–1239
17. Papayannopoulou T, Nakamoto B (1993) Peripheralization of hemopoietic progenitors in primates treated with anti-VLA4 integrin. Proc Natl Acad Sci USA 90:9374–9378
18. Levesque J, Takamatsu Y, Nilsson S, Haylock D, Simmons P (2001) Vascular cell adhesion molecule-1 (CD106) is cleaved by neutrophil proteases in the bone marrow following hematopoietic progenitor cell mobilization by granulocyte colony-stimulating factor. Blood 98:1289–1297
19. Hosokawa K, Arai F, Yoshihara H et al (2010) Knockdown of N-cadherin suppresses the long-term engraftment of hematopoietic stem cells. Blood 116:554–563
20. Jung Y, Wang J, Song J et al (2007) Annexin II expressed by osteoblasts and endothelial cells regulates stem cell adhesion, homing, and engraftment following transplantation. Blood 110:82–90
21. Adams GB, Chabner KT, Alley IR et al (2006) Stem cell engraftment at the endosteal niche is specified by the calcium-sensing receptor. Nature 439:599–603
22. Lapidot T, Petit I (2002) Current understanding of stem cell mobilization: the roles of chemokines, proteolytic enzymes, adhesion molecules, cytokines, and stromal cells. Exp Hematol 30:973–981
23. Foudi A, Jarrier P, Zhang Y et al (2006) Reduced retention of radioprotective hematopoietic cells within the bone marrow microenvironment in CXCR4–/– chimeric mice. Blood 107:2243–2251
24. Méndez-Ferrer S, Lucas D, Battista M, Frenette P (2008) Haematopoietic stem cell release is regulated by circadian oscillations. Nature 452:442–447
25. Broxmeyer H, Orschell C, Clapp D et al (2005) Rapid mobilization of murine and human hematopoietic stem and progenitor cells with AMD3100, a CXCR4 antagonist. J Exp Med 201:1307–1318
26. Peled A, Kollet O, Ponomaryov T et al (2000) The chemokine SDF-1 activates the integrins LFA-1, VLA-4, and VLA-5 on immature human CD34(+) cells: role in transendothelial/stromal migration and engraftment of NOD/SCID mice. Blood 95:3289–3296
27. Morstyn G, Brown S, Gordon M et al (1994) Stem cell factor is a potent synergistic factor in hematopoiesis. Oncology 51:205–214
28. King AG, Horowitz D, Dillon SB et al (2001) Rapid mobilization of murine hematopoietic stem cells with enhanced engraftment properties and evaluation of hematopoietic progenitor cell mobilization in rhesus monkeys by a single injection of SB-251353, a specific truncated form of the human CXC chemokine GRObeta. Blood 97:1534–1542
29. Calvi LM, Adams GB, Weibrecht KW et al (2003) Osteoblastic cells regulate the haematopoietic stem cell niche. Nature 425:841–846
30. Levesque J, Hendy J, Takamatsu Y, Simmons P, Bendall L (2003) Disruption of the CXCR4/CXCL12 chemotactic interaction during hematopoietic stem cell mobilization induced by GCSF or cyclophosphamide. J Clin Invest 111:187–196

31. De Clercq E, Yamamoto N, Pauwels R et al (1992) Potent and selective inhibition of human immunodeficiency virus (HIV)-1 and HIV-2 replication by a class of bicyclams interacting with a viral uncoating event. Proc Natl Acad Sci USA 89:5286–5290
32. Hendrix C, Flexner C, MacFarland R et al (2000) Pharmacokinetics and safety of AMD-3100, a novel antagonist of the CXCR-4 chemokine receptor, in human volunteers. Antimicrob Agents Chemother 44:1667–1673
33. Liles W, Broxmeyer H, Rodger E et al (2003) Mobilization of hematopoietic progenitor cells in healthy volunteers by AMD3100, a CXCR4 antagonist. Blood 102:2728–2730
34. Flomenberg N, Devine S, Dipersio J et al (2005) The use of AMD3100 plus G-CSF for autologous hematopoietic progenitor cell mobilization is superior to G-CSF alone. Blood 106:1867–1874
35. Devine S, Vij R, Rettig M et al (2008) Rapid mobilization of functional donor hematopoietic cells without G-CSF using AMD3100, an antagonist of the CXCR4/SDF-1 interaction. Blood 112:990–998
36. Robinson JA, Demarco S, Gombert F, Moehle K, Obrecht D (2008) The design, structures and therapeutic potential of protein epitope mimetics. Drug Discov Today 13:944–951
37. Schmitt S, Weinhold N, Dembowsky K, et al (2010) First results of a phase-II study with the new CXCR4 antagonist POL6326 to mobilize hematopoietic stem cells (HSC) in multiple myeloma (MM). In: Dunbar S (ed) American Society of Hematology, Orlando. Blood 116(21)
38. Nagler A, Shimoni A, Avivi I, et al (2010) BKT140 is a novel CXCR4 antagonist with stem cell mobilization and antimyeloma effects: an open-label first human trial in patients with multiple myeloma undergoing stem cell mobilization for autologous transplantation. In: Dunbar S (ed) American Society of Hematology, Orlando. Blood 116(21)
39. Chung D, Chang L-W, Huang Y-H, et al (2009) TG-0054, a novel and potent stem cell mobilizer, displays excellent PK/PD and safety profile in phase I trial. In: Dunbar C (ed) American Society for Hematology, New Orleans. Blood 116(21)
40. Sayyed SG, Hagele H, Kulkarni OP et al (2009) Podocytes produce homeostatic chemokine stromal cell-derived factor-1/CXCL12, which contributes to glomerulosclerosis, podocyte loss and albuminuria in a mouse model of type 2 diabetes. Diabetologia 52:2445–2454
41. Rivera J, Proia R, Olivera A (2008) The alliance of sphingosine-1-phosphate and its receptors in immunity. Nat Rev Immunol 8:753–763
42. Rosen H, Gonzalez-Cabrera PJ, Sanna MG, Brown S (2009) Sphingosine 1-phosphate receptor signaling. Annu Rev Biochem 78:743–768
43. Alvarez SE, Milstien S, Spiegel S (2007) Autocrine and paracrine roles of sphingosine-1-phosphate. Trends Endocrinol Metab 18:300–307
44. Rosen H, Goetzl EJ (2005) Sphingosine 1-phosphate and its receptors: an autocrine and paracrine network. Nat Rev Immunol 5:560–570
45. Peest U, Sensken S, Andréani P, Hänel P, Van Veldhoven P, Gräler M (2008) S1P-lyase independent clearance of extracellular sphingosine 1-phosphate after dephosphorylation and cellular uptake. J Cell Biochem 104:756–772
46. Schwab S, Pereira J, Matloubian M, Xu Y, Huang Y, Cyster J (2005) Lymphocyte sequestration through S1P lyase inhibition and disruption of S1P gradients. Science 309:1735–1739
47. Ishii I, Fukushima N, Ye X, Chun J (2004) Lysophospholipid receptors: signaling and biology. Annu Rev Biochem 73:321–354
48. Im DS, Heise CE, Ancellin N et al (2000) Characterization of a novel sphingosine 1-phosphate receptor, Edg-8. J Biol Chem 275:14281–14286
49. Graler MH, Grosse R, Kusch A, Kremmer E, Gudermann T, Lipp M (2003) The sphingosine 1-phosphate receptor S1P4 regulates cell shape and motility via coupling to Gi and G12/13. J Cell Biochem 89:507–519
50. Goetzl EJ, Wang W, McGiffert C, Huang MC, Graler MH (2004) Sphingosine 1-phosphate and its G protein-coupled receptors constitute a multifunctional immunoregulatory system. J Cell Biochem 92:1104–1114
51. Liu Y, Wada R, Yamashita T et al (2000) Edg-1, the G protein-coupled receptor for sphingosine-1-phosphate, is essential for vascular maturation. J Clin Invest 106:951–961
52. Peters SL, Alewijnse AE (2007) Sphingosine-1-phosphate signaling in the cardiovascular system. Curr Opin Pharmacol 7:186–192

53. Graeler MH, Kong Y, Karliner JS, Goetzl EJ (2003) Protein kinase C epsilon dependence of the recovery from down-regulation of S1P1 G protein-coupled receptors of T lymphocytes. J Biol Chem 278:27737–27741
54. Matloubian M, Lo C, Cinamon G et al (2004) Lymphocyte egress from thymus and peripheral lymphoid organs is dependent on S1P receptor 1. Nature 427:355–360
55. Lee MJ, Evans M, Hla T (1996) The inducible G protein-coupled receptor edg-1 signals via the G(i)/mitogen-activated protein kinase pathway. J Biol Chem 271:11272–11279
56. Windh RT, Lee MJ, Hla T, An S, Barr AJ, Manning DR (1999) Differential coupling of the sphingosine 1-phosphate receptors Edg-1, Edg-3, and H218/Edg-5 to the G(i), G(q), and G(12) families of heterotrimeric G proteins. J Biol Chem 274:27351–27358
57. Van Brocklyn JR, Graler MH, Bernhardt G, Hobson JP, Lipp M, Spiegel S (2000) Sphingosine-1-phosphate is a ligand for the G protein-coupled receptor EDG-6. Blood 95:2624–2629
58. Lee JF, Gordon S, Estrada R et al (2009) Balance of S1P1 and S1P2 signaling regulates peripheral microvascular permeability in rat cremaster muscle vasculature. Am J Physiol Heart Circ Physiol 296:H33–42
59. Spiegel S, Milstien S (2002) Sphingosine 1-phosphate, a key cell signaling molecule. J Biol Chem 277:25851–25854
60. Allende M, Yamashita T, Proia R (2003) G-protein-coupled receptor S1P1 acts within endothelial cells to regulate vascular maturation. Blood 102:3665–3667
61. Brinkmann V, Davis MD, Heise CE et al (2002) The immune modulator FTY720 targets sphingosine 1-phosphate receptors. J Biol Chem 277:21453–21457
62. Graler M, Goetzl E (2004) The immunosuppressant FTY720 down-regulates sphingosine 1-phosphate G-protein-coupled receptors. FASEB J 18:551–553
63. Chiba K, Yanagawa Y, Masubuchi Y et al (1998) FTY720, a novel immunosuppressant, induces sequestration of circulating mature lymphocytes by acceleration of lymphocyte homing in rats. I. FTY720 selectively decreases the number of circulating mature lymphocytes by acceleration of lymphocyte homing. J Immunol 160:5037–5044
64. Hla T, Maciag T (1990) An abundant transcript induced in differentiating human endothelial cells encodes a polypeptide with structural similarities to G-protein-coupled receptors. J Biol Chem 265:9308–9313
65. Lee MJ, Thangada S, Claffey KP et al (1999) Vascular endothelial cell adherens junction assembly and morphogenesis induced by sphingosine-1-phosphate. Cell 99:301–312
66. Lee JF, Zeng Q, Ozaki H et al (2006) Dual roles of tight junction-associated protein, zonula occludens-1, in sphingosine 1-phosphate-mediated endothelial chemotaxis and barrier integrity. J Biol Chem 281:29190–29200
67. Wei SH, Rosen H, Matheu MP et al (2005) Sphingosine 1-phosphate type 1 receptor agonism inhibits transendothelial migration of medullary T cells to lymphatic sinuses. Nat Immunol 6:1228–1235
68. Kimura T, Boehmler A, Seitz G et al (2004) The sphingosine 1-phosphate receptor agonist FTY720 supports CXCR4-dependent migration and bone marrow homing of human CD34+ progenitor cells. Blood 103:4478–4486
69. Whetton AD, Lu Y, Pierce A, Carney L, Spooncer E (2003) Lysophospholipids synergistically promote primitive hematopoietic cell chemotaxis via a mechanism involving Vav 1. Blood 102:2798–2802
70. Yanai N, Matsui N, Furusawa T, Okubo T, Obinata M (2000) Sphingosine-1-phosphate and lysophosphatidic acid trigger invasion of primitive hematopoietic cells into stromal cell layers. Blood 96:139–144
71. Ratajczak MZ, Lee H, Wysoczynski M et al (2010) Novel insight into stem cell mobilization-plasma sphingosine-1-phosphate is a major chemoattractant that directs the egress of hematopoietic stem progenitor cells from the bone marrow and its level in peripheral blood increases during mobilization due to activation of complement cascade/membrane attack complex. Leukemia 24:976–985
72. Massberg S, Schaerli P, Knezevic-Maramica I et al (2007) Immunosurveillance by hematopoietic progenitor cells trafficking through blood, lymph, and peripheral tissues. Cell 131:994–1008

73. Halin C, Scimone M, Bonasio R et al (2005) The S1P-analog FTY720 differentially modulates T cell homing via HEV: T cell-expressed S1P1 amplifies integrin activation in peripheral lymph nodes but not in Peyer's patches. Blood 106(4):1314–1322
74. Maeda Y, Seki N, Sato N, Sugahara K, Chiba K (2010) Sphingosine 1-phosphate receptor type 1 regulates egress of mature T cells from mouse bone marrow. Int Immunol 22:515–525
75. Pereira JP, Cyster JG, Xu Y (2010) A role for S1P and S1P1 in immature-B cell egress from mouse bone marrow. PLoS One 5:e9277
76. Allende ML, Tuymetova G, Lee BG, Bonifacino E, Wu YP, Proia RL (2010) S1P1 receptor directs the release of immature B cells from bone marrow into blood. J Exp Med 207:1113–1124
77. Golan K, Vagima Y, Ludin A, et al (2010) The chemotactic lipid S1P regulates hematopoietic progenitor cell egress and mobilization via its major receptor S1P1 and by SDF-1 inhibition in a p38/Akt/mTOR dependent manner. In: Dunbar S (ed) American Society for Hematology, Orlando
78. Harun N, Thien M, Juarez J, Bradstock K, Bendall L. S1P1 agonists for use as adjunct mobilizing agents. In: Dunbar S (ed) American Society for Hematology, Orlando
79. Kim C, Wan W, Liu R, et al (2010) A novel paradigm in stem cell trafficking: the ratio of peripheral blood sphingosine-1 phosphate (S1P) to bone marrow ceramide-1 phosphate (C1P) regulates mobilization and homing of hematopoietic stem cells. In: Dunbar S (ed) American Society for Hematology, Orlando
80. Weiss L (1988) Cell and tissue biology. A textbook of histology, 6th edn. Urban & Schwarzenberg, Baltimore
81. Billich A, Bornancin F, Devay P, Mechtcheriakova D, Urtz N, Baumruker T (2003) Phosphorylation of the immunomodulatory drug FTY720 by sphingosine kinases. J Biol Chem 278:47408–47415
82. Budde K, Schmouder RL, Brunkhorst R et al (2002) First human trial of FTY720, a novel immunomodulator, in stable renal transplant patients. J Am Soc Nephrol 13:1073–1083
83. Sanna MG, Liao J, Jo E et al (2004) Sphingosine 1-phosphate (S1P) receptor subtypes S1P1 and S1P3, respectively, regulate lymphocyte recirculation and heart rate. J Biol Chem 279:13839–13848
84. LaMontagne K, Littlewood-Evans A, Schnell C et al (2006) Antagonism of sphingosine-1-phosphate receptors by FTY720 inhibits angiogenesis and tumor vascularization. Cancer Res 66:221–231
85. Panetti TS (2002) Differential effects of sphingosine 1-phosphate and lysophosphatidic acid on endothelial cells. Biochim Biophys Acta 1582:190–196
86. Paugh SW, Cassidy MP, He H et al (2006) Sphingosine and its analog, the immunosuppressant 2-amino-2-(2-[4-octylphenyl]ethyl)-1,3-propanediol, interact with the CB1 cannabinoid receptor. Mol Pharmacol 70:41–50
87. Xin C, Ren S, Eberhardt W, Pfeilschifter J, Huwiler A (2006) The immunomodulator FTY720 and its phosphorylated derivative activate the Smad signalling cascade and upregulate connective tissue growth factor and collagen type IV expression in renal mesangial cells. Br J Pharmacol 147:164–174
88. Honig SM, Fu S, Mao X et al (2003) FTY720 stimulates multidrug transporter- and cysteinyl leukotriene-dependent T cell chemotaxis to lymph nodes. J Clin Invest 111:627–637
89. Payne SG, Oskeritzian CA, Griffiths R et al (2007) The immunosuppressant drug FTY720 inhibits cytosolic phospholipase A2 independently of sphingosine-1-phosphate receptors. Blood 109:1077–1085
90. Jo E, Sanna MG, Gonzalez-Cabrera PJ et al (2005) S1P1-selective in vivo-active agonists from high-throughput screening: off-the-shelf chemical probes of receptor interactions, signaling, and fate. Chem Biol 12:703–715
91. Whetzel AM, Bolick DT, Srinivasan S et al (2006) Sphingosine-1 phosphate prevents monocyte/endothelial interactions in type 1 diabetic NOD mice through activation of the S1P1 receptor. Circ Res 99:731–739
92. Battaglia M, Gregori S, Bacchetta R, Roncarolo MG (2006) Tr1 cells: from discovery to their clinical application. Semin Immunol 18:120–127

93. Morris ES, MacDonald KP, Hill GR (2006) Stem cell mobilization with G-CSF analogs: a rational approach to separate GVHD and GVL? Blood 107:3430–3435
94. Pan L, Delmonte J Jr, Jalonen CK, Ferrara JL (1995) Pretreatment of donor mice with granulocyte colony-stimulating factor polarizes donor T lymphocytes toward type-2 cytokine production and reduces severity of experimental graft-versus-host disease. Blood 86:4422–4429
95. Hartung T, Docke WD, Gantner F et al (1995) Effect of granulocyte colony-stimulating factor treatment on ex vivo blood cytokine response in human volunteers. Blood 85:2482–2489
96. Smith A, Jungnam J, Rao S, et al (2007) Significant alterations in T-cell TH1 and TH2 cytokine gene profiles associated with G-CSF mobilization do not occur in T-cells mobilized with AMD3100, vol. 110 (11). American Society of Hematology, p 3277
97. Liu G, Burns S, Huang G et al (2009) The receptor S1P1 overrides regulatory T cell-mediated immune suppression through Akt-mTOR. Nat Immunol 10:769–777
98. Liu G, Yang K, Burns S, Shrestha S, Chi H (2010) The S1P(1)-mTOR axis directs the reciprocal differentiation of T(H)1 and T(reg) cells. Nat Immunol 11:1047–1056

Chapter 4
Should We Stay or Should We Go Now?

Cell Adhesion and Mobilization Pathways of Hematopoietic Cells

Eike C. Buss and Anthony D. Ho

Introduction

Understanding cell adhesion properties is essential for an optimal exploitation of mobilization mechanisms, as these are two sides of the same coin. It is also noteworthy that several mobilization strategies influence directly and indirectly different adhesion molecules, resulting in the release of different blood cell populations. The adhesion of hematopoietic progenitor cells (HPCs) is not exclusive, as many of these mechanisms are shared with other cell types. Adhesion is a localized process with certain features of adhesion molecules at given locations of the microarchitecture. The same molecules can have different properties at other microarchitecture locations. The interplay between homing, engraftment, adhesion, and mobilization is a dynamic process that can be influenced with interaction of various molecules. Most of the drugs that were developed to mobilize bone marrow cells interact with adhesion processes. To achieve selective mobilizations, a precise understanding of the adhesion mechanisms is indispensable.

E.C. Buss (✉) • A.D. Ho
Department of Internal Medicine V, Heidelberg University Hospital,
Im Neuenheimer Feld 410, 69120 Heidelberg, Germany
e-mail: Eike_Buss@med.uni-heidelberg.de

S. Fruehauf et al. (eds.), *Novel Developments in Stem Cell Mobilization: Focus on CXCR4*, DOI 10.1007/978-1-4614-1960-0_4,

Cell Adhesion Mechanisms

The SDF-1- CXCR4 Axis

One well-characterized mechanism of cell adhesion is the CXCR4/SDF-1 interaction. This pathway was first detected in the 1990s with description of the chemokine SDF-1 (synonym: CXCL12) [1] and explored further in several biological systems, especially in hematopoiesis [2]. It was also studied in other tissues, organs, and tumors such as pancreas cancer, lymphomas, prostate cancer, and it also plays an important role in developmental biology.

The CXCR4 receptor is a G-protein-coupled receptor tyrosine kinase. It delivers signals through G-protein-dependent and -independent pathways, the latter involving its serine-rich cytoplasmic tail [3]. After binding of its exclusive ligand SDF-1, CXCR4 activates several signaling cascades that result in intracellular calcium release and phosphorylation of ERK1/2. Present evidence indicates that adhesion vs. mobilization of hematopoietic cells is dependent on SDF-1 concentrations in the blood and the bone marrow space that acts via CXCR4 signaling [4]. This challenges the previous notion of mobilization by CXCR4 interacting agents by a pure antagonist process. CXCR4 can be probably considered more as a signaling receptor than an adhesion molecule and SDF-1 can be viewed as a chemokine directing cell movement, as it was originally described, and not as an anchoring factor [4].

There are cross reactions to numerous other systems. An example is the connection with the CXCR7 system. This chemokine receptor seems to be the only other designated receptor for SDF-1. If confirmed, this might change the special notion of a monogamous relationship of SDF-1 with CXCR4. There are several reports about a functional signaling of CXCR7 via SDF-1 action. Given the recent research efforts in this field, it seems unlikely, that this mechanism has a significant impact on hematopoietic cells [5].

Interplay of the Sympathetic Nervous System with the SDF-1- CXCR4 Axis

Recently, the significant influence of the sympathetic nervous system on hematopoiesis has been reported. The association of G-CSF effects with catecholamines on the adhesion of hematopoietic stem cells (HSCs) to bone marrow osteoblasts vs. release and mobilization was described by Katayama et al. [6, 7]. In a second step, the group of Frenette analyzed the mechanisms of mobilization induced by the central nervous system [8]. The central signal is via exposure of the visual sensory organs to light that, in turn, trigger activity of the sympathetic nervous system. Catecholamines are released from sympathetic nerve endings in the bone marrow and signals are transmitted via adrenergic ß3-receptors on mesenchymal stromal cells. This signaling leads to the degradation of transcription factor SP1 which results in cessation of SDF-1 synthesis. The resulting changes can be followed in the bone marrow concentrations of SDF-1, decreasing quickly after onset of light. With a delay of about 6 h the number of progenitors in the peripheral blood, assessed as CFUs, increases to an apex in the middle of the daylight period. Unfortunately, the study did not assess the SDF-1 levels in the peripheral blood of the experimental animals, which would have been interesting for comparison with other studies examining changes in SDF-1 homeostasis and its connection with adhesion, mobilization, and engraftment. The specificity of the ß3-receptor was validated thoroughly in the studies by Mendez-Ferrer et al. [8, 9]. In comparison to this experimentally investigated adhesion mechanism in mice, the human SDF-1 homeostasis is shifted by about 12 h with a maximum of progenitors in the early evening. In addition, it could be shown that collections later in the day result in higher yields of mobilized stem and progenitor cells [10].

In an important follow-up study Frenette and colleagues further examined the nature of the signal receiving mesenchymal stem cells and could pin them down to a nestin-rich mesenchymal cell that is SDF-1-rich and receives sympathetic signals via β3-receptors [9]. Furthermore, in this murine model they could demonstrate the proximity and adherence of rare mouse HSCs to the nestin-rich mesenchymal cells. These cells could be found close to osteoblasts, to sinusoids, and in the space in between, supporting theories of stem cell niches in all of these locations. Administration of G-CSF or broad β or specific β3-agonists inhibited proliferation of nestin-GFP$^+$ MSCs, whereas sympathectomy led to increased proliferation of these cells. The adhesion properties were further examined in detail. By PCR of sorted cells it could be shown, that they contain high levels of SDF-1, of stem cell associated protein c-kit, angiopoietin-1, IL-7 and of adhesion factors VCAM and osteopontin. Expression levels of SDF-1, VCAM, and osteopontin were lower in GFP–MSC by magnitudes. The expression was significantly downregulated after administration of G-CSF. This corresponds with the study of Katayama from 2006 [6] in which G-CSF-induced mobilization correlated with downregulation of SDF-1 expression in the osteoblasts, albeit this was not examined in the privileged MSCs at the time. According to the recent results, direct sympathetic innervation would be exclusively reserved for the privileged MSCs, whereas osteoblasts and other cells could receive cues by secreted catecholamines and possibly from nestin-rich MSCs.

To examine the role of catecholamines and the sympathetic nervous system on maintenance and mobilization, Spiegel, Lapidot, and colleagues examined the catecholamine system directly on hematopoietic stem and progenitor cells [11]. They could demonstrate catecholamine receptors directly on human blood progenitor cells by FACS analysis for dopamine receptors 3 and 5 and the β2 receptor. Expression was higher on more immature CD34$^+$CD38^{low} progenitors and higher on G-CSF-mobilized progenitor cells as compared to cord blood cells. It could be further upregulated on the cord blood progenitors by treatments with G-CSF and GM-CSF. Furthermore, the functional relevance of these receptors was demonstrated by preincubation with dopamine agonists and catecholamines and subsequent injection into immunodeficient, pre-irradiated NOD/SCID mice. This pretreatment has also led to increased homing and engraftment in the recipients.

These observations demonstrate that there is a direct signaling via catecholamine receptors on hematopoietic cells with functional relevance and that exogenous cues, such as G-CSF and GM-CSF also act indirectly via alterations in catecholamine receptor homeostasis. The in vivo treatments have also led to increased proliferation of immature blood progenitor cells within the bone marrow and to increased motility. It could be shown that the signal transduction of the catecholamine receptors results in activation of Wnt-signaling. Treatment of cord blood $CD34^+$ cells with GM-CSF and epinephrine is associated with accumulation of β-catenin. This effect could be neutralized by treatment with medium enriched for the cysteine-rich domain of Frzb that has a Wnt-binding domain and thereby antagonistic activity.

The role of SDF-1 and functions of the CXCR4-receptor were recently reported by Dar and colleagues [4]. They described in detail SDF-1 homoeostasis in AMD3100-induced mobilizations. It could be shown that AMD3100 administration leads to an increased SDF-concentration in the peripheral blood, concomitantly with the mobilization of progenitor cells, both by a factor of approximately 2. This effect could be inhibited by prior administration of Anti-CXCR4 antibodies. This could be further refined by experiments with direct injection of a truncated, biotinylated preparation of SDF-1, that does not bind to heparan sulfate, thus excluding CXCR4-independent binding and release processes. With this method, a release of SDF-1 from the bone marrow as well as an increase in the peripheral blood could also be demonstrated. That AMD3100 was able to induce a release of SDF-1 could be supported by in vitro results which showed a release of SDF-1 from osteoblast cultures and endothelial cells after incubation with AMD3100. Compatible with the results from other studies, it could be shown that noradrenaline led to progenitor cell mobilization which was accompanied by SDF-1 release. In support of this notion, administration of the β2-antagonist ICI inhibited mobilization and SDF-1 release.

Adhesion via CD44

Another important player in adhesion between HPC and their niche is the molecule CD44 that is expressed by HPC and interacts mostly with hyaluronic acid in the bone marrow niche. CD44 can be used as a flow cytometric marker for HSCs and is also found on cancer stem cells, including leukemia stem cells. Importantly, tumor cells preferentially express CD44-variant isoforms (CD44v) instead of the standard form expressed by healthy cells [12]. This allows the design of antibodies against variant isoforms that might be associated with specific cancers. Recently, we could show that in blood progenitor cells ($ALDH^+/CD34^+$) from cord blood and mobilized peripheral blood almost no CD44v expressions could be measured in contrast to a low expression on progenitors from bone marrow cells. Immature AML cells showed partially markedly increased expression of the variant isoform CD44v7. CD44v7 expression was also increased by co-cultivation of healthy progenitor cells with MSCs [13].

CD44 is pivotal in the homing, transmigration, and adhesion process of HPC and leukemic cells [12]. The initial step in homing is partial binding to CD62L on endothelial cells as well as leukocytes and thrombocytes. The second step is firm attachment on deposited hyaluronic acid and engagement of more adhesion receptors, especially VLA-4 (α4 β1) on the HPC. After extravasation the CD44–hyaluronic acid binding results in firm attachment to the niche via hyaluronic acid. The intracellular signaling is via the Rho pathway, the first activated signaling molecule is the Rho guanine exchange factor (GEP) [14]. This signaling cascade results in strengthening of the binding of CD44 to the actin cytoskeleton via ankyrin. Furthermore, hyaluronic acid binding is accompanied by an association of CD44 with VLA-4 and both molecules share intracellular signaling pathways, namely src-kinases. Among others this results in transient reduced interaction of VLA-4 with paxillin, putatively allowing the CD44 VLA-4 complex to move to the leading end of the migrating cell [15].

Cadherin-Mediated Adhesion

Cadherins are a superfamily of calcium-binding membrane glycoproteins. E-cadherin is mainly found in epithelial cells and maintains tissue architecture. N-cadherin is mostly expressed in the nervous system, smooth muscle, stromal, and endothelial cells. Cell–cell adhesion by cadherins is achieved by homophilic binding of cadherin molecules of neighboring cells in a calcium-dependent manner. Intracellularly they are connected to actin via α-catenin and β-catenin [16]. These signaling molecules also lead to indirect connections to signaling pathways like the Wnt-pathway.

There have been controversies about the role of cadherins in adhesion of hematopoietic cells. Some reports did not find evidence for expression and functional significance of N-cadherins in stem cell adhesion [17, 18], whereas other authors demonstrated that knockdown of N-cadherin by retroviral transduction of N-cadherin shRNA resulted in the suppression of hematopoiesis [19]. Divergent reports could be reconciled by differences in gene-product doses in different studies and apparently the current monoclonal N-cadherin antibody might not be suitable for flow cytometry [19].

Our group has recently shown moderate expression of N-cadherin and cadherin-11 on HPC by RT-PCR, Western Blot, and flow cytometry. Both molecules were not expressed in differentiated cells. Direct imaging showed the colocalization of N-cadherin with β-catenin at the junction of HPC and MSCs. The functional relevance of these observations could be demonstrated by siRNA knock-down or blocking by antibodies, both of which resulted in reduced adhesion of progenitors to MSCs as well as reduced LTC-IC maintenance in HPC–MSC cocultures [20].

Homing and Adhesion via VLA-4

VLA-4 (α4 β1 integrin) is an essential factor for homing and redistribution of blood cells. VCAM-1 and fibronectin are the major ligands for VLA-4 and are essential for homing of circulating blood cells onto endothelial surfaces [21]. The orchestrated adhesion is regulated by an "inside-out" signaling of integrins with conformational changes of the extracellular domains. This is elicited by cytokine or chemokine stimulations of the VLA-4 bearing cell [22, 23], leading subsequently to altered adhesiveness of the VLA-4 receptor.

The role of integrins in the homeostasis of HSC has been demonstrated in murine models. Homozygote α4-integrin knockout was lethal for fetuses in mice and chimeric mice created from wild-type embryonic stem cells. Embryonic stem cells with the α4-integrin knockout demonstrated the essential role of this surface receptor for the hematopoietic development. Whereas development of blood cells with α4-integrin knockout could be found in the fetal liver, hematopoiesis could not be established in the subsequent blood forming organs and in adult hematopoiesis [24, 25]. A cell-type specific Tie2Cre + $a4^{f/f}$ floxed phenotype allowed conditional knockout of VLA-4 in hematopoietic and endothelial cells. After the conditional knockout, these mice showed a significantly increased amount of circulating immature blood cells. Transplantation studies with these cells revealed that the disruption of hematopoiesis was due to the lack of VLA-4 on the blood progenitor cells and not on the endothelial cells [26]. Thus, the VLA-4 function is essential for homing and redistribution of HPC during the fetal period. These processes can be influenced by neutralizing antibodies and by small molecule antagonists. The humanized mouse antihuman function-blocking α4-integrin antibody natalizumab, e.g., is approved for therapy of multiple sclerosis. Its administration has resulted in a significant mobilization of HPCs to the peripheral blood [27, 28]. The levels of circulating progenitor cells were elevated sixfold one day after the first dose of natalizumab, and similar levels were continuously maintained under monthly natalizumab infusions.

Influence of Mobilization Treatments on Adhesion Mechanisms

A better understanding of the mechanisms involved in the adhesion between HPC and the marrow niche represents a prerequisite for mobilization of HPC for clinical transplantations. All available mobilization agents have a significant impact on the mechanisms of adhesion.

Mobilization Treatments

Clinical mobilization of HPC can be performed by G-CSF stimulation without additional chemotherapy. This is regular in clinical practice when PB HPCs need to be obtained from healthy donors for allogeneic transplantations. In these settings, G-CSF is typically given subcutaneously daily at a dose of 10 μg/kg body weight for 4–5 successive days [29]. Leukapheresis follows 12 h after the last injection. If the collection was insufficient, G-CSF administration is continued. Compared to bone marrow harvests, G-CSF mobilized blood contains higher $CD34^+$ cell doses.

Its major advantage is the more rapid reconstitution compared to bone marrow grafts [30, 31]. Usually, G-CSF administration is well tolerated, however, donors may suffer from mild symptoms, such as bone pain, headache, fatigue, and nausea [29]. There are cases in which patients are mobilized with G-CSF alone for autologous transplantation as well, due to toxicity or ineffectiveness of common chemotherapeutical treatments [32]. The majority of clinical mobilization protocols are conducted today for autologous transplantation. This trend toward more use of blood stem transplantations is also observed for allogeneic transplantations [33].

Mobilization with Chemotherapy

Autologous transplantations using mobilized HSC have been shown to be an effective treatment for patients with multiple myeloma and patients with relapsed Hodgkin's and non-Hodgkin's lymphomas. Other indications have not been so well defined and are less common [34]. One protocol that has been often used for multiple myeloma consists of Cyclophosphamide Day 1, Adriamycin Days 1–4 and Dexamethasone Days 1–4. G-CSF is administered starting from day 9 [35], which also serves as a treatment for the disease. In order to achieve successful leukapheresis, it is essential to determine the optimal starting time point for the leukapheresis procedure. The decision is usually based on the WBC and $CD34^+$ counts in PB, of which the latter is considered a more reliable factor. Leukapheresis procedures will be initiated as soon as day 11 (counting from the first day of chemotherapy), or when $>20\times10^6$ $CD34^+$ cells/L are detected in the PB [36]. G-CSF administration is continued in the same doses as noted above until an adequate amount of stem cells is collected.

Alternative Mobilizing Agents

(See also Table 4.1).

GM-CSF

GM-CSF was successfully applied for HSC mobilization and the cells were subsequently used for autologous transplantation at the late 1980s and early 1990s [37, 38]. In a comparative study of mobilization in healthy donors, G-CSF alone mobilized about ten times more colony-forming HPCs than GM-CSF alone [39]. Notably, the total number of immature $CD34^+$ cells collected in the leukapheresis process was much higher following G-CSF treatment compared to GM-CSF treatment. The combination of G-CSF and GM-CSF for mobilization led to similar collection

Table 4.1 Mobilizing agents

Generic name	Trade names in use	Biological entity	Description	Usage	Half-life (h)	Reference
Filgrastim	Neupogen™	r-Hu-G-CSF	First cloned recombinant G-CSF without glycosylation (produced by *E. coli*)	Clinical standard	3–4	[55]
Lenograstim	Granocyte™	r-Hu-G-CSF	Second recombinant G-CSF with glycosylation (produced by chinese hamster ovary cells)	Clinical standard	3–4	[55]
Peg-Filgrastim	Neulasta™	r-Hu-G-CSF	Pegylated G-CSF without glycosylation (produced by *E. coli*)	Increasingly replacing Fil/ Lenograstim	33	[35]
Molgramostim	Leukomax ™	r-Hu-GM-CSF	Recombinant human GM-CSF (*E. coli*)	No longer used for mobilization in clinical practice		[37] [39]
Sargramostim	Leukine™	r-Hu-GM-CSF	Recombinant human GM-CSF (yeast)	No longer used for mobilization in clinical practice		[39]
Ancestim	StemGen™	r-metHu-SCF	Recombinant methionyl human stem cell factor (*E. coli*)	Limited clinical usage in combination with G-CSF		[44] [45]
Plerixafor (AMD3100)	Mozobil™	–	Synthetic small molecule, CXCR4-antagonist	In use for clinical mobilization		[56] [57, 58]
GROβ (CXCL2, MIP2-α)	–	GROβ (CXCL2, MIP2-α)	Natural chemokine	Experimentally well-explored mobilization potential		[47]
AMD3465	–	–	Synthetic small molecule, CXCR4-antagonist	Experimental mobilization potential		[50]
BIO5192	–	–	Synthetic small molecule, VLA4-antagonist	Experimental mobilization potential		[49]
T-140	–	–	Engineered small peptide analogue	Experimental mobilization potential		[51]
POL6326	–	–	Polyphemusin II derivate, CXCR4-antagonist	Clinical mobilization studies		[54]

results compared to G-CSF alone and resulted in significant higher number of $CD34^+/CD38^-$ cells collected than with G-CSF mobilization alone. These cells are considered to be more immature. Nevertheless, mobilization with GM-CSF is not longer performed in clinical practice today, due to toxicity and relative inefficiency compared to G-CSF.

Peg-Filgrastim

Recently, a pegylated formulation of G-CSF (i.e., Peg-Filgrastim or Neulastim) with a half-life of 33 h has become available for clinical usage. In recent studies, multiple myeloma and non-Hodgkin's lymphoma patients were mobilized with only a single dose of Peg-Filgrastim (6–12 mg), following a chemotherapy regimen [35, 40]. Mobilization efficacy was comparable to non-pegylated G-CSF. Peg-Filgrastim was also demonstrated to be effective in healthy donors [41]. The success of this drug is promising, enabling shortening of the mobilization protocol, at least in healthy donors. Still, side effects with flu-like symptoms can persist for days once the drug has been injected.

SCF

Combination of G-CSF and stem cell factor (SCF) results in a synergistic effect on mobilization of HPCs in nonhuman primates [42]. It should be noted that mobilization trials with a combined G-CSF and SCF administration (i.e., ancestim, r-metHuSCF, Amgen, Inc., USA) led to severe mast-cell mediated reactions [43]. Nonetheless, several studies have shown that with an appropriate co-medication, SCF can be used safely and in combination with G-CSF is able to achieve mobilization in patients who have failed G-CSF mobilization or are expected to be poor mobilizers [44, 45].

AMD3100

This agent is described in detail in other chapters of this book.

Experimental Antagonists

Several new antagonists, most of which targeting the receptor CXCR4, have been studied experimentally and might have the potential to be utilized clinically (see also Table 4.1).

GROβ

GROβ (CXCL2, MIP2 is the murine homologue) is a natural chemokine and ligand for the receptor CXCR2. Other ligands for CXCR2 include IL-8, and the modified GROβΔ4. All of these chemokines are capable of a rapid HPCs mobilization [46]. The detailed description by Fukuda et al. shows that mouse progenitor cells mobilized by GROβΔ4 alone or with G-CSF contained significantly more immature SKL cells in comparison to G-CSF mobilization. Furthermore, these cells seem to engraft better with significantly shorter times to recovery of WBCs and platelets [47]. The transplanted SKL cells resulted also in better competitive long-term repopulation activity including secondary and tertiary recipients. The authors recently compared some of the features of the mobilized HPC using AMD3100 or GROβ administration in mice. AMD3100 or GROβ alone yielded about 51% and 58% donor chimerism respectively, following a secondary transplantation of mobilized cells [46]. However, treatments with combinations of AMD3100 plus G-CSF or GROβ + G-CSF yielded about 84% and 85% donor chimerism respectively, following a secondary transplantation of mobilized cells [46]. These results have suggested a comparable mobilization capacity of AMD3100 or GROβ. In one abstract publication, the combination of all three agents has led to a synergistic mobilization in mice with about 75 times higher concentrations of CFU-GM (progenitor cells) than with G-CSF alone [48].

BIO5192

A small molecule inhibitor of the integrin VLA-4 (BIO5192, 1 mg/kg i.v.) was evaluated for its mobilization potential in mice. A rapid mobilization was detected upon a single dose administration. Combined with AMD3100, a significantly augmented mobilization of HSC has been reported [49].

AMD3465

AMD3465 is a second generation CXCR4 antagonist, which has been shown to induce mobilization of leukocytes in mice and dogs [50]. It is yet to be examined how its administration results in mobilization of human HPCs.

T-140

The CXCR4 antagonist T-140 (4F-benzoyl-TN14003) is a modified pentapeptide that has high affinity to the CXCR4-receptor and probably acts as an inverse agonist.

The combination of T-140 with G-CSF seemed to be superior to the combination of AMD3100 with G-CSF. Furthermore, a comparison for long-term repopulation potential showed a survival advantage for T-140 mobilized cells compared to AMD3100 mobilized cells in a murine model. These results suggest that T-140 potentially mobilizes more immature HPCs than AMD3100 [51].

POL6326

Another CXCR4 inhibitor was obtained by a protein epitope mimetics (PEM) technology by derivation from the naturally occurring β-hairpin peptide polyphemusin II. Preclinical studies of precursor molecules showed reliable high efficacy mobilizations of hematopoietic cells [52, 53]. The substance intended for clinical application is currently in a phase II study for autologous stem cell mobilization for multiple myeloma that is ongoing at our institution [54].

Conclusions

Adhesion of HSCs to its bone marrow niche is via multiple mechanisms. The present focus of interest has been the SDF-1/CXCR4 interaction and a number of novel agents targeting this pathway have been developed. Other important players are CD44 and its ligands, N-cadherin, and other cadherins with homophilic and heterophilic interactions and integrins, especially VLA-4. One important signaling mechanism that influences the adhesion properties is via the sympathetic nervous system and β-receptors. All of these adhesion mechanisms can be pharmacologically manipulated and thereby utilized for mobilization of HSCs.

Acknowledgments This work was supported by the German Federal Ministry of Education and Research (BMBF) within the supporting program "Cell Based Regenerative Medicine" (START-MSC2) and by the program "Maintenance and Differentiation of Stem Cells in Development and Disease" (SFB 873) of the German Research Foundation (DFG).

References

1. Peled A, Petit I, Kollet O, Magid M, Ponomaryov T, Byk T, Nagler A, Ben-Hur H, Many A, Shultz L, Lider O, Alon R et al (1999) Dependence of human stem cell engraftment and repopulation of NOD/SCID mice on CXCR4. Science 283:845–848
2. Wright DE, Bowman EP, Wagers AJ, Butcher EC, Weissman IL (2002) Hematopoietic stem cells are uniquely selective in their migratory response to chemokines. J Exp Med 195: 1145–1154
3. Cronshaw DG, Nie Y, Waite J, Zou YR (2010) An essential role of the cytoplasmic tail of CXCR4 in G-protein signaling and organogenesis. PLoS One 5:e15397
4. Dar A, Schajnovitz A, Lapid K, Kalinkovich A, Itkin T, Ludin A, Kao WM, Battista M, Tesio M, Kollet O, Cohen NN, Margalit R et al (2011) Rapid mobilization of hematopoietic

progenitors by AMD3100 and catecholamines is mediated by CXCR4-dependent SDF-1 release from bone marrow stromal cells. Leukemia 25(8):1286–1296, Erratum 1378
5. Hartmann TN, Grabovsky V, Pasvolsky R, Shulman Z, Buss EC, Spiegel A, Nagler A, Lapidot T, Thelen M, Alon R (2008) A crosstalk between intracellular CXCR7 and CXCR4 involved in rapid CXCL12-triggered integrin activation but not in chemokine-triggered motility of human T lymphocytes and CD34+ cells. J Leukoc Biol 84:1130–1140
6. Katayama Y, Battista M, Kao WM, Hidalgo A, Peired AJ, Thomas SA, Frenette PS (2006) Signals from the sympathetic nervous system regulate hematopoietic stem cell egress from bone marrow. Cell 124:407–421
7. Larsson J, Scadden D (2006) Nervous activity in a stem cell niche. Cell 124:253–255
8. Mendez-Ferrer S, Lucas D, Battista M, Frenette PS (2008) Haematopoietic stem cell release is regulated by circadian oscillations. Nature 452:442–447
9. Mendez-Ferrer S, Michurina TV, Ferraro F, Mazloom AR, Macarthur BD, Lira SA, Scadden DT, Ma'ayan A, Enikolopov GN, Frenette PS (2010) Mesenchymal and haematopoietic stem cells form a unique bone marrow niche. Nature 466:829–834
10. Lucas D, Battista M, Shi PA, Isola L, Frenette PS (2008) Mobilized hematopoietic stem cell yield depends on species-specific circadian timing. Cell Stem Cell 3:364–366
11. Spiegel A, Shivtiel S, Kalinkovich A, Ludin A, Netzer N, Goichberg P, Azaria Y, Resnick I, Hardan I, Ben-Hur H, Nagler A, Rubinstein M et al (2007) Catecholaminergic neurotransmitters regulate migration and repopulation of immature human CD34+ cells through Wnt signaling. Nat Immunol 8:1123–1131
12. Zoller M (2011) CD44: can a cancer-initiating cell profit from an abundantly expressed molecule? Nat Rev Cancer 11:254–267
13. Taubert I, Schubert M, Hellwig I, Zepeda-Moreno A, Ran D, Pietsch L, Eckstein V, Zoeller M, Ho AD (2010) Importance of CD44 and CD44v7 in the interaction of HPC and LSC with their niche. Int J Canc Res Treat [Onkologie] 33S6:V734
14. Bourguignon LY (2008) Hyaluronan-mediated CD44 activation of RhoGTPase signaling and cytoskeleton function promotes tumor progression. Semin Cancer Biol 18:251–259
15. Marhaba R, Freyschmidt-Paul P, Zoller M (2006) In vivo CD44-CD49d complex formation in autoimmune disease has consequences on T cell activation and apoptosis resistance. Eur J Immunol 36:3017–3032
16. Pokutta S, Weis WI (2007) Structure and mechanism of cadherins and catenins in cell–cell contacts. Annu Rev Cell Dev Biol 23:237–261
17. Kiel MJ, Acar M, Radice GL, Morrison SJ (2009) Hematopoietic stem cells do not depend on N-cadherin to regulate their maintenance. Cell Stem Cell 4:170–179
18. Kiel MJ, Radice GL, Morrison SJ (2007) Lack of evidence that hematopoietic stem cells depend on N-cadherin-mediated adhesion to osteoblasts for their maintenance. Cell Stem Cell 1:204–217
19. Hosokawa K, Arai F, Yoshihara H, Iwasaki H, Nakamura Y, Gomei Y, Suda T (2010) Knockdown of N-cadherin suppresses the long-term engraftment of hematopoietic stem cells. Blood 116:554–563
20. Wein F, Pietsch L, Saffrich R, Wuchter P, Walenda T, Bork S, Horn P, Diehlmann A, Eckstein V, Ho AD, Wagner W (2010) N-cadherin is expressed on human hematopoietic progenitor cells and mediates interaction with human mesenchymal stromal cells. Stem Cell Res 4:129–139
21. Imai Y, Shimaoka M, Kurokawa M (2010) Essential roles of VLA-4 in the hematopoietic system. Int J Hematol 91:569–575
22. Kinashi T (2007) Integrin regulation of lymphocyte trafficking: lessons from structural and signaling studies. Adv Immunol 93:185–227
23. Grabovsky V, Feigelson S, Chen C, Bleijs DA, Peled A, Cinamon G, Baleux F, Arenzana-Seisdedos F, Lapidot T, van Kooyk Y, Lobb RR, Alon R (2000) Subsecond induction of alpha4 integrin clustering by immobilized chemokines stimulates leukocyte tethering and rolling on endothelial vascular cell adhesion molecule 1 under flow conditions. J Exp Med 192:495–506
24. Arroyo AG, Yang JT, Rayburn H, Hynes RO (1996) Differential requirements for alpha4 integrins during fetal and adult hematopoiesis. Cell 85:997–1008

25. Arroyo AG, Yang JT, Rayburn H, Hynes RO (1999) Alpha4 integrins regulate the proliferation/differentiation balance of multilineage hematopoietic progenitors in vivo. Immunity 11:555–566
26. Priestley GV, Ulyanova T, Papayannopoulou T (2007) Sustained alterations in biodistribution of stem/progenitor cells in Tie2Cre+alpha4(f/f) mice are hematopoietic cell autonomous. Blood 109:109–111
27. Bonig H, Wundes A, Chang K-H, Lucas S, Papayannopoulou T (2008) Increased numbers of circulating hematopoietic stem/progenitor cells are chronically maintained in patients treated with the CD49d blocking antibody natalizumab. Blood 111:3439–3441
28. Zohren F, Toutzaris D, Klarner V, Hartung HP, Kieseier B, Haas R (2008) The monoclonal anti-VLA-4 antibody natalizumab mobilizes CD34+ hematopoietic progenitor cells in humans. Blood 111:3893–3895
29. Cashen AF, Lazarus HM, Devine SM (2007) Mobilizing stem cells from normal donors: is it possible to improve upon G-CSF? Bone Marrow Transplant 39:577–588
30. Beyer J, Schwella N, Zingsem J, Strohscheer I, Schwaner I, Oettle H, Serke S, Huhn D, Stieger W (1995) Hematopoietic rescue after high-dose chemotherapy using autologous peripheral-blood progenitor cells or bone marrow: a randomized comparison. J Clin Oncol 13:1328–1335
31. Schmitz N, Linch DC, Dreger P, Goldstone AH, Boogaerts MA, Ferrant A, Demuynck HM, Link H, Zander A, Barge A (1996) Randomised trial of filgrastim-mobilised peripheral blood progenitor cell transplantation versus autologous bone-marrow transplantation in lymphoma patients. Lancet 347:353–357
32. Anderson JE, Tefferi A, Craig F, Holmberg L, Chauncey T, Appelbaum FR, Guardiola P, Callander N, Freytes C, Gazitt Y, Razvillas B, Deeg HJ (2001) Myeloablation and autologous peripheral blood stem cell rescue results in hematologic and clinical responses in patients with myeloid metaplasia with myelofibrosis. Blood 98:586–593
33. Baldomero H, Gratwohl M, Gratwohl A, Tichelli A, Niederwieser D, Madrigal A, Frauendorfer K (2011) The EBMT activity survey 2009: trends over the past 5 years. Bone Marrow Transplant 46:485–501
34. Jantunen E, Kuittinen T (2008) Blood stem cell mobilization and collection in patients with lymphoproliferative diseases: practical issues. Eur J Haematol 80:287–295
35. Fruehauf S, Klaus J, Huesing J, Veldwijk MR, Buss EC, Topaly J, Seeger T, Zeller WJ, Moehler T, Ho AD, Goldschmidt H (2007) Efficient mobilization of peripheral blood stem cells following CAD chemotherapy and a single dose of pegylated G-CSF in patients with multiple myeloma. Bone Marrow Transplant 39:743–750
36. Wuchter P, Ran D, Bruckner T, Schmitt T, Witzens-Harig M, Neben K, Goldschmidt H, Ho AD (2010) Poor mobilization of hematopoietic stem cells-definitions, incidence, risk factors, and impact on outcome of autologous transplantation. Biol Blood Marrow Transplant 16:490–499
37. Haas R, Ho AD, Bredthauer U, Cayeux S, Egerer G, Knauf W, Hunstein W (1990) Successful autologous transplantation of blood stem cells mobilized with recombinant human granulocyte-macrophage colony-stimulating factor. Exp Hematol 18:94–98
38. Gianni AM, Siena S, Bregni M, Tarella C, Stern AC, Pileri A, Bonadonna G (1989) Granulocyte-macrophage colony-stimulating factor to harvest circulating haemopoietic stem cells for autotransplantation. Lancet 2:580–585
39. Lane TA, Law P, Maruyama M, Young D, Burgess J, Mullen M, Mealiffe M, Terstappen LW, Hardwick A, Moubayed M et al (1995) Harvesting and enrichment of hematopoietic progenitor cells mobilized into the peripheral blood of normal donors by granulocyte-macrophage colony-stimulating factor (GM-CSF) or G-CSF: potential role in allogeneic marrow transplantation. Blood 85:275–282
40. Russell N, Mesters R, Schubert J, Boogaerts M, Johnsen HE, Canizo CD, Baker N, Barker P, Skacel T, Schmitz N (2008) A phase 2 pilot study of pegfilgrastim and filgrastim for mobilizing peripheral blood progenitor cells in patients with non-Hodgkin's lymphoma receiving chemotherapy. Haematologica 93:405–412
41. Hill GR, Morris ES, Fuery M, Hutchins C, Butler J, Grigg A, Roberts A, Bradstock K, Szer J, Kennedy G, Morton J, Durrant S (2006) Allogeneic stem cell transplantation with peripheral blood stem cells mobilized by pegylated G-CSF. Biol Blood Marrow Transplant 12:603–607

42. Andrews RG, Briddell RA, Knitter GH, Rowley SD, Appelbaum FR, McNiece IK (1995) Rapid engraftment by peripheral blood progenitor cells mobilized by recombinant human stem cell factor and recombinant human granulocyte colony-stimulating factor in nonhuman primates. Blood 85:15–20
43. Stiff P, Gingrich R, Luger S, Wyres MR, Brown RA, LeMaistre CF, Perry J, Schenkein DP, List A, Mason JR, Bensinger W, Wheeler C et al (2000) A randomized phase 2 study of PBPC mobilization by stem cell factor and filgrastim in heavily pretreated patients with Hodgkin's disease or non-Hodgkin's lymphoma. Bone Marrow Transplant 26:471–481
44. Moskowitz CH, Stiff P, Gordon MS, McNiece I, Ho AD, Costa JJ, Broun ER, Bayer RA, Wyres M, Hill J, Jelaca-Maxwell K, Nichols CR et al (1997) Recombinant methionyl human stem cell factor and filgrastim for peripheral blood progenitor cell mobilization and transplantation in non-Hodgkin's lymphoma patients—results of a phase I/II trial. Blood 89:3136–3147
45. To LB, Bashford J, Durrant S, MacMillan J, Schwarer AP, Prince HM, Gibson J, Lewis I, Swart B, Marty J, Rawling T, Ashman L et al (2003) Successful mobilization of peripheral blood stem cells after addition of ancestim (stem cell factor) in patients who had failed a prior mobilization with filgrastim (granulocyte colony-stimulating factor) alone or with chemotherapy plus filgrastim. Bone Marrow Transplant 31:371–378
46. Pelus LM (2008) Peripheral blood stem cell mobilization: new regimens, new cells, where do we stand. Curr Opin Hematol 15:285–292
47. Fukuda S, Bian H, King AG, Pelus LM (2007) The chemokine GRObeta mobilizes early hematopoietic stem cells characterized by enhanced homing and engraftment. Blood 110:860–869
48. Pelus L, Clapp D, Bridger G (2006) Suprasynergistic peripheral blood stem cell mobilization in normal and Fanconi anemia knockout mice by the combination of G-CSF plus the CXCR4 antagonist AMD3100 and the CXCR2 agonist GRO ß. ASH annual meeting abstracts 108
49. Ramirez P, Rettig MP, Uy GL, Deych E, Holt MS, Ritchey JK, DiPersio JF (2009) BIO5192, a small molecule inhibitor of VLA-4, mobilizes hematopoietic stem and progenitor cells. Blood 114:1340–1343
50. Bodart V, Anastassov V, Darkes MC, Idzan SR, Labrecque J, Lau G, Mosi RM, Neff KS, Nelson KL, Ruzek MC, Patel K, Santucci Z et al (2009) Pharmacology of AMD3465: a small molecule antagonist of the chemokine receptor CXCR4. Biochem Pharmacol 78:993–1000
51. Abraham M, Biyder K, Begin M, Wald H, Weiss ID, Galun E, Nagler A, Peled A (2007) Enhanced unique pattern of hematopoietic cell mobilization induced by the CXCR4 antagonist 4F-benzoyl-TN14003. Stem Cells 25:2158–2166
52. DeMarco SJ, Henze H, Lederer A, Moehle K, Mukherjee R, Romagnoli B, Robinson JA, Brianza F, Gombert FO, Lociuro S, Ludin C, Vrijbloed JW et al (2006) Discovery of novel, highly potent and selective beta-hairpin mimetic CXCR4 inhibitors with excellent anti-HIV activity and pharmacokinetic profiles. Bioorg Med Chem 14:8396–8404
53. Lederer A, DeMarco SJ, Henze H, Romagnoli B, Mukherjee R, Zumbrunn J, Brianza F, Gombert FO, Ludin C, Vrijbloed JW, Obrecht JP, Lociuro S et al (2007) Discovery of highly potent and selective CXCR4 inhibitors using protein epitope mimetics (PEM) technology. Chimia 61:147–150
54. Schmitt S, Weinhold N, Dembowsky K, Neben K, Witzens-Harig M, Braun M, Klemmer J, Wuchter P, Ludin C, Ho AD, Goldschmidt H (2010) First results of a phase-II study with the new CXCR4 antagonist POL6326 to mobilize hematopoietic stem cells (HSC) in multiple myeloma (MM). ASH annual meeting abstracts 116:824.
55. Martin-Christin F (2001) Granulocyte colony stimulating factors: how different are they? How to make a decision? Anticancer Drugs 12:185–191
56. Broxmeyer HE, Orschell CM, Clapp DW, Hangoc G, Cooper S, Plett PA, Liles WC, Li X, Graham-Evans B, Campbell TB, Calandra G, Bridger G et al (2005) Rapid mobilization of murine and human hematopoietic stem and progenitor cells with AMD3100, a CXCR4 antagonist. J Exp Med 201:1307–1318

57. DiPersio JF, Micallef IN, Stiff PJ, Bolwell BJ, Maziarz RT, Jacobsen E, Nademanee A, McCarty J, Bridger G, Calandra G (2009) Phase III prospective randomized double-blind placebo-controlled trial of plerixafor plus granulocyte colony-stimulating factor compared with placebo plus granulocyte colony-stimulating factor for autologous stem-cell mobilization and transplantation for patients with non-Hodgkin's lymphoma. J Clin Oncol 27:4767–4773
58. DiPersio JF, Stadtmauer EA, Nademanee A, Micallef IN, Stiff PJ, Kaufman JL, Maziarz RT, Hosing C, Fruehauf S, Horwitz M, Cooper D, Bridger G et al (2009) Plerixafor and G-CSF versus placebo and G-CSF to mobilize hematopoietic stem cells for autologous stem cell transplantation in patients with multiple myeloma. Blood 113:5720–5726

Chapter 5
Role of the CXCR4/CXCL12 Axis in Hematopoietic Stem Cell Trafficking

Amnon Peled and Arnon Nagler

Abstract During embryogenesis, CXCR4, a chemokine receptor, and its ligand, stromal cell-derived factor-1 (SDF-1/CXCL12), are critically involved in the development of the hematopoietic organs such as the liver and the bone marrow (BM), by regulating hematopoietic stem cell (HSC) homing retention, survival, and mobilization. In adult life, the CXCR4 axis serves as the key factor for retention of hematopoietic cells including HSCs in the BM. Under physiological conditions, the exit of HSC is controlled by the circadian loop and it is an infrequent event. Tissue damage or infections increase levels of chemokines such as CXCL12 or cytokines such as G-CSF in the periphery and facilitate the exit of HSC and progenitors, which can contribute to tissue repair. Reducing the levels of CXCL12 signaling within the BM can be done either by CXCR4 antagonists or by the sequential administration of G-CSF. G-CSF, which is widely used to mobilize HSC, stimulates neutrophils activation, proteases secretion, and consequently degradation of CXCR4 and CXCL12 and indirectly increase HSC motility and release from the BM. Improved and more direct agents that will increase stem cell motility combined with superior CXCR4 antagonists may even further improve stem cell collection for transplantation. In this review, we update current knowledge about the role of CXCR4/CXCL12 in stem cell retention and mobilization.

Keywords CXCR4 • CXCL12/SDF-1 • Stem cell mobilization • WHIM

A. Peled (✉)
Hadassah Hebrew University Hospital, Goldyne Savad Institute of Gene Therapy, P.O. Box 12000, Jerusalem 91120, Israel
e-mail: Peled@hadassah.org.il

A. Nagler
Chaim Sheba Medical Center, Tel-Hashomer, Israel

S. Fruehauf et al. (eds.), *Novel Developments in Stem Cell Mobilization: Focus on CXCR4*, DOI 10.1007/978-1-4614-1960-0_5,

During mammalian development, hematopoietic stem cells (HSCs), rare and pluripotent self-renewing cells that give rise to all hematopoietic lineages, exit the yolk sac blood islands, the dorsal aorta of the aorta–gonad–mesonephros (AGM) region and the placenta, and home into the liver, spleen, and later on into the bone marrow (BM). In order to home correctly to their target tissue, HSCs must interact with the BM vascular endothelium. Following their interaction with the BM endothelial cells, the stem cells migrate into the BM microenvironment and are localized in the stem cell niche where they self-renew and differentiate into the different lineages [1]. The murine HSCs home and engraft the BM with extremely high efficiency [2]. Furthermore, it was demonstrated that murine HSCs migrate only in response to the stromal-derived factor-1 (SDF-1/CXCL12), the ligand for the CXC chemokine receptor 4 (CXCR4). CXCR4 expression by HSCs was confirmed by reverse transcription polymerase chain reaction (RT-PCR) analysis. Although HSCs also expressed mRNA for CCR3 and CCR9, they failed to migrate to these receptor ligands [3]. The chemokine receptor, CXCR4, and its ligand, CXCL12, belong to a large family of chemoattractant cytokines, which are small (5–20 kDa) proteins that regulate leukocyte trafficking by mediating the migration and adhesion of leukocytes [4–8]. The chemokine receptors are G-protein-coupled, seven transmembrane spanning molecules [9]. Being G-protein-coupled receptors (GPCRs), chemokine receptors characteristically signal through hetero-trimeric G-proteins, primarily involving Gi [10]. Despite the apparent redundancy within the chemokine system, CXCL12 is the only known ligand for CXCR4 [11]. CXCL12 and CXCR4 have highly conserved amino acid (aa) sequences between human and mouse (e.g., 98% and 94% identity, respectively). CXCL12/SDF-1 was originally cloned and designated as a pre-B-cell growth-stimulating factor (PBSF) [12]. Later, it was named stromal cell-derived factor-1 (SDF-1) and characterized as a highly efficacious $CD34^+$ progenitor stem cell and lymphocyte chemo-attractant secreted by the murine BM stroma cell line MS-5 [13, 14].

CXCR4 was the first chemokine receptor shown to be essential for life in mice [15–17]. Genetic disruption of CXCL12 and CXCR4 in mice results in a similar, lethal phenotype with ventricular septal defects, defective gastric vasculogenesis, cerebellar development defects, and abnormal hematopoiesis [16–19]. More specifically, the number of B-cell progenitors in CXCL12 and CXCR4 knockout embryos was severely reduced in fetal liver and BM; myeloid progenitors were reduced in the liver and were absent in the BM, indicating that PBSF/SDF-1 is responsible for both myelopoiesis and B-cell lymphopoiesis and BM myelopoiesis [18, 19]. The BM from an E15.5 CXCR4-deficient embryo was hypocellular with marked reduction in hematopoiesis. The entire marrow was composed predominantly of stromal cells and osteoblasts with a severe reduction in all hematopoietic lineages [19].

At the age of E18.5, the CXCR4-deficient BM also exhibited a severe reduction in myelopoiesis and normal numbers of maturing erythrocytes and megakaryocytes. Interestingly, adoptive transfer experiments done with c-kit$^+$ Sca-1$^+$ lin$^{low/-}$ CXCR4–/– fetal liver long-term repopulating stem cells revealed a deficiency in long-term, albeit not short-term lymphoid and myeloid repopulation in adult BM. The fact that stromal cell-derived factor/pre-B cell growth stimulating factor–/– fetal liver cells yielded short-term normal multilineage reconstitution implies that CXCR4 is essential for either self-renewal of stem cells or for their retention and proper localization in the BM [20].

To further study the role of the CXCL12/CXCR4 axis in the trafficking and engraftment of long-term repopulating HSCs, a long-term competitive repopulation assay was performed. HSCs that are generated in AGM and expand in fetal liver are released from the hematopoietic organs including fetal liver, and colonize the BM or spleen via the peripheral blood (PB). A long-term competitive repopulation assay revealed that, in CXCL12–/– embryos, the number of HSCs were comparable in fetal liver and increased in the PB, but were severely reduced in the BM compared to control embryos. Furthermore, enforced expression of CXCL12 in vascular endothelial cells could completely rescue the reduction of HSCs in CXCL12–/– BM and spleen. These results demonstrate that CXCL12 is essential for the colonization of the BM by HSCs from the peripheral circulation during embryogenesis. HSCs were found to be in contact with the cells expressing high amounts of CXCL12 such as reticular cells surrounding sinusoidal endothelial cells or osteoblasts near the endosteum. Induced deletion of CXCR4 in c-kit$^+$ Sca-1$^+$ Lin$^-$HSCs in adult mice resulted in the severe reduction of HSC numbers in the BM. Thus, CXCL12–CXCR4 signaling plays an essential role in maintaining the quiescent HSC pool and appears to be a key component of HSC niches, including both vascular and endosteal niches in the adult BM [21].

Human hematopoietic progenitor CD34$^+$ cells were shown in vivo and in vitro to roll along BM endothelial cells displaying selectins such as P-selectin, E-selectin, and adhesion molecules such as VCAM-1 as well as the chemokine CXCL12 [22]. Activation of CD34$^+$ cells, which bear the chemokine receptor CXCR4 with CXCL12, led to firm adhesion and transendothelial migration, which was dependent on LFA-1/ICAM-1 (intracellular adhesion molecule-1) and VLA-4/VCAM-1 (vascular adhesion molecule-1). Furthermore, CXCL12-induced polarization and extravasation of CD34$^+$/CXCR4$^+$ cells through the extracellular matrix underlining the endothelium was dependent on both VLA-4 and VLA-5 [23]. In addition, CXCR4 regulates the interaction of hematopoietic progenitors with the BM stroma; furthermore, the addition of CXCR4 antagonists to long-term hematopoietic cultures reduces significantly the number of cobblestone areas [24].

CXCR4/CXCL12 axis was found to be critical for nonobese diabetic/severe combined immunodeficiency (NOD/SCID) mouse BM engraftment by human SCID repopulating CD34$^+$ stem cells. Furthermore, using the same model system, SCID repopulating CD34$^+$ CD38$^{-/low}$CXCR4$^+$ stem cells home and accumulate rapidly, within a few hours, in the BM of total irradiated mice and were dependent on the CXCR4/CXCL12 axis [25]. A lentiviral gene transfer technique as well as pretreatment with stem cell factor (SCF) or culture medium increased CXCR4 expression on human CD34$^+$ progenitors and improved SDF-1-induced migration of HPC and progenitors [23, 26]. This resulted in significantly higher levels of in vivo repopulation of NOD/SCID mice including primitive CD34$^+$/CD38$^{-/low}$ cells [26, 27]. Overall, these results suggested that CXCR4 expression is important for human stem cell homing, retention, and multilineage repopulation of the BM.

To investigate whether the CXCR4-dependent migratory ability of peripheral blood-derived $CD34^+$ cells of patients undergoing autologous peripheral blood stem cell (PBSC) transplantation is related to the homing efficiency of these cells, the migration in vitro of these cells in response to CXCL12 was determined and correlated with in vivo hematopoietic recovery. Significantly faster hematologic recovery was observed in those patients who received transplanted $CD34^+$ cells that showed high spontaneous and CXCL12-induced migration in vitro ($P<0.05$). Moreover, $CD34^+$ cells from healthy granulocyte colony-stimulating factor (G-CSF)-mobilized donors exhibited significantly higher spontaneous and CXCL12-induced ($P<0.01$) migration than $CD34^+$ cells from patients mobilized with chemotherapy and G-CSF. Interestingly, the lower migratory capacity in vitro of patient-derived $CD34^+$ cells was not due to a lower expression of CXCR4, but probably reflected decreased motogenic behavior of the cells. These results indicate that the migratory capacity of the cells is important for hematopoietic recovery. An exponential relationship between CXCR4 expression and the number of $CD34^+$ cells that mobilized to the PB was found ($P<0.001$), suggesting that CXCR4 expression plays a role in the mobilization of $CD34^+$ cells [28]. In another study which included 35 patients that underwent G-CSF HPC collection and autologous transplant, those transplanted with a relatively lower $CD34^+$ cell dose achieved fast engraftment, a higher responsiveness to CXCL12 and high chemotactic index, which could have compensated for the lower cell dose. However, to apply the chemotactic index to CXCL12 as a prognostic factor of the rate of engraftment requires validation in a larger number of patients [29]. Another study tested the CXCR4 expression on transplanted PB $CD34^+$ cells in relation to engraftment after autologous transplantation in a cohort of multiple myeloma patients. Cryopreserved samples from stem cell collections of 27 myeloma patients were analyzed for CD34 and CXCR4 expression and time to engraftment was measured. The median percentage of $CD34^+$ cells co-expressing CXCR4 was 37% (3.7–97%). Both CD34 doses correlated with neutrophil engraftment ($P<0.005$), while the $CD34^+/CXCR4^+$ dose did not. However, patients given a higher dose of $CD34^+/CXCR4^+$ cells ($\geq 1.75\times 10^6$/kg) showed a faster time to platelet recovery ($P<0.05$) than those given a lower dose ($\leq 0.42\times 10^6$/kg). Further studies of CD34/CXCR4 expression by mobilized HSCs and the relationship to platelet recovery post-transplantation in a larger cohort of patients are warranted [30]. The described studies have suggested that the expression of CXCR4 may be an important characteristic of HSC/HPC. Hoffman et al. studied the dynamic expression of CXCR4 during growth factor-induced mobilization of HSCs in a clinically relevant nonhuman primate model, Papio anubis (baboons). It was found that an overwhelming number of $CD34^+$ cells within the mobilized peripheral blood grafts were cell surface CXCR4 negative and were capable of rescuing lethally irradiated baboons. Therefore, it was concluded that it is unlikely that the cell surface expression of CXCR4 in vitro is an absolute requirement for HSCs homing and engraftment. Furthermore, the data indicate that the lack of cell surface CXCR4 expression is possibly a trait of relatively more primitive HSCs characterized by a higher proliferative capacity [31]. In addition, it was also demonstrated that human cord and fetal blood $CD34^+CD38^-CXCR4^-$ and $CXCR4^+$ cells, sorted with neutralizing anti-CXCR4 monoclonal antibody (mAb), have a similar NOD/SCID repopulation potential [32]. However, CXCR4 expression is dynamic, and CXCR4-cells harbor intracellular CXCR4, which can be rapidly induced to cell surface expression within a few hours. Interestingly, co-injection of purified cells with 10 μg anti-CXCR4 mAb significantly reduced engraftment of all $CD34^+$ subsets, and 50 μg completely abrogated engraftment of NOD/SCID by all $CD34^+$ cells [33]. In 1999, Ma et al. reported that the chemokine receptor CXCR4 is required for the retention of the B lineage and granulocytic precursors within the murine fetal liver and BM microenvironment. It was demonstrated that in CXCR4-deficient embryos, pro-B cells are present in the blood, but hardly detectable in the liver. Similarly, myeloid cells were elevated in the blood and reduced in the liver compared to wild-type embryos [34]. Furthermore, the numbers of pro-B and pre-B cells were reduced in the BM and were abnormally high in the blood. Similarly, in CXCL12–/– embryos [20] showed that the number of HSCs was increased in the PB, but was severely reduced in the BM.

BM-derived SDF-1-responsive cell types include monocytes and macrophages, B and T lymphocytes, platelets and megakaryocytes, and $CD34^+$ cells, including both hematopoietic progenitors and stem cells. Intravenous injection of a replication-incompetent adenovector expressing the CXCL12 gene (AdSDF-1) elevated serum levels of SDF-1 in Balb/c and SCID mice and induced a marked leukocytosis within 3–5 days, predominantly involving monocytes, and a threefold increase in platelets. In addition, AdenoCXCL12–/– mobilized colony-forming units-granulocyte macrophages (CFU-GM) and cells with a long-term repopulating potential [35]. G-CSF-induced HSC mobilization and is widely used for clinical transplantation. In 2002, Petit et al. showed that G-CSF induced a reduction of SDF-1 in the BM, whereas SDF-1 levels in the blood were not affected. CXCL12 degradation by neutrophil elastase correlated with stem cell mobilization, and blocking elastase function reduced G-CSF-dependent mobilization. Surprisingly, neutralizing CXCR4 or CXCL12 function by neutralizing antibodies inhibited G-CSF-dependent mobilization of human and murine stem cell mobilization, indicating that CXCL12/CXCR4 signaling may also be involved in cell egress from the BM [36]. In previous studies done in the laboratory of Bendall, it was shown that granulocyte precursors accumulating in the BM during mobilization significantly increased their active proteases. In 2003, it was reported by the same group that mobilization of HPCs by G-CSF coincided in vivo with the cleavage of the N terminus of the chemokine receptor CXCR4 on HPCs. Following cleavage of CXCR4, the HPCs lost their ability to migrate in response to SDF-1. Furthermore, the concentration of SDF-1 decreased in vivo in the BM of mobilized mice, and this decrease coincided with the accumulation of serine proteases capable of directly cleaving and inactivating CXCL12 [37]. Thus, the proteolytic degradation of CXCL12 together with that of CXCR4 could represent a critical step leading to the mobilization of HPCs into the PB in response to G-CSF.

Mobilization of murine HPCs by increasing continuous peripheral levels of N-terminal modification of CXCL12 has been described by Moore et al. However, adenoviral delivery was required for effect and could not be demonstrated with native protein. The CTCE-0021 is a cyclized CXCR4 agonist CXCL12-based peptide, with comparable bioactivity and improved stability relative to CXCL12alpha [38]. CTCE-0021 dose-dependently and rapidly elevated blood neutrophils. Furthermore, CTCE-0021 also rapidly mobilized CFU-GM, burst-forming unit erythroid (BFU-E), and CFU-granulocyte–erythrocyte–monocyte–megakaryocyte (CFU-GEMM). Mobilization induced by CTCE-0021 was associated with rapid down-regulation of CXCR4 expression on HPCs, but did not change protease levels implicated in HPC mobilization. The CXCR4 antagonist, bicyclam AMD3100, was first identified as a blocker of HIV-1 entry and membrane fusion via the CXCR4 co-receptor, but not via CCR5.

The first pharmacokinetic and safety study with AMD3100 in human volunteers was reported in 2000 [39]. Twelve healthy volunteers were given AMD3100 as a single 15-min intravenous infusion at 10, 20, 40, or 80 μg/kg. Five subjects also received a single subcutaneous injection of AMD3100 (40 or 80 μg/kg). Three subjects received two escalating oral doses each (80 and 160 μg/kg). All subjects tolerated their dose(s) well without any grade 2 toxicity or dose adjustment. Six subjects experienced mild, transient symptoms, primarily gastrointestinal in nature and not dose-related. All subjects experienced a dose-related elevation of the white blood cell count, from 1.5 to 3.1 times the baseline, which returned to the baseline 24 h after dosing.

In another phase I study published in 2003, ten individuals received each a single dose of AMD3100 (80 μg/kg subcutaneously), which induced rapid, generalized leukocytosis associated with an increase in PB $CD34^+$ cells. Subsequent dose–response studies showed a maximum increase in circulating $CD34^+$ cells from 2.6 ± 0.3 to 40.4 ± 3.4/μL at 9 h after 240 μg/kg AMD3100. Serial administration of AMD3100 resulted in consistent, reversible increases in PB $CD34^+$ cells with no observed accumulation of $CD34^+$ cells. AMD100 was well tolerated and caused only mild, transient toxicity [40].

In an additional phase I study allografts from HLA-matched sibling donors were mobilized and collected without G-CSF using AMD3100. Donors ($N=25$) were treated with AMD3100 at a dose of 240 μg/kg by subcutaneous injection, and leukapheresis was then initiated just 4 h later. The median baseline PB $CD34^+$ count just before AMD3100 administration was 2/μL (range, 1–7/μL). At 4 h after a single dose of AMD3100, the $CD34^+$ count rose to a median of 16/μL (range, 4–54/μL), representing a median eightfold increase (Fig. 5.1). The baseline PB $CD34^+$ count was 3/μL (range, 1–8/μL) just before initiation of G-CSF; this rose to a median of 46/μL on day 5, representing a median 15.3-fold increase from baseline. This fold increase after 5 days of G-CSF was significantly greater than the rise 4 h after AMD3100 ($P<0.001$). There were significantly fewer $CD34^+$ cells/kg (2.9×10^6 vs. 4.2×10^6; $P=0.006$), but greater numbers of $CD3^+$ cells/kg (4.7×10^8 vs. 1.5×10^8; $P=0.006$) and $CD4^+$ cells/kg (3.1×10^8 vs. 1.1×10^8; $P=0.002$) in the AMD3100-mobilized products compared with the G-CSF-mobilized allografts. However, the differences in $CD8^+$, $CD19^+$, and $CD56^+$ cell content were not significant.

Two-thirds of the donors collected an allograft with a $CD34^+$ cell dose sufficient for transplantation after just one dose of AMD3100. No donor experienced more than grade 1 toxicity. The most common grade 1 toxicities included lightheadedness

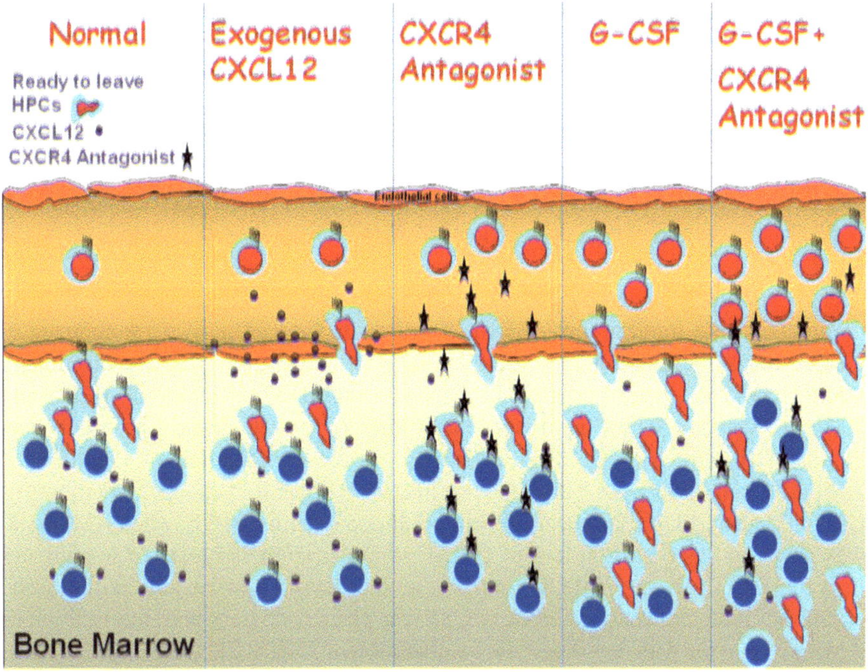

Fig. 5.1 Under physiological condition stem and progenitor cells are released to the circulation at a low pace and are controlled by the circadian loop (*Normal*). Stem and progenitor cells can be induced to leave the BM by increasing the levels of CXCL12 in the periphery (*Exogenous CXCL12*). Reducing the levels of CXCL12 signaling and the retention signals within the BM can be done by CXCR4 antagonists (*CXCR4 antagonist*). Following treatment with G-CSF, CXCL12 and CXCR4 are cleaved and increased number of "ready to go" cells is formed, some of these cells are released into the circulation. Co treatment with G-CSF and CXCR4 antagonist will lead to reduced retention signals and increased number of "ready to go cells" that will exit the BM (*G-CSF+CXCR4 antagonist*)

(44%); nausea, bloating, or flatulence (36%); injection site discomfort or warm sensation (28%); perioral paresthesias, loose stools, or diaphoresis (20%); and headache (16%). These toxicities typically resolved in a few hours and did not require any intervention. After a myeloablative regimen, 20 patients with hematologic malignancies received allografts collected after AMD3100 alone. All patients engrafted neutrophils (median day 10) and platelets (median day 12) promptly. Acute graft-versus-host disease (GVHD) grades 2 through 4 occurred in 35% of patients. One patient died due to complications related to acute GVHD. No unexpected adverse events were observed in any of the recipients.

Direct antagonism of CXCR4 by AMD3100 or other more potent CXCR4 antagonist may provide in the future more rapid and possibly less toxic and cumbersome alternative to traditional G-CSF-based mobilization in normal donors [41].

To further investigate the potential clinical utility of AMD3100 for CD34^{+} cell mobilization and collection, a phase I study was carried out in normal volunteers pretreated with a standard 5-day G-CSF regimen. Following 4 days of treatment with G-CSF, AMD3100 was administered alone or in combination with G-CSF. AMD3100 (160 μg/kg × 1 on day 5) significantly increased both G-CSF-stimulated (10 μg/kg/day) mobilization of $CD34^+$ cells (3.8-fold) and leukapheresis yield of $CD34^+$ cells. Moreover, collection of $CD34^+$ cells was comparable between individuals mobilized by a single-dose regimen of AMD3100 (240 μg/kg) and individuals mobilized with a 5-day regimen of G-CSF. AMD3100-mobilized leukapheresis products contained significantly greater numbers of T and B cells compared to G-CSF-stimulated leukapheresis products [42].

In an additional study testing the mobilizing effects of G-CSF plus AMD3100, healthy volunteers received 4 days of G-CSF (10 μg/kg/day s.c.) and then were randomized into three groups of two donors each. One group was randomized to receive the same amount of G-CSF on day 5, the second group received only AMD3100 (160 μg/kg s.c.) on day 5, and the third group received G-CSF and AMD3100 on day 5. HPC numbers per milliliter were evaluated just before the last treatment on day 5 of G-CSF, AMD3100, or the combination of G-CSF plus AMD3100, and also 1–48 h after the last treatment. Peak fold change in numbers of CFU-GM and CFU-GEMM per milliliter of blood occurred at 6 h, when AMD3100 was given on day 5 after 4 days of G-CSF administration and resulted in a greater than fourfold increase in HPCs compared with 5 days of administration of G-CSF. No further increase was seen when G-CSF was given for 5 days with the addition of AMD3100 on the fifth day. Thus, the combination of AMD3100 with G-CSF greatly enhanced mobilization of human HPCs. Donors whose HPCs were mobilized by multiple injections of G-CSF, or one injection of AMD3100 after multiple injections of G-CSF as noted directly above, were apheresed. The total number of HPCs apheresed and progenitors/kg donor after apheresis was tested using colony assay and scid repopulating cells (SRC). Significantly enhanced numbers of HPCs and colony-forming cells were observed in apheresed samples from donors who were mobilized with the combination of G-CSF plus AMD3100 compared with either G-CSF or AMD3100. AMD3100 alone mobilized SRC similarly to G-CSF although it failed to mobilize colony-forming cells [43].

A phase I study assessing the safety and clinical effects of AMD3100 in patients with multiple myeloma (MM) and non-Hodgkin's lymphoma (NHL) was first reported by DiPersio JF in 2005 [44]. Thirteen patients (MM, $n=7$; NHL, $n=6$) received AMD3100 at a dose of either 160 μg/kg ($n=6$) or 240 μg/kg ($n=7$). WBC and PB $CD34^+$ cell counts were analyzed at 4 and 6 h following injection. AMD3100 caused a rapid and statistically significant increase in the total WBC and PB $CD34^+$ counts at both 4 and 6 h following a single injection. The absolute $CD34^+$ cell count increased from a baseline of 2.6 ± 0.7/μL (mean ± SE) to 15.6 ± 3.9/μL and 16.2 ± 4.3/μL at 4 h ($P=0.002$) and 6 h after injection ($P=0.003$), respectively. The absolute $CD34^+$ cell counts observed at 4 and 6 h following AMD3100 were higher in the 240 μg/kg group (19.3 ± 6.9 and 20.4 ± 7.6/μL, respectively) compared with the 160 μg/kg group (11.3 ± 2.7 and 11.3 ± 2.5/μL, respectively). The drug was well tolerated and only grade 1 toxicities were encountered. AMD3100 was safe, however, not effective enough by itself for the rapid mobilization of $CD34^+$ cells in patients who received prior chemotherapy. Indeed, in 2005, Calandra et al. reported that the use of AMD3100 plus G-CSF for autologous hematopoietic progenitor cell mobilization is superior to G-CSF alone.

Another phase II study of 11 refractory or relapsed NHL patients, receiving 16 μg/kg daily of G-CSF for 4 days followed by 240 μg/kg of AMD3100 given subcutaneously on a new schedule of 9–10 h before apheresis collection on day 5 assessed the effect of AMD3100 on the mobilization of $CD34^+$ cells, dendritic cells (DCs), and lymphoma cells. Administration of G-CSF and AMD3100 was continued daily until > or $=2\times10^6$ $CD34^+$ cells/kg were collected. Adequate collection of the target of $CD34^+$ cells was achieved in all but 1 patient within 2 days, and 10/11 patients were transplanted within 2 months. All transplanted patients engrafted with a mean of 10 and 12 days for neutrophils and platelets, respectively. The addition of AMD3100 to G-CSF resulted in a >2.5-fold increase in $CD34^+$ cells/μL ($P=0.0001$). The average yield of $CD34^+$/kg was $3.0\pm1.5\times10^6$ (1.08–6.9) [45].

AMD3100 was further given with G-CSF to NHL, MM, and Hodgkin's lymphoma (HL) patients who could not collect sufficient cells for autologous transplant following administration of G-CSF. These poor mobilizers have been included in an AMD3100 Single Patient Use protocol, referred to as a Compassionate Use Protocol (CUP). A cohort of 115 data-audited poor mobilizers in CUP was assessed, with the objective being to collect > or $=2\times10^6$ $CD34^+$ cells per kg following AMD3100 plus G-CSF mobilization. The rates of successful $CD34^+$ cell collection were NHL 60.3%, MM 71.4%, and HL 76.5%, the average number of $CD34^+$ cells per kg was $3.51\pm2.9\times10^6$. Thirty-three percent of these patients failed to collect more than 2.0×10^6 kg of $CD34^+$ cells and the median apheresis days were 3. Following transplant, median times to neutrophil and PLT engraftment were 11 days and 18 days, respectively. Engraftment was durable (3 and 6 months post-transplant follow-up). There were no drug-related serious adverse events. Of the adverse events that were considered to be related to AMD3100, two (1.6%) were severe (one patient—headache, one patient—nightmares). Other AMD3100-related adverse events were mild (84.8%) or moderate (13.6%). The most common AMD3100-related adverse events were gastrointestinal reactions, injection site reactions, and paresthesias. AMD3100 plus G-CSF offers a new treatment to collect $CD34^+$ cells for autologous transplant from poor mobilizers [45].

Chemotherapy plus G-CSF is an alternative (peripheral blood stem cells) PBSC mobilization strategy for use in patients undergoing auto-stem cell transplant (SCT). A pilot study explored the safety of AMD3100 mobilization when incorporated into a conventional stem cell mobilization regimen of chemotherapy and G-CSF [46]. Forty (26 MM and 14 NHL) patients were treated with AMD3100. G-CSF was administered s.c. at 10 μg/kg/day after chemotherapy until the day before the last day of apheresis. All patients received AMD3100 240 μg/kg/day s.c. for up to 5 days. Twenty-four patients (60%) experienced AEs that were considered to be related to the study treatment, the majority of which were mild in severity. Of the three patients who experienced study treatment-related AEs that were moderate or severe in intensity, two discontinued study treatment: one patient experienced severe back pain, considered to be definitely related to the study drug, and the second patient experienced severe anxiety that was considered to be part of an acute systemic reaction possibly related to the study drug. This latter reaction occurred within 1 h of AMD3100 injection and required medical follow-up with nasal oxygen for mild hypoxia. The patient continued with the apheresis the next morning. Common adverse events that occurred within 30 days after the administration of AMD3100 and before chemoablation and transplantation included nausea, diarrhea, injection site reactions, bone pain, paresthesias, headache, and dizziness.

The addition of AMD3100 to a chemo-mobilization regimen resulted in an increase in the PB $CD34^+$ cells. The mean rate of increase in the PB $CD34^+$ cells was 2.8 cells/μL/h pre- and 13.3 cells/μL/h post-AMD3100 administrations. Engraftment parameters were acceptable after myeloblative chemotherapy, with the median day for neutrophil and platelet engraftment being day 11 (range 8–20 days) and day 13 (range 7–77 days), respectively. The data obtained from the analysis of the cohorts suggest that AMD3100 can be added to chemotherapy-based mobilization regimens and may accelerate the rate of increase in $CD34^+$ cells on the second day of apheresis.

An additional European phase II study tested whether a combination of G-CSF and AMD3100 mobilizes more primitive PB progenitor cells than G-CSF alone [47]. Patients with MM and NHL ($n=15$; phase II study) were investigated for co-expression of primitive and lineage-associated markers, their proliferative activity in vitro and repopulation potential after clinical transplantation. A significant increase in primitive $CD34^+$ $CD38^-$ cells was observed in intraindividual comparisons of all patients after administration of G-CSF+AMD3100 (PB 2.8-fold, range 1.6–4.0-fold; leukapheresis product 2.7-fold, 1.2–8.8-fold) compared with G-CSF alone. When using a long-term culture-initiating cell (LTCIC) assay, this increase was confirmed. After transplantation of G-CSF+AMD3100-mobilized PBPC, the time to leukocyte reconstitution $>1\times10^3$/μL and platelet reconstitution $>2\times10^4$/μL was 14 (10–19 days) and 13 days (10–15 days), respectively. A complete and stable hematologic reconstitution (platelets $>1.5\times10^5$/μL) was observed in 91% of all patients within 35 days. This may indicate that AMD3100 together with G-CSF lead to a significant increase in primitive HSCs with high repopulation potential.

A phase III prospective randomized double-blind placebo-controlled trial of AMD3100 plus G-CSF compared with placebo plus G-CSF for autologous stem-cell mobilization and transplantation for patients with NHL was published in 2009 [48]. Patients with non-Hodgkin's lymphoma requiring an autologous hematopoietic stem-cell transplantation in first or second complete or partial remission were eligible. Patients received G-CSF(10 μg/kg) subcutaneously daily for up to 8 days. Beginning on the evening of day 4, and continuing daily for up to 4 days, patients received either AMD3100 (240 μg/kg) or placebo subcutaneously. Starting on day 5, patients began daily apheresis for up to 4 days or until > or = 5×10^6 $CD34^+$ cells/kg were collected. The primary end point was the percentage of patients who collected > or = 5×10^6 $CD34^+$ cells/kg in four or fewer apheresis days. Eighty-nine (59%) of 150 patients in the AMD3100 group and 29 (20%) of 148 patients in the placebo group met the primary end point ($P<.001$). One hundred thirty-five patients (90%) in the AMD3100 group and 82 patients (55%) in the placebo group underwent transplantation after initial mobilization. Median time to engraftment was similar in both groups. The most common AMD3100-associated adverse events were gastrointestinal disorders and injection site reactions. AMD3100 and G-CSF were well tolerated and resulted in a significantly higher proportion of patients with NHL achieving the optimal $CD34^+$ cell target for transplantation in fewer apheresis days, compared with G-CSF alone.

Another phase III, multicenter, randomized (1:1), double-blind, placebo-controlled study evaluated the safety and efficacy of AMD3100 with G-CSF in mobilizing HSCs in patients with multiple myeloma [49]. Patients received G-CSF (10 μg/kg) subcutaneously daily for up to 8 days. Beginning on day 4 and continuing daily for up to 4 days, patients received either AMD3100 (240 μg/kg) or placebo subcutaneously. Starting on day 5, patients began daily apheresis for up to 4 days or until more than or equal to 6×10^6 $CD34^+$ cells/kg were collected. The primary endpoint was the percentage of patients who collected more than or equal to 6×10^6 $CD34^+$ cells/kg in less than or equal to 2 aphereses. A total of 106 of 148 (71.6%) patients in the AMD3100 group and 53 of 154 (34.4%) patients in the placebo group met the primary endpoint ($P < 0.001$). A total of 54% of AMD3100-treated patients reached target after one apheresis, whereas 56% of the placebo-treated patients required four aphereses to reach target. The most common adverse events related to AMD3100 were gastrointestinal disorders and injection site reactions. AMD3100 and G-CSF were well tolerated, and significantly more patients collected the optimal $CD34^+$ cell/kg target for transplantation earlier compared with G-CSF alone.

The CXCR4 antagonists BKT140, CTCE-0214, POL6326, or TG-0054 also induce a rapid and robust mobilization of hematopoietic cells, including hematopoietic stem and progenitor cells, pre-B cells, as well as mature cells, such as neutrophils, monocytes, macrophages, T cells, and NK cells in a variety of animal models and humans. This is further supported by the fact that CXCR4 plays a critical role in the retention of hematopoietic cells within the BM [40, 43, 50].

The warts, hypogammaglobulinemia, infections, and myelokathexis (WHIM) syndrome is characterized by susceptibility to the human papilloma virus infection-induced warts and carcinomas; neutropenia, B-cell lymphopenia and hypogammaglobulinemia-related infections, and BM myelokathexis (myeloid hyperplasia with apoptosis). This is a rare immunodeficiency syndrome caused by autosomal dominant mutations truncating the C terminus of the chemokine receptor CXCR4. WHIM mutations potentiate CXCR4 signaling, and thereby increase the retention signals within the BM, causing severe neutropenia [51, 52]. Current clinical management of WHIM includes treatment with G-CSF to mobilize neutrophils. The use of potent CXCR4 antagonists such as Mozobil is currently being studied in a clinical study [53].

Overall, it is evident that CXCR4 is critical for the retention of hematopoietic stem and progenitors in the BM. Furthermore, CXCR4 is also critical for neutrophils, monocytes, macrophages, T cells, and NK cells retention in the BM. Stem and progenitor cells can be induced to leave the BM by either increasing the levels of CXCL12 in the periphery or reducing the levels of CXCL12 signaling within the BM. Reducing the levels of CXCL12 signaling within the BM can be done by CXCR4 antagonists or by the sequential administration of G-CSF. G-CSF stimulates neutrophils and granulocyte progenitor activation, proteases secretion, and consequently degradation of CXCR4 and CXCL12. However, in contrast to CXCR4, the antagonist G-CSF also increases the motility of cells within the BM. It is therefore not surprising that CXCR4 antagonists are powerful synergistic factors with G-CSF. Our studies clearly demonstrated that mobilized progenitor cells are activated and motile and secrete high levels of MMP-2 [24]. We suggest that under normal conditions, there is a small pool of "ready to go cells" which are localized close to the endothelium. These stem and progenitor cells are released to the circulation at a low pace and are controlled by the circadian loop. Following preconditioning, the BM with cytokines such as G-CSF or following severe damage to organs such as the heart, there is a larger pool of "ready to go" cells which are released to the circulation by reducing their retention signals through CXCR4 by way of either increasing the levels of SDF-1 in the periphery or reducing the levels of CXCL12/ CXCR4 in the BM. Improved and more direct agents that will increase stem cell motility combined with better CXCR4 antagonists may even further perfect stem cell collection for transplantation (Fig. 5.1).

References

1. Ueno H, Weissman IL (2010) The origin and fate of yolk sac hematopoiesis: application of chimera analyses to developmental studies. Int J Dev Biol 54(6–7):1019–1031
2. Benveniste P, Cantin C, Hyam D, Iscove NN (2003) Hematopoietic stem cells engraft in mice with absolute efficiency. Nat Immunol 4(7):708–713
3. Wright DE, Bowman EP, Wagers AJ, Butcher EC, Weissman IL (2002) Hematopoietic stem cells are uniquely selective in their migratory response to chemokines. J Exp Med 195(9): 1145–1154
4. Butcher EC, Picker LJ (1996) Lymphocyte homing and homeostasis. Science 272(5258): 60–66
5. Rossi D, Zlotnik A (2000) The biology of chemokines and their receptors. Annu Rev Immunol 18:217–242
6. Murphy PM, Baggiolini M, Charo IF, Hebert CA, Horuk R, Matsushima K, Miller LH, Oppenheim JJ, Power CA (2000) International union of pharmacology. XXII. Nomenclature for chemokine receptors. Pharmacol Rev 52(1):145–176
7. Locati M, Otero K, Schioppa T, Signorelli P, Perrier P, Baviera S, Sozzani S, Mantovani A (2002) The chemokine system: tuning and shaping by regulation of receptor expression and coupling in polarized responses. Allergy 57(11):972–982
8. Moser B, Wolf M, Walz A, Loetscher P (2004) Chemokines: multiple levels of leukocyte migration control. Trends Immunol 25(2):75–84
9. Murphy PM (2002) International union of pharmacology. XXX. Update on chemokine receptor nomenclature. Pharmacol Rev 54(2):227–229
10. Thelen M (2001) Dancing to the tune of chemokines. Nat Immunol 2(2):129–134
11. Horuk R (2001) Chemokine receptors. Cytokine Growth Factor Rev 12(4):313–335
12. Nagasawa T, Kikutani H, Kishimoto T (1994) Molecular cloning and structure of a pre-B-cell growth-stimulating factor. Proc Natl Acad Sci U S A 91(6):2305–2309
13. Bleul CC, Farzan M, Choe H, Parolin C, Clark-Lewis I, Sodroski J, Springer TA (1996) The lymphocyte chemoattractant SDF-1 is a ligand for LESTR/fusin and blocks HIV-1 entry. Nature 382(6594):829–833

14. Aiuti A, Webb IJ, Bleul C, Springer T, Gutierrez-Ramos JC (1997) The chemokine SDF-1 is a chemoattractant for human CD34+ hematopoietic progenitor cells and provides a new mechanism to explain the mobilization of CD34+ progenitors to peripheral blood. J Exp Med 185(1): 111–120
15. Arenberg DA, Keane MP, DiGiovine B, Kunkel SL, Morris SB, Xue YY, Burdick MD, Glass MC, Iannettoni MD, Strieter RM (1998) Epithelial-neutrophil activating peptide (ENA-78) is an important angiogenic factor in non-small cell lung cancer. J Clin Invest 102(3):465–472
16. Tachibana K, Hirota S, Iizasa H, Yoshida H, Kawabata K, Kataoka Y, Kitamura Y, Matsushima K, Yoshida N, Nishikawa S, Kishimoto T et al (1998) The chemokine receptor CXCR4 is essential for vascularization of the gastrointestinal tract. Nature 393(6685):591–594
17. Zou YR, Kottmann AH, Kuroda M, Taniuchi I, Littman DR (1998) Function of the chemokine receptor CXCR4 in haematopoiesis and in cerebellar development. Nature 393(6685):595–599
18. Nagasawa T, Hirota S, Tachibana K, Takakura N, Nishikawa S, Kitamura Y, Yoshida N, Kikutani H, Kishimoto T (1996) Defects of B-cell lymphopoiesis and bone-marrow myelopoiesis in mice lacking the CXC chemokine PBSF/SDF-1. Nature 382(6592):635–638
19. Ma Q, Jones D, Borghesani PR, Segal RA, Nagasawa T, Kishimoto T, Bronson RT, Springer TA (1998) Impaired B-lymphopoiesis, myelopoiesis, and derailed cerebellar neuron migration in CXCR4- and SDF-1-deficient mice. Proc Natl Acad Sci U S A 95(16):9448–9453
20. Kawabata K, Ujikawa M, Egawa T, Kawamoto H, Tachibana K, Iizasa H, Katsura Y, Kishimoto T, Nagasawa T (1999) A cell-autonomous requirement for CXCR4 in long-term lymphoid and myeloid reconstitution. Proc Natl Acad Sci U S A 96(10):5663–5667
21. Sugiyama T, Kohara H, Noda M, Nagasawa T (2006) Maintenance of the hematopoietic stem cell pool by CXCL12–CXCR4 chemokine signaling in bone marrow stromal cell niches. Immunity 25(6):977–988
22. Peled A, Grabovsky V, Habler L, Sandbank J, Arenzana-Seisdedos F, Petit I, Ben-Hur H, Lapidot T, Alon R (1999) The chemokine SDF-1 stimulates integrin-mediated arrest of CD34(+) cells on vascular endothelium under shear flow. J Clin Invest 104(9):1199–1211
23. Peled A, Kollet O, Ponomaryov T, Petit I, Franitza S, Grabovsky V, Slav MM, Nagler A, Lider O, Alon R, Zipori D et al (2000) The chemokine SDF-1 activates the integrins LFA-1, VLA-4, and VLA-5 on immature human CD34(+) cells: role in transendothelial/stromal migration and engraftment of NOD/SCID mice. Blood 95(11):3289–3296
24. Abraham M, Beider K, Wald H, Weiss ID, Zipori D, Galun E, Nagler A, Eizenberg O, Peled A (2009) The CXCR4 antagonist 4F-benzoyl-TN14003 stimulates the recovery of the bone marrow after transplantation. Leukemia 23(8):1378–1388
25. Peled A, Petit I, Kollet O, Magid M, Ponomaryov T, Byk T, Nagler A, Ben-Hur H, Many A, Shultz L, Lider O et al (1999) Dependence of human stem cell engraftment and repopulation of NOD/SCID mice on CXCR4. Science 283(5403):845–848
26. Kahn J, Byk T, Jansson-Sjostrand L, Petit I, Shivtiel S, Nagler A, Hardan I, Deutsch V, Gazit Z, Gazit D, Karlsson S et al (2004) Overexpression of CXCR4 on human CD34+ progenitors increases their proliferation, migration, and NOD/SCID repopulation. Blood 103(8):2942–2949
27. Ohno N, Kajiume T, Sera Y, Sato T, Kobayashi M (2009) Short-term culture of umbilical cord blood-derived CD34 cells enhances engraftment into NOD/SCID mice through increased CXCR4 expression. Stem Cells Dev 18(8):1221–1226
28. Voermans C, Kooi ML, Rodenhuis S, van der Lelie H, van der Schoot CE, Gerritsen WR (2001) In vitro migratory capacity of CD34+ cells is related to hematopoietic recovery after autologous stem cell transplantation. Blood 97(3):799–804
29. Marquez-Curtis LA, Turner AR, Larratt LM, Letcher B, Lee SF, Janowska-Wieczorek A (2009) CD34+ cell responsiveness to stromal cell-derived factor-1alpha underlies rate of engraftment after peripheral blood stem cell transplantation. Transfusion 49(1):161–169
30. Hicks C, Isaacs A, Wong R, Chong BH (2011) CXCR4 expression on transplanted peripheral blood CD34(+) cells: relationship to engraftment after autologous transplantation in a cohort of multiple myeloma patients. Ann Hematol 90(5):547–555

31. Mahmud N, Patel H, Hoffman R (2004) Growth factors mobilize CXCR4 low/negative primitive hematopoietic stem/progenitor cells from the bone marrow of nonhuman primates. Biol Blood Marrow Transplant 10(10):681–690
32. Rosu-Myles M, Gallacher L, Murdoch B, Hess DA, Keeney M, Kelvin D, Dale L, Ferguson SS, Wu D, Fellows F, Bhatia M (2000) The human hematopoietic stem cell compartment is heterogeneous for CXCR4 expression. Proc Natl Acad Sci U S A 97(26):14626–14631
33. Kollet O, Petit I, Kahn J, Samira S, Dar A, Peled A, Deutsch V, Gunetti M, Piacibello W, Nagler A, Lapidot T (2002) Human CD34(+)CXCR4(−) sorted cells harbor intracellular CXCR4, which can be functionally expressed and provide NOD/SCID repopulation. Blood 100(8):2778–2786
34. Ma Q, Jones D, Springer TA (1999) The chemokine receptor CXCR4 is required for the retention of B lineage and granulocytic precursors within the bone marrow microenvironment. Immunity 10(4):463–471
35. Hattori K, Heissig B, Tashiro K, Honjo T, Tateno M, Shieh JH, Hackett NR, Quitoriano MS, Crystal RG, Rafii S, Moore MA (2001) Plasma elevation of stromal cell-derived factor-1 induces mobilization of mature and immature hematopoietic progenitor and stem cells. Blood 97(11):3354–3360
36. Petit I, Szyper-Kravitz M, Nagler A, Lahav M, Peled A, Habler L, Ponomaryov T, Taichman RS, Arenzana-Seisdedos F, Fujii N, Sandbank J et al (2002) G-CSF induces stem cell mobilization by decreasing bone marrow SDF-1 and up-regulating CXCR4. Nat Immunol 3(7):687–694
37. Levesque JP, Hendy J, Takamatsu Y, Simmons PJ, Bendall LJ (2003) Disruption of the CXCR4/CXCL12 chemotactic interaction during hematopoietic stem cell mobilization induced by GCSF or cyclophosphamide. J Clin Invest 111(2):187–196
38. Pelus LM, Bian H, Fukuda S, Wong D, Merzouk A, Salari H (2005) The CXCR4 agonist peptide, CTCE-0021, rapidly mobilizes polymorphonuclear neutrophils and hematopoietic progenitor cells into peripheral blood and synergizes with granulocyte colony-stimulating factor. Exp Hematol 33(3):295–307
39. Hendrix CW, Flexner C, MacFarland RT, Giandomenico C, Fuchs EJ, Redpath E, Bridger G, Henson GW (2000) Pharmacokinetics and safety of AMD-3100, a novel antagonist of the CXCR-4 chemokine receptor, in human volunteers. Antimicrob Agents Chemother 44(6):1667–1673
40. Liles WC, Broxmeyer HE, Rodger E, Wood B, Hubel K, Cooper S, Hangoc G, Bridger GJ, Henson GW, Calandra G, Dale DC (2003) Mobilization of hematopoietic progenitor cells in healthy volunteers by AMD3100, a CXCR4 antagonist. Blood 102(8):2728–2730
41. Devine SM, Vij R, Rettig M, Todt L, McGlauchlen K, Fisher N, Devine H, Link DC, Calandra G, Bridger G, Westervelt P et al (2008) Rapid mobilization of functional donor hematopoietic cells without G-CSF using AMD3100, an antagonist of the CXCR4/SDF-1 interaction. Blood 112(4):990–998
42. Liles WC, Rodger E, Broxmeyer HE, Dehner C, Badel K, Calandra G, Christensen J, Wood B, Price TH, Dale DC (2005) Augmented mobilization and collection of CD34+ hematopoietic cells from normal human volunteers stimulated with granulocyte-colony-stimulating factor by single-dose administration of AMD3100, a CXCR4 antagonist. Transfusion 45(3):295–300
43. Broxmeyer HE, Orschell CM, Clapp DW, Hangoc G, Cooper S, Plett PA, Liles WC, Li X, Graham-Evans B, Campbell TB, Calandra G et al (2005) Rapid mobilization of murine and human hematopoietic stem and progenitor cells with AMD3100, a CXCR4 antagonist. J Exp Med 201(8):1307–1318
44. Flomenberg N, Devine SM, Dipersio JF, Liesveld JL, McCarty JM, Rowley SD, Vesole DH, Badel K, Calandra G (2005) The use of AMD3100 plus G-CSF for autologous hematopoietic progenitor cell mobilization is superior to G-CSF alone. Blood 106(5):1867–1874
45. Calandra G, McCarty J, McGuirk J, Tricot G, Crocker SA, Badel K, Grove B, Dye A, Bridger G (2008) AMD3100 plus G-CSF can successfully mobilize CD34+ cells from non-Hodgkin's lymphoma, Hodgkin's disease and multiple myeloma patients previously failing mobilization with chemotherapy and/or cytokine treatment: compassionate use data. Bone Marrow Transplant 41(4):331–338

46. Dugan MJ, Maziarz RT, Bensinger WI, Nademanee A, Liesveld J, Badel K, Dehner C, Gibney C, Bridger G, Calandra G (2010) Safety and preliminary efficacy of plerixafor (Mozobil) in combination with chemotherapy and G-CSF: an open-label, multicenter, exploratory trial in patients with multiple myeloma and non-Hodgkin's lymphoma undergoing stem cell mobilization. Bone Marrow Transplant 45(1):39–47
47. Fruehauf S, Veldwijk MR, Seeger T, Schubert M, Laufs S, Topaly J, Wuchter P, Dillmann F, Eckstein V, Wenz F, Goldschmidt H et al (2009) A combination of granulocyte-colony-stimulating factor (G-CSF) and plerixafor mobilizes more primitive peripheral blood progenitor cells than G-CSF alone: results of a European phase II study. Cytotherapy 11(8):992–1001
48. DiPersio JF, Micallef IN, Stiff PJ, Bolwell BJ, Maziarz RT, Jacobsen E, Nademanee A, McCarty J, Bridger G, Calandra G (2009) Phase III prospective randomized double-blind placebo-controlled trial of plerixafor plus granulocyte colony-stimulating factor compared with placebo plus granulocyte colony-stimulating factor for autologous stem-cell mobilization and transplantation for patients with non-Hodgkin's lymphoma. J Clin Oncol 27(28): 4767–4773
49. DiPersio JF, Stadtmauer EA, Nademanee A, Micallef IN, Stiff PJ, Kaufman JL, Maziarz RT, Hosing C, Fruehauf S, Horwitz M, Cooper D et al (2009) Plerixafor and G-CSF versus placebo and G-CSF to mobilize hematopoietic stem cells for autologous stem cell transplantation in patients with multiple myeloma. Blood 113(23):5720–5726
50. Abraham M, Biyder K, Begin M, Wald H, Weiss ID, Galun E, Nagler A, Peled A (2007) Enhanced unique pattern of hematopoietic cell mobilization induced by the CXCR4 antagonist 4F-benzoyl-TN14003. Stem Cells 25(9):2158–2166
51. Hernandez PA, Gorlin RJ, Lukens JN, Taniuchi S, Bohinjec J, Francois F, Klotman ME, Diaz GA (2003) Mutations in the chemokine receptor gene CXCR4 are associated with WHIM syndrome, a combined immunodeficiency disease. Nat Genet 34(1):70–74
52. Balabanian K, Lagane B, Pablos JL, Laurent L, Planchenault T, Verola O, Lebbe C, Kerob D, Dupuy A, Hermine O, Nicolas JF et al (2005) WHIM syndromes with different genetic anomalies are accounted for by impaired CXCR4 desensitization to CXCL12. Blood 105(6):2449–2457
53. McDermott DH, Lopez J, Deng F, Liu Q, Ojode T, Chen H, Ulrick J, Kwatemaa N, Kelly C, Anaya-O'Brien S, Garofalo M et al (2011) AMD3100 is a potent antagonist at CXCR4(R334X), a hyperfunctional mutant chemokine receptor and cause of WHIM syndrome. J Cell Mol Med 15(10):2071–2081

Part II
Clinical Studies on Stem Cell Mobilization

Chapter 6
Early Studies of AMD3100/Plerixafor in Healthy Volunteers

David C. Dale and W. Conrad Liles

Abbreviations

CXCR4	Chemokine (C-X-C motif) receptor type 4
SDF-1	Stromal cell-derived factor-1
CCR5	Chemokine (C-C motif) receptor type 5
HIV	Human immunodeficiency virus
FDA	Food and drug administration
µg	Micrograms
kg	Kilograms
SC	Subcutaneously
FACS	Fluorescence-activated cell sorter
c-kit	Cytokine receptor (CD117) for kit ligand or stem cell factor
CFU-GM	Colony-forming unit–granulocyte/macrophage
BFU-E	Erythroid burst forming units
CFU-GEMM	Colony-forming unit–granulocyte, erythrocyte, macrophage, megakaryocyte
G-CSF	Granulocyte colony-stimulating factor
mL	Milliliter
10 L	10 liter

D.C. Dale, MD (✉)
University of Washington, 1959 NE Pacific St., Rm AA522, Box 356422,
Seattle, WA 98195, USA
e-mail: dcdale@u.washington.edu

W.C. Liles, MD, PhD
University Health Network/University of Toronto, Toronto General Hospital 13E 220,
200 Elizabeth St., TGH EN13-220, Toronto, ON, Canada
e-mail: conrad.liles@uhn.on.ca

S. Fruehauf et al. (eds.), *Novel Developments in Stem Cell Mobilization: Focus on CXCR4*, DOI 10.1007/978-1-4614-1960-0_6,

HSCT	Hematopoietic stem cell transplantation
CFUs	Colony-forming units
NOD-SCID	Nonobese diabetic severe combined immunodeficient
SRC	Stem cell repopulating cell

Introduction

Approval of CXCR4 antagonist AMD3100 or plerixafor for hematopoietic stem cell mobilization followed a series of basic and clinical studies on the retention and release of hematopoietic cells from the bone marrow. The first observation was the importance of the ligand pair SDF1-CXCR4 in the trafficking of hematopoietic progenitor cells [1]. About the same time, it was learned that CXCR4 and CCR5 are coreceptors for the entry of HIV into human cells [2]. Soon after AMD3100/plerixafor was identified as a promising CXCR4 antagonist that appeared to inhibit HIV entry into host target cells, its effects were examined in preclinical models [3, 4] and then in ten men with HIV infection [5]. These studies showed that administration of AMD3100/plerixafor was well tolerated and caused significant leukocytosis, with increases in neutrophils, lymphocytes and monocytes. The only concern was premature ventricular contractions in 2 of 40 subjects during the study [5]. These results prompted investigations addressing specific details of the leukocytosis induced by AMD3100/plerixafor in healthy subjects.

Dose Response Studies

Investigations in normal healthy subjects were initiated at the University of Washington Clinical Research Center in 2000 under a series of protocols approved by the UW Human Subjects Committee/Investigational Review Board and the Federal Food and Drug Administration (FDA).

The initial study involved 26 healthy human volunteers (age 24–33 years, 13 men and 13 women) [6]. The first ten subjects received AMD3100/plerixafor at a dose of 80 μg/kg as a single subcutaneous injection. Subsequently, a second group was tested over a range of doses from 10 to 240 μg/kg, administered SC (SC) as a single dose. In the final phase of this initial study, three subjects received the 80 μg/kg dose on three consecutive days [6]. Throughout this study, observations were made on the peripheral blood total leukocyte count and differential white blood cell counts at 1, 3, 6, 9, and 24 h after the injection. In addition, $CD34^+$ cells were enumerated by FACS analysis utilizing a standard protocol for cell labeling and flow cytometry. For some studies, numbers of colony-forming cells, i.e., granulocyte macrophage colony-forming cells, granulocyte-erythroid-macrophage-megakaryocytic colony-forming cells, and erythroid burst forming units, were enumerated by standard methods [7]. High specific activity tritiated thymidine studies were also performed to determine the percentage of the hematopoietic colony-forming cells in cell cycle [7].

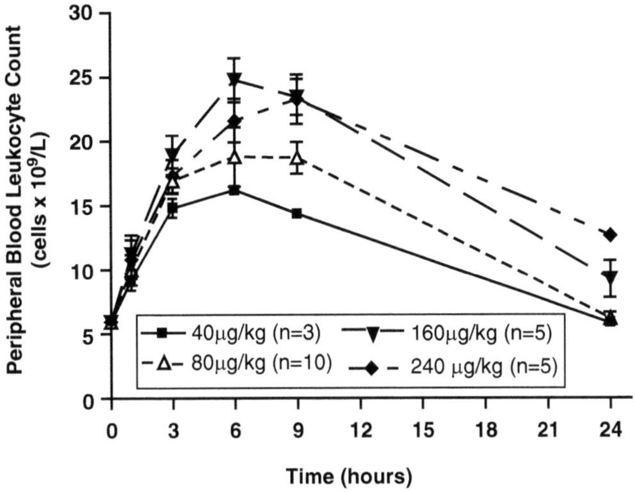

Fig. 6.1 Leukocyte Counts in Response to Single-Dose Administration of AMD3100.* Time course of mobilization of CD34⁺ cells into peripheral blood induced by single dose administration of AMD3100 to normal human volunteers. Ten normal human volunteers received a single 80 µg/kg subcutaneous dose of AMD3100. Peripheral venous blood was withdrawn at time intervals following drug administration and the concentration of CD34⁺ cells was determined by FACS. Each value represents the mean ± SEM ($n = 10$) (from [8], with permission)

Administration of a single dose of AMD3100 caused a dose-dependent leukocytosis in the healthy subjects. Figure 6.1 shows the peripheral blood leukocyte counts for each dose of AMD3100. At all doses, the maximum increase occurred approximately 6–9 h after administration of AMD3100. Neutrophils, lymphocytes, monocytes, eosinophils, and basophils all increased (see Fig. 6.2) [7, 8]. The responses were very consistent across the group of subjects. There was no significant change in circulating levels of erythrocytes or platelets at any dose of AMD3100/plerixafor administered (see Table 6.1).

This initial study focused first on determining if peripheral blood CD34⁺ cells increased in response to AMD3100 and then on the timing and magnitude of the response at various doses of the drug [3]. CD34⁺ cells increased at all doses, and the peak of the response occurred somewhat later at the higher doses. As shown in Fig. 6.3, CD34⁺ cells increased at all doses, with a relatively narrow standard error of the mean, reflecting consistency across subjects. With the 80 µg/kg dose, the number of peripheral blood CD34⁺ cells increased approximately fourfold. There was a tenfold increase in CD34⁺ cells at 9 h following the 240 µg/kg dose. Administration of AMD3100/plerixafor at a dose of 80 µg/kg for three consecutive days induced approximately the same response in peripheral blood CD34⁺ cell counts each day, with no appreciable increment or decrement in the observed responses (see Fig. 6.4). Each day, the peak occurred approximately 6–9 h following administration of AMD3100/plerixafor. Greater than 70% of the CD34⁺ cells mobilized by the 80 µg/kg dose of AMD3100/plerixafor were c-kit positive (CD117⁺) (see Table 6.2).

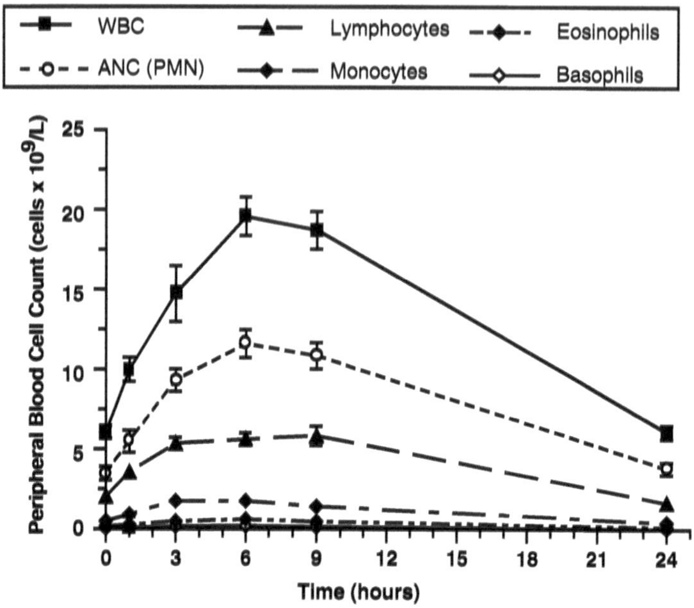

Fig. 6.2 Differential Leukocyte Count Following Administration of AMD3100.* Ten normal human volunteers received a single 80 μg/kg subcutaneous dose of AMD3100. Peripheral venous blood was withdrawn for determination of the leukocyte differential count at time intervals following drug administration. Each value represents the mean ± SEM ($n = 10$). WBC, white blood cell count; ANC, absolute neutrophil count; PMN, polymorphonuclear neutrophils (from [8], with permission)

Table 6.1 Blood count before and after a single injection of AMD3100

	WBC (×10³/μL)	Hct (%)	Plts (×10³/μL)
80 μg/kg AMD3100			
Baseline	6.29 ± 0.45	39.5 ± 1.4	215 ± 17
6 h post AMD	19.49 ± 1.27	37.6 ± 1.2	208 ± 15
9 h post AMD	18.71 ± 1.23	38.5 ± 1.3	215 ± 17
240 μg/kg AMD3100			
Baseline	6.17 ± 0.50	42.8 ± 1.4	246 ± 27
6 h post AMD	21.62 ± 1.71	39.6 ± 1.2	241 ± 20
9 h post AMD	23.28 ± 1.92	39.2 ± 0.9	239 ± 32

From [8], with permission

Measurement of blood myeloid progenitor cells after AMD3100/plerixafor administration mirrored the changes in the peripheral blood CD34⁺ cells, with similar results observed for the culture of cells in either agar or methyl cellulose (see Table 6.3). Importantly for future studies, there was a significant increase in CFU-GM, BFU-E and CFU-GEMM. Furthermore, the colony-forming cells were quiescent as determined by "thymidine suicide" assays, suggesting that AMD3100/plerixafor mobilizes quiescent pluripotent hematopoietic stem cells [7].

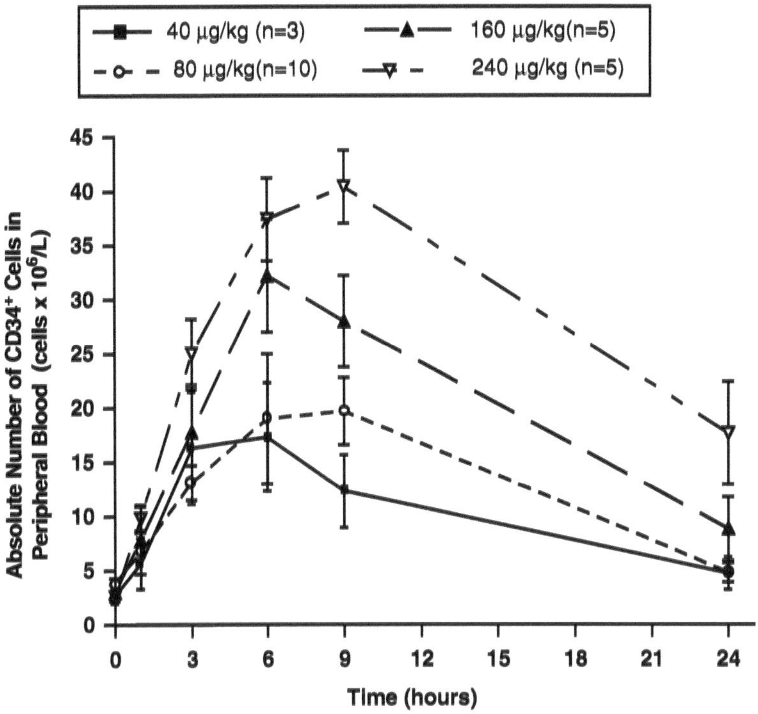

Fig. 6.3 Dose–response analysis of AMD3100-induced mobilization of CD34⁺ cells into peripheral blood.* Normal human volunteers received a single subcutaneous injection of AMD3100 at the following doses: 40 μg/kg ($n=3$); 80 μg/kg ($n=10$); 160 μg/kg ($n=5$); and 240 μg/kg ($n=5$). Peripheral venous blood was withdrawn at time intervals following drug administration, and the concentration of $CD34^+$ cells was determined by FACS. Each value represents the mean ± SEM (from [6], with permission)

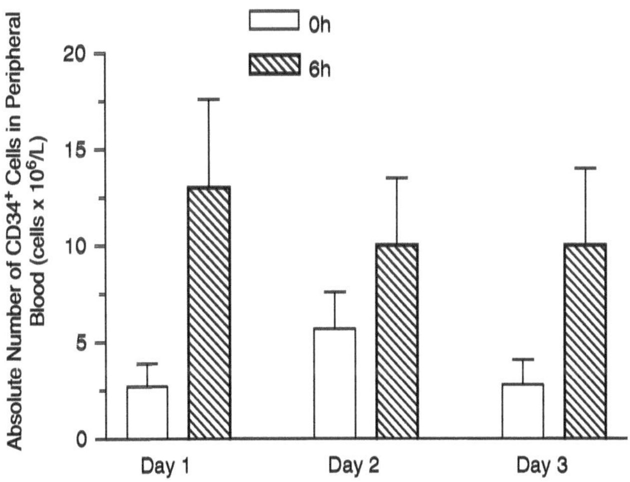

Fig. 6.4 Peripheral Blood $CD34^+$ Cell Count Following Serial Administration of AMD3100.* Three normal human volunteers received a single subcutaneous dose of AMD3100 (80 μg/kg) for 3 consecutive days. Peripheral venous blood was withdrawn immediately prior to and 6 h after each dose of AMD3100 for determination of the concentration of $CD34^+$ cells by FACS. Each value represents the mean ± SEM ($n=3$) (from [8], with permission)

Table 6.2 Immunophenotype of $CD34^+$ cells mobilized 6 h following administration of AMD3100 (80 μg/kg SC) to normal volunteers

Cell type	Percentage of total $CD34^+$ cells
$CD34^+/CD33^+$	57.0 ± 16.4
$CD34^+/CD38^{dim}$	64.2 ± 11.9
$CD34^+/CD38^{bright}$	35.8 ± 11.9
$CD34^+/CD117^+$	72.6 ± 7.0

Mean ± SEM, $n = 10$
From [8], with permission

Table 6.3 Peripheral blood myeloid progenitor cell mobilizing effects of AMD3100 (80 μg/kg SC) in normal human volunteers

	Myeloid progenitor cells (fold change from time = 0 h)			
	Agar	Methyl cellulose		
	CFU-GM	CFU-GM	BFU-E	CFU-GEMM
$T = 1$ h	2.8 ± 0.3*	4.9 ± 0.5*	2.1 ± 0.2*	2.6 ± 0.3*
$T = 3$ h	8.5 ± 0.3*	11.3 ± 1.6*	3.2 ± 0.3*	5.1 ± 0.8*
$T = 6$ h	17.9 ± 0.7*	19.7 ± 2.4*	5.5 ± 0.7*	9.7 ± 1.4*
$T = 9$ h	10.3 ± 2.0*	8.9 ± 1.1*	3.8 ± 0.3*	4.5 ± 0.8*
$T = 24$ h	2.1 ± 1.0	1.4 ± 0.1*	1.2 ± 0.1	1.3 ± 0.2

Mean ± SEM; $n = 10$; *$p < 0.005$ compared to baseline [$T = 0$ h]
From [6], with permission

The subjects in this initial study were carefully monitored for adverse effects [6]. The most common event observed was redness or stinging at the AMD3100/plerixafor injection site. These reactions were all mild and transient and did not interrupt the study at any dose level. Other adverse events included headache, perioral paresthesias, nausea, and a sensation of abdominal distention. Monitoring by self-reporting of symptoms (e.g., tachycardia, palpitations), physical examination, and electrocardiography revealed no evidence for cardiac arrhythmias in any of the subjects. Standard blood tests, including assessment of renal and hepatic function, revealed no significant changes.

This study was very encouraging for the development of AMD3100/plerixafor as an agent for mobilization of pluripotent hematopoietic progenitor cells, either when administered alone or in conjunction with granulocyte colony-stimulating factor (G-CSF).

Mobilization of $CD34^+$ Cells with AMD3100/Plerixafor and G-CSF

After establishing that AMD3100/plerixafor mobilized $CD34^+$ cells, we undertook a second series of studies in normal volunteers to determine if AMD3100/plerixafor could be used to augment G-SCF-induced $CD34^+$ cell mobilization [9]. Two cohorts of healthy human subjects were investigated. The first cohort of 18 healthy subjects

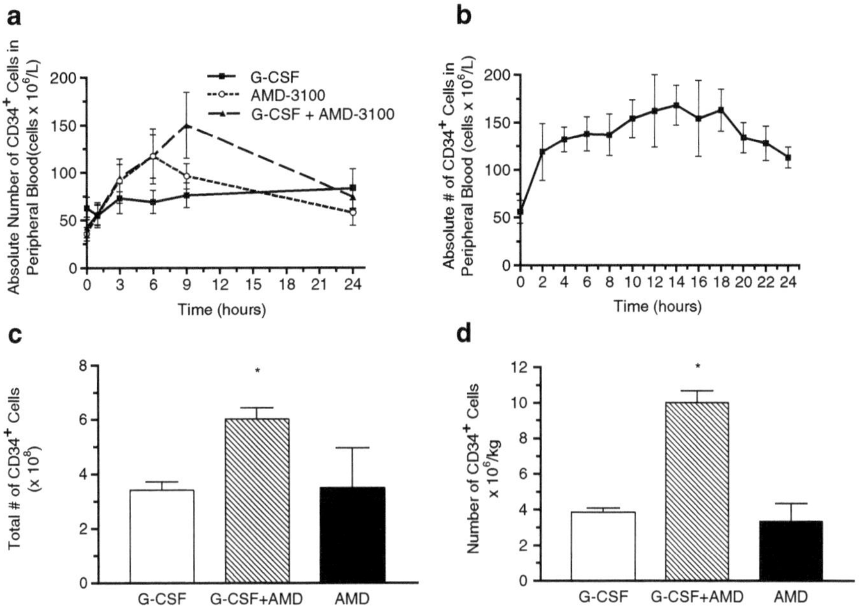

Fig. 6.5 Mobilization and Collection of CD34⁺ Cells Following Administration of G-CSF alone, AMD3100 alone, and G-CSF plus AMD3100 to Healthy Human Volunteers.* Panel (**a**) 18 healthy human volunteers received recombinant human G-CSF (10 μg/kg/day) subcutaneously (SC) for 4 days, followed by randomization on day 5 to one of three groups ($n=6$/group): (1) G-CSF only (10 μg/kg SC×1); (2) AMD3100 only (160 μg/kg SC×1); and (3) G-CSF plus AMD3100. Peripheral blood CD34⁺ counts (mean±SEM) were determined at the designated time intervals following drug administration on day 5. Panel (**b**) Three healthy human volunteers received recombinant human G-CSF (10 μg/kg/day SC) for 4 days, followed by G-CSF plus AMD3100 (240 μg/kg SC×1). Peripheral blood CD34⁺ cell counts (mean±SEM) were determined at 2 h intervals for the ensuing 24 h. Panel (**c**) ten healthy human volunteers were randomized to three groups: (1) G-CSF (10 μg/kg/day SC)×5d ($n=3$); (2) G-CSF (10 μg/kg/day SC)×4 days, then G-CSF plus AMD3100 (160 μg/kg SC×1) on day 5 ($n=3$); and (3) AMD3100 (240 μg/kg SC)×1 ($n=4$). An 18-L leukapheresis was performed beginning 4 h after final drug administration. Data show total number of CD34⁺ cells in the respective leukapheresis products (mean±SEM; *$P<0.05$ compared to leukapheresis products obtained from individuals mobilized with G-CSF only). Panel (**d**) Data from panel **c** depicted as CD34⁺ cells/kg (mean±SEM; *$P<0.05$ compared to leukapheresis products obtained from individuals mobilized with G-CSF only) (from [9], with permission)

received G-CSF (10 μg/kg/day) SC for 4 days. These subjects were then randomized to receive: (1) G-CSF alone (10 μg/kg) subcutaneously; (2) AMD3100/plerixafor alone (160 μg/kg) subcutaneously; (3) or a combination of G-CSF (10 μg/kg) and AMD3100/plerixafor (160 μg/kg) SC on day 5. Peripheral blood CD34⁺ cells were enumerated at 1, 3, 6, 9 and 24 h following drug(s) administration. To assure that a maximum response had been achieved and assess the timing of the response, an additional cohort of three healthy subjects received G-CSF (10 μg/kg/day) SC for 4 days followed by G-CSF (10 μg/kg) and AMD3100/plerixafor (240 μg/kg) SC on day 5, and peripheral blood levels of CD34⁺ cells were monitored at 2-h intervals.

Results of these experiments are shown in Fig. 6.5. Addition of AMD3100/plerixafor at a dose of 160 μg/kg to G-CSF on day 5 increased peripheral blood $CD34^+$ cells significantly [9]. At 9 h following combined administration, circulating $CD34^+$ cells increased to 150×10^6/L. All of the other regimens increased circulating $CD34^+$ cells in a dose-dependent fashion. In this protocol, AMD3100/plerixafor at a dose of 160 μg/kg ($CD34^+$ cell count: $117.3 \times 10^6 \pm 23.6 \times 10^6$/L) was more effective than G-CSF at a dose of 10 μg/kg ($CD34^+$ cell count: $69.3 \times 10^6 \pm 10.6 \times 10^6$/L) on day 5. A 5-day regimen of G-CSF (10 μg/kg/day subcutaneously) plus AMD3100/plerixafor (240 μg/kg SC on day 5) yielded the highest results. The peak value for circulating $CD34^+$ cells was $168.0 \times 10^6 \pm 45.0 \times 10^6$/L at 14 h (see Fig. 6.5).

The next step was to determine how many $CD34^+$ cells could be harvested from peripheral blood by leukapheresis after administration of AMD3100/plerixafor alone vs. administration of G-CSF alone vs. administration of the combination of AMD3100/plerixafor plus G-CSF [9]. For this phase of the study, healthy human volunteers received either a single dose of AMD3100/plerixafor (240 μg/kg subcutaneously), G-CSF (10 μg/kg/day × 5 days subcutaneously), or G-CSF (10 μg/kg/day × 5 days subcutaneously) plus AMD3100/plerixafor (160 μg/kg SC on day 5). Addition of AMD3100/plerixafor to G-CSF yielded the largest harvest of circulating $CD34^+$ cells (see Fig. 6.5). The combined regimen of G-CSF plus AMD3100/plerixafor yielded a harvest of $6.02 \times 10^8 \pm 0.42 \times 10^6$ $CD34^+$ cells using a standard 10-L volume leukapheresis with blood flow rates of 50–100 mL/min. These results demonstrated that AMD3100/plerixafor represented a potentially valuable independent agent for $CD34^+$ cell mobilization and that AMD3100/plerixafor in conjunction with G-CSF was clearly a very promising mobilization strategy [9].

Immunophenotypes of Cells Collected by Leukapheresis Following Mobilization with AMD3100/Plerixafor

To estimate the potential for either inducing graft-versus-host disease and/or "graft-versus-leukemia" effects if the lymphocyte-rich leukapheresis products collected after administration of AMD3100/plerixafor were used for allogeneic hematopoietic stem cell transplantation (allo-HSCT), the immunophenotypes of the mobilized cells were examined using flow cytometric methodology [9]. AMD3100/plerixafor-mobilized leukapheresis cell collections contained significantly greater numbers of T ($CD3^+$) and B ($CD19^+$) cells and increased numbers of almost all other lymphocyte subtypes compared to leukapheresis cell collections obtained after G-CSF alone (see Table 6.4). The clinical significance of these findings, particularly for the

Table 6.4 Immunocompetent cells contained in Leukapheresis products collected following mobilization with G-CSF alone, AMD3100 alone, and G-CSF plus AMD3100

Cells × 10^9	G-CSF[a] (n=3)	G-CSF ± AMD3100[b] (n=3)	AMD3100[c] (n=4)
$CD2^+$	14.6 ± 4.4	25.4 ± 1.1*	40.3 ± 6.9*
$CD3^+$	12.9 ± 4.1	23.6 ± 1.2*	37.4 ± 6.3*
TCR^+	12.1 ± 4.3	22.2 ± 0.9*	35.5 ± 5.7*
$TCR_{\gamma/\delta}+$	0.7 ± 0.4	0.7 ± 0.1	1.5 ± 0.6
$CD3^+/CD4^+$	7.7 ± 2.8	12.6 ± 0.2*	20.9 ± 1.9*
$CD4^+/CD45RA^+$	2.2 ± 0.8	4.9 ± 1.1	8.2 ± 1.7*
$CD4^+/CD45RO^+$	5.5 ± 2.1	7.7 ± 1.0	12.8 ± 1.5*
$CD3^+/CD8^+$	3.9 ± 1.5	9.0 ± 0.8*	13.2 3.6*
$CD3^+/CD4^-/CD8^-$	1.3 ± 0.3	2.0 ± 0.2	3.2 ± 1.2
$CD19^+$	2.3 ± 0.6	8.7 ± 0.3*	9.9 ± 3.6*
$CD45^+/CD14^+$	21.5 ± 3.1	35.7 ± 3.8*	15.4 ± 3.7
$CD16^+/CD56^+/CD3^-$	1.8 ± 0.6	1.8 ± 0.2	2.9 ± 0.5

Each value represents the mean ± SEM (# of cells × 10^9)
*$P<0.05$ compared with G-CSF alone
From [9], with permission
Mobilization regimens:
[a]G-CSF: 10 μg/kg SC qd × 5 days
[b]G-CSF: 10 μg/kg SC qd × 4 days, then G-CSF + AMD3100: 160 μg/kg SC × 1 on day 5
[c]AMD3100: 240 μg/kg SC × 1

use of AMD3100/plerixafor as an adjunct therapy in both autologous and allogeneic HSCT, awaited clinical investigations.

Characterization of $CD34^+$ Cells Mobilized with AMD3100/Plerixafor

Using in vitro colony-forming assays, the effects of administration of AMD3100/plerixafor on the subtypes of circulating hematopoietic progenitor cells were further examined [7]. In studies measuring CFU-GM and CFU-GEMM serially over a 2-day period, it was clear that addition of AMD3100/plerixafor to G-CSF increased both subtypes of colony-forming cells (see Fig. 6.6). The peak in CFUs occurred 6 h after administration of the combination of G-CSF at 10 μg/kg for 5 days and AMD3100/plerixafor (160 μg/kg administered on day 5, concomitant with the final dose of G-CSF). Examination of the colony-forming cells from the leukapheresis products also showed a substantially greater number of CFU-GM, BFU-E, and CFU-GEMM when the product was collected after the combination of G-CSF plus AMD3100/plerixafor, either expressed as total progenitors in the leukapheresis products or as progenitors per kilogram of body weight of the subject.

These studies also examined the capacity of hematopoietic stem cells collected after administration of G-CSF alone, administration of AMD3100/plerixafor alone, or after combined administration of the two agents to engraft in nonobese

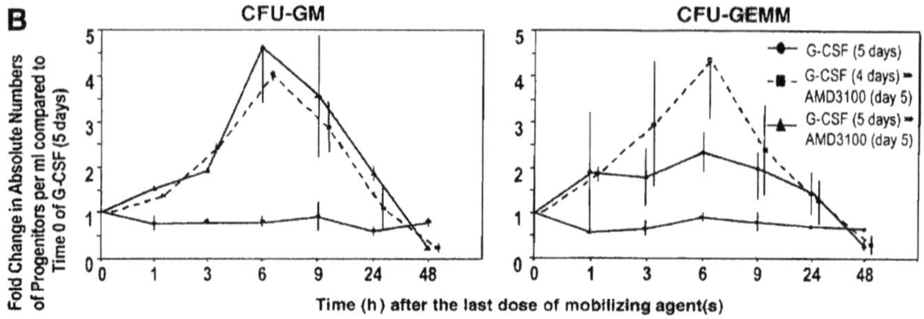

Fig. 6.6 Influence of AMD3100 with G-CSF on mobilization of circulating HPC in healthy human volunteers.* Six volunteers received 4 days of G-CSF (10 μg/kg/day SC×1). The volunteers were randomized into three groups of two donors each. Group I received G-CSF (10 μg/kg SC×1) on day 5. Group II received AMD3100 (160 μg/kg SC×1) on day 5. Group III received G-CSF (10 μg/kg SC×1) and AMD3100 (160 μg/kg SC×1) on day 5. The results shown are the mean plus range of fold increases of the absolute numbers of CFU-GM and CFU-GEMM per ml of blood for two healthy volunteers each at 1, 3, 6, 9, 24, and 48 h after the last injection on day 5. The fold changes are based on the following numbers of G-CSF Day 5, 0 h control progenitor cells/ml: Group I: G-CSF (CFU-GM: 34403 and 27194; CFU-GEMM: 14363 and 10083); Group II: G-CSF (4 days) plus AMD3100 (day 5) CFU-GM: 11968 and 2675; CFU-GEMM: 3366 and 510), and Group III: G-CSF (5 days) plus AMD3100 (day 5) CFU-GM: 2698 and 2380; CFU-GEMM: 1028 and 1238) (from [7], with permission)

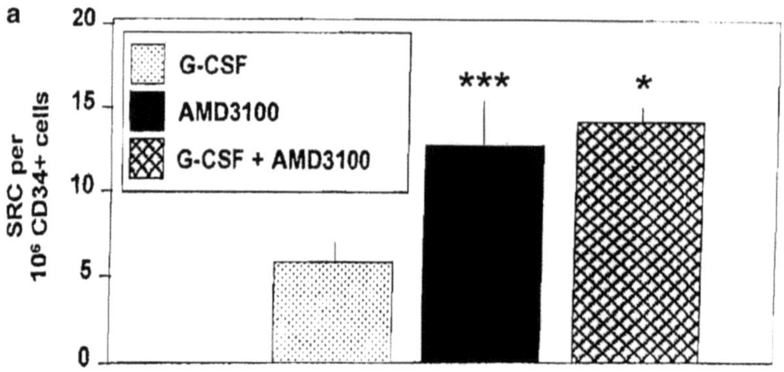

Fig. 6.7 Influence of AMD3100, G-CSF, and the Combination of G-CSF plus AMD3100 on Mobilization of NOD-SCID Repopulating Cells (SRC) from Normal Human Volunteers and Surface Expression of Adhesion Molecules and Chemotaxis of $CD34^+$ Cells. Frequency of SRC per 10^6 $CD34^+$ cells (mean ± 1 SEM). Human volunteers received AMD3100 (80 μg/kg SC×1) (N=4), or G-CSF (10 μg/kg SC×4 days) and then on the fifth day were given either G-CSF (10 μg/kg SC×1) (N=8) or G-CSF (10 μg/kg SC×1) plus AMD3100 (80 μg/kg SC×1) (N=3) and blood collected 6 h after the last injection of AMD3100, G-CSF or G-CSF plus AMD3100. Each set of test samples was assayed simultaneously in limiting dilutions in conditioned NOD-SCID mice. For every sample, four different cell concentrations were used and four mice were transplanted with each cell concentration. Mice were assayed for chimerism 8 weeks later, and those demonstrating >0.2% chimerism (total $CD45^+$ cells in bone marrow) were considered positive. Percentage of negative mice were used to calculate SRC frequencies (from [7], with permission)

diabetic severe combined immunodeficient (NOD-SCID) mice using a stem cell repopulating cell (SRC) assay [7]. The studies showed that adding AMD3100/plerixafor to G-CSF increased the number of SRCs in the leukapheresis products approximately fourfold compared to G-CSF alone (see Fig. 6.7). These results suggested that hematopoietic stem cells collected after AMD3100/plerixafor, either alone or in combination with G-CSF, were potentially more effective at repopulating marrow after ablation or injury than hematopoietic stem cells collected by leukapheresis after administration of G-CSF alone.

Pharmacokinetic–Pharmacodynamic Modeling

During the course of the studies, blood samples were regularly collected to assess AMD3100/plerixafor blood concentrations for pharmacokinetic studies [10]. This line of investigation showed that the absorption and distribution of AMD3100/plerixafor is best described by a 2-compartment model with first-order absorption of the drug. The clearance of the drug was estimated to be 5.17 ± 0.49 L/h, and the central volume of distribution was 16.9 ± 3.79 L. These data provide a background for understanding proper utilization of AMD3100/plerixafor for hematopoietic progenitor cell mobilization in other populations.

Discussion

Within the first year of initiating these experimental studies, we recognized the potential of AMD3100/plerixafor for hematopoietic progenitor cell mobilization. It was very fortunate for the drug's development that this new agent was well tolerated by the normal subjects participating in these studies. The results were clear-cut and established a solid foundation for clinical trials.

Several key findings arose from these studies.

- AMD3100/plerixafor induces a clear dose-dependent increase in peripheral blood leukocyte counts.
- AMD3100/plerixafor causes a consistent and significant elevation in peripheral blood $CD34^{+}$ counts in normal human volunteers. It is noteworthy, however, that only healthy volunteers, age 18–55 years were included in these studies. It would be necessary to conduct clinical investigations in specific populations of patients with diverse underlying diseases, comorbidities, and therapies to determine the utility and applicability of AMD3100/plerixafor for clinical hematopoietic stem cell mobilization.
- AMD3100/plerixafor is well tolerated when administered SC in single doses up to 240 μg/kg. Only a few subjects received multiple doses in these investigations. The effect of multiple doses or chronic therapy with AMD3100/plerixafor was not investigated.

- AMD3100/plerixafor causes a marked broad leukocytosis. These effects appeared to be transient. When $CD34^+$ cells are collected by leukapheresis after administration of AMD3100/plerixafor, the cell products contain larger numbers of potential immunoeffector cells than products obtained after administration of G-CSF. The benefits or detriments of the larger numbers of immunoeffector cells in AMD3100/plerixafor-mobilized products will require evaluation in diverse clinical settings.
- These studies in healthy subjects demonstrate that a relatively low percentage of the colony-forming cells mobilized by administration of AMD3100/plerixafor are actively in cell cycle. Further studies indicated that these relatively quiescent progenitor cell populations have a greater capacity for repopulation in NOD-SCID mice than cells collected after G-CSF administration. The clinical and biological significance of these findings are not known, but these findings may be very important for stem cell therapy and transplantation.
- The exact mechanisms responsible for the synergy of AMD3100/plerixafor and G-CSF in $CD34^+$ cell mobilization were not investigated in these studies conducted in normal human volunteers. Bone marrow examinations were not performed. The results suggest that G-CSF expands the myeloid progenitor pool, thereby allowing AMD3100/plerixafor to release a larger number of cells into the peripheral blood.

Acknowledgments This work was supported by a contract with AnorMED Inc, and NIH grants MO1RR 00037, RO1 DK53674, PO1, RO1 HL 56416, DK53574, HL67384, RO1 HL 63219 PO1 HL53586, DK49218, RO1 DK 53674, and T32 DK07519. The authors gratefully acknowledge the contributions of their collaborators and coinvestigators at AnorMED Inc, the University of Washington, and Indiana University.

References

1. Kollet O, Spiegel A, Peled A, Petit I, Byk T, Hershkoviz R, Guetta E, Barkai G, Nagler A, Lapidot T (2001) Rapid and efficient homing of human CD34(+)CD38(−/low)CXCR4(+) stem and progenitor cells to the bone marrow and spleen of NOD/SCID and NOD/SCID/B2m(null) mice. Blood 97(10):3283–3291
2. Bleul CC, Wu L, Hoxie JA, Springer TA, Mackay CR (1997) The HIV coreceptors CXCR4 and CCR5 are differentially expressed and regulated on human T lymphocytes. Proc Natl Acad Sci USA 94(5):1925–1930
3. Esté JA, Cabrera C, De Clercq E, Struyf S, Van Damme J, Bridger G, Skerlj RT, Abrams MJ, Henson G, Gutierrez A, Clotet B, Schols D (1999) Activity of different bicyclam derivatives against human immunodeficiency virus depends on their interaction with the CXCR4 chemokine receptor. Mol Pharmacol 55(1):67–73
4. Egberink HF, De Clercq E, Van Vliet AL, Balzarini J, Bridger GJ, Henson G, Horzinek MC, Schols D (1999) Bicyclams, selective antagonists of the human chemokine receptor CXCR4, potently inhibit feline immunodeficiency virus replication. J Virol 73(8):6346–6352
5. Hendrix CW, Flexner C, MacFarland RT, Giandomenico C, Fuchs EJ, Redpath E, Bridger G, Henson GW (2000) Pharmacokinetics and safety of AMD-3100, a novel antagonist of the

CXCR-4 chemokine receptor in human volunteers. Antimicrob Agents Chemother 44(6):1667–1673
6. Liles WC, Broxmeyer HE, Rodger E, Wood B, Hübel K, Cooper S, Hangoc G, Bridger GJ, Henson GW, Calandra G, Dale DC (2003) Mobilization of hematopoietic progenitor cells in healthy volunteers by AMD3100, a CXCR4 antagonist. Blood 102:2728–2730
7. Broxmeyer HE, Orschell CM, Clapp DW, Hangoc G, Cooper S, Plett PA, Liles WC, Li X, Graham-Evans B, Campbell TB, Calandra G, Bridger G, Dale DC, Srour EF (2005) Rapid mobilization of murine and human hematopoietic stem and progenitor cells with AMD3100, a CXCR4 antagonist. J Exp Med 201:1307–1318
8. Hübel K, Liles WC, Broxmeyer HE, Rodger E, Wood B, Cooper S, Hangoc G, MacFarland R, Bridger GJ, Henson GW, Calandra G, Dale DC (2004) Leukocytosis and mobilization of CD34+ hematopoietic progenitor cells by AMD3100, a CXCR antagonist. Support Canc Ther 1:165–172
9. Liles WC, Rodger E, Broxmeyer HE, Dehner C, Badel K, Calandra G, Christensen J, Wood B, Price TH, Dale DC (2005) Augmented mobilization and collection of CD34+ hematopoietic cells from normal human volunteers stimulated with G-CSF by single-dose administration of AMD3100, a CXCR4 antagonist. Transfusion 45:295–300
10. Lack NA, Green B, Dale DC, Calandra GB, Lee H, MacFarland RT, Badel K, Liles WC, Bridger G (2005) A pharmacokinetic/pharmacodynamic model for the mobilization of CD34+ hematopoietic progenitor cells by AMD3100. Clin Pharmacol Ther 77:427–436

Chapter 7
The Current Role of Plerixafor in Stem Cell Mobilization for Hematopoietic Stem Cell Transplantation*

Amy R. MacKenzie, Matias E. Valsecchi, and Neal Flomenberg

Abstract Granulocyte colony-stimulating factor has been the traditional agent used for mobilization of stem cells for hematopoietic stem cell (HSC) transplantation. Recently, plerixafor, an inhibitor of the interaction between CX chemokine receptor 4 (CXCR4) and stromal derived factor-1α (SDF-1) has been evaluated in clinical trials and approved by the FDA. This agent has very modest toxicity but appears to be quite potent at HSC mobilization. The rationale for the use of this agent and the clinical trials in which it was evaluated are the subject of this review.

Keywords Plerixafor • CXCR4 • SDF-1 • Stem cell mobilization • Stem cell transplantation

Introduction

Consistent and robust mobilization of $CD34^+$ hematopoietic stem cells (HSCs) is an essential step to optimize the outcomes of autologous stem cell transplantation. While transplantation becomes feasible at cell doses between 1 and 2×10^6 $CD34^+$ cells/kg, increasing the dose of infused HSCs improves bone marrow recovery both qualitatively and quantitatively. Platelet engraftment, for example, is particularly sensitive to HSC dose and rapid platelet recovery is most reproducible at doses above 5×10^6 $CD34^+$ cells/kg.

---

*Amy R. MacKenzie and Matias E. Valsecchi contributed equally to the preparation of this review.

A.R. MacKenzie • M.E. Valsecchi • N. Flomenberg (✉)
Thomas Jefferson University, 834 Chestnut Street, Suite 320, Philadelphia, PA 19107, USA
e-mail: Neal.Flomenberg@Jefferson.edu

S. Fruehauf et al. (eds.), *Novel Developments in Stem Cell Mobilization: Focus on CXCR4*, DOI 10.1007/978-1-4614-1960-0_7,

In a number of hematologic malignancies, including multiple myeloma (MM), non-Hodgkin's lymphoma (NHL), and Hodgkin's lymphoma (HL), high-dose chemotherapy with stem cell rescue may offer the only chance for a durable remission. Historically, pretransplant mobilization of HSCs was most commonly performed using granulocyte colony-stimulating factor (G-CSF) with or without chemotherapy. However, after 5 days of apheresis, an unacceptably high number of patients (5–40%) fail to mobilize $\geq 2 \times 10^6$ $CD34^+$ cells/kg, which is commonly considered to be the minimum number of HSCs needed for prompt and consistent engraftment [1, 2]. Inadequate numbers of HSCs can lead to delayed or failed engraftment, prolonged thrombocytopenia or neutropenia, increased infectious complications, and, subsequently, prolonged hospital stay or death [3, 4].

Mobilization with G-CSF is thought to be mediated through disruption of a variety of pathways and molecules involved in signaling and adhesion including stromal derived factor-1α (SDF-1) and CX chemokine receptor 4 (CXCR4). The interaction between this ligand and receptor has been shown to regulate survival, trafficking, and homing of HSCs in the marrow [5, 6]. Although mobilization can be achieved with G-CSF with or without chemotherapy in many patients, more recent data suggest that direct disruption of this chemokine–receptor interaction using a novel agent, plerixafor, produces superior results.

Plerixafor (previously AMD3100) was initially developed as an anti-HIV agent via its ability to block CXCR4 [7]. A profound leukocytosis was noted as an aside in this research, but has come to be the desired main effect in current clinical applications. Plerixafor is a slowly reversible inhibitor of CXCR4 and its interaction with SDF-1 in the bone marrow microenvironment has led to mobilization of $CD34^+$ cells in both healthy volunteers and cancer patients [8].

Preclinical models have been established in murine, canine, and primate species. Administration of a single subcutaneous injection of plerixafor to C3H/HeJ mice was, in a dose-dependent manner, able to mobilize HSCs in this strain which is known to be a difficult strain to mobilize [9]. HSCs were mobilized from bone marrow in this murine model and the animals responded to G-CSF together with plerixafor in a synergistic fashion [10]. As in humans, canines responded to plerixafor administration with a leukocytosis and rapid mobilization of $CD34^+$ cells. Successful engraftment was established in both allogeneic and autologous canine transplant settings [11]. In a study of Rhesus macaques, retroviral gene vectors were used to evaluate the long-term repopulating capacity of HSCs mobilized with plerixafor vs. G-CSF. Cells were also compared on the basis of cell-cycling status, surface phenotype, and homing to SDF. The results showed a statistically significant increase in the number of plerixafor-mobilized $CD34^+$ cells expressing the chemokine receptor CXCR4 and the cell-adhesion molecule VLA-4 (very late antigen-4) compared with G-CSF-mobilized $CD34^+$ cells. These markers, and the tendency for plerixafor-mobilized cells to migrate toward SDF-1α, more closely resemble cells in the steady-state bone marrow. These data indicate that plerixafor mobilizes a population of HSCs with long-term repopulating capacity and characteristics intrinsically different from those of HSCs mobilized with G-CSF. These cells may prove to be more efficacious in the transplant setting [12, 13].

Based on these encouraging preclinical studies, a number of human clinical trials were conducted. We describe below a number of studies that led to FDA approval of plerixafor as a mobilizing agent for human HSCs and highlight some future potential applications of this drug in clinical transplantation.

Autologous Stem Cell Transplantation

Plerixafor + G-CSF

In December 2008, the FDA approved the use of plerixafor, in combination with G-CSF (filgrastim) to mobilize HSCs from peripheral blood of patients with NHL and MM, who would subsequently undergo an autologous bone marrow transplant. This decision was based on evidence from phase I, II, and III clinical trials. In this section, the pharmacological properties, the safety profile, and the clinical efficacy derived from those clinical trials of plerixafor in combination with G-CSF are described.

Phase I Studies

Conventional pharmacokinetic–pharmacodynamic studies, as well as phase Ib trials, were conducted in both healthy volunteers and NHL and MM patients. Plerixafor was tested alone or in combination with G-CSF.

In a study of 29 healthy volunteers [14], five escalating doses of plerixafor alone (40, 80, 160, 240, and 320 μg/kg) were studied. The results showed a *pharmacokinetic* model compatible with two-compartment, first-order kinetics. Plerixafor is very hydrophilic and is predominantly excreted by the kidneys. It is eliminated from the plasma in a biexponential manner, with a terminal half life of 3–6 h. Dose adjustment is required when renal clearance is less than 50 mL/h. Obesity may affect the volume of distribution and final effects of the drug; however, formal studies addressing this issue are not available. Area under the curve (AUC) graphs with different drug concentrations are depicted in Fig. 7.1. *Pharmacodynamic* (dose–response) analyses, using the concentration of $CD34^+$ cells in peripheral blood samples as the monitored outcome, suggested a delay in the concentration–effect relationship as a result of drug distribution and/or indirect mechanism of effect. The drug shows an onset of action lag period of approximately 6 h (Fig. 7.2). This phenomenon is easily explained by the fact that plerixafor first needs to enter the bone marrow, block the interaction between $CD34^+$ cells and the surrounding stroma, and initiate a series of events which will ultimately result in the movement of HSCs from the marrow into the peripheral blood stream. Moreover, the pharmacodynamic observations are consistent with a classical ligand–receptor interaction, where incremental doses are associated with increased effects to the point when all receptors are saturated (typical sigmoid

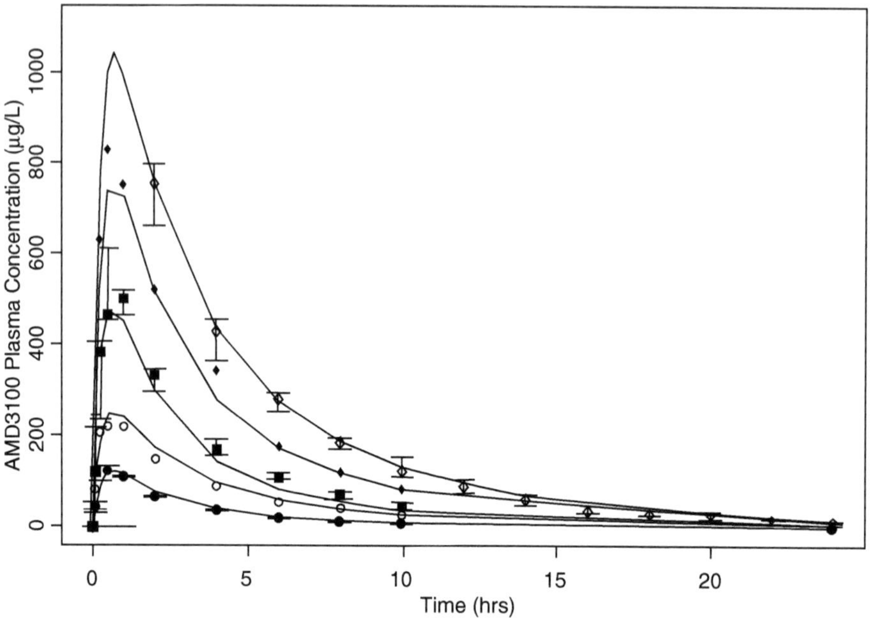

Fig. 7.1 Plasma concentration vs. time profile of AMD3100 in healthy human volunteers. The *points* represent the experimental data (median). The *errors bars* represent the interquartile range (shown for representative data sets) for 40 μg/kg (*solid circles*), 80 μg/kg (*open circles*), 160 μg/kg (*squares*), 240 μg/kg (*solid diamonds*), and 320 μg/kg (*open diamonds*). The *lines* represent the population-predicted concentrations from the pharmacokinetic model (reproduced with permission from [14])

dose–response curve). Importantly, most of the subjects' white blood cells returned to baseline after 24 h of the drug administration (Fig. 7.2). These observations were similar to the kinetics of the leukocytosis observed in healthy volunteers when plerixafor was being developed as a potential agent for treatment of HIV+ patients [7].

The time course of $CD34^+$ cell mobilization after plerixafor injection in normal individuals was described by Liles et al. [15]. In this study, 26 healthy humans were exposed to single dose (80 μg/kg) ($n=10$), escalating doses (40–240 μg/kg) ($n=13$), or daily doses for three consecutive days (80 μg/kg each day) ($n=3$). The study showed a clear dose–response dependent effect with a peak of tenfold increase in peripheral blood $CD34^+$ cells at 9 h (40.4 ± 3.4/μL cells) after injection of 240 μg/kg. With consecutive daily administration, similar effects were observed each day suggesting that $CD34^+$ cells could be repeatedly mobilized with each day's plerixafor dose without further beneficial or detrimental effects on the cell mobilization response from continued administration.

An additional phase I study investigated the effects of plerixafor in combination with a standard G-CSF regimen on mobilization and collection of $CD34^+$ cells from

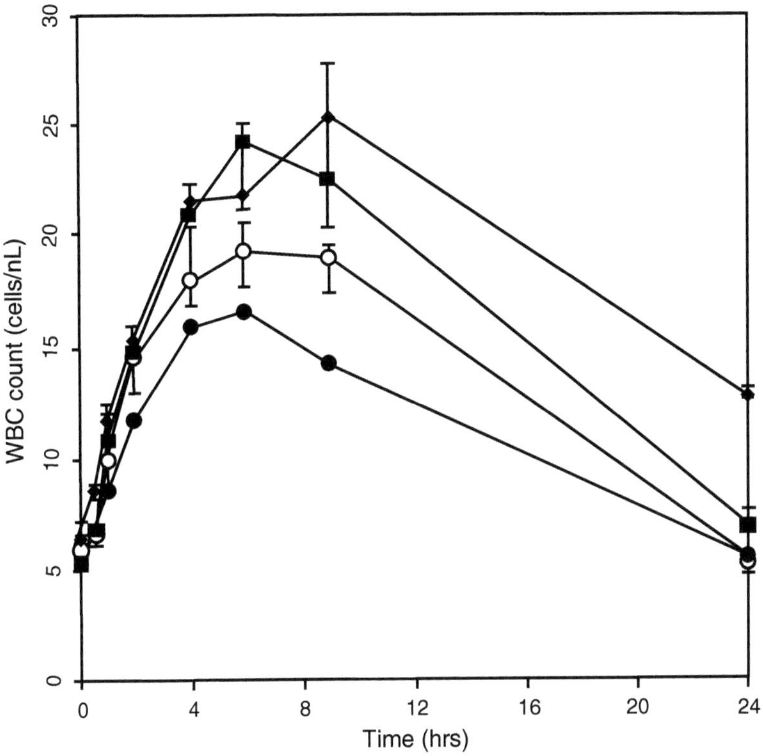

Fig. 7.2 Total white blood cell counts vs. time. The *points* represents the experimental data (median). The *error bars* represent the interquartile range (shown for representative data sets) for 40 μg/kg (*solid circles*), 80 μg/kg (*open circles*), 160 μg/kg (*squares*), and 240 μg/kg (*diamonds*) (reproduced with permission from [14])

healthy subjects [16]. In a cohort of ten subjects who received either 5 days of G-CSF (10 μg/kg/day) ($n=3$) or 4 days of G-CSF and then a single dose of plerixafor 160 μg/kg on day 5 ($n=3$) or a single dose of plerixafor 240 μg/kg alone with no G-CSF ($n=4$), the addition of plerixafor to filgrastim resulted in a significant improvement in the collection of CD34$^+$ cells by leukapheresis ($p<0.05$) suggesting a synergistic effect from the use of the two drugs in combination. Interestingly, in this study, the administration of single dose of plerixafor (240 μg/kg) resulted in similar cell yield as five consecutive days of G-CSF (Fig. 7.3).

These trials served to prove that plerixafor could be easily administrated, had a predictable dose–response curve, and was well tolerated. Most of the adverse effects observed were mild and transitory. However, the studies were conducted exclusively in normal, healthy volunteers who, unlike patients with hematologic malignancies, had neither been exposed to chemotherapy nor the effects of neoplastic cell infiltration of the bone marrow. With the intention to shift the study of plerixafor to patients who had been previously treated with chemotherapy, Devine and colleagues

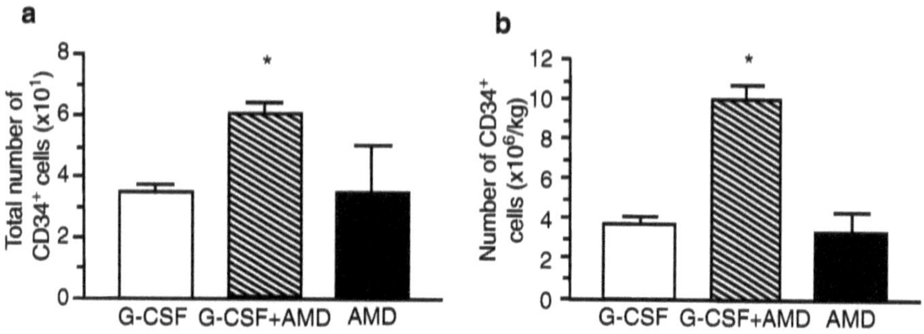

Fig. 7.3 (**a**) Ten healthy human volunteers were randomly assigned to three groups: G-CSF (10 μg/kg/day SC)×5 days ($n=3$); G-CSF (10 μg/kg/day SC)×4 days, and then G-CSF plus AMD3100 (160 μg/kg SC×1) on day 5 ($n=3$); and AMD3100 (240 μg/kg SC)×1 ($n=4$). An 18-L leukapheresis procedure was performed beginning 4 h after final drug administration. Data show total number of CD34⁺ cells in the respective leukapheresis products (mean±SEM; *$p<0.05$ compared to leukapheresis products obtained from individuals mobilized with G-CSF only). (**b**) Data from A depicted as CD34⁺ cells per kg of donor body weight (mean±SEM; *$p<0.05$ compared to leukapheresis products obtained from individuals mobilized with G-CSF only) (reproduced with permission from [16])

[17] designed a phase Ib clinical trial in patients with MM and NHL. Importantly, the study served as a proof of concept that the drug was similarly efficacious in these populations.

In this study, 13 patients (7 with MM and 6 with NHL) were enrolled. The primary endpoints were safety and efficacy of 160 and 240 μg/kg doses of plerixafor alone. A threefold increase above baseline circulating CD34⁺ cells was selected as the threshold for efficacy. Inclusion criteria included, among others, normal white blood cells, last dose of chemotherapy between 4 and 8 weeks from enrollment, and no patients could received hematopoietic growth factors the previous 35 days. Patients were stratified into different cohorts according to underlying diagnosis and dose received. The median number of cycles of chemotherapy received was 6. The drug was extremely well tolerated and all side effects were self-limited and grade 1 in the WHO scale. The most common toxicities were skin erythema and abdominal discomfort. Regarding the hematological effects, the mean baseline WBC counts and circulating CD34⁺ cell counts were 4,732±648/μL and 2.6±0.7/μL, respectively, and these counts increased to a mean of 13,568±1,971/μL ($p<0.001$) and 16.2±4.3/μL ($p=0.003$), respectively, 6 h after receiving plerixafor (Fig. 7.4) with kinetics that were similar to those seen previously in normal volunteers [14]. These changes were significant irrespective of the dose used. However, a mean sevenfold increase of circulating CD34⁺ cells was noted after a dose of 240 μg/kg. There was not a statistically significant change in the number of platelets or erythrocytes or in the relative proportion of WBC subsets.

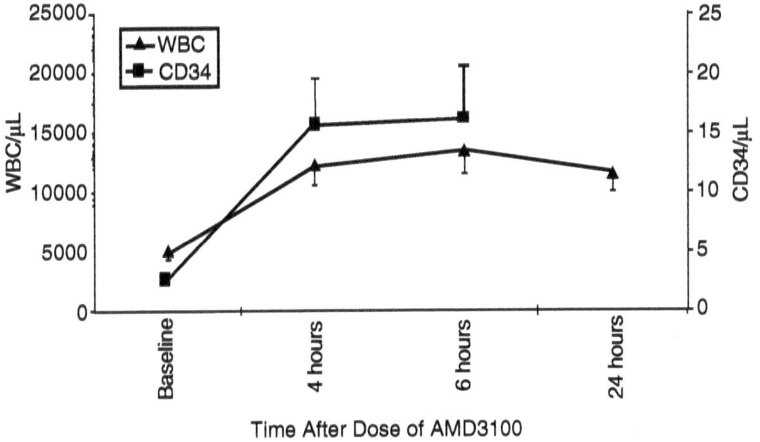

Fig. 7.4 Total WBC count and peripheral blood CD34⁺ cell count observed in patients receiving AMD3100 at 160 μg/kg or 240 μg/kg at baseline and 4, 6, and 24 h (WBC count only at 24 h) after the dose. Each value represents the mean ± SE ($n = 13$) (reproduced with permission from [17])

Phase II Studies

Phase I studies demonstrated that plerixafor had minimal side effects and was able to effectively mobilize $CD34^+$ HSCs in healthy as well as heavily pretreated patients. The next key step was to demonstrate that plerixafor could, meaningfully improve the number of $CD34^+$ cells collected and/or reduce the number of apheresis procedures necessary for stem cell collection. Subsequent to collection, it would be important to additionally demonstrate that HSCs exposed to plerixafor maintained adequate homing and engraftment capacity after myeloablative chemotherapy and autologous stem cell transplantation in human subjects.

The first clinical trial in patients with NHL and MM to test the hypothesis that stem cells mobilized by a combination of G-CSF and plerixafor engrafted as well as their counterparts mobilized with G-CSF alone was published in 2005 (study 2101) [18] The study included patients with MM and NHL in first or second complete or partial remission, with optimal ECOG performance status (0–1), who had received up to three lines of chemotherapy and who also had acceptable renal, hepatic, hematological, cardiac, and pulmonary organ function to safely undergo a conventional autologous stem cell transplant. The primary outcome of the study was to prove that the experimental arm (plerixafor) mobilized more progenitor cells per unit blood volume of apheresis than conventional treatment (G-CSF alone). Secondary outcomes focused on the number of apheresis procedures needed to obtain an optimal number of 5×10^6 cells/kg and to determine whether the patients on the experimental arm had at a 90% rate of successful engraftment following autologous transplantation defined by the achievement of three consecutive days of absolute neutrophil count above 500 cells/μL by day 21 posttransplant. The investigators considered that a 50% increase in the number of HSCs collected would be sufficient to be clinically meaningful.

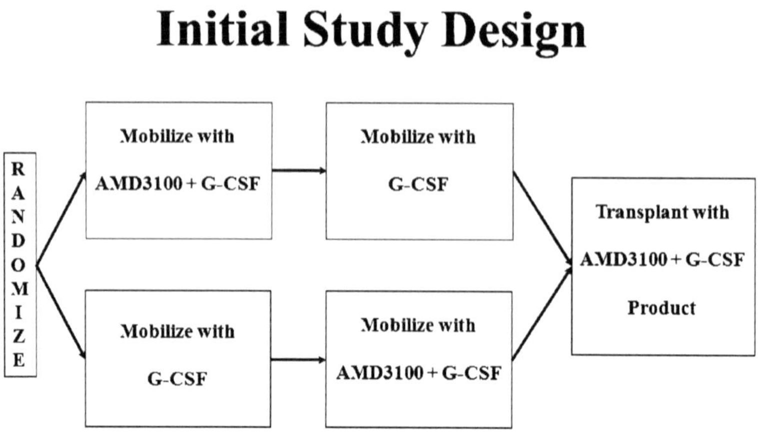

Fig. 7.5 Initial study design of the study 2101. Each patient was mobilized twice with either AMD3100+G-CSF or G-CSF alone first and then, after wash-out, remobilized with the other regimen (reproduced with permission from [18])

In order to test this hypothesis and maximize patient safety, the trial included a cross-over design such that each subject was mobilized twice, once with G-CSF alone and once with G-CSF+plerixafor. Each subject thus served as his/her own control (Fig. 7.5). Moreover, the cells mobilized with G-CSF alone provided a potential rescue product in the event that exposure to plerixafor reduced the ability of HSCs to promote long-term count recovery after autologous transplantation. Patients had a 2 week "wash-out" or "restabilization" period between the two mobilization and collection procedures allowing the effects of the preceding treatment to dissipate. Originally the patients were randomly assigned with regard to the sequence of the two mobilization regimens, but after the 13th patient, the protocol was amended and all the remaining patients received initial mobilization with G-CSF alone.

The backbone mobilization regimen consisted of (up to) an 8-day treatment period during which patients received G-CSF at a dose of 10 μg/kg of actual body weight each day. Beginning on day 5, patients underwent up to four consecutive days of apheresis with continued daily G-CSF treatment alone or with the addition of plerixafor. The first eight patients received 160 μg/kg of plerixafor while subsequent patients received 240 μg/kg. Patients subsequently underwent stem cell transplantation following myeloablative conditioning regimens. The minimal dose of $CD34^+$ cells required to undergo transplant was 2×10^6 cells/kg, but investigators were permitted to combine cells retrieved from both mobilization regimens if the minimal target was not achieved from a single mobilization regimen.

A total of 25 patients (10 with MM and 15 with NHL) were enrolled in this study. With the exception of two patients, all patients showed a significant increase in the number of HSCs collected using the combination, with a median of 2.9-fold improvement. These results are consistent with previous observations in phase I studies. Moreover, and directly related to the primary outcome of the study, in every

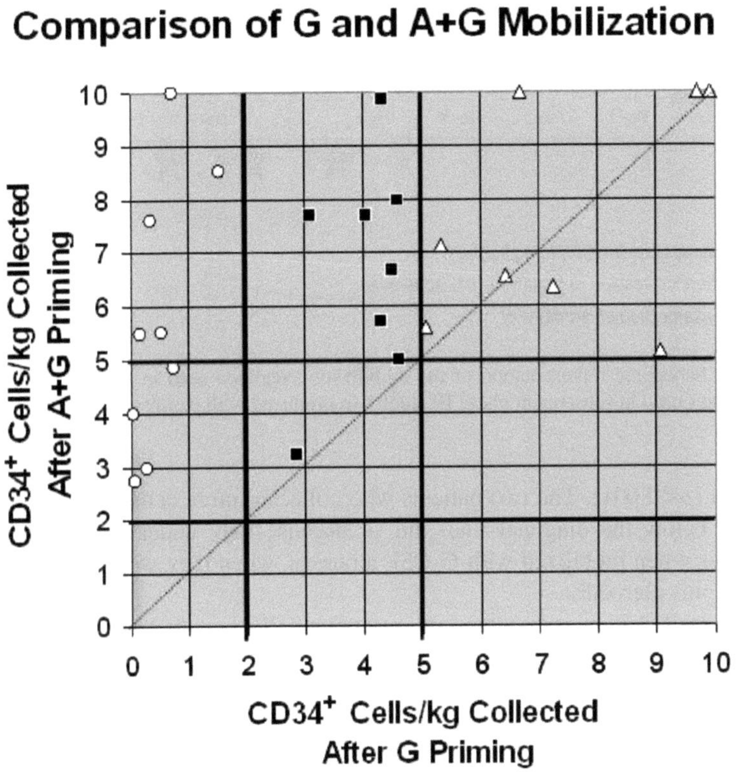

Fig. 7.6 The mobilization of CD34⁺ cells/kg (×10^6) after G or A+G mobilization. Values above 10×10^6 were reduced to 10×10^6 to reduce the scale of the figure and to allow the data points with lower values to be better separated and visualized. *Open circles* indicate patients mobilizing less than 2×10^6 CD34⁺ cells/kg; (*filled squares*) those mobilizing at least 2×10^6 but less than 5×10^6 CD34⁺ cells/kg; and (*triangles*) those mobilizing at least 5×10^6 CD34⁺ cells/kg. The line of identity ($y=x$) is shown as a *dotted diagonal line* (reproduced with permission from [18])

case, the quantity of HSCs collected per day of apheresis after plerixafor + G-CSF mobilization was more than in the case of G-CSF alone. In 84% of the cases (21/25) this was more than a 50% increase—the proportion a priori considered clinically relevant. In addition, in nine cases, G-CSF alone was not able to mobilize the minimally required number of cells (2×10^6 CD34⁺ cells/kg) but in each of these cases, the addition of plerixafor overcame that problem. The reverse pattern (successful mobilization with G-CSF alone but failure with the combination) was not seen in any patient. Regarding the optimal number of stem cells mobilized and collected (5×10^6 CD34⁺ cells/kg), only 8 patients (32%) obtained that threshold with G-CSF alone but 20 (80%) achieved it with G-CSF+plerixafor. The pattern of HSC mobilization with each treatment is clearly represented in Fig. 7.6 demonstrating superior collection of CD34⁺ cells when plerixafor was added to the mobilization

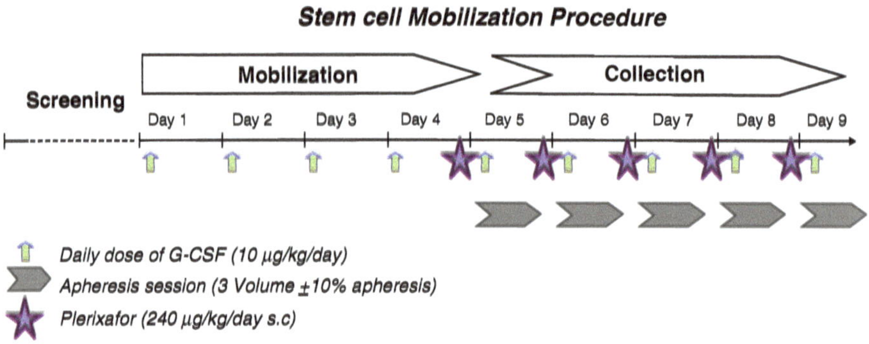

Fig. 7.7 Schematic representation of the mobilization regimen used in study 2105. The same scheme was used in subsequent phase III studies (reproduced with permission from [19])

regimen ($p<0.001$). The two patients who collected more cells with G-CSF alone (falling below the diagonal line) did so because they underwent more days of apheresis when mobilized with G-CSF alone vs. when they were mobilized using G-CSF plus plerixafor.

This trial demonstrates that patients potentially benefit from the addition of plerixafor in three ways. They are more likely to reach the minimally required cell dose required for transplant, they may require fewer apheresis sessions to reach this cell collection goal, and/or they may also undergo their transplant with a more robust cell dose. Finally, 19 patients in this trial underwent subsequent transplant using only plerixafor+G-CSF mobilized cells and 95% of these patients (18/19) showed a consistent pattern of early engraftment with neutrophil recovery in a median of 10 days and platelet recovery in a median of 16 days. No cases of late graft failure were noted. Only six patients experienced serious side effects but none of them occurred during the mobilization phase and all were felt to be transplantation related complications.

Another phase II, single arm, multicenter, clinical trial (study 2105) that included 49 patients produced very similar results to study 2101 and confirmed that 240 μg/kg was the optimal dose. It also demonstrated that administration of plerixafor 10–11 h pre-apheresis (i.e., the evening before) was logistically feasible and effective [19]. Moreover, this study established that plerixafor was very active even in those patients who fulfill the criteria to be at high risk for "poor mobilization" such as patients who had received ten or more total cycles of chemotherapy, had received platinum-based chemotherapy, had been exposed to bone marrow radiation, or had ≤10 circulating $CD34^+$ cells/μL. These patients usually have a failure rate on the order of 30% [4].

The study itself had similar inclusion criteria as study 2101 and the mobilization regimen consisted of G-CSF at 10 μg/kg subcutaneously for up to 9 days and plerixafor (240 μg/kg) starting on the evening of the fourth day (Fig. 7.7). The apheresis was initiated 10–11 h after each dose of plerixafor, starting on day 5. This has the practical advantage that patients can receive plerixafor during the evening and return

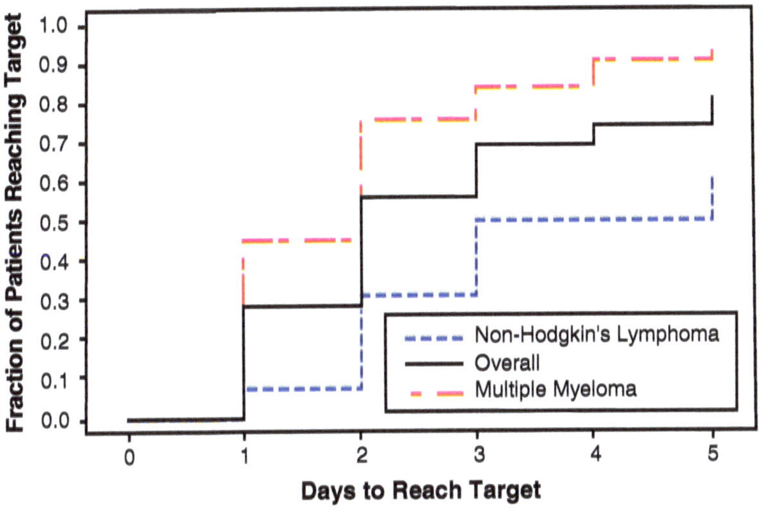

Fig. 7.8 Number of apheresis days to reach cell count target of 5×10^6 CD34$^+$/kg for all patients, and the non-Hodgkin's and MM subsets (reproduced with permission from [19])

for apheresis early the next morning, making the entire process more convenient for the patients as well as the apheresis and cryopreservation laboratory staff. As in the 2101 study, investigators aimed to demonstrate that plerixafor was safe and effective as demonstrated by a ≥twofold increase in the circulating CD34$^+$ cells, a reduction in the number of days of apheresis and a successful rate of engrafted patients (neutrophil engraftment). The results showed a median increase in the CD34$^+$ mobilization of 2.5-fold (range: 1.3–6.0) and a median of two apheresis sessions (range: 1–5) to collect the desirable 5×10^6 CD34$^+$ cells/kg target cell dose (Fig. 7.8). In total, 77.6% of the patients (38/49) collected $\geq 5 \times 10^6$ CD34$^+$ cells/kg and 96% (47/49) reached the minimal dose of 2×10^6 CD34$^+$ cells/kg. All patients underwent transplantation with a median time of ANC and platelet engraftment of 11 and 14.5 days, respectively; 44 patients survived >12 months with durable engraftment. The most common side effects were gastrointestinal. Six patients developed severe lymphopenia associated with the apheresis, but the drug was again well tolerated. However, one of the most interesting aspects of the 2105 study is that 57% (28/49) of these patients met the previously noted criteria for being considered heavily pretreated (high likelihood for poor mobilization). The median increase in circulating CD34$^+$ cells in this particular group was 2.6-fold and 67% collected $\geq 5 \times 10^6$ CD34$^+$ cells/kg. Furthermore, all of them reached the threshold of 2×10^6 CD34$^+$ cells/kg and engraftment time was exactly the same as the less heavily pretreated patients.

Following the same line of thought, study 2102 further pursued the activity of plerixafor in poor mobilizers in a single center, phase II study [20]. This study enrolled patients with MM who had either previously received a mobilization regimen (G-CSF alone or chemotherapy + G-CSF) from which $<2 \times 10^6$ CD34$^+$ cells/kg were collected (*proven poor mobilizers*), or patients who had received chemotherapy and G-CSF as mobilization regimen and who had peripheral $CD34^+$ cell counts of 5–12 cells/μL or had pre-mobilization platelet counts of 100,000–150,000/μL. These last patients were predicted to yield a total apheresis collection of $<1 \times 10^6$ $CD34^+$ cells/kg (*predicted poor mobilizers*). Inclusion and exclusion criteria were similar to the two previous studies as were the primary and secondary outcomes. In addition, these authors investigated whether the addition of plerixafor would result in greater tumor cell mobilization in the HSC products. The regimen used was similar to those utilized in the previous studies, but, in this case, 240 μg/kg of plerixafor was given subcutaneously from day 1 of the cycle. A total of 20 patients were enrolled and again a median threefold increase in circulating $CD34^+$ cells was observed from a baseline median of 2.1 cells/μL pre-plerixafor to 6 cells/μL after administration of the drug. Moreover, 75% (15/20) of the patients achieved cumulative apheresis yields of $\geq 2 \times 10^6$ $CD34^+$ cells/kg. Seventeen patients had autologous transplantation with a median of 13 days to neutrophil engraftment. Twelve patients were assessed after 1 year and all of them showed durable engraftment. Interestingly, none of the ten patients studied for tumor cell content in their apheresis products tested positive after 2 days of consecutive apheresis. However, conclusions were somewhat limited by the small number of cases investigated and by the fact that authors used flow cytometry which has a sensitivity of <1/100 cells (in comparison to 1/100,000 cells when using PCR).

Another study also tried to assess whether the use of plerixafor resulted in mobilization of tumor cells. In this case, Gazitt and colleagues [21] investigated 11 refractory or relapsed NHL patients who received 16 μg/kg of G-CSF for 4 days followed by 240 μg/kg of plerixafor starting on the fourth evening. The main objectives were to assess mobilization of tumor cells, dendritic cell subtypes, and $CD34^+$ cells. Unfortunately, the assessment of lymphoma cell mobilization was limited in that pre-apheresis testing was not performed. However, no malignant cells were detected. Regarding dendritic cell mobilization, no consistent trend was observed in the type of dendritic cells mobilized and no correlation was found between the number of dendritic cells and $CD34^+$ cells mobilized. However, once again, this phase II study showed a consistent mean increase of approximately 2.5-fold in $CD34^+$ cells/μL (from 35 to 81 cells/μL; $p<0.0001$) with a median of 3×10^6 $CD34^+$ cells/kg collected in 1–2 days of apheresis. Ten patients had successful autologous stem cell transplantation with a median engraftment of 10 (range 9–12) and 12 (range 9–15) days for neutrophils and platelets, respectively. No drug-related serious adverse events were documented.

These four phase II clinical trials—performed in different centers with different authors and in different clinical scenarios—repeatedly and consistently showed that, in patients with NHL and MM, plerixafor boosts the $CD34^+$ cells yields by a median order of ≥2.5-fold while requiring significantly fewer apheresis sessions and without adversely affecting engraftment. Even more important, the addition of plerixafor can "rescue" many poor mobilizers who otherwise would have never been able to receive autologous transplantation. The clinical utility of this agent is also enhanced by the fact that it was consistently well tolerated with few and mild side effects.

A final phase II trial (study 2106) expanded the use of plerixafor beyond MM and NHL. Cashen and colleagues [22] published a study in which 22 patients with relapsed or refractory Hodgkin lymphoma (HL) were treated with a similar mobilization regimen as utilized in the other phase II studies, receiving up to 9 days of G-CSF plus 240 μg/kg of plerixafor starting on the fourth evening. Study patients were compared to historical controls mobilized only with G-CSF from Washington University (St. Louis, MO). The authors reported that 68% of the participants (15/22) achieved a collection of $\geq 5 \times 10^6$ $CD34^+$ cells/kg and 95% (21/22) reached $\geq 2 \times 10^6$ $CD34^+$ cells/kg. The median number of apheresis procedures was 2 and a median 3.2-fold increase in peripheral $CD34^+$ cells after plerixafor administration was documented. Twenty-one patients were transplanted with G-CSF + plerixafor-mobilized cells and all showed rapid and durable engraftment. Compared with 98 historical controls, the addition of plerixafor produced a statistically significant improvement in the collection of $\geq 5 \times 10^6$ $CD34^+$ cells/kg, in the median number of $CD34^+$ cells collected, and a reduction in the apheresis days. These results in HL patients are thus very similar to those obtained in MM and NHL.

Together, the phase II studies of plerixafor built a compelling case of efficacy and safety. These studies led to phase III trials of plerixafor in NHL and MM patients in an effort to secure FDA approval for this agent.

Phase III Studies

Two phase III, multicenter, randomized (1:1), double-blind, placebo-controlled studies were performed to compare the safety and efficacy of plerixafor and G-CSF with placebo and G-CSF in mobilization of $CD34^+$ cells. The studies were very similar in design with few exceptions (Table 7.1).

The first trial [23] was open to patients with NHL who required (and were eligible for) an autologous HSC transplant in first or second complete or partial remission. Patients were included between the ages of 18 and 78 with good performance status, no cytopenias, and normal liver and kidney function. The primary end point of this trial was the proportion of patients able to mobilize $\geq 5 \times 10^6$ $CD34^+$ cells/kg in ≤4 apheresis days. Secondary efficacy end points were the proportion of patients able to mobilize $\geq 2 \times 10^6$ $CD34^+$ cells/kg in ≤4 apheresis days, the number of apheresis days to reach $\geq 5 \times 10^6$ $CD34^+$ cells/kg, the fold increase in the number of peripheral blood $CD34^+$ cells prior to and after intervention (days 4 and 5, respectively), the number of days to platelet and neutrophil engraftment, and the proportion of patients maintaining a durable graft at 100 days, 6 months, and 12 months posttransplant. Patients who failed to mobilize $\geq 0.8 \times 10^6$ $CD34^+$ cells/kg after 2 apheresis days or $\geq 2 \times 10^6$ $CD34^+$ cells/kg in ≤4 apheresis days were allowed to enter a rescue protocol with G-CSF plus plerixafor 240 μg/kg after a 7-day rest period.

All patients were given G-CSF 10 μg/kg subcutaneously daily in the morning for up to 8 days. Beginning on the evening of day 4, patients received either 240 μg/kg plerixafor as a subcutaneous injection or placebo daily for up to 4 days. Apheresis was started on the morning of day 5 and continued for up to 4 days or until $\geq 5 \times 10^6$

Table 7.1 Summary of two phase III clinical studies of plerixafor for hematopoietic stem cell mobilization in patients with non-Hodgkin's lymphoma or multiple myeloma (reproduced with permission from Choi HY et al. (2010) Ann Pharmacother 44(1):117–126)

Parameter	Non-Hodgkin's lymphoma	Multiple myeloma
Study design	MC, R, DB, PC	MC, R, DB, PC
Subjects	$N=298$ adults requiring aHSC transplantation	$N=302$ adults requiring aHSC transplantation
Treatment regimen	G-CSF (10 μg/kg) subcutaneous injection in the morning for 4 days, then plerixafor 240 μg/kg or placebo in the evening of day 4, apheresis beginning fifth day after G-CSF dose in the morning, continue G-CSF and plerixafor (or placebo) up to four apheresis or until 5×10^6 $CD34^+$ cells/kg were collected	G-CSF (10 μg/kg) subcutaneous injection in the morning for 4 days, then plerixafor 240 μg/kg or placebo in the evening of day 4, apheresis beginning fifth day after G-CSF dose in the morning, continue G-CSF and plerixafor (or placebo) up to four aphereses or until 6×10^6 $CD34^+$ cells/kg were collected
Primary endpoint	Percentage of patients who achieved 5×10^6 $CD34^+$ cells/kg in ≤4 apheresis days	Percentage of patients who achieved 6×10^6 $CD34^+$ cells/kg in ≤2 apheresis days
Follow-up period	12 months after transplantation	12 months after transplantation

Results	Plerixafor + G-CSF ($n=150$)	Placebo + G-CSF ($n=148$)	Plerixafor + G-CSF ($n=148$)	Placebo + G-CSF ($n=154$)
Patients who met primary end point (%)	59.3*	19.6	71.6*	34.4
Patients who achieved minimum collection (%)[a]	86.7*	47.3	95.9	92.9
Patients who underwent transplantation (%)	90.0*	55.4	95.9	88.3
Mean number ± SD of $CD34^+$ cells transplanted ($\times10^6$ cells/kg)	6.06 ± 2.98*	4.09 ± 1.56	5.84 ± 2.64	4.41 ± 2.22
Patients who underwent tandem transplantation (%)	NA	NA	21.6	15.6
Graft durability rate				
After 100 days[b]	94.8	95.1	98.6	97.8
After 6 months[b]	97.6	98.7	98.5	98.4
After 12 months[c]	98.2	100.0	99.2	99.2

aHSC autologous hematopoietic stem cell, *DB* double blind, *G-CSF* granulocyte colony-stimulating factor, *MC* multicenter, *NA* not applicable, *PC* placebo controlled, *R* randomized

[a]Minimum collection for transplantation was 2×10^6 cells/kg

[b]For all patients who underwent transplantation

[c]For all patients who underwent transplantation and had laboratory data at the study visit

*$p<0.001$ compared to placebo + G-CSF

CD34+ cells/kg were successfully collected. Patients were to proceed to transplant (performed according to local guidelines) within 5 weeks of stem cell collection. G-CSF was initiated on day 5 or 6 after transplant until ANC was $\geq 0.5 \times 10^9$/L for 3 days or $\geq 1.0 \times 10^9$/L for 1 day (considered neutrophil engraftment).

A total of 298 patients were randomized; 150 were initially randomized to G-CSF plus plerixafor, and 148 to G-CSF plus placebo. In the plerixafor arm, 147 patients underwent apheresis and ten of these received the rescue protocol because of poor mobilization. One hundred and thirty-five of the 137 remaining patients in this arm received a transplant and 112 patients were available for final analysis 12 months posttransplant. Of the 148 patients randomized to G-CSF plus placebo, 142 underwent apheresis, 52 of whom went on to the rescue protocol. Of the 90 remaining patients, 82 proceeded to transplant and 68 completed the 12 months follow-up. Following transplant, patients who did not complete the study either withdrew electively, were lost to follow-up, or died. A substantially greater percentage of patients in the placebo arm entered the rescue protocol than in the plerixafor arm: 36.6% vs. 6.8%, respectively.

The proportion of patients in the plerixafor arm achieving the primary end point was significantly higher than in the placebo arm (59.3% vs. 19.6%; $p<0.001$). In addition, a significantly higher proportion of patients achieved the minimum cell dose ($\geq 2 \times 10^6$ CD34+ cells/kg) in ≤4 apheresis days in the plerixafor group compared to the placebo group (86.7% vs. 47.3%; $p<0.001$); the number of cells collected in a single day was also significantly greater in the plerixafor arm ($p<0.001$). The median number of cells mobilized in the plerixafor arm was 5.69×10^6 CD34+ cells/kg vs. 1.98×10^6 CD34+ cells/kg in the placebo arm and the fold increase in CD34+ cells before and after intervention was fivefold with plerixafor and 1.4-fold for placebo ($p<0.001$). Treatment with plerixafor plus G-CSF did not have a deleterious effect on days to engraftment, durability of engraftment or mortality in the 12 months after transplant. There was no improvement in overall survival with the use of plerixafor.

Of the 68 patients who failed initial mobilization in this trial, 62 opted to be remobilized as part of the rescue protocol (10 in plerixafor group and 52 in the placebo group) [24]. If an adequate number of stem cells were mobilized, patients were then offered transplantation. From a total of 68 patients who originally failed mobilization, 37 of 62 patients achieved yields of $>2 \times 10^6$ CD34+ cells/kg in four or fewer days of apheresis and 7 (11%) achieved $>5 \times 10^6$ CD34+ cells/kg. After combining cells from the two collections (clinical trial and rescue protocol), 52 patients were able to proceed to transplantation with a median time for neutrophil engraftment of 11 days and 20 for platelets. Only one patient did not complete the rescue protocol due to adverse events (bone pain, headaches, nausea, and vomiting). The overall importance of this analysis is related to the fact that plerixafor + G-CSF can safely and effectively remobilize patients who had previously failed an initial mobilization effort. This is also in accordance with the data reflected by the phase II study (study 2101) from Flomenberg and colleagues [18].

The second phase III trial [25] was similar in design to the first study but assessed patients with MM rather than NHL. The study group consisted of transplant-eligible multiple myeloma patients in first or second complete or partial remission. Inclusion criteria were the same, but patients were stratified in this trial based on platelet count and planned transplant type (single vs. tandem). The primary efficacy endpoint was the proportion of patients collecting $\geq 6 \times 10^6$ $CD34^+$ cells/kg (vs. 5 in the NHL trial) in ≤ 2 apheresis days (vs. ≤ 4 apheresis days in the NHL trial). Secondary end points were the same (aside from the higher number of $CD34^+$ cells). The stem cell mobilization protocol was identical to the NHL trial. Patients who did not successfully mobilize were again allowed to enter a rescue protocol.

A total of 302 patients were randomized, 148 to the plerixafor arm and 154 to the placebo arm. In the plerixafor arm, 144 patients underwent collection, none of whom entered the rescue protocol. One hundred and forty-two patients proceeded to transplant and 129 completed the 12-month follow-up. Of the patients in the placebo arm, 150 underwent collection, 7 of whom entered the rescue protocol. One hundred and thirty-six patients underwent transplant and 121 completed the 12 months follow-up. All rescue patients went to transplant and had durable grafts at 12 months.

As in the NHL trial, a significantly greater proportion of patients in the plerixafor group reached the primary efficacy endpoint of $\geq 6 \times 10^6$ $CD34^+$ cells/kg in ≤ 2 apheresis days as compared to the placebo group (71.6% vs. 34.4%; $p<0.001$). Again, patients mobilized $\geq 6 \times 10^6$ $CD34^+$ cells/kg more quickly in the plerixafor arm (median of 1 day) than in the placebo arm (median of 4 days) ($p<0.001$). A greater proportion of plerixafor-treated patients achieved the secondary end points of collecting $\geq 6 \times 10^6$ $CD34^+$ cells/kg in ≤ 4 apheresis days (75.7% vs. 51.3%, $p<0.001$). There was a statistically insignificant trend with regard to collecting $\geq 2 \times 10^6$ $CD34^+$ cells/kg in ≤ 4 apheresis days (95.3% vs. 88.3%, $p=0.31$). The median number of cells collected (median 109 cells/μL vs. 33 cells/μL, $p<0.001$) and the fold increase in collection on days 4 and 5 (pre- and postintervention) were again significantly higher in the plerixafor arm compared to the placebo arm (4.8-fold vs. 1.7-fold, $p<0.001$). Both groups had equivalent engraftment rates (99.3% with plerixafor and 100% with placebo) as well as time to neutrophil engraftment (11 days) and platelet engraftment (18 days). Overall survival at 12 months was the same.

Adverse events (AEs) were similar between the two trials (Table 7.2). The most common AEs associated with plerixafor were gastrointestinal (especially diarrhea and nausea) and injection site erythema. Two patients in the NHL study experienced serious AEs (hypotension/dizziness and thrombocytopenia) after plerixafor administration. Three patients in the plerixafor arm of the study experienced AEs (seizure, systemic reaction not specified, and central line infection) that were significant but did not lead to withdrawal. One patient in the plerixafor arm of the multiple myeloma study experienced severe fatigue and diarrhea and the drug was stopped after three doses.

Compassionate Use and Rescue Studies

In patients undergoing their first mobilization attempt, the data indicate that plerixafor + G-CSF is a superior mobilization regimen when compared to G-CSF alone.

Table 7.2 Summary of common adverse reactions observed during the two phase III clinical studies (reproduced with permission from Choi HY et al. (2010) Ann Pharmacother 44(1):117–126)

Adverse reaction	Plerixafor + G-CSF, % ($n=298^{a}$)	Placebo + G-CSF, % ($n=302^{b}$)
Diarrhea	37*	17
Nausea	34**	22
Injection site erythema	34*	0
Fatigue	27	25
Headache	22	21
Joint pain	12	12
Dizziness	11	6
Insomnia	7	5
Flatulence	7	3
Vomiting	6	6

G-CSF Granulocyte colony-stimulating factor
[a]Number of patients includes 150 non-Hodgkin's lymphoma patients and 148 multiple myeloma patients
[b]Number of patients includes 148 non-Hodgkin's lymphoma patients and 154 multiple myeloma patients
*$p<0.001$ compared to placebo + G-CSF
**$p<0.05$ compared to placebo + G-CSF

Decrease in the number of apheresis sessions as well as a more robust cell dose upon collection are compelling reasons to include plerixafor in autologous mobilization regimens. As there are a number of patients who fail to mobilize sufficient $CD34^{+}$ cells on the first attempt with G-CSF alone or G-CSF plus chemotherapy, it is reasonable to examine plerixafor in a rescue or compassionate use setting as well. While there have not been randomized trials to evaluate this, retrospective review, single institution experiences, and cohort studies have been published describing the compassionate use of plerixafor.

Pusic and colleagues [26] did a retrospective review of 1,834 patients who underwent mobilization of stem cells for autologous transplantation between November 1995 and October 2006 at the Washington University, St. Louis. This review was undertaken to examine institutional mobilization practices as well as factors influencing the success or failure of mobilization. A total of 1,040 patients met inclusion criteria for review: multiple myeloma, NHL, or HL patients who had at least one attempt at HSC mobilization with G-CSF, alone or in combination with chemotherapy. Mobilization regimens were similar to previously used protocols: G-CSF 10 μg/kg subcutaneously daily for 4 days prior to apheresis, then continued in conjunction with apheresis daily for 5 days or until $\geq 2\times 10^{6}$ $CD34^{+}$ cells/kg were collected. The specific chemotherapy regimen used in mobilization was at the discretion of the treating physician and was variable over the 11 years examined. Mobilization failure was defined as $<2\times 10^{6}$ $CD34^{+}$ cells/kg within five apheresis days. Patients who failed initial collection were remobilized after 10–30 days with either G-CSF and/or GM-CSF, G-CSF/chemotherapy (G/C), or G-CSF plus plerixafor (G/P).

81.3% (846 of 1,040) patients were mobilized successfully in their initial mobilization attempt, collecting $\geq 2\times 10^{6}$ $CD34^{+}$ cells/kg after five apheresis days.

Of these successfully mobilizing patients, 52.7% (548 of 1,040) collected 2–5 × 10^6 CD34$^+$ cells/kg, and 28.7% (298 of 1,040) collected >5 × 10^6 CD34$^+$ cells/kg. More patients receiving G/C mobilized >5 × 10^6 CD34$^+$ HSC than patients receiving G-CSF alone (56.3% vs. 26.8%). However, failure rates were the same between the two regimens (18.8% G/C vs. 18.6% G-CSF alone, $p = 0.984$). G/C led to the greatest number of patients collecting the optimal amount, i.e., >5 × 10^6 CD34$^+$ HSC, in all three groups of patients. MM patients had the highest yield regardless of regimen. Higher pre-apheresis CD34$^+$ cell counts were a significant predictor of day 1 HSC cell collection ($p < 0.0001$), and infusion of >10 × 10^6 CD34$^+$ cells/kg was associated with faster engraftment than a lower dose of HSC cells, <2 × 10^6 CD34$^+$ cells/kg.

In the remobilization analysis, all patients from the database were included. Of the 1,834 patients, 350 failed initial mobilization, and 269 of those patients underwent remobilization. Following remobilization, 23% of these 269 patients successfully mobilized ≥2 × 10^6 CD34$^+$ cells/kg. However, the rates of successful remobilization varied with the regimen utilized. Successful remobilization occurred in 18.4% of patients receiving G-CSF ± GM-CSF and 26.5% of patients receiving G/C vs. 72.2% in patients receiving G/P. When cells from first and second mobilization were pooled, G/P consistently had the lowest failure rate (16.7% vs. 28.1% for G-CSF ± GM-CSF) and G/C had the highest pooled failure rate at 47.1% ($p = 0.03$, comparison among all three groups).

Since a considerable number of auto-transplant candidates fail to mobilize an adequate number of HSCs, a number of compassionate use trials have been performed in the USA and Europe investigating plerixafor as a rescue drug for patients who have failed prior mobilization efforts.

In a recent paper by Duarte [27], 56 patients from Spain and the UK who were previous mobilization failures were enrolled in a compassionate use program (CUP). The CUP was started in 2008 to allow patients who were not previously eligible for plerixafor registration trials to undergo attempted mobilization with plerixafor. Patients in this trial received a median of two lines of treatment prior to transplant and underwent an average of 1.3 failed mobilization regimens per patient. The primary end point was collection of ≥2 × 10^6 CD34$^+$ cells/kg at any point in the collection. Secondary end points were HSC mobilization efficacy after plerixafor, neutrophil and platelet engraftment, toxicity and adverse events. Patients received G-CSF as a subcutaneous injection at a dose of 10 μg/kg daily for 4 days. At 11:00 pm the evening prior to the fifth day, patients received 240 μg/kg of plerixafor subcutaneously. Apheresis was started on day 5 and continued until patients collected ≥2 × 10^6 cells/kg. Patients underwent a median of two apheresis procedures. Seventy-five percent of previous failures were successfully rescued using G-CSF plus plerixafor and ultimately 35 patients (63%) underwent transplant with an average of 3.1 ± 1.2 (1.9–7.7) × 10^6 CD34$^+$ cells/kg. Remarkably, 71% of patients met the secondary end point of collecting ≥10 × 10^6 CD34$^+$ cells/kg.

In Germany [28], 60 patients (a mix of previously failed mobilizations and predicted poor mobilizers) from 23 centers were treated with plerixafor 9–11 h pre-apheresis. Forty-seven (78.3%) patients received G-CSF for 4 days prior to plerixafor; nine patients (15%) received plerixafor and/or G-CSF for less than

4 days. For the remaining four patients, no data regarding concomitant G-CSF use was available. In patients receiving 4 days of G-CSF prior to initiating plerixafor, NHL patients mobilized a median of 2.79×10^6 $CD34^+$ cells/kg, MM patients a median of 4.47×10^6 $CD34^+$ cells/kg, and HD patients a median of 2.41×10^6 $CD34^+$ cells/kg. In patients receiving less than 4 days of G-CSF prior to initiating plerixafor, the median number of cells collected in NHL patients was 2.52×10^6 $CD34^+$ cells/kg, in MM 5.6×10^6 $CD34^+$ cells/kg, and in patients with other diagnoses 2.75×10^6 $CD34^+$ cells/kg. There was no significant difference in yield with the shorter treatment time ($p=0.157$). All patients, irrespective of underlying disease, needed a median of two apheresis treatments. Forty of the successfully mobilized patients proceeded to transplant. Median time to engraftment was 12 days and this was not significantly different between the groups who received four or less than 4 days of G-CSF prior to initiating plerixafor.

Other compassionate reports have been similar: Calandra and colleagues [29], for example, reported that 66% of patients with NHL, MM, and HD who had previously failed to mobilize sufficient numbers of $CD34^+$ cells with chemotherapy or cytokine therapy for transplant could be successfully remobilized with plerixafor and G-CSF. Patients were eligible for the CUP if they were appropriate transplant candidates but had been unsuccessful in apheresis collection or cell mobilization. As in other trials, patients needed to demonstrate peripheral blood counts normally associated with reasonable bone marrow function, good liver and kidney function, left ventricular ejection fraction greater than 40%, and forced expiratory volume >60% predicted. Given the nature of the protocol, there were some exemptions for lower WBC or platelet counts, lower creatinine clearance, and some extension of the age limits. The mobilization protocol was as documented in the aforementioned European CUP trial [27].

A total of 200 patients were initially enrolled in CUP including patients with acute myeloid leukemia (AML) and solid tumors. Outcomes and safety data on a subgroup of 115 patients with NHL, MM, and HD were analyzed from sites whose data were audited as part of the trial. Sites that were audited met the following criteria: most patients enrolled in CUP, more than three patients in each disease group, and/or sites conducting a company-sponsored plerixafor study.

Patients had received a median number of two prior chemotherapy regimens and 75% of patients had peripheral blood $CD34^+$ counts <10 cells per microliter. Sixty-six percent of patients collected $\geq 2 \times 10^6$ cells/kg and over 75% of patients were able to proceed to transplant. Of the 87 transplanted patients, 50 received cells mobilized only with plerixafor + G-CSF. The remaining 37 patients used cells mobilized in the CUP plus cells mobilized from prior collection efforts. Follow-up data were available on 36 patients at the 1-year posttransplant time point (as many patients left their CUP physician to return to the referring physician and were not available for follow-up). Ninety-four percent of these patients showed laboratory evidence of graft durability. Safety data and time to engraftment were similar to other trials [18]. The most common AEs were diarrhea, injection site erythema, and nausea/vomiting. Although the number of patients available for long-term follow-up was small, the high percentage of graft durability is very encouraging in a patient population who would not have gone to transplant in the absence of this compassionate use protocol and is consistent with the other mobilization trials.

An area of concern regarding the safety of plerixafor arose in the setting of mobilization of patients with AML. Andreef and colleagues [30] demonstrated the presence of circulating blasts (ranging up to 80%) in patients with AML in complete morphologic remission receiving plerixafor and G-CSF for mobilization. Similarly, an AML patient treated with plerixafor was found to have a dramatic reduction in $CD34^+$ cells in the bone marrow, suggesting a high degree of mobilization of blast cells to the periphery [31]. Therefore, based on these data, the use of plerixafor to mobilize AML patients prior to autologous transplantation is not recommended due to concerns regarding the risk of mobilizing occult tumor cells into the stem cell product. Since AML cells approximate a malignant equivalent of normal early hematopoietic elements, it is not surprising that they may be similarly mobilized to the periphery by a highly efficacious mobilization regimen.

Plerixafor + Chemotherapy

Even though the majority of the clinical trials of plerixafor mobilization focused on patients receiving G-CSF alone, it is clinically well-recognized that the administration of chemotherapy, most often high-dose cyclophosphamide with or without other agents, prior to growth factor, enhances $CD34^+$ mobilization. The particular type of regimen used varies according to the primary diagnosis but this strategy has often been utilized for patients who have already failed mobilization with G-CSF alone or for patients who, due to large tumor burden, may benefit from additional cytoreduction before transplant. The drawbacks of chemotherapy utilization are mainly related to the toxicities and complications derived from the use of chemotherapy itself as well as the increase in the duration and the cost of the mobilization regimen. However, chemotherapy-based mobilization is widely used and for some transplant programs represents the standard of care. An important question is whether the addition of plerixafor to a chemotherapy + G-CSF regimen will improve efficacy further. While the role of plerixafor in chemotherapy-based mobilization regimens is less well studied, at least one phase II clinical trial has been performed.

A prospective, multicenter, open-label, sequential phase II study (study 2104) [32] was conducted to evaluate the safety and feasibility of combining plerixafor with chemotherapy in patients with NHL and MM. The authors designed a trial in which four cohorts were planned. Patients were not randomized but rather enrolled in a sequential manner. Patients in cohorts A and B received mobilizing chemotherapy followed by daily G-CSF and initiated apheresis when the circulating $CD34^+$ count exceeded 20 cells/μL. Daily plerixafor was initiated after the first apheresis (though with different schedules in the two cohorts) so as to allow a comparison of the $CD34^+$ cell yields on the first 2 days of collection, one with and one without plerixafor. Cohort C enrolled patients who previously failed mobilization with chemotherapy and G-CSF, and cohort D was designed to explore the potential ability of earlier plerixafor administration to accelerate when collection could be initiated. For this last cohort, patients received chemotherapy followed by daily G-CSF. Plerixafor was added on day 6 and continued for a minimum of 3 days thereafter. Apheresis was initiated when the circulating $CD34^+$ count exceeded 20 cells/μL.

A total of 40 patients received a plerixafor dose of 240 μg/kg and the HSCs collected in all aphereses were used for transplantation. The primary endpoint was related to safety since the key issue was to prove that plerixafor would not be detrimental in the face of previously administered chemotherapy. The secondary endpoints varied according to the cohort group. For cohorts A and B, this was the mean fold increase in $CD34^+$ cells between first and second aphereses. For cohort C, this was efficacy of plerixafor as a rescue agent and for cohort D this was whether plerixafor could accelerate the time for collection by allowing effective collections to begin before full WBC recovery. Through the use of these four cohorts, the authors hoped to demonstrate that any enhancement in number the HSCs collected was due to plerixafor administration and not to a delayed effect of chemotherapy.

In general, the drug was well tolerated with similar adverse events as previously described in clinical trials that did not employ chemotherapy for mobilization. Three patients experienced moderate to severe adverse events (severe back pain and anxiety attack), but in no case was massive leukocytosis observed. Regarding efficacy-related endpoints, cohorts A and B demonstrated a significant increase in the number of $CD34^+$ cells collected (mean 2.06-fold increase), between the first (pre-plerixafor) and the second (post-plerixafor) apheresis. Only one patient failed to mobilize with chemotherapy and was included in cohort C. This patient was successfully rescued with plerixafor. A total of five patients were enrolled in cohort D and four of them reached >20 $CD34^+$ cells/μL on day 9 (3 days after the beginning of plerixafor) but none were able to have apheresis before white blood count recovery. All patients who received plerixafor underwent successful transplantation with a median time to neutrophil recovery of 11 days (range 8–20), and, in 35 cases evaluated, durable engraftment was demonstrated 12 months posttransplant.

Although data concerning the addition of plerixafor to chemotherapy-based mobilization regimens is limited, this study demonstrated that plerixafor can safely be added to chemotherapy-based mobilization regimens with a mean increase in the $CD34^+$ cell yields consistent with what has been observed in trials using growth factors alone for mobilization. It is expected that other clinical trials will soon expand our knowledge in this area.

Plerixafor as a Single Mobilization Agent

Filgrastim, though generally well tolerated, does have potential side effects such as bone pain and fever that can be uncomfortable for a subset of patients. In addition, it contributes to the costs of the mobilization regimen. This prompted the exploration of plerixafor alone without the concomitant use of G-CSF and/or chemotherapy. Phase I studies in healthy volunteers (described above) suggested that a single dose of plerixafor is able to mobilize similar numbers of $CD34^+$ cells as 5 days of G-CSF. However, it is also true that healthy individuals generally have higher circulating peripheral blood $CD34^+$ cells than cancer patients who have been exposed to several rounds of chemotherapy. This raised the question as to whether plerixafor alone is a feasible mobilization strategy for these patients.

A phase II trial (study 2108, [33]) planned to enroll 20 patients with MM to be mobilized with 240 μg/kg/day for four consecutive days. The trial was terminated after enrollment of nine patients. All patients mobilized $\geq 2\times 10^6$ $CD34^+$ cells/kg (range: $2.27–6.64\times 10^6$ cells/kg). All patients received a transplant with median neutrophil and platelet engraftment times of 10.5 days and 21 days, respectively. Adverse events were mild and consistent with other studies. However, five of nine patients did not mobilize sufficient cells, $\geq 4\times 10^6$ $CD34^+$ cells/kg for two transplants (tandem transplant), a common practice in the treatment of MM. For this reason, the authors concluded that the approach would generate little enthusiasm in the transplant community. Nonetheless, the results do indicate that plerixafor alone is able to mobilize sufficient cells for at least a single autologous transplant. At the present time, in the autologous transplant setting, the use of plerixafor alone for mobilization would appear to be limited to patients who are intolerant of G-CSF.

Resource Utilization and Patient Tolerance

Administration of plerixafor represents an incremental expense to the mobilization process which is relatively easy to measure. Potential associated cost reductions are more complex and, in some cases, more challenging to measure. Reduction in the number of apheresis sessions and associated charges to third party payers are easily measured, but the cost savings to collection and cryopreservation centers (with fixed salary, space, and other costs as well as variable costs for supplies and disposables) is more difficult to pinpoint. Similarly, while it is clear that fewer patients will require remobilization and more will proceed to transplant, the impact of these outcomes on the overall costs of caring for these patients is more difficult to quantitate to assess the overall medico-economic impact of utilizing plerixafor. Higher cell doses may lead to more rapid platelet recovery leading to reduction in transfusion expenses, but these potential savings have yet to be formally demonstrated. Measurement of how addition of plerixafor thus impacts patient morbidity, treatment tolerance, time missed from work (and its associated costs to society), and patient satisfaction/sense of well being is even more difficult. A number of investigators have attempted to address these challenging issues.

Reduction in the number of days of apheresis with adequate numbers of cells mobilized is one of the effects of plerixafor that potentially has the greatest impact on reduction in patient morbidity. Outcomes were assessed by Jagasia [34], regarding cost analysis and toxicity profile of stem cell mobilization in NHL ($n=115$) and MM ($n=121$) patients. Those who were able to collect $\geq 2\times 10^6$ $CD34^+$ cells/kg (with high-dose cyclophosphamide and G-CSF) on the planned day of collection in one or two apheresis sessions without a negative clinical event were considered to have an "ideal outcome." Only 25% of NHL patients and 18% of MM patients met such criteria. Patients with a nonideal outcome included patients who experienced febrile neutropenia, hospitalization, bone pain, gastrointestinal toxicity, and line infections. Ideal outcomes were associated with significantly lower costs than non-ideal outcomes. Clearly, less than optimal stem cell mobilization takes a toll on both patients and the health care system alike. Patients who can be mobilized more quickly and efficiently with plerixafor stand to experience fewer adverse effects as a result of prolonged or repeated apheresis sessions.

Gertz and colleagues [35] also retrospectively reviewed patients to evaluate the burden of unsuccessful mobilization. Of 1,775 patients undergoing mobilization, 47% of collections were determined to be less than optimal (either $<2\times10^6$ $CD34^+$ cells/kg or failed). This correlated with increased resource consumption, increased transfusional support, more frequent admissions to the hospital, and increased number of apheresis procedures.

These studies represent an important first step in the process of understanding how the application of a new, efficacious agent such as plerixafor alters the costs of caring for potential transplant patients. Whether it will be more cost effective to treat all prospective patients with plerixafor as part of their primary mobilization or to focus on approaches which will more reliably identify the subset of patients who are at highest risk to fail primary mobilization without plerixafor and treat only that subset up front is a question which remains to be addressed. Economical analyses and endpoints are likely to be increasingly common in future studies.

Allogeneic Stem Cell Transplantation

Almost all of the clinical investigations carried out with plerixafor have been in the autologous transplant setting and this currently represents the only FDA approved indication for this drug. However, studying this agent in the allogeneic transplant setting is a logical next step. In the allogeneic setting, one is far less concerned about whether the marrow is contaminated with malignancy or whether the stem and progenitor cell pool have been compromised from prior chemotherapy and/or radiotherapy. In contrast, the effects of plerixafor on immune cell function have the capability to influence other outcome variables in allogeneic BMT including engraftment/graft rejection, graft vs. host disease, and immune reconstitution.

The standard approach to collect mobilized products for allografting is with G-CSF stimulation [36], sparing the donors a bone marrow harvest. To date, only a single trial [37] has investigated an alternate approach using plerixafor. This study included patients with hematological malignancies suitable for transplantation who had an appropriate HLA-identical sibling donor. In this case, subjects exposed to the experimental arm were not the patients (or at least not directly the patients) but rather the healthy donors. Donors were mobilized using 240 μg/kg of plerixafor on the morning of day 1 and underwent leukapheresis at midday with a minimal target of 2×10^6 $CD34^+$ cells/kg of actual recipient weight. There was no maximal target; if 2×10^6 $CD34^+$ cells/kg was collected then no further apheresis procedures were performed. Conversely, if the target was not reached, then a second attempt was planned 72 h later (day 3) with the same approach and the cells were pooled. Initially, donors were scheduled to undergo a 7-day wash-out period and then to have a backup product collected using a standard G-CSF mobilization approach. Collection of backup products was stopped after the eighth transplant since all allografts had demonstrated prompt and durable engraftment. All transplanted patients received cyclophosphamide 60 mg/kg IV daily for two doses on days −3 and −2, followed by a single dose of total body irradiation (550 cGy) on day −1 as conditioning, single agent cyclosporine for acute graft vs. host disease (GVHD) prophylaxis and supportive care with G-CSF starting day +1 posttransplant.

A total of 25 HLA-identical sibling donor/recipient pairs were enrolled, 20 of whom (80%) had AML as the primary diagnosis. All donors received at least one dose of plerixafor and they demonstrated a median of eightfold increase in the peripheral $CD34^+$ cells. One donor could not undergo plasmapheresis due to line-related issues, but of the other 24, 16 (66%) achieved the target number of cells in the first day. Six of the other eight donors reached the threshold in the second attempt giving a total failure rate of 8.3% (2/24).

These data are encouraging, but it should be noted that some investigators would consider a failure rate of 8.3% high for allogeneic donors mobilized with G-CSF. It is also noteworthy that in the donors who also underwent backup mobilization with G-CSF, the median fold increase of $CD34^+$ cells after 5 days was 15.3 with G-CSF vs. 8.0 with plerixafor ($p<0.001$). Interestingly, immunophenotyping of the plerixafor and G-CSF products demonstrated a significantly higher proportion of $CD3^+$ and $CD4^+$ cells in the plerixafor products. The adverse events experienced by the donors were mild and similar to the ones previously described in the autologous transplant setting.

Twenty patients received allografts (five patients could not receive a transplant for diverse reasons) with a median time to neutrophil and platelet engraftment of 10 and 12 days, respectively. Donor chimerism ranged from 95 to 100% in whole bone marrow specimens. Seventy-five percent (15/20) of the transplanted patients experienced acute GVHD but only one case was severe (grade 4) leading to death. The rest responded to conventional steroid-based therapy. Six patients experienced extensive chronic GVHD. The median $CD3^+$ and $CD4^+$ cell counts were greater than 200/μL at all times studied which may be a consequence of the higher numbers of these cells in the plerixafor products. Regarding overall survival and relapse, five patients relapsed, four of them died and a total of 14 patients remained alive at the time the study was reported.

This trial raises a number of important questions which may form the basis of future trials. Use of plerixafor as an alternative to G-CSF in the allogeneic setting will depend on whether this agent can mobilize allogeneic donors with as high a success rate as G-CSF and whether use of plerixafor has any positive or negative effects on transplant outcomes. A first step is for plerixafor to successfully mobilize almost all allogeneic donors in whom it is utilized. The 8% failure rate in this study needs to be lowered. The question has been raised as to whether plerixafor-mobilized CD34$^+$ cells may be qualitatively different than their G-CSF mobilized counterparts and whether, based on a higher representation of less mature CD34$^+$ cells, fewer cells will be required for optimal engraftment. Alternatively use of higher doses or other routes of plerixafor administration may prove more efficacious when the drug is used as a single agent. Studies have typically added plerixafor to G-CSF after a typical (4–5 day) period of G-CSF administration for mobilization. Perhaps fewer days of G-CSF priming will be necessary in the allogeneic transplant setting when G-CSF is combined with plerixafor.

Immunologic endpoints also need to be assessed in studies of plerixafor mobilization. There was a twofold higher CD3$^+$ and CD4$^+$ cell content in the plerixafor-mobilized allografts in this trial. However, GVHD did not appear increased raising the question as to whether lymphocytes exposed to plerixafor may also exhibit qualitative differences from those mobilized with G-CSF. CD4$^+$ lymphocyte recovery was consistent and rapid. Graft rejection, GVHD, rates of relapse (as a surrogate marker of GVL effects), and immunologic reconstitution need to be important end points in future allogeneic trials.

Summary and Discussion

Based on the clinical trials described above, plerixafor has been approved by the FDA for use together with G-CSF in the mobilization of autologous HSCs in patients with MM and NHL. As is the case for most newly FDA approved drugs, additional or alternate uses of plerixafor may emerge over time. It is worth emphasizing the fact that consistent results were obtained in multiple trials in several different clinical scenarios, conducted by different investigators in different medical centers. Several consistent observations have been generated in the course of this research. To summarize:

- Plerixafor plus G-CSF is superior to G-CSF alone for the initial mobilization of patients with MM and NHL.
- Plerixafor plus G-CSF appears to be equally or more efficacious than other regimens used as salvage for patients with MM and NHL who have failed another mobilization approach.
- Superiority of plerixafor plus G-CSF vs. G-CSF alone is reflected in a clinically meaningful increase in the number of HSCs collected, more patients reaching the minimum number of HSCs acceptable for auto-transplant, more patients reaching an optimal number of HSCs desired for auto-transplant, and fewer days of apheresis required to reach these cell dose targets.
- As a consequence of the above activities, plerixafor may allow more MM and NHL patients to proceed to transplant than would be possible without this drug.
- Plerixafor is generally well tolerated in this setting with few serious or unexpected adverse events.

- A more limited body of data suggest that patients with Hodgkin's lymphoma behave similarly to their NHL counterparts.
- While plerixafor may have utility in chemotherapy-based mobilization, the optimal role and schedule for this agent in this setting have yet to be established.
- Mobilization of AML blasts into the peripheral blood has been observed in several patients with AML thought to be in remission. For this reason, plerixafor should not be used for stem cell mobilization in patients with AML.
- A small number of trials have addressed whether addition of plerixafor results in mobilization of more circulating tumor cells at the time of stem cell collection. The limited data available do not currently increase concerns about tumor mobilization (other than AML) though more studies are needed to definitively address this issue.
- Plerixafor is being explored as a mobilization agent in the allogeneic setting as well.
- Beyond the scope of this review, plerixafor is being evaluated for use via the intravenous route. In addition, plerixafor is being studied as an adjunct/sensitizing agent in the treatment of AML testing the concept that dissociating AML cells from marrow stroma may lead to loss of protective effects mediated by the stromal microenvironment.

Clinical studies of plerixafor have all focused on quantitative issues, specifically how many $CD34^+$ cells were collected. Little has been investigated with regard to qualitative differences. The $CD34^+$ population is heterogeneous and only a small subfraction represents true stem cells. There is no reason to presume a priori that the $CD34^+$ cells isolated using plerixafor are qualitatively identical to those mobilized with G-CSF alone. We have presumed that our ideas about optimal $CD34^+$ cell number developed from our experience with G-CSF will apply to plerixafor-mobilized products. However, if the cells are qualitatively different, then the optimal numbers required in various clinical applications may differ as well. There is at least one study [8] suggesting that fewer human $CD34^+$ cells are required to engraft NOD/SCID mice when plerixafor is used for mobilization vs. when G-CSF is used for mobilization. If confirmed, it would raise the question as to whether smaller numbers of plerixafor-mobilized $CD34^+$ cells will behave similar clinically to higher numbers of their G-CSF mobilized counterparts.

In conclusion, plerixafor is an agent which has demonstrated clear-cut evidence of efficacy with little toxicity. In the absence of cost considerations, there would be little downside to recommending its fairly routine use in autologous PBSC mobilization in diseases other than AML. Going forward, medico-economic analyses will demonstrate whether it is most cost effective to use this agent on a routine basis or to try to identify those patients most likely to fail to mobilize an optimal product in its absence. Given its safety and efficacy, further research on the route of administration, dose, schedule, and use in the allogeneic transplant setting are likely to identify additional applications of this novel stem cell mobilizing agent.

References

1. Pavone V, Gaudio F, Console G, Vitolo U, Iacopino P, Guarini A, Liso V, Perrone T, Liso A (2006) Poor mobilization is an independent prognostic factor in patients with malignant lymphomas treated by peripheral blood stem cell transplantation. Bone Marrow Transplant 37:719–724
2. Bensinger W, DiPersio JF, McCarty JM (2009) Improving stem cell mobilization strategies: future directions. Bone Marrow Transplant 43:181–195
3. Shpall EJ (1999) The utilization of cytokines in stem cell mobilization strategies. Bone Marrow Transplant 23(Suppl 2):S13–S19
4. Kuittinen T, Nousiainen T, Halonen P, Mahlamaki E, Jantunen E (2004) Prediction of mobilisation failure in patients with non-Hodgkin's lymphoma. Bone Marrow Transplant 33:907–912
5. Ponomaryov T, Peled A, Petit I, Taichman RS, Habler L, Sandbank J, Arenzana-Seisdedos F, Magerus A, Caruz A, Fujii N, Nagler A, Lahav M, Szyper-Kravitz M, Zipori D, Lapidot T (2000) Induction of the chemokine stromal-derived factor-1 following DNA damage improves human stem cell function. J Clin Invest 106:1331–1339
6. Petit I, Szyper-Kravitz M, Nagler A, Lahav M, Peled A, Habler L, Ponomaryov T, Taichman RS, Arenzana-Seisdedos F, Fujii N, Sandbank J, Zipori D, Lapidot T (2002) G-CSF induces stem cell mobilization by decreasing bone marrow SDF-1 and up-regulating CXCR4. Nat Immunol 3:687–694
7. Hendrix CW, Collier AC, Lederman MM, Schols D, Pollard RB, Brown S, Jackson JB, Coombs RW, Glesby MJ, Flexner CW, Bridger GJ, Badel K, MacFarland RT, Henson GW, Calandra G, AMD3100 HIV Study Group (2004) Safety, pharmacokinetics, and antiviral activity of AMD3100, a selective CXCR4 receptor inhibitor, in HIV-1 infection. J Acquir Immune Defic Syndr 37:1253–1262
8. Hess DA, Bonde J, Craft TP, Wirthlin L, Hohm S, Lahey R, Todt LM, Dipersio JF, Devine SM, Nolta JA (2007) Human progenitor cells rapidly mobilized by AMD3100 repopulate NOD/SCID mice with increased frequency in comparison to cells from the same donor mobilized by granulocyte colony stimulating factor. Biol Blood Marrow Transplant 13:398–411
9. Broxmeyer HE, Orschell CM, Clapp DW, Hangoc G, Cooper S, Plett PA, Liles WC, Li X, Graham-Evans B, Campbell TB, Calandra G, Bridger G, Dale DC, Srour EF (2005) Rapid mobilization of murine and human hematopoietic stem and progenitor cells with AMD3100, a CXCR4 antagonist. J Exp Med 201:1307–1318
10. Martin C, Bridger GJ, Rankin SM (2006) Structural analogues of AMD3100 mobilise haematopoietic progenitor cells from bone marrow in vivo according to their ability to inhibit CXCL12 binding to CXCR4 in vitro. Br J Haematol 134:326–329
11. Burroughs L, Mielcarek M, Little MT, Bridger G, Macfarland R, Fricker S, Labrecque J, Sandmaier BM, Storb R (2005) Durable engraftment of AMD3100-mobilized autologous and allogeneic peripheral-blood mononuclear cells in a canine transplantation model. Blood 106:4002–4008
12. Larochelle A, Krouse A, Metzger M, Orlic D, Donahue RE, Fricker S, Bridger G, Dunbar CE, Hematti P (2006) AMD3100 mobilizes hematopoietic stem cells with long-term repopulating capacity in nonhuman primates. Blood 107:3772–3778
13. Peled A, Grabovsky V, Habler L, Sandbank J, Arenzana-Seisdedos F, Petit I, Ben-Hur H, Lapidot T, Alon R (1999) The chemokine SDF-1 stimulates integrin-mediated arrest of CD34(+) cells on vascular endothelium under shear flow. J Clin Invest 104:1199–1211
14. Lack NA, Green B, Dale DC, Calandra GB, Lee H, MacFarland RT, Badel K, Liles WC, Bridger G (2005) A pharmacokinetic-pharmacodynamic model for the mobilization of $CD34^+$ hematopoietic progenitor cells by AMD3100. Clin Pharmacol Ther 77:427–436
15. Liles WC, Broxmeyer HE, Rodger E, Wood B, Hubel K, Cooper S, Hangoc G, Bridger GJ, Henson GW, Calandra G, Dale DC (2003) Mobilization of hematopoietic progenitor cells in healthy volunteers by AMD3100, a CXCR4 antagonist. Blood 102:2728–2730

16. Liles WC, Rodger E, Broxmeyer HE, Dehner C, Badel K, Calandra G, Christensen J, Wood B, Price TH, Dale DC (2005) Augmented mobilization and collection of CD34⁺ hematopoietic cells from normal human volunteers stimulated with granulocyte-colony-stimulating factor by single-dose administration of AMD3100, a CXCR4 antagonist. Transfusion 45:295–300
17. Devine SM, Flomenberg N, Vesole DH, Liesveld J, Weisdorf D, Badel K, Calandra G, DiPersio JF (2004) Rapid mobilization of CD34⁺ cells following administration of the CXCR4 antagonist AMD3100 to patients with multiple myeloma and non-Hodgkin's lymphoma. J Clin Oncol 22:1095–1102
18. Flomenberg N, Devine SM, Dipersio JF, Liesveld JL, McCarty JM, Rowley SD, Vesole DH, Badel K, Calandra G (2005) The use of AMD3100 plus G-CSF for autologous hematopoietic progenitor cell mobilization is superior to G-CSF alone. Blood 106:1867–1874
19. Stiff P, Micallef I, McCarthy P, Magalhaes-Silverman M, Weisdorf D, Territo M, Badel K, Calandra G (2009) Treatment with plerixafor in non-Hodgkin's lymphoma and multiple myeloma patients to increase the number of peripheral blood stem cells when given a mobilizing regimen of G-CSF: implications for the heavily pretreated patient. Biol Blood Marrow Transplant 15:249–256
20. Tricot G, Cottler-Fox MH, Calandra G (2010) Safety and efficacy assessment of plerixafor in patients with multiple myeloma proven or predicted to be poor mobilizers, including assessment of tumor cell mobilization. Bone Marrow Transplant 45:63–68
21. Gazitt Y, FreytesCO AC, Badel K, Calandra G (2007) Improved mobilization of peripheral blood CD34⁺ cells and dendritic cells by AMD3100 plus granulocyte-colony-stimulating factor in non-Hodgkin's lymphoma patients. Stem Cells Dev 16:657–666
22. Cashen A, Lopez S, Gao F, Calandra G, MacFarland R, Badel K, DiPersio J (2008) A phase II study of plerixafor (AMD3100) plus G-CSF for autologous hematopoietic progenitor cell mobilization in patients with Hodgkin lymphoma. Biol Blood Marrow Transplant 14:1253–1261
23. DiPersio JF, Micallef IN, Stiff PJ, Bolwell BJ, Maziarz RT, Jacobsen E, Nademanee A, McCarty J, Bridger G, Calandra G, 3101 Investigators (2009) Phase III prospective randomized double-blind placebo-controlled trial of plerixafor plus granulocyte colony-stimulating factor compared with placebo plus granulocyte colony-stimulating factor for autologous stem-cell mobilization and transplantation for patients with non-Hodgkin's lymphoma. J Clin Oncol 27:4767–4773
24. Micallef IN, Stiff PJ, DiPersio JF, Maziarz RT, McCarty JM, Bridger G, Calandra G (2009) Successful stem cell remobilization using plerixafor (mozobil) plus granulocyte colony-stimulating factor in patients with non-hodgkin lymphoma: results from the plerixafor NHL phase 3 study rescue protocol. Biol Blood Marrow Transplant 15:1578–1586
25. DiPersio JF, Stadtmauer EA, Nademanee A, Micallef IN, Stiff PJ, Kaufman JL, Maziarz RT, Hosing C, Fruehauf S, Horwitz M, Cooper D, Bridger G, Calandra G, 3102 Investigators (2009) Plerixafor and G-CSF versus placebo and G-CSF to mobilize hematopoietic stem cells for autologous stem cell transplantation in patients with multiple myeloma. Blood 113:5720–5726
26. Pusic I, Jiang SY, Landua S, Uy GL, Rettig MP, Cashen AF, Westervelt P, Vij R, Abboud CN, Stockerl-Goldstein KE, Sempek DS, Smith AL, DiPersio JF (2008) Impact of mobilization and remobilization strategies on achieving sufficient stem cell yields for autologous transplantation. Biol Blood Marrow Transplant 14:1045–1056
27. Duarte RF, Shaw BE, Marin P, Kottaridis P, Ortiz M, Morante C, Delgado J, Gayoso J, Goterriz R, Martinez-Chamorro C, Mateos-Mazon JJ, Ramirez C, de la Rubia J, Achtereekte H, Gandhi PJ, Douglas KW, Russell NH (2011) Plerixafor plus granulocyte CSF can mobilize hematopoietic stem cells from multiple myeloma and lymphoma patients failing previous mobilization attempts: EU compassionate use data. Bone Marrow Transplant 46:52–58
28. Hubel K, Fresen MM, Salwender H, Basara N, Beier R, Theurich S, Christopeit M, Bogner C, Galm O, Hartwig R, Heits F, Lordick F, Rosler W, Wehler D, Zander AR, Albert MH, Dressler S, Ebinger M, Frickhofen N, Hertenstein B, Kiehl M, Liebler S, von Lilienfeld-Toal M, Weidmann E, Weigelt C, Lange F, Kroger N (2010) Plerixafor with and without chemotherapy in poor mobilizers: results from the German compassionate use program. Bone Marrow Transplant 2010. doi:10.1038/bmt.2010.249

29. Calandra G, McCarty J, McGuirk J, Tricot G, Crocker SA, Badel K, Grove B, Dye A, Bridger G (2008) AMD3100 plus G-CSF can successfully mobilize CD34+ cells from non-Hodgkin's lymphoma, Hodgkin's disease and multiple myeloma patients previously failing mobilization with chemotherapy and/or cytokine treatment: compassionate use data. Bone Marrow Transplant 41:331–338
30. Andreeff M, Konoplev S, Wong R-Y et al (2006) Massive mobilization of AML cells into circulation by disruption of leukemia/stroma cell interactions using CXCR4 antagonist AMD3100: first evidence in patients and potential for abolishing bone marrow microenvironment-mediated resistance [abstract]. Blood 108:176a
31. Fierro FA, Brenner S, Oelschlaegel U et al (2009) Combining SDF-1/CXCR4 antagonism and chemotherapy in relapsed acute myeloid leukemia. Leukemia 23:393–396
32. Dugan MJ, Maziarz RT, Bensinger WI, Nademanee A, Liesveld J, Badel K, Dehner C, Gibney C, Bridger G, Calandra G (2010) Safety and preliminary efficacy of plerixafor (Mozobil) in combination with chemotherapy and G-CSF: an open-label, multicenter, exploratory trial in patients with multiple myeloma and non-Hodgkin's lymphoma undergoing stem cell mobilization. Bone Marrow Transplant 45:39–47
33. Flomenberg N, Comenzo RL, Badel K, Calandra G (2010) Plerixafor (Mozobil) alone to mobilize hematopoietic stem cells from multiple myeloma patients for autologous transplantation. Biol Blood Marrow Transplant 16:695–700
34. Jagasia MH, Savani BN, Neff A, Dixon S, Chen H, Pickard AS (2010) Outcome, toxicity profile and cost analysis of autologous stem cell mobilization. Bone Marrow Transplant. doi:10.1038/bmt.2010.254
35. Gertz MA, Wolf RC, Micallef IN, Gastineau DA (2010) Clinical impact and resource utilization after stem cell mobilization failure in patients with multiple myeloma and lymphoma. Bone Marrow Transplant 45:1396–1403
36. Copelan EA (2006) Hematopoietic stem-cell transplantation. N Engl J Med 354:1813–1826
37. Devine SM, Vij R, Rettig M, Todt L, McGlauchlen K, Fisher N, Devine H, Link DC, Calandra G, Bridger G, Westervelt P, Dipersio JF (2008) Rapid mobilization of functional donor hematopoietic cells without G-CSF using AMD3100, an antagonist of the CXCR4/SDF-1 interaction. Blood 112:990–998

Chapter 8
Experience with Apheresis Procedures After Plerixafor Mobilisation

Kenneth Douglas

Current Apheresis Protocols for Autologous HPC-A Procurement: An Overview

General Introduction

On reviewing current protocols for procurement of autologous Haematopoietic Progenitor Cells by apheresis—commonly known as "Peripheral Blood Stem Cells (PBSC)" or "Peripheral Blood Progenitor cells (PBPC)", but more correctly termed "HPC-A" using FACT/JACIE terminology [1]—it is immediately striking how diverse current clinical practice actually is. Individual centres, even within one country or even within one city, may be using different mobilisation regimes, different apheresis platforms (i.e. different machines), different "trigger" peripheral blood markers for apheresis and different threshold levels of these markers, different target $CD34^+$ cell doses and different protocols for how much of the patient's blood to process during each apheresis. Although plerixafor undoubtedly represents a significant advance in autologous HPC-A procurement, the challenge for many centres has been incorporating the drug into very diverse local protocols. This chapter aims to review published experience regarding how plerixafor may best be incorporated into existing apheresis protocols. However, given the logistical obstacles to practising "evidence-based Apheresis Medicine" and the general lack of randomised controlled

K. Douglas (✉)
Clinical Apheresis Unit, Beatson West of Scotland Cancer Centre, Glasgow G12 0YN, UK
e-mail: Kenneth.Douglas@nhs.net

S. Fruehauf et al. (eds.), *Novel Developments in Stem Cell Mobilization: Focus on CXCR4*, DOI 10.1007/978-1-4614-1960-0_8,

studies in this subspecialty [2, 3], this chapter is necessarily a rather subjective overview, and the author discusses published and unpublished experience from his own centre in addition to the existing published experience from elsewhere.

Current Apheresis Platforms

Historically only a few companies have marketed apheresis platforms (i.e. "cell separator machines", which are extracorporeal blood centrifuges) for HPC-A procurement, and at the time of writing there are only a few platforms which have US or European regulatory approval for PBSC collection. CaridianBCT market the COBE Spectra® platform in both the USA and Europe for HPC-A procurement: this platform has now been in use for more than 20 years with only minor modifications, having proven to be both robust and versatile in clinical practice. However, CaridianBCT have more recently developed a new platform, known as Spectra Optia® or more commonly just "Optia", which is intended to replace the older COBE Spectra®, incorporating recent technological advances such as a smaller and lighter machine, a touch-screen graphical user interface and an automated interface monitoring system. Optia is currently CE-marked for HPC-A procurement within the European Economic Area, but has not been marketed for this indication in the USA as yet pending FDA approval. Fresenius also market an apheresis platform, known as Com.Tec®, which is widely used in Germany and mainland Europe. Other platforms include Baxter Amicus® and Haemonetics MCS+®. Published experience appears broadly similar for all of the apheresis platforms above in terms of collection efficiency and procedure run times: however, it should be noted that relatively few direct comparative studies have been published. As yet, none of the existing platforms has a clear advantage over the others, and many apheresis units have more than one type of apheresis platform in use. Features of current apheresis platforms, including potential advantages and disadvantages with references to such published studies as exist, are summarised in Table 8.1.

Even on a single platform, there may be alternative software settings and disposable "kits" that may be used for HPC-A procurement. This is the case with COBE Spectra (see Table 8.1), where there are two different settings approved for HPC-A procurement in the USA and Europe, each with its own disposable "kit" of single-use plastic tubing: the "autoPBSC" setting (sometimes confusingly called "Version 6" after the first software version for Spectra to offer this option); and the "MNC" setting (sometimes called "Version 4.1"). These two settings are actually quite different: the "autoPBSC" setting is a highly automated procedure, which requires less operator intervention during the procedure but considerably more complex initial data entry, while "MNC" is more labour-intensive for the operator during the procedure but has much simpler initial data entry. The single published comparison between these two settings on Spectra showed better performance for "MNC" in terms of collection efficiency and failed mobilisation rates [4], but this is achieved at the expense of higher levels of granulocyte contamination of the product, which

Table 8.1 A summary of existing commonly used apheresis platforms and software settings, including potential advantages and disadvantages

Apheresis platform (±software setting)	Manufacturer	Potential advantages	Potential disadvantages
COBE Spectra®, MNC software setting	CaridianBCT	• Widely used platform (>90% of world market) • Higher collection efficiency than autoPBSC setting [4] • Faster per blood volume processed than autoPBSC setting [4] • Less complex initial data entry than autoPBSC setting—more consistent procedural results	• Higher granulocyte contamination of product than autoPBSC setting [4]—can lead to higher cryopreservation volumes, particularly with plerixafor [5] • Requires more operator input during procedure than autoPBSC setting
COBE Spectra®, autoPBSC software setting	CaridianBCT	• Widely used platform (>90% of world market) • Lower granulocyte contamination of product than MNC setting [4]—lower cryopreservation volumes • Requires less operator input during procedure than MNC setting	• Lower collection efficiency than MNC setting [4] • Slower per blood volume processed than MNC setting [4] • More complex initial data entry than MNC setting—less consistent procedural results
Spectra Optia®	CaridianBCT	• Comparable or higher collection efficiency to MNC on COBE Spectra® [6] • Less granulocyte contamination than COBE Spectra—lower cryopreservation volumes [7] • Automated interface management—less operator input during procedure	• Relatively new platform—limited experience to date • Not yet approved by FDA for use in USA
Fresenius Com.Tec® and predecessors (Fresenius AS®)	Fresenius Kabi	• Less platelet loss than COBE Spectra using Fresenius AS [8] • Com.Tec has automated interface management—less operator input during procedure [10]	• Trend to lower collection efficiency than COBE Spectra for Fresenius AS in one study [8] • More platelet loss experienced with Fresenius Com.Tec than with Baxter Amicus in one study [9]
Baxter Amicus®	Baxter Fenwal	• Low platelet loss—less than Fresenius Com.Tec in one comparative study [9] and less than autoPBSC setting on COBE Spectra in another [11] • Good collection efficiency: higher than autoPBSC setting on COBE Spectra in one comparative study [11]	• Slower to process one blood volume than autoPBSC setting on COBE Spectra in one comparative study [11]
Haemonetics MCS+®	Haemonetics	• Discontinuous flow cell separator [12], therefore only one point of vascular access required (good for patients with difficult venous access)	• Discontinuous flow cell separator [12], therefore slower per blood volume processed than other machines listed [13]

can impact on cryopreservation volumes. This has been found to be a particular problem with the "MNC" setting on COBE Spectra when plerixafor is used with G-CSF but without prior chemotherapy, as high granulocyte counts in the peripheral blood lead to high cell counts in the apheresis product and high cryopreservation volume [5].

"Trigger" Peripheral Blood CD34⁺ Counts (and Other Peripheral Blood Markers) for Initiation of HPC-A Collection

Established clinical practice in HPC-A collection is that autologous HPC-A are collected in one of two ways: either by chemomobilisation, using mobilising chemotherapy (e.g. cyclophosphamide) followed by G-CSF at a dose of 5–10 μg/kg/day; or using G-CSF alone without prior mobilising chemotherapy, generally at a dose of 10 μg/kg/day. Both approaches are effective, with published clinical experience suggesting increased efficacy in terms of mobilising optimum $CD34^+$ cell doses using chemomobilisation, but with increased toxicity for the patient due to the chemotherapy [14–17]. Broadly speaking, many US cancer centres use chemomobilisation for lymphoma patients, because lymphoma salvage chemotherapy regimes are well suited as mobilising chemotherapy for HPC-A procurement so that the patient does not have to receive any additional chemotherapy for purposes of HPC-A collection, but use G-CSF-only mobilisation for myeloma patients to limit treatment-related toxicity. By contrast, most European centres use chemomobilisation not only for lymphoma patients (where lymphoma salvage regimes are used as mobilising chemotherapy), but also for myeloma patients, where intravenous cyclophosphamide at varying doses between 1 and 7 g/m^2 is used for purposes of HPC-A mobilisation.

Regardless of the mobilising regimes used (G-CSF alone or chemotherapy plus G-CSF), not all patients will mobilise sufficient HPC into the peripheral blood to allow collection of a transplantable HPC-A cell dose. To avoid exposing a patient to the discomfort and potential toxicities of apheresis (which include citrate toxicity, vasovagal episodes and platelet depletion) when there is little or no prospect of achieving a transplantable cell dose, virtually all centres measure peripheral blood markers—most commonly a peripheral blood $CD34^+$ cell count performed by FACS—before initiating autologous HPC-A collection. It is generally accepted that a peripheral $CD34^+$ count of greater than 20 μL^{-1} predicts a high likelihood of achieving a transplantable cell dose over 3 or fewer consecutive days of apheresis [18, 19], and virtually all centres using peripheral $CD34^+$ count monitoring will initiate apheresis at this level. However, many centres (the author's own included) will initiate apheresis at lower peripheral $CD34^+$ cell counts in patients who mobilise HPC-A poorly, sometimes processing more of the patient's blood to compensate for the lower peripheral blood stem cell concentration (often known as "Large Volume Leukapheresis" [20, 21]).

Although peripheral blood $CD34^+$ count performed by FACS is now the most widely used "trigger" for the initiation of apheresis, some centres still measure levels of peripheral blood "progenitor cell" counts performed by automated cell counters such as Sysmex [22], or just total and differential white cell count parameters in the peripheral blood [23], as less costly alternatives to peripheral $CD34^+$ count as apheresis triggers. However, these are less accurate predictors of successful HPC-A collection than peripheral $CD34^+$ count.

How Much Blood to Process? Dose Prediction on the Basis of Peripheral CD34⁺ Counts

Although there is a strong positive correlation between peripheral $CD34^+$ count taken immediately prior to apheresis and the $CD34^+$ cell dose in the apheresis product [18, 19], this correlation is imprecise with a fair degree of "scatter". Confounding variables include patient total blood volume (which is weight- and height-dependent) and whether the peripheral $CD34^+$ count is rising or falling at the time of collection; but probably most importantly, how much blood is processed through the cell separator machine. Although it might be expected that peripheral blood $CD34^+$ counts would fall significantly during an apheresis procedure due to depletion of circulating HPC by the cell separator machine, in fact clinical experience has been that the fall is less than expected due to the recruitment of fresh HPC from the bone marrow into the bloodstream in the course of the procedure [24]. Broadly speaking, processing larger volumes of the patient's blood will therefore yield larger doses of HPC [20, 21, 24–26]. If an approximate anticipated Collection Efficiency (i.e. what percentage of the HPC going through the machine actually end up in the apheresis product) is already known for the apheresis platform and setting being used (e.g. MNC setting on COBE Spectra), then it is possible to predict the HPC dose in the product, using the formula: Predicted HPC dose per kg = (anticipated Collection Efficiency) × (Volume of blood processed) × (HPC concentration in peripheral blood)/(patient's weight). The author's centre has found Collection Efficiency to be surprisingly predictable for the "MNC" setting on COBE Spectra at around 52%, and has developed a dose prediction formula as follows [27]: Predicted $CD34^+$ cell dose $\times 10^6$/kg = (4.75 × (predicted final inlet volume in mL) × (peripheral $CD34^+$ count per μL))/(patient's weight in kg × 10,000). This formula assumes a relatively standard Inlet: Anticoagulant setting of 13.5:1, with the volume of citrate anticoagulant calculated in to the equation leading to an apparent "lowering" of collection efficiency to 47.5%. "Final Inlet Volume" is the predicted final volume of citrated blood expected to be processed by the machine at the end of the procedure based on initial data entry for height, weight and gender, and is available via the machine's "Predicted End Run Results" screen at the start of a collection procedure. "Peripheral $CD34^+$ count" is a single count performed on a sample taken immediately pre-apheresis on the morning of collection (in other words, the "anticipated Collection Efficiency" of 52% used for the calculation is based on pre-run $CD34^+$ count alone; what has been

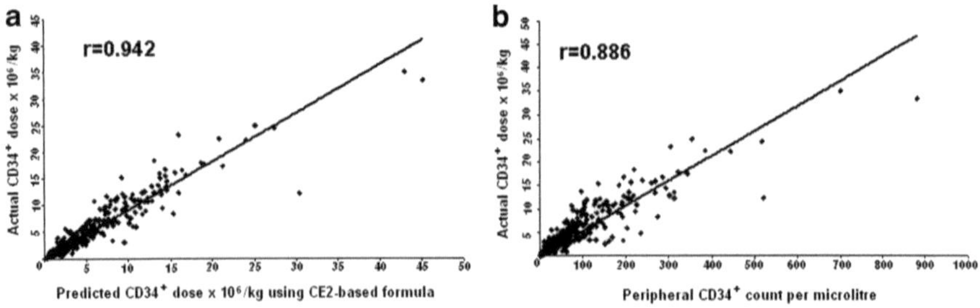

Fig. 8.1 Dose prediction using formula based on "CE2" Collection Efficiency is more accurate than dose prediction based on "Collection Ratio" (original diagram). (**a**) Correlation between predicted dose (using CE2-based formula) and actual dose in 440 consecutive HPC-A collection procedures at the author's centre. (**b**) Correlation between peripheral $CD34^+$ count alone and actual dose (as in "Collection Ratio"-based dose prediction) for the same 440 procedures, showing weaker correlation

called "CE2" [6]). Spectra defaults to process twice the patient's estimated total blood volume, but this can be modified upwards by the operator for patients with lower peripheral $CD34^+$ counts, with re-calculation of the expected cell dose. Figure 8.1 demonstrates a significantly closer correlation between predicted and actual $CD34^+$ dose in the product using this formula than is found using peripheral $CD34^+$ count alone, on a series of 440 consecutive collection procedures. The author has found this formula to be particularly useful for collections performed after plerixafor, where large volume leukapheresis is often indicated both to maximise cell dose in a poor mobiliser, and to limit the total number of plerixafor doses and of aphereses.

Simpler algorithms have also been used for $CD34^+$ dose prediction based on pre-run peripheral $CD34^+$ count. Another way of expressing the "Collection Efficiency" of an apheresis platform is by determining the average "Collection Ratio" expected for the platform and software setting in question, defined as: Collection Ratio = ($CD34^+$ cells/kg bodyweight in apheresis product)/(pre-run peripheral $CD34^+$ count) [4, 25, 26]. The anticipated $CD34^+$ cell dose can then be calculated at the start of a procedure by using the simple formula: Predicted $CD34^+$ cell dose = Collection Ratio × Peripheral $CD34^+$ count. However, because Collection Ratio disregards the volume of blood process during apheresis, dose prediction using Collection Ratio is less accurate than dose prediction based on CE2 [27].

Cryopreservation Issues

Unlike allogeneic HPC-A products which are usually transplanted "fresh", autologous HPC-A are generally cryopreserved in liquid nitrogen for a period of months (and occasionally years) prior to re-infusion at the time of transplant. To allow cryopreservation without significant loss of cell viability, the cryoprotectant chemical dimethyl sulfoxide (DMSO) is added to HPC-A products prior to cryopreservation, at a concentration either of 10% or of 5% [28, 29]. DMSO is potentially toxic to the patient at the time of re-infusion, with reported uncommon side-effects including cardiac toxicity, anaphylaxis, seizures and rare but potentially fatal encephalopathy [30–32]: for these reasons, most institutions limit maximum DMSO volume re-infused to 1 mL/kg in any 24-h period, this being equivalent to 10 mL/kg of a PBSC product containing 10% DMSO.

The eventual cryopreservation volume of a HPC-A product, which is generally equivalent to the re-infusion volume, is *not* the same as the initial product volume. This is because of the need to dilute the HPC-A product prior to cryopreservation, so as to avoid loss of viability due to depletion of nutrients in an excessively cellular product. Most centres dilute HPC-A products to a maximum Total Nucleated Cell (TNC) concentration of 200×10^6/mL, using either autologous plasma or Human Albumin Solution [33]. However, because the degree of dilution required is based on the TNC rather than the $CD34^+$ cell count in the product, HPC-A products that have a low ratio of $CD34^+$ cells to other white cells will require more dilution. Although generally referred to as "a stem cell collection" by most healthcare and laboratory professionals, HPC-A products are of course composed predominantly of other white cells (mononuclear cells such as lymphocytes and monocytes, plus varying degrees of granulocyte contamination), with actual $CD34^+$ "haematopoietic progenitor cells" or "haematopoietic stem cells" making up a relatively small proportion of TNC.

It has become clear in clinical practice that, as might be expected, the patient's peripheral blood counts at the time of HPC-A collection have a significant impact on the TNC in the apheresis product, and this in turn has a significant impact on cryopreservation volume. Broadly speaking, when HPC-A collection is carried out on a patient with a high total peripheral white cell count and relatively low peripheral $CD34^+$ count, then this will lead to high cryopreservation volumes (mainly due to increased granulocyte contamination of the product); conversely, collection on lower total peripheral white cell count and relatively high peripheral $CD34^+$ count will lead to low cryopreservation volumes. It might be expected that the apheresis platform used would also affect cryopreservation volumes. Although it is not currently possible to separate out $CD34^+$ cells from other mononuclear cells (lymphocytes or monocytes) by centrifugation alone at spin speeds that do not damage the cells, it *is* possible to separate out granulocytes by centrifugation, and it is known that some platforms perform better than others in terms of granulocyte contamination of the HPC-A product.

Plerixafor has conventionally been used along with G-CSF, but without prior mobilising chemotherapy (i.e. the patient is mobilised in a similar way to an allogeneic HPC-A donor, using G-CSF 10 μg/kg/day for 4 days, except that plerixafor is also given on the evening of Day 4 [34–37]). This means that the patient's total white cell count at the time of apheresis will typically be in the range of $25–55 \times 10^9$/L, due to G-CSF related leucocytosis unopposed by the effects of prior chemotherapy, with a slight additional rise in the leucocyte count due to plerixafor. This is substantially higher than would be seen for chemomobilisation (either with or without plerixafor), where white cell count will typically be in the range of $8–20 \times 10^9$/L at the time of

HPC-A procurement. In the experience of the author's own centre, median white cell count in a series of 21 patients mobilised with plerixafor (mostly without prior mobilising chemotherapy) was 29.8×10^9/L compared with a median white cell count of 15.1 in a series of 25 chemomobilised patients [7]. This might be expected to impact on cryopreservation volumes, and this has indeed been the experience of several centres. This problem is compounded further by the fact that patients mobilised with plerixafor will by definition have mobilised PBSC poorly by conventional means, and will therefore tend to have relatively low peripheral CD34$^+$ counts even when plerixafor is used. HPC-A products procured using G-CSF plus plerixafor without prior mobilising chemotherapy tend to be large-volume, dilute and granulocyte-rich, and this inevitably leads to large cryopreservation volumes [5].

In the experience of the author's centre, the issue of higher cryopreservation volumes when mobilising HPC-A with G-CSF plus plerixafor but without prior mobilising chemotherapy has not been insurmountable: it is generally possible to re-infuse the cryopreserved product over two or three days, although there are some impacts on liquid nitrogen storage space, lab staff time and BMT Unit nursing staff time. Potential solutions to cryopreservation volume issues with plerixafor include first using a cell separator platform that minimises granulocyte contamination of the HPC-A product, and second incorporating plerixafor into chemomobilisation protocols so that the patient's total white cell count is lower at the time of collection. Both of these approaches potentially appear effective, as discussed in section "Impact of Plerixafor on Apheresis for Autologous HPC Procurement: Initial Published Experience and Clinical Protocols" below.

What Are the Definitions of "Mobilisation Failure" and of "Poor Mobilisation"? Target HPC-A CD34$^+$ Cell Doses and Engraftment

It is now well established that total CD34$^+$ cell dose in the HPC-A product is the best predictor for successful engraftment, with higher CD34$^+$ cell doses correlating with higher probabilities of successful and durable neutrophil and platelet engraftment following high-dose chemotherapy and autologous HPC-A transplant [38–41]. However, the effect of CD34$^+$ dose on engraftment is not linear, but an asymptotic curve [41]: in other words, the impact of increasing transplanted CD34$^+$ cell doses on engraftment time becomes progressively less as CD34$^+$ dose increases, until the graph eventually flattens off completely. A theoretical autologous transplant with an infinitely high dose of CD34$^+$ cells would still result in neutrophil and platelet engraftment times of around 8 days, due to the minimum times taken for production of mature blood cells from HPC-A after successful re-engraftment in the bone marrow. The question of "where to stop" in terms of *optimum* CD34$^+$ dose for autologous transplant—in other words, at what level do further increases in transplanted CD34$^+$ dose become clinically meaningless—remains unresolved and hotly debated [42–45]. In terms of *minimum acceptable* CD34$^+$ dose for autologous transplant, there is more consensus: a CD34$^+$ dose of 2×10^6/kg is generally regarded as giving a high probability of successful and durable neutrophil and platelet engraftment for the majority of patients [46], although some centres (the author's included) may set a slightly higher minimum acceptable dose of 2.5×10^6/kg to reduce the risk of failed platelet engraftment.

Generally speaking, when carrying out HPC-A collection for autologous transplantation, three separate threshold levels of CD34$^+$ dose are potentially important:

1. *Minimum acceptable target CD34$^+$ dose*: this is the cell dose below which the patient will not proceed with autologous transplant by local policy, because the risk of failed or delayed neutrophil or platelet engraftment is considered too high.
2. *"Stop dose"*: this is the cell dose at which level the patient will not be put back on the machine for a further day's apheresis, because the quality-of-life and financial costs of further apheresis are felt to outweigh the clinical benefits. The "stop dose" may vary with the patient's clinical diagnosis; with how many aphereses have already been carried out (most centres will "cap" the number of aphereses per patient at somewhere between 3 and 5, due to cost and increasing cryopreservation volume); and with whether there is a likelihood of the patient undergoing more than one autologous transplant (in which case "stop dose" will be higher).
3. *Optimum dose*: this is the cell dose beyond which further HPC-A collection would offer no further clinical benefit. It is a useful concept for purposes such as research use of "surplus" autologous PBSC: cells should generally only be taken for research purposes if and when the patient has had a true "optimum dose" cryopreserved for his or her own use.

Note that "stop dose" is not the same as "optimum dose". For patients who are truly "good mobilisers" with very high peripheral CD34$^+$ counts, most centres will hope to collect the optimum dose in a single apheresis procedure. However, providing the patient achieves the "stop dose", a second day's apheresis will not be undertaken. For "intermediate mobilisers", where the "stop dose" is not achieved in a single apheresis, apheresis will continue daily until either the "stop dose" is achieved, or the patient has reached the maximum permissible number of aphereses according to local policy (typically a maximum number of between 3 and 5 consecutive apheresis days). For "poor mobilisers"—patients with peripheral CD34$^+$ counts that are low but not so low as to make apheresis worthless—there is little prospect of the patient reaching the "stop dose", and the target becomes the "minimum acceptable dose" instead. The patient will generally undergo apheresis daily until either the minimum acceptable dose has been reached, or the maximum permissible number of aphereses has been reached. Patients may be considered to be "absolute failed mobilisers" if their peripheral CD34$^+$ counts are so low that apheresis would be worthless, and no apheresis is undertaken.

It is possible to incorporate all of the considerations above into a local decision-making flowchart, based on the patient's peripheral CD34$^+$ count per microlitre on the morning of apheresis, and the cumulative CD34$^+$ cell dose x 10^6/kg collected to date. Figure 8.2 shows the decision-making flowchart used by the Scottish National Blood Transfusion Service for autologous HPC-A collection.

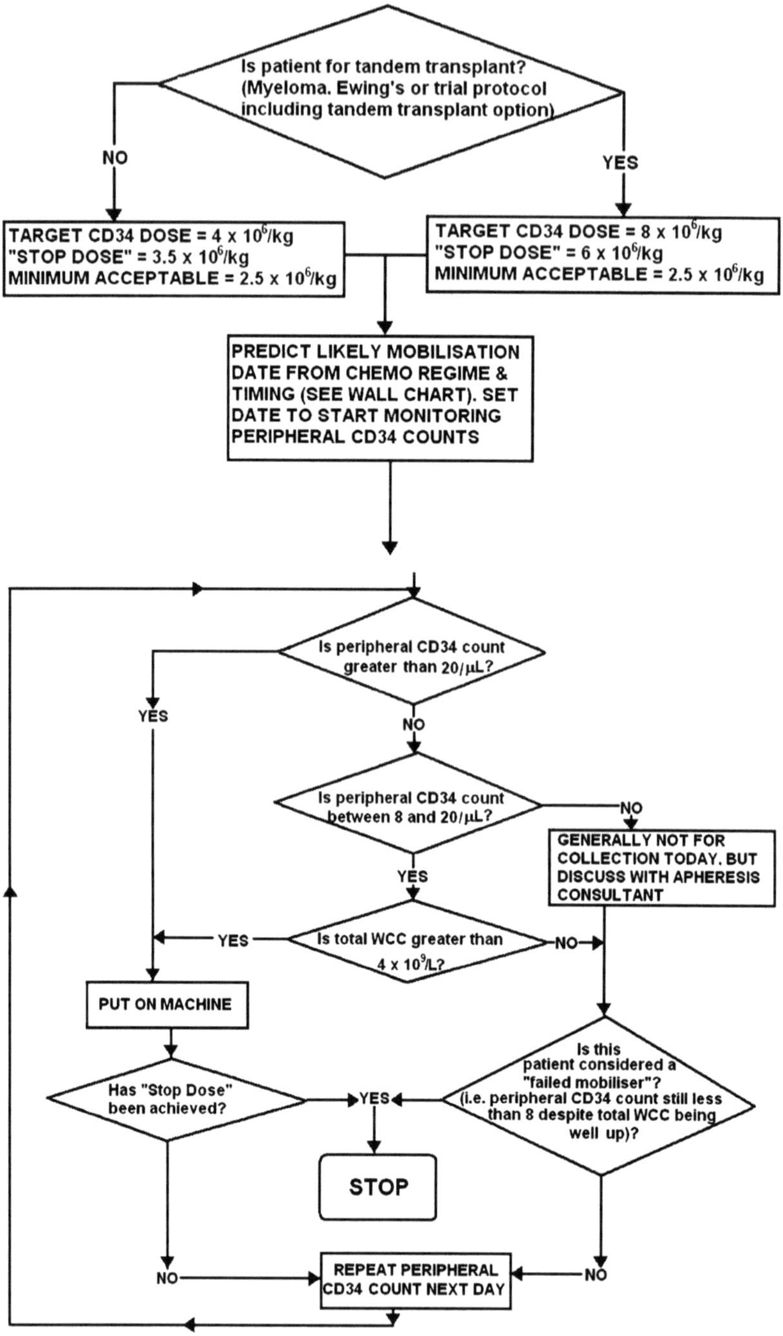

Fig. 8.2 Flowchart used for apheresis decision-making in non-plerixafor collections at the author's centre. Taken from current Scottish National Blood Transfusion (SNBTS) West of Scotland Standard Operating Procedure for autologous HPC-A procurement, and used by permission

Patients can be divided into several different groups in terms of the autologous $CD34^+$ dose achieved:

1. Optimal mobilisation: the patient has achieved the optimum $CD34^+$ dose.
2. Adequate but not optimal mobilisation: the patient has achieved the minimum target cell dose, but optimum dose has not been achieved after several days' apheresis.
3. Failed mobilisation but apheresis attempted: the patient's peripheral $CD34^+$ count has been high enough for apheresis to be initiated, but the minimum target dose has not been achieved after several days' apheresis.
4. Absolute failed mobilisation: the patient's peripheral $CD34^+$ count has been so low that apheresis has not been attempted.

Novel mobilisation agents such as plerixafor clearly have the potential to move patients up the "ladder" of mobilisation success as described above, at any level: however, for most apheresis clinicians and HPC transplant physicians, the priority will be getting patients from Category 3 or 4 (failed or absolute failed mobilisation) into Category 2 (adequate but not optimal mobilisation), so that the patient is able to proceed to autologous HPC transplant. Section "Impact of Plerixafor on Apheresis for Autologous HPC Procurement: Initial Published Experience and Clinical Protocols" below discusses published experience to date with clinical protocols using plerixafor to achieve this goal.

Impact of Plerixafor on Apheresis for Autologous HPC Procurement: Initial Published Experience and Clinical Protocols

Pre-licensing Experience with Plerixafor, from Clinical Studies and from US and European Compassionate Use Programmes

As discussed above, established practice in HPC-A collection is that autologous HPC-A are collected either by chemomobilisation, or using G-CSF alone. Both approaches are effective for most but not all patients, with somewhat better results in terms of $CD34^+$ dose achieved when using chemomobilisation, but at the expense of increased toxicity. It is also important to note that cyclophosphamide and other chemotherapy drugs are not currently licensed for purposes of HPC-A procurement, so this is off-licence use.

All of the pre-licensing clinical studies assessing plerixafor as a HPC-A mobilisation agent, and also the US and European Compassionate Use Programmes, used a mobilisation regime where plerixafor was incorporated into a G-CSF mobilisation protocol without prior mobilising chemotherapy (see Fig. 8.3). This was not because it had been anticipated that plerixafor would be difficult to incorporate into chemomobilisation protocols, but simply that there are considerable regulatory obstacles

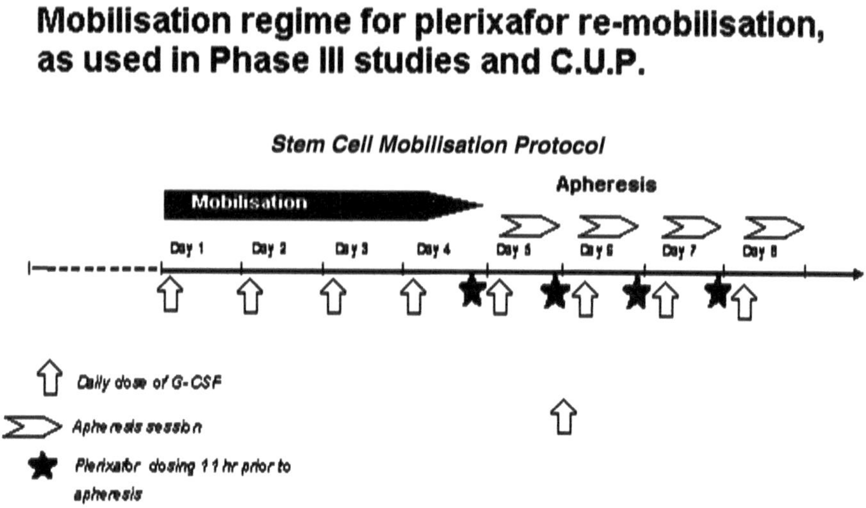

Fig. 8.3 Schedule used for HPC-A mobilisation with G-CSF and plerixafor in pivotal pre-licensing studies, and in most C.U.P. patients (Genzyme diagram, used by permission)

to the inclusion of off-licence use of chemotherapeutic agents (for purposes of HPC-A procurement) into clinical research protocols. However, it would be fair to say that this has initially skewed the way that the drug has been used post-licensing, and it is only relatively recently that there has been any published experience relating to the use of plerixafor in combination with chemomobilisation.

Prior to the licensing of plerixafor for autologous HPC-A collection, the drug was assessed in pivotal Phase III studies in patients with myeloma or NHL [34, 35]. Patients were randomised to receive either G-CSF plus plerixafor (see Fig. 8.3 for regime used), or G-CSF alone at the same dosage. In terms of the primary end point of "optimal" HPC-A mobilisation, it was found that plerixafor significantly increased the proportion of myeloma patients achieving a $CD34^{+}$ dose of 6×10^{6}/kg in 2 or fewer aphereses (70.3% versus 34.4% for placebo; $p<0.001$), and significantly increased the proportion of lymphoma patients achieving a $CD34^{+}$ dose of 5×10^{6}/kg in 4 aphereses or less and subsequently engrafting successfully following autograft (57.3% versus 18.9% for placebo; $p<0.001$). In terms of secondary end points, a significantly greater proportion of patients in the plerixafor groups in both studies proceeded to transplant, and a significantly smaller proportion of patients failed to achieve a minimum transplant dose of 2×10^{6}/kg $CD34^{+}$ cells.

Considerable "real-world" experience in the use of plerixafor for patients failing to mobilise HPC-A by conventional means came from Genzyme's Compassionate Use Programmes (C.U.P.s) in the USA and (later) in Europe. Prior to regulatory approval of plerixafor for HPC-A collection, Genzyme USA had made the drug available on a named-patient basis between 2006 and 2007 to patients previously failing to mobilise HPC-A by conventional means, as part of a Compassionate Use Programme. The published experience from 115 patients with lymphoma or myeloma in the US C.U.P., all of whom had previously failed to mobilise HPC-A by conventional means, was that a minimum transplantable HPC-A dose of 2×10^6/kg was achieved by 60.3% of patients with NHL, 71.4% of myeloma patients, and 75% of patients with Hodgkin's Lymphoma [36]. When compared with published historical experience of re-mobilisation success rates of 20–50% without plerixafor in patients failing prior PBSC mobilisation [47, 48], this suggested a high degree of efficacy for plerixafor as a mobilisation agent. There were no drug-related serious adverse events. This very positive clinical experience with plerixafor was subsequently replicated in a European Compassionate Use Programme, in which the drug was made available by Genzyme Europe on a named-patient basis between May 2008 and July 2009 for myeloma or lymphoma patients failing HPC-A mobilisation by conventional means. In a series of 56 consecutive Spanish and UK patients from the European C.U.P., the overall success rate in mobilising a minimum transplantable $CD34^+$ dose of 2×10^6/kg was 75% [37].

Ongoing data collection from the US and European C.U.P., including subgroup analysis, is continuing to generate useful "real-world" published clinical experience with plerixafor, some of which is discussed below. Broadly speaking, delayed re-mobilisation of patients failing HPC-A mobilisation by conventional means using a G-CSF-plus-plerixafor protocol (as shown in Fig. 8.3) has been found to be reliable and easy to schedule, with strikingly low toxicity. However, as discussed in section "Cryopreservation Issues" above, there is the potential disadvantage that apheresis is carried out at a time when the patient's white cell count is markedly elevated, and this can cause issues with excessive cryopreservation volume [5].

An Overview of Post-licensing Experience, Including Logistical Aspects of Plerixafor Use

Perhaps unsurprisingly, most initial experience with plerixafor following its regulatory approval, first in the US and subsequently in Europe, tended to involve use along with G-CSF but without prior mobilising chemotherapy, as in the pre-licensing studies and the C.U.P. patients. However, towards the end of the European C.U.P., some European clinicians had requested permission from Genzyme to incorporate the drug into chemomobilisation protocols, predominantly for patients with higher-grade lymphomas for whom it would have been undesirable to have long periods without chemotherapy for purposes of HPC-A mobilisation. Incorporation of plerixafor into chemotherapy-based re-mobilisation protocols (often involving lymphoma "salvage" chemotherapy regimes) allowed re-mobilisation of patients failing prior HPC-A mobilisation by conventional means, without necessitating a prolonged time gap with no chemotherapy. Published experience with an initial series of 13 European C.U.P. patients from Italy, Austria and the UK where plerixafor had been incorporated into chemomobilisation regimes confirmed this to be a safe and effective way of using the drug. All 13 patients mobilised a minimum transplant dose of greater than 2×10^6/kg $CD34^+$ cells in 1–3 aphereses, and there were no drug-related serious adverse events. At the time of publication, five patients had undergone autologous transplant and had engraftment data available: engraftment had been prompt and durable in all cases. The median fold-increase in peripheral CD34$^+$ count from pre-plerixafor levels on the morning of the day of plerixafor administration, to the morning of Day +1 post-plerixafor, was 4.7. Although the exact regime varied from centre to centre, in general plerixafor was started on a "pre-emptive" basis based on a poor peripheral CD34$^+$ count on what would otherwise have been the predicted day of first apheresis, depending on the chemotherapy regime used, with the actual first apheresis being the following day [49]. A number of German patients in the European C.U.P. also received plerixafor in combination with chemo-mobilisation, generally with good outcomes: this series has now been published as part of the total German experience from the C.U.P. [50].

A number of US and European centres have investigated the use of plerixafor in what has been variously described as a "pre-emptive", "on-demand" or "immediate rescue" manner [51–57]. Rather than allowing a patient to fail a complete mobilisation episode, and then attempting re-mobilisation using G-CSF plus plerixafor (± mobilising chemotherapy) four or more weeks later, as was generally done for C.U.P. patients, plerixafor can be administered *immediately* in the course of a single mobilisation episode to a patient who appears to be failing HPC-A mobilisation by conventional means, on the basis of poor peripheral CD34$^+$ counts and/or poor CD34$^+$ doses in apheresis products. Potential advantages in using plerixafor in a "pre-emptive" manner are first that it is likely to be more cost-effective (the drug is used only for patients where it is needed, and it may be more effective in combination with mobilising chemotherapy so that fewer plerixafor doses are given on average), second that the costs of re-mobilising the patient (which include financial, toxicity and quality-of-life "costs") are avoided, and finally that patients are able to proceed immediately with their planned autologous HPC-A transplant without a need for rescheduling following delayed re-mobilisation, with obvious quality-of-life benefits for the patient as well as efficiency savings for the Transplant Unit. Experience to date with "pre-emptive" use of plerixafor is discussed in more detail in section "Evolving Patterns of Plerixafor Use: From Re-mobilisation to Pre-emptive Use" below.

There has also been interest in the use of plerixafor (sometimes "up-front") in specific patient groups, where HPC-A mobilisation by conventional means is currently sometimes problematic. These groups include children with neuroblastoma and similar solid tumours (see section "Special Patient Groups: (1) Children Undergoing Apheresis for Autologous HPC-A Procurement," below), adult patients with dialysis-dependent renal failure (see section "Special Patient Groups: (2) Adult Patients with Dialysis-Dependent Renal Failure" below), patients pretreated with fludarabine or with lenalidomide, and patients with low baseline platelet counts due to heavy pretreatment with chemotherapy.

The progressively evolving patterns of plerixafor use, moving from second-line use for re-mobilisation of previous failed mobilisers, to pre-emptive use, and then to potential "up-front" first-line use in selected patient groups, are summarised in Fig. 8.4.

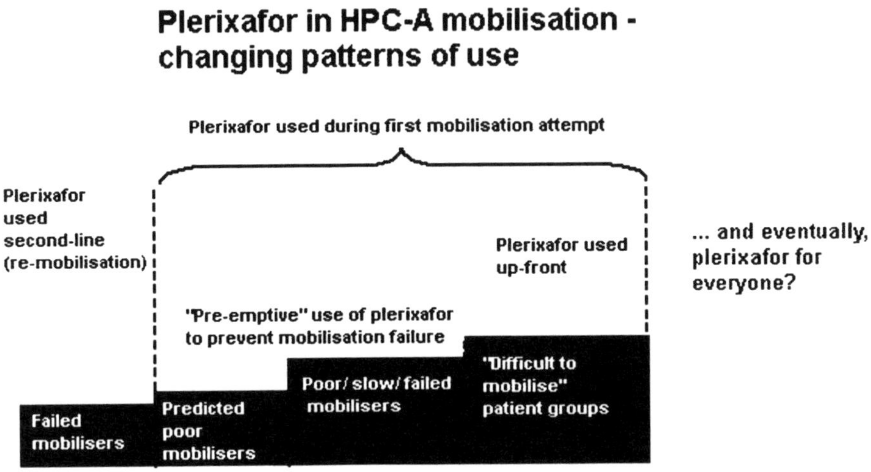

Fig. 8.4 Evolving patterns of plerixafor use (original diagram)

Evolving Patterns of Plerixafor Use: From Re-mobilisation to "Pre-emptive" Use

As discussed above, the conventional approach to plerixafor use is to wait until a patient has completely failed a HPC-A mobilisation episode, and then to re-mobilise the patient four or more weeks later using plerixafor along with G-CSF (± mobilising chemotherapy). However, this involves rescheduling of the patient's initial planned dates for autologous transplant, which is not ideal either for the patient or for the Transplant Unit. Also, it may not be the most cost-effective way of using plerixafor. Would it not perhaps be better to introduce plerixafor immediately during the course of a mobilisation episode, if the patient seems likely to fail to achieve a transplantable HPC-A dose, either on the basis of poor peripheral $CD34^+$ counts or because of poor $CD34^+$ doses in the apheresis products? This question has been investigated by several centres to date, with some results having been published in abstract form. It has proven feasible to use plerixafor "pre-emptively" both in combination with G-CSF-only mobilisation, and in combination with chemomobilisation.

The first clinical data on "pre-emptive" plerixafor use relate to pre-emptive use of the drug with G-CSF mobilisation. Results from the Mayo Clinic in the USA were presented in abstract form at the ASH Annual Scientific Meeting in 2009, with further data presented in abstract at the Tandem meeting in 2010 [51, 52]. A risk-adapted approach to plerixafor use was adopted for 147 consecutive patients with myeloma or lymphoma undergoing G-CSF-only mobilisation. Peripheral $CD34^+$ count was checked on Day 5 of G-CSF. Patients with Day 5 peripheral $CD34^+$ count of less than 10 per microlitre did not undergo apheresis that day but received plerixafor pre-emptively that evening, with apheresis the following morning. Additionally, patients undergoing apheresis on Day 5 of G-CSF but achieving a $CD34^+$ cell dose of less than

0.5×10^6/kg, also received plerixafor pre-emptively on the evening of Day 5 with further apheresis the following morning. Historical data from a series of 80 patients undergoing G-CSF-only mobilisation without plerixafor was used as a comparator group. In the historical comparator group, there was a 28% mobilisation failure rate overall, and patients with Day 5 peripheral CD34⁺ count below 10 per microlitre were at greater than 50% risk of mobilisation failure. In the plerixafor group, some 72% of patients had a Day 5 peripheral CD34⁺ count below 10 per microlitre, but the overall mobilisation failure rate was just 5%. The University of Kansas Medical Center presented similar results in abstract form at the 2010 Tandem meeting [53]. In a series of 50 patients with lymphoma or myeloma undergoing G-CSF-only mobilisation, a similar risk-adapted approach was adopted, with plerixafor being introduced pre-emptively either if Day 5 peripheral CD34⁺ count was below 20 per microlitre, or if the CD34⁺ cell yield on the first apheresis day was less than half of the desired target cell dose. Sixteen patients (32%) received pre-emptive plerixafor, of whom only 2 patients failed to achieve a transplantable CD34⁺ dose. This represented an overall failed mobilisation rate of just 2/80 or 3%, which compared very favourably with historical pre-plerixafor failed mobilisation rates at the same institution of 18–19%. Similar experiences with "pre-emptive" plerixafor following G-CSF-only mobilisation have also been reported by other US centres [54, 55]: one of these series has now been published in full including economic analysis, and is discussed in section "Financial Aspects of Incorporating Plerixafor into Apheresis Protocols" below [55].

Similar results from ongoing data analysis of patients from the European C.U.P. were published in abstract form at the EBMT Annual Scientific Meeting in 2010 [56]. For a series of 38 C.U.P. patients, peripheral CD34⁺ count results were available on Day 4 of G-CSF (i.e. pre-plerixafor samples from the morning of the day of plerixafor administration) as well as peripheral CD34⁺ count results from Day 5 of G-CSF (which was Day +1 post-plerixafor and the first day of apheresis). This made it possible to carry out a "virtual study", using historical data from 175 patients with myeloma or lymphoma mobilised with G-CSF-only protocols at the same centres as a control group. The control patients also had peripheral CD34⁺ count results available both from Day 4 and from Day 5 of G-CSF. Two questions could therefore be asked: first, what levels of Day 4 peripheral CD34⁺ count predict for mobilisation failure when plerixafor is not used, and second, what effect does intervention with plerixafor on the evening of Day 4 have on this predicted mobilisation failure? It was found that where plerixafor was not used, a Day 4 peripheral CD34⁺ count below 20 per microlitre predicted only a 65% chance of mobilising a minimum transplantable CD34⁺ dose of 2×10^6/kg, and in the subgroup of patients with a Day 4 peripheral CD34⁺ count below 10 per microlitre, this fell to just a 53% chance of mobilising a minimum transplantable dose. With the addition of plerixafor, the proportions of patients achieving a minimum transplantable cell dose improved substantially: 89% for the CUP patients overall, and 87% for CUP patients with a Day 4 peripheral CD34⁺ count below 10 per microlitre. These data suggest that "pre-emptive" use of plerixafor in patients undergoing G-CSF-only mobilisation of autologous HPC-A, whose peripheral CD34⁺ count on Day 4 of G-CSF is below 10 per microlitre, is likely to improve the chances of achieving a transplantable cell dose from just over 50% to almost 90%. Clearly, there are now good grounds to investigate this further in a prospective RCT.

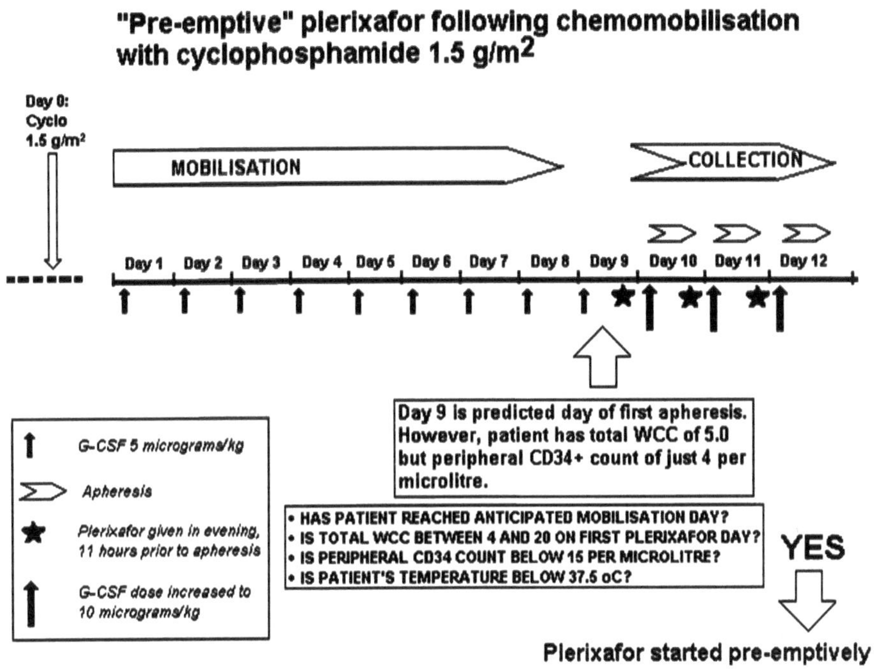

Fig. 8.5 Schedule used for HPC-A chemomobilisation with pre-emptive plerixafor in a hypothetical patient receiving cyclophosphamide 1.5 g/m² with G-CSF for HPC-A procurement (original diagram)

It is also possible to use plerixafor pre-emptively for patients failing chemomobilisation: indeed, this was the approach adopted in the published case series by D'Addio et al. discussed above, although the exact intervention protocol for pre-emptive plerixafor use varied between centres [49]. The author's centre has used plerixafor pre-emptively on a routine basis since European licensing in July 2009, predominantly in combination with chemomobilisation. This has been carried out according to a pre-agreed local protocol, with plerixafor being introduced pre-emptively if the following combination of factors are met: the patient is no more than 1 day before the anticipated day of first mobilisation based on the mobilising chemotherapy regime used (a table is in use locally to predict first apheresis day based on local historical data for that chemotherapy regime—see Table 8.3, which is given as an Appendix to this chapter); the peripheral CD34⁺ count on day of first plerixafor administration is less than 15 per microlitre; the patient's total white cell count on day of first plerixafor administration is more than 4 but less than 20×10^9/L; and the patient is clinically infection-free with temperature of 37.5°C or less. Figure 8.5 summarises this in diagrammatic form for a hypothetical patient undergoing mobilisation after cyclophosphamide 1.5 g/m². To date, data are available for 14 adult patients where plerixafor was used pre-emptively following chemomobilisation on the protocol above. A transplantable CD34⁺ cell dose was achieved in 12 cases (86%), in between 1 and 3 aphereses. The two patients failing to achieve a transplantable cell dose both underwent successful re-mobilisation using G-CSF plus plerixafor after a delay of

4 weeks or more. These results have been presented in abstract form at EBMT 2011 as part of our total single-centre plerixafor experience [57], which is discussed in more detail in section "Financial Aspects of Incorporating Plerixafor into Apheresis Protocols" below. At least one other UK centre has experienced very similar outcomes with pre-emptive plerixafor use following chemomobilisation in a large series of myeloma patients mobilised with cyclophosphamide 3 g/m^2 (Professor Nigel Russell, Nottingham; personal communication).

Potential Solutions to the Problem of Higher Cryopreservation Volumes

As discussed in section "Cryopreservation Issues" above, if plerixafor is incorporated into G-CSF-only mobilisation protocols without prior mobilising chemotherapy, then cryopreservation volumes are often high due to the patient's significantly elevated total WCC at the time of collection, which leads in turn to a high TNC in the product and a high cryopreservation volume. Potential solutions to cryopreservation volume issues with plerixafor include first using a cell separator platform that minimises granulocyte contamination of the HPC-A product, and second incorporating plerixafor into chemomobilisation protocols so that the patient's total white cell count is lower at the time of collection. In the author's experience, both of these approaches are entirely feasible.

The author's centre was involved both in initial pre-marketing evaluation of the novel Spectra Optia® apheresis platform for PBSC collection, and in the European Compassionate Use Programme for plerixafor. We became aware that cryopreservation volume was a frequent issue when collecting PBSC post-plerixafor using the MNC setting on COBE Spectra. On introduction of Spectra Optia for PBSC collection, we noted that the effect of plerixafor on cryopreservation volume seemed much less marked, and we decided to audit this more closely. Data were collected from a series of 21 consecutive apheresis procedures from 16 patients, where plerixafor had been used as part of the conditioning regime. In this group of patients, Spectra Optia (Version 5 software) was used for 10 procedures and COBE Spectra (MNC setting) for 11 procedures. As a comparator group, a series of 26 temporally matched apheresis procedures from 18 consecutive patients were audited, where plerixafor had not been used. In the non-plerixafor group, Spectra Optia was used for 7 procedures and COBE Spectra for 19 procedures. Total cryopreservation volume was determined for each PBSC collection, as well as the patient's total WCC at the time of collection. As expected, the plerixafor patients had significantly higher total WCC at the time of apheresis (median WCC of 29.8 compared with median WCC of 15.1 for non-plerixafor patients; $p<0.001$). However, although cryopreservation volume was relatively high for post-plerixafor collections carried out using COBE Spectra (median volume 756 mL; range 524–2,400 mL), this was not the case for post-plerixafor collections carried out using Optia (median volume 351 mL; range 170–716 mL; $p<0.001$). Optia appears to limit cryopreservation volumes in HPC-A products because of lower granulocyte contamination in the PBSC product, with this effect being most marked when apheresis is carried out on a high total WCC (as is the case when plerixafor is used along with G-CSF but without mobilising chemotherapy). This data was presented in abstract form at ASH 2010 [7].

A potential alternative (or additional) way of limiting cryopreservation volumes in post-plerixafor collections is to incorporate plerixafor into chemomobilisation, rather than using the drug along with G-CSF without prior mobilising chemotherapy. Most apheresis centres have found that patients undergoing chemomobilisation have lower total WCC at the time of apheresis than patients undergoing G-CSF-only mobilisation: this is not unexpected, as peak peripheral $CD34^+$ counts are generally seen around the time that WCC first returns to normal levels on regeneration from chemotherapy, whereas with G-CSF-only mobilisation, peak peripheral $CD34^+$ counts are generally seen on Day 5 of G-CSF, at which time patients will generally have significant leucocytosis. At the author's centre, historical data before plerixafor became available for clinical use showed median total WCC at the time of apheresis to be approximately 12×10^9/L for chemomobilisation patients, compared with approximately 35×10^9/L for G-CSF-only mobilisation patients. Although plerixafor will slightly increase total WCC over and above the effect of G-CSF, this effect is relatively slight. It might be expected therefore that the use of plerixafor on a pre-emptive basis after chemomobilisation would limit cryopreservation volumes by reducing the patient's total WCC at the time of apheresis. This does indeed appear to have been the case in our own initial experience (unpublished data).

Financial Aspects of Incorporating Plerixafor into Apheresis Protocols

Due largely to its "ultra-orphan" status, plerixafor is an expensive drug in terms of unit cost, retailing at the time of writing at around £5,000 per 24 mg vial in the UK (approximately equivalent to $8,000 in US currency or to 6,000 Euros). However, patients who require plerixafor for autologous HPC-A procurement will require relatively few doses in the entire course of their treatment, generally only between 1 and 3 doses for the great majority of patients where the drug is used. Also, the majority of patients will mobilise autologous HPC-A by conventional means without the addition of plerixafor, so that the cost of the drug becomes substantially lower when averaged out among all patients in an autologous HPC-A transplant programme.

The cost of plerixafor may be partially or entirely offset first by reduction in the costs of re-mobilisation of HPC-A (or alternatively, the costs of autologous bone marrow harvest) for patients failing PBSC mobilisation by conventional means, and second by reduction in the costs of expensive third-line therapeutic options (such as lenalidomide or bortezomib) for patients unable to undergo autologous PBSC transplant due to HPC-A mobilisation failure.

Some attempts at economic costings for plerixafor have been published over the past 2 years. A group from the Medical University of South Carolina has published a cost-saving decision-making algorithm [55] based on mathematical modelling of observed outcomes ($CD34^+$ dose obtained depending on peripheral $CD34^+$ counts on Day 4 and Day 5 of G-CSF mobilisation) in a group of 50 patients with myeloma or NHL mobilised without the use of plerixafor, and assuming that the introduction of plerixafor on Day 4 would have led to an approximately threefold increase in peripheral $CD34^+$ count on Day 5 (which was exactly what was seen in the two pivotal pre-licensing studies [34, 35]). This model predicts that the introduction of plerixafor on a "pre-emptive" basis would become cost-effective for patients where the target $CD34^+$ dose was 3×10^6/kg (for instance, most NHL patients) if Day 4 peripheral $CD34^+$ count was below 15 per microlitre, and that use of "pre-emptive" plerixafor would become cost-effective for patients where the target $CD34^+$ dose was 6×10^6/kg (for instance, younger myeloma patients scheduled for tandem transplant) if Day 4 peripheral $CD34^+$ count was below 28 per microlitre. Predicted cost-effectiveness was on the basis of apheresis days saved and re-mobilisation episodes prevented.

Two studies have been published in abstract form in which total costs of mobilisation with G-CSF plus plerixafor (based on data from patients in the US C.U.P.) were compared against total costs of chemomobilisation along with G-CSF but without plerixafor [58, 59]. In both studies, overall costs were very similar, but a significantly higher proportion of patients achieved a transplantable $CD34^+$ cell dose using G-CSF plus plerixafor, suggesting that "up-front" plerixafor would be cost-neutral but more effective when compared against chemomobilisation. A similar study published in abstract form comparing the costs of mobilisation with G-CSF plus plerixafor against G-CSF-only mobilisation (data from patients from the US C.U.P. versus a historical control group) suggests that the use of G-CSF plus plerixafor is more costly (by about $5,000 US on average) but much more effective, with 100% of patients in the G-CSF plus plerixafor group achieving a transplantable $CD34^+$ dose versus only 60% in the G-CSF-only group. If an assumption was made that patients failing G-CSF-only would require re-mobilisation with G-CSF plus plerixafor, then the cost differential fell to only $1,998 in favour of the G-CSF-only group [60].

The author's centre has recently presented in abstract form a total single-centre experience with plerixafor use in 40 mobilisation episodes in 37 patients between June 2008 and December 2010, including 14 European C.U.P. patients and a further 23 patients post-licensing for whom plerixafor was generally used pre-emptively following chemomobilisation [57]. This represented 16% of all mobilisation episodes at our centre over this time period. For patients receiving plerixafor, the success rate in achieving local institutional minimum $CD34^+$ dose of 2.5×10^6/kg for subsequent autologous transplant was 92% (34/37 attempts) at first mobilisation using plerixafor, and rose to 100% (3/3 attempts) at re-mobilisation using plerixafor in the 3 patients failing at first attempt, i.e. ultimately a 100% autologous HPC-A mobilisation success rate. Median $CD34^+$ dose ultimately achieved was 3.33×10^6/kg (2.57–8.42), after a median of 2 aphereses per patient (range 1–5) and a mean of 1.73 plerixafor doses per patient (range 1–5). Most patients in the autologous transplant programme (84%) did not require plerixafor. The additional cost of plerixafor per patient in the programme to achieve 100% mobilisation success was therefore (£5,000 × 0.16 × 1.73) = £1,384. This compares with a historical failed HPC-A mobilisation rate at our centre of approximately 15%. Even allowing a relatively conservative figure of £8,000 for the total cost of re-mobilising a patient failing initial HPC-A mobilisation using chemotherapy without plerixafor (which would generally have been our approach in the past), plerixafor is likely to be virtually cost-neutral. Given that plerixafor is significantly more effective than re-mobilisation with either G-CSF alone or chemotherapy plus G-CSF (historically only around 40% effective in re-mobilising patients failing initial HPC-A mobilisation at our centre), it is difficult to argue against its general incorporation into autologous HPC-A mobilisation protocols.

"How to Do plerixafor": A Personal View

Having reviewed above the current published evidence relating to the incorporation of plerixafor into apheresis protocols for HPC-A collection, the author feels it may be helpful to summarise "how to do plerixafor" from an entirely subjective and personal viewpoint.

Of the three ways in which plerixafor has been used (delayed re-mobilisation with plerixafor plus G-CSF for previous failed mobilisers; "pre-emptive" use with G-CSF-only mobilisation; "pre-emptive" use after chemomobilisation), each has both advantages and disadvantages, and there is unlikely to be a single, one-size-fits-all method of using the drug that will be suitable for all patients. I summarise potential advantages and disadvantages of each method in Table 8.2.

In my opinion, there is little point in attempting to identify "likely poor mobilisers" in advance, based on such known risk factors for poor mobilisation as cumulative prior chemotherapy, exposure to fludarabine or lenalidomide, age or prior radiotherapy. Some patients who are predicted to mobilise poorly actually mobilise successfully without requiring plerixafor, while conversely some patients who would be predicted to mobilise well actually mobilise poorly (or fail altogether) without plerixafor. For this reason, it is best from the patient's point of view, and also probably more cost-effective, to have plerixafor universally available for pre-emptive use if required in all lymphoma or myeloma patients undergoing autologous HPC-A mobilisation. From a logistical point of view, this requires having a local protocol with pre-agreed criteria for plerixafor use, and a stock of the drug "on the shelf" in the hospital pharmacy which can be accessed at short notice for patients who are failing HPC-A mobilisation by conventional means. This clearly requires close collaboration with pharmacy and management colleagues.

I prefer to use plerixafor pre-emptively along with chemomobilisation, rather than combining the drug with G-CSF without prior mobilising chemotherapy, for two reasons: first because this is probably the most effective way of using the drug in terms of its impact on $CD34^+$ cell doses achieved, and second because use with chemomobilisation helps to prevent excessive cryopreservation volumes for the

Table 8.2 Potential advantages and disadvantages for published methods of plerixafor use

Method	Advantages	Disadvantages
"Delayed re-mobilisation" with G-CSF plus plerixafor	• Timing of apheresis sessions is completely predictable—very helpful for Apheresis Unit • Successful in achieving a transplantable CD34+ dose for most patients, with a median of two doses of plerixafor • Toxicities are low	• PBSC collection done on a high WCC, so product is more cellular—high cryopreservation volumes • Theoretically, potential danger of hyperleucocytosis and its side-effects (splenic rupture, arterial thrombosis etc) • Probably less cost-effective than "immediate-rescue" use
"Pre-emptive" use of plerixafor for poor mobilisers following chemomobilisation	• More cost-effective: some patients predicted to mobilise poorly (e.g. heavily pretreated) actually do OK and don't need plerixafor • No delay for the patient—able to proceed to transplant on planned date • Bigger plerixafor effect on CD34 count: possibly fewer plerixafor doses required on average to achieve transplantable cell dose • Collection done on lower WCC—gets round cryopreservation volume issues	• Plerixafor toxicities may be higher if added to pre-existing toxicities of chemo, especially gastrointestinal toxicities • Not as predictable in terms of apheresis scheduling • Potential problem with collections falling on weekend days (there are problems with weekend aphereses at many centres)
"Pre-emptive" use of plerixafor for poor mobilisers in the course, of G-CSF only mobilisation	• More cost-effective: some patients predicted to mobilise poorly (e.g. heavily pretreated) actually do OK and do not need plerixafor • No delay for the patient—able to proceed to transplant on planned date • Predictable apheresis scheduling—good for the apheresis unit • Low toxicity (especially GI) compared to post-chemotherapy immediate rescue use	• Collection on higher white cell count, leading to higher cryopreservation volumes and higher DMSO exposure for patient at time of re-infusion • May be somewhat less effective than post-chemotherapy pre-emptive use, particularly for very heavily pretreated patients (no direct comparisons done to date, however)

HPC-A product as discussed above. For successful use of plerixafor pre-emptively following chemomobilisation, it is vital to know the anticipated day of first apheresis depending on the mobilising chemotherapy regime used. This involves either standardising chemomobilisation by using the same regime for all patients with a single diagnosis, or developing local guidance such as a mobilisation chart giving anticipated mobilisation timings for all mobilising chemotherapy regimes based on historical audit data from your own centre. At the Beatson West of Scotland Cancer Centre, lymphoma patients are generally mobilised using the patient's scheduled lymphoma salvage chemotherapy (such as IVE or ESHAP), while myeloma patients are generally mobilised using cyclophosphamide 1.5 g/m^2, which has relatively low toxicity while still being effective in mobilising good CD34⁺ cell doses for the majority of patients.

For apheresis procedures following plerixafor, I would advocate processing a minimum of 3 blood volumes per apheresis, so as to maximise the benefit of the drug for the patient and reduce the number of aphereses required (which obviously also reduces direct drug costs by reducing the number of plerixafor doses required). It is important to start apheresis as early in the day as possible, so as to have time for a "long run" as well as time to resolve any venous access difficulties or other unforeseen problems. Because of this, if your centre (like ours) has a turnaround time of more than 1 h for peripheral $CD34^+$ counts, then I would suggest that apheresis should be commenced in all patients on the morning after plerixafor without necessarily waiting for the peripheral $CD34^+$ count. It is not necessary to use central venous access for all patients—a high proportion of patients, even older children, can undergo successful apheresis using peripheral venous access—however, it is advisable to assess venous access in all patients before the start of the mobilisation regime, with central access being arranged well in advance of collection for patients with inadequate peripheral veins. It makes sense to use an apheresis platform and a software setting that maximises collection efficiency while also minimising granulocyte contamination in the HPC-A product: I have found Spectra Optia® to be a very successful apheresis platform for HPC-A collection post-plerixafor, but I must admit that my personal experience is limited to the CaridianBCT apheresis platforms, COBE Spectra® and Spectra Optia®.

In general terms, I would currently only recommend "up-front" use of plerixafor in one specific patient group, namely adult patients with dialysis-dependent renal failure. For this group of patients, international experience has shown plerixafor along with G-CSF to be highly effective with relatively low toxicity, and also to be simple to schedule around haemodialysis sessions [61]; whereas the alternative approaches of G-CSF alone or of chemomobilisation both have the disadvantage of lower efficacy (especially G-CSF alone), and for chemomobilisation also the disadvantages of higher toxicity and poorer predictability.

Special Patient Groups: (1) Children Undergoing Apheresis for Autologous HPC-A Procurement, and (2) Adult Patients with Dialysis-Dependent Renal Failure

Technical Aspects of Apheresis for HPC-A Procurement in Children

High-dose chemotherapy with autologous HPC-A support is increasingly used in the treatment of paediatric solid tumours, as well as in some subtypes of lymphoma and in relapsed acute promyelocytic leukaemia in children, due to improved survival outcomes compared with conventional dose chemotherapy ± radiotherapy [17, 62–64]. In children as in adults, HPC-A are generally preferred to bone marrow

(HPC-M) for autologous transplantation, due to more rapid and reliable engraftment, lower tumour cell contamination and less invasive procurement [62]; and apheresis for HPC procurement has been shown to be safe and feasible even in very young children, although it does present some technical challenges (reviewed in Sevilla et al. [65]). The extracorporeal volume of the disposable kit ("circuit") for most apheresis platforms is in the region of 150–350 mL: while the great majority of adult patients will tolerate this degree of hypovolaemia for the 3–4 h of a collection procedure, it would be an unacceptably large volume for smaller children. Because of this, common practice is to prime the disposable kit with blood (using a donated red cell unit provided by the Blood Transfusion Service) prior to connecting a smaller child to the cell separator machine for an apheresis procedure. This is a sensible precaution if the extracorporeal volume of the circuit is 10% or more of the child's calculated total blood volume, and is mandatory if the extracorporeal volume of the circuit is 15% or more of the child's calculated total blood volume [65]. Most apheresis platforms are designed to operate using citrate as a regional anticoagulant: this is still possible even in smaller children, but severe citrate toxicity (hypotension; tetany) is seen more often in very small children of 10 kg or less unless calcium supplementation is administered prophylactically (usually intravenous calcium gluconate, sometimes guided by measurement of ionised calcium levels peri-procedure).

Although the majority of children, as for adults, will mobilise transplantable doses of HPC-A using conventional approaches of G-CSF alone or chemomobilisation along with G-CSF, poor HPC-A mobilisation remains a significant problem in paediatric haemato-oncology. This is firstly because many children have been heavily pretreated with chemotherapy, often including substantial quantities of alkylating agent, prior to HPC-A procurement, secondly because ex vivo "purging" of the HPC-A product (for instance, by $CD34^+$ selection) is sometimes carried out for some paediatric solid tumours such as neuroblastoma, with some cell loss during the process necessitating higher starting doses of $CD34^+$ cells, and thirdly because many autologous HSC transplant protocols for children involve tandem transplantation (discussed in Fish and Grupp, 2008 [62]). Although approaches such as large volume apheresis have been used with success in some children [66], citrate toxicity can be a problem, and there is still a substantial subgroup of children who do not achieve transplantable autologous HPC-A doses by conventional means. It is therefore not surprising that there has been considerable interest in the use of plerixafor for autologous HPC-A procurement in children.

Experience to Date with Plerixafor for HPC-A Collection in Children

Although plerixafor is not currently licensed for autologous HPC-A procurement in children, it has been used off-licence in a number of paediatric cancer centres worldwide, with some of this experience now having been published, including four peer-reviewed papers [67–70] as well as five abstracts [71–75]. Taking all 9 publications together, there is published experience of plerixafor use in a total of 34 patients to date, including 24 patients with solid tumours (medulloblastoma/PNET: $n=11$; Ewing's sarcoma: $n=6$; neuroblastoma: $n=4$; osteogenic sarcoma: $n=1$; Wilms' Tumour: $n=1$; desmoplastic small cell tumour: $n=1$) and 10 patients with haematological malignancy (NHL: $n=8$; HL: $n=1$; ALL: $n=1$). Plerixafor was successful in mobilising a transplantable $CD34^+$ dose in 30/34 patients (88%) and in 30/37 mobilisation episodes (81%), with 3 patients having been successfully re-mobilised using plerixafor after an initial failed attempt using plerixafor [67, 75]. Of the papers and abstracts that discussed transplantation outcomes [68–70, 72–75], 22/29 children receiving plerixafor for autologous HPC-A mobilisation ultimately proceeded to transplant (76%), with engraftment being reported to be satisfactory in all cases. Reported toxicities were all minor, including injection site reaction ($n=5$), insomnia ($n=2$), vomiting ($n=2$), nausea ($n=1$), bone pain ($n=1$), arthralgia ($n=1$) and oral paraesthesia ($n=1$).

Although there may of course be a degree of publication bias, these results are very encouraging, and suggest that plerixafor is both safe and effective in children. Clearly, however, the publication of a large case series in full remains desirable.

It might be expected that the renal clearance of plerixafor in children may exceed adult values, particularly in children less than 12 years of age. This is because renally excreted drugs such as plerixafor are usually cleared more rapidly in children because of their higher kidney-size to body-size ratio compared to adults [76]. Although all published clinical use of plerixafor to date in children has used a standard dosage of 240 μg/kg/day, a multicentre study sponsored by Genzyme is currently recruiting in the European Union, investigating the use of plerixafor for HPC-A mobilisation for autologous transplantation in children, with the drug being given at varying dose levels and blood being sampled for pharmacokinetic studies (Dr. Nicky Whitaker, Genzyme Europe, personal communication).

Plerixafor for HPC-A Collection in Patients with Dialysis-Dependent Renal Failure

Clinical experience with younger myeloma patients presenting in end-stage renal failure suggests a potential benefit from autologous HPC-A transplant, with 20–35% of patients recovering renal function post transplant, albeit with substantially higher early transplant-related mortality than patients with normal renal function [77]. However, HPC-A collection from myeloma patients on dialysis can be challenging, as cyclophosphamide (the chemotherapy drug generally used for HPC-A mobilisation in myeloma) is renally excreted with potentially increased toxicity in patients with renal failure; while the alternative approach of HPC-A mobilisation with G-CSF alone without prior chemotherapy has a lower success rate in terms of achieving a transplantable $CD34^+$ cell dose. There are also significant challenges in the scheduling of apheresis around dialysis sessions. There is therefore a need for new approaches to PBSC mobilisation in this patient population.

The international experience to date with plerixafor use in myeloma patients with advanced renal failure has very recently been published [61]. In a series of 21 patients from 15 centres in Europe and the USA, all of whom had advanced renal failure and 20 of whom were still on dialysis at the time of HPC-A collection, plerixafor resulted in successful collection of a transplantable $CD34^+$ dose in 20/21 patients (95%). The one remaining patient was successfully re-mobilised with plerixafor at a higher dosage. Fifteen patients (71%) proceeded to autologous HSC transplant, with recovery of renal function in three cases. The dosage of plerixafor was reduced to 160 μg/kg in the first instance for 15 patients, with the remaining six patients receiving standard plerixafor dosage of 240 μg/kg. Reported plerixafor toxicities were all minor (predominantly gastrointestinal toxicity). Importantly, plerixafor appeared to be relatively straightforward to schedule around dialysis. As a small, highly polar and highly water-soluble molecule, plerixafor would be expected to be removed efficiently both by haemodialysis and by peritoneal dialysis (although no actual data are available to date to confirm this). For most patients in the published international series, a schedule was therefore used in which plerixafor was started (following a short course of G-CSF) in the evening after a dialysis day (typically a Monday), with apheresis being carried out the following morning. Further plerixafor was given if required that evening (typically Tuesday), with further apheresis the following morning (typically Wednesday), with a haemodialysis session immediately after apheresis that afternoon. This avoided the need for any extra haemodialysis sessions. For the single patient in this series who was on peritoneal dialysis, dialysis was discontinued prior to each dose of plerixafor (given in the evening), and recommenced immediately after completion of apheresis the following day. Plerixafor appears to be particularly effective in this patient group, with considerable logistical advantages over alternative mobilisation strategies.

Appendix

Table 8.3 Table of usual day of first PBSC collection depending on mobilising chemotherapy

Chemotherapy regime	Recommended day to start chemo	Start GCSF (first day of chemo = day 0)	Average rebound day
CHOP	Friday	3	10
Cyclo 1.5 g/m² or 2 g/m²	Monday	1	9
Cyclo 3 g/m² or 4 g/m²	Friday	1	10
Cyclo 6 g/m² or 7 g/m²	Wednesday	7	14
Cytarabine 6 g/m²	Friday	4 or 7	17–19
DAT	No preference	16	20
DHAP	Wednesday	8	13
ESHAP	Wednesday	7	13
IVAC	Wednesday	6	14
IVE	Wednesday	5	13
MACE	No preference	13	16–26
H.D. Methotrexate	Tuesday	4	8–10
MIDAC	No preference	10	24
TIP	Friday	6	11
VIDE	Tuesday	5	14

Please consider date of commencing chemotherapy carefully

NB Many centres have *no* weekend or public holiday processing service available

Example of a chart used to determine anticpated day of first apheresis after various mobilising chemotherapy regimes. Based on Scottish National Blood Transfusion Service (SNBTS) West of Scotland document, and used by permission

References

1. FACT/JACIE Standards, 4th edn. International Standards for Cellular Therapy Product Collection, Processing and Administration. Available from website of Joint Accreditation Committee of ISCT and EBMT (JACIE), at http://www.jacie.org/portal/en/public/document-centre. Accessed 1 November 2011
2. Szczepiorkowski ZM, Shaz BH, Bandarenko N, Winters JL (2007) The new approach to assignment of ASFA categories—introduction to the fourth special issue: clinical applications of therapeutic apheresis. J Clin Apher 22:96–105
3. Szczepiorkowski ZM, Winters JL, Bandarenko N, Kim HC, Linenberger ML, Marques MB, Sarode R, Schwartz J, Weinstein R, Shaz BH (2010) Guidelines on the use of therapeutic apheresis in clinical practice—evidence-based approach from the Apheresis Applications Committee of the American Society for Apheresis. J Clin Apher 25:83–177
4. Cooling L, Hoffmann S, Herrst M, Muck C, Armelagos H, Davenport R (2010) A prospective randomized trial of two popular mononuclear cell collection sets for autologous peripheral blood stem cell collection in multiple myeloma. Transfusion 50:100–119
5. Tanhehco YC, Adamski J, Sell M, Cunningham K, Eisenmann C, Magee D, Stadtmauer EA, O'Doherty U (2010) Plerixafor mobilization leads to a lower ratio of CD34+ cells to total nucleated cells which results in greater storage costs. J Clin Apher 25(4):202–208
6. Reinhardt P, Brauninger S, Bialleck H, Thorausch K, Smith R, Schrezenmeier H, Seifried E, Wiesneth M, Bonig H (2011) Automatic interface-controlled apheresis collection of stem/progenitor cells: results from an autologous donor validation trial of a novel stem cell apheresis device. Transfusion 51(16):1321–1330
7. Copland M, Alcorn M, Patton D, Doig A, Farrell E, Currie C, Sinclair JE, Parker AN, Douglas KW (2010) Significantly lower cryopreservation volumes for PBSC collections using Spectra Optia® Version 5 Software compared with the MNC setting on COBE® Spectra, particularly when using plerixafor for mobilisation. Blood 116(21) (ASH Abstracts Book): Abstract No. 825
8. Herrmann O, Cassens U, Krakowitzky P, Stahl D, Sibrowski W (2001) Prospective study on the comparison of two apheresis systems for collecting Peripheral Blood Stem Cells. Infus Ther Transfus Med 28:183–187
9. Altuntas F, Kocyigit I, Ozturk A, Kaynar L, Sari I, Oztekin M, Somaz M, Eser B, Cetin M, Unal A (2007) Comparison of the Fenwal Amicus and Fresenius Com.Tec cell separators for autologous peripheral blood stem cell collection. Transfus Apher Sci 36:159–167
10. Del Fante C, Perotti C, Viarengo G, Bellotti L, Parisi C, Marchesi A, Tinelli C, Salvaneschi L (2006) Clinical impact of a new automated system employed for peripheral blood stem cell collection. J Clin Apher 21(4):227–232
11. Ikeda K, Ohto H, Kanno T, Ogata T, Noji H, Ogawa K, Maruyama Y (2007) Automated programs for collection of mononuclear cells and progenitor cells by two separators for peripheral blood progenitor cell transplantation: comparison by a randomised crossover study. Transfusion 47(7):1234–1240
12. Valbonesi M, Carlier P, Bo A, Stura P, Massazza S, Sanfilippo B, Varinelli I (2001) The MCS+ revision A2 for highly efficient PBSC collection. Transfus Apher Sci 24(3):293–296
13. Abdelkefi A, Maamar M, Torjman L, Ladeb S, Lakhal A, Ben Othman T, Slama H, Jenhani F, Mojaat N, Ben Hamed L, Bouhoula S, Hsairi M, Boukef K, Ben Abdeladhim A (2006) Prospective randomised comparison of the COBE Spectra Version 6 and Haemonetics MCS(+) cell separators for haematopoietic progenitor cells leucapheresis in patients with multiple myeloma. J Clin Apher 21(2):111–115
14. Jillella AP, Ustun C, Robach E, Sertkaya D, DiPiro C, Kallab AM, Brick WG, Dainer PM, Kutlar A, Townsend AR, Burgess RE (2003) Infectious complications in patients receiving mobilization chemotherapy for autologous peripheral blood stem cell collection. J Hematother Stem Cell Res 12:155–160

15. De La Rubia J, Bladé J, Lahueta JJ (2006) Effect of chemotherapy with alkylating agents on the yield of CD34+ cells in patients with multiple myeloma. Results of the Spanish Myeloma Group (GEM) study. Hematologica 91:621–627
16. Gertz MA, Kumar SK, Lacy MQ, Dispenzieri A, Hayman SR, Buadi FK, Dingli D, Gastineau DA, Winters JL, Litzow MR (2009) Comparison of high-dose CY and growth factor with growth factor alone for mobilization of stem cells for transplantation in patients with multiple myeloma. Bone Marrow Transplant 43:619–625
17. Watanabe H, Watanabe T, Suzuya H, Wakata Y, Kaneko M, Onishi T, Okamoto Y, Abe T, Kawano Y, Kagami S, Takaue Y (2006) Peripheral blood stem cell mobilization by granulocyte colony-stimulating factor alone and engraftment kinetics following autologous transplantation in children and adolescents with solid tumor. Bone Marrow Transplant 37:661–668
18. Elliott C, Samson DM, Armitage S, Lyttelton MP, McGuigan D, Hargreaves R, Giles C, Abrahamson G, Abboudi Z, Brennan M, Kanfer EJ (1996) When to harvest peripheral blood stem cells after mobilization therapy: prediction of CD34 positive cell yield by preceding day CD34 positive concentration in peripheral blood. J Clin Oncol 14:970–973
19. Möhle R, Murea S, Pförsich M et al (1996) Estimation of the progenitor cell yield in a leukapheresis product by previous measurement of CD34+ cells in the peripheral blood. Vox Sang 71:90–96
20. Majado MJ, Minguela A, Gonzalez-Carcia C, Salido E, Blanquer M, Funes C, Insausti CL, Garcia-Hernandez AM, Moraleda JM, Morales A (2009) Large-volume-apheresis facilitates autologous transplantation of hematopoietic progenitors in poor mobilizer patients. J Clin Apher 24:12–17
21. Moog R, Moog R (2008) Management strategies for poor peripheral blood stem cell mobilization. Transfus Apher Sci 38:229–236
22. Padmanabhan A, Reich-Slotky R, Jhang JS, Dael S, Crowder T, Colovai AI, Schwartz J (2009) Use of the haematopoietic progenitor cell parameter in optimising timing of peripheral blood stem cell harvest. Vox Sang 97(2):153–159
23. Gao Y, Lim S, Gao F, Ng J, Phoon Y, Tham C, Quek R, Tao M (2009) Analysing white blood cell subpopulations as quick and simple predictors for autologous stem cell collection. J Clin Oncol 27(15S) (ASCO Abstract Book): Abstract No. 7101
24. Ford CD, Greenwood J, Strupp A, Lehman CM (2002) Change in CD34+ cell concentration during peripheral blood progenitor cell collection: effects on collection efficiency and efficacy. Transfusion 42(7):904–911
25. Cassens U, Barth IM, Baumann C, Fischer RJ, Kienast J, Vormoor J, Sibrowski W (2004) Factors affecting the efficacy of peripheral blood progenitor cells collections by large-volume leukaphereses with standardized processing volumes. Transfusion 44:1593–1602
26. Smolowicz AG, Villman K, Tidefelt U (1997) Large-volume apheresis for the harvest of peripheral blood progenitor cells for autologous transplantation. Transfusion 37:188–192
27. Douglas KW, McGarvey M, Robertson S, Sinclair JE, Taylor S, Green RHA (2008) "Will I have enough cells for a transplant, doctor?" Validation of a CD34+ dose prediction formula using patient weight, peripheral CD34+ count, and predicted end run results in a series of 440 consecutive PBSC collection procedures using the MNC program on COBE Spectra. J Clin Apher 23(1):21–22 (ASFA Abstract Book)
28. Stiff PJ, Koester AR, Weidner MK et al (1987) Autologous bone marrow transplantation using unfractionated cells cryopreserved in dimethylsulfoxide and hydroxyethyl starch without controlled-rate freezing. Blood 70:975–978
29. Clarke DM, Yadock DJ, Nicoud IB, Mathew AJ, Heimfeld S (2009) Improved post-thaw recovery of peripheral blood stem/progenitor cells using a novel intracellular-like cryopreservation solution. Cytotherapy 11(4):472–479
30. Chen-Plotkin AS, Vossel KA, Martin A, Samuels MA, Chen MH (2007) Encephalopathy, stroke and myocardial infarction with DMSO use in stem cell transplantation. Neurology 68:859–861
31. Marcacci G, Corazzelli G, Becchimanzi C, Arcamone M, Capobianco G, Russo F, Frigeri F, Pinto A (2009) DMSO-associated encephalopathy during autologous peripheral stem cell infusion: a predisposing role of preconditioning exposure to CNS-penetrating agents? Bone Marrow Transplant 44:133–135

32. Zenhäusern R, Tobler A, Leoncini L, Hess OM, Ferrari P (2000) Fatal cardiac arrhythmia after infusion of dimethyl sulfoxide-cryopreserved hematopoietic stem cells in a patient with severe primary cardiac amyloidosis and end-stage renal failure. Ann Hematol 79(9):523–526
33. Berz D, McCormack EM, Winer ES et al (2007) Cryopreservation of hematopoietic stem cells (Review). Am J Hematol 82:463–472
34. DiPersio JF, Micallef IN, Stiff PJ, Bolwell BJ, Maziarz RT, Jacobsen E, Nademanee A, McCarty J, Bridger G, Calandra G (2009) Phase III prospective randomized double-blind placebo-controlled trial of plerixafor plus granulocyte colony-stimulating factor compared with placebo plus granulocyte colony-stimulating factor for autologous stem-cell mobilization and transplantation for patients with non-Hodgkin's lymphoma. J Clin Oncol 27: 4767–4773
35. DiPersio JF, Stadtmauer EA, Nademanee A, Micallef INM, Stiff PJ, Kaufman JL, Maziarz RT, Hosing C, Fruehauf S, Horwitz M, Cooper D, Bridger G, Calandra G (2009) Plerixafor and G-CSF versus placebo and G-CSF to mobilize hematopoietic stem cells for autologous stem cell transplantation in patients with multiple myeloma. Blood 113:5720–5726
36. Calandra G, McCarty J, McGuirk J, Tricot G, Crocker S-A, Badel K, Grove B, Dye A, Bridger G (2008) AMD3100 plus G-CSF can successfully mobilize CD34+ cells from non-Hodgkin's lymphoma, Hodgkin's disease and multiple myeloma patients previously failing mobilization with chemotherapy and/or cytokine treatment: compassionate use data. Bone Marrow Transplant 41:331–338
37. Duarte RF, Shaw BE, Marín P, Kottaridis P, Ortiz M, Morante C, Delgado J, Gayoso J, Gotteriz R, Martinez-Chamorro C, Mateos-Mazon JJ, Ramirez C, de la Rubia J, Achtereekte H, Gandhi PJ, Douglas KW, Russell NH (2011) Plerixafor plus granulocyte CSF can mobilize hematopoietic stem cells from multiple myeloma and lymphoma patients failing previous mobilization attempts: EU Compassionate Use data. Bone Marrow Transplant 46(1):52–58
38. Stewart DA, Guo D, Luider J, Auer I, Klassen J, Ching E, Morris D, Chaudhry A, Brown C, Russell JA (1999) Factors predicting engraftment of autologous blood stem cells: CD34+ subsets inferior to the total CD34+ cell dose. Bone Marrow Transplant 23(12):1237–1243
39. Abrahamsen JF, Wentzel-Larsen T, Bruserud Ø (2004) Autologous transplantation: the viable transplanted CD34+ cell dose measured post-thaw does not predict engraftment kinetics better than the total CD34+ dose measured pre-freeze in patients that receive more than 2 x 10^6 CD34+ cells/kg. Cytotherapy 6(4):356–362
40. Schwella A, Siegert W, Beyer J, Rick O, Zingsem J, Eckstein R, Serke S, Huhn D (1995) Autografting with blood progenitor cells: predictive value of preapheresis blood cell counts on progenitor cell harvest and correlation of the reinfused cell dose with hematopoietic reconstitution. Ann Hematol 71(5):227–234
41. Jansen EM, Hanks SG, Terry C, Akard L, Thompson JM, Dugan MJ, Jansen J (2007) Prediction of engraftment after autologous peripheral blood progenitor cell transplantation: CD34, colony-forming-unit-granulocyte-macrophage, or both? Transfusion 47:817–823
42. Ketterer N, Salles G, Raba M et al (1998) High CD34+ cell counts decrease hematologic toxicity of autologous peripheral blood progenitor cell transplantation. Blood 91:3148–3155
43. Shpall EJ, Champlin R, Glaspy JA (1998) Effect of CD34+ peripheral blood progenitor cell dose on hematopoietic recovery. Biol Blood Marrow Transplant 4:84–92
44. Schulman KA, Birch R, Zhen B, Pania N, Weaver CH (1999) Effect of CD34+ dose on resource utilization in patients after high-dose chemotherapy with peripheral blood stem cell support. J Clin Oncol 17:1227–1233
45. Limat S, Wornonoff-Lemsi MC, Deconinck E et al (2000) Cost-effectiveness of CD34+ dose in peripheral blood progenitor cell transplantation for non-Hodgkin's lymphoma patients: a single centre study. Bone Marrow Transplant 25:997–1002
46. Alegre A (2009) Optimal mobilization method and CD34+ dose calculation for autologous PBSC transplant in myeloma patients: two important unresolved questions (Review). Bone Marrow Transplant 43:593–595
47. Goterris R, Hernandez-Boluda JC, Teruel A, Gomez C, Lis MJ, Terol MJ et al (2005) Impact of different strategies of secondline stem cell harvest on the outcome of autologous transplantation in poor peripheral blood stem cell mobilizers. Bone Marrow Transplant 36:847–853

48. Weaver CH, Tauer K, Zhen B, Schwartzberg LS, Hazelton B, Weaver Z et al (1998) Second attempts at mobilization of peripheral blood stem cells in patients with initial low CD34+ cell yields. J Hematother 7:241–249
49. D'Addio A, Curti A, Worel N, Douglas K, Motta MR, Rizzi S, Dan E, Taioli S, Giudice V, Agis H, Kopetzky G, Soutar R, Casadei B, Baccarani M, Lemoli RM (2011) The addition of plerixafor is safe and allows adequate PBSC collection in multiple myeloma and lymphoma patients who are poor mobilizers after chemotherapy and G-CSF. Bone Marrow Transplant 46:356–363
50. Hübel K, Fresen MM, Salwender H, Basara N, Beier R, Theurick S, Christopeit M, Bogner C, Galm O, Hartwig R, Heits F, Lordick F, Rösler W, Wehler D, Zander AR, Albert MH, Dressler S, Ebinger M, Frickhofen N, Hertenstein B, Kiehl M, Liebler S, von Lilienfeld-Toal M, Weidmann E, Weigelt C, Lange F, Kröger N (2011) Plerixafor with and without chemotherapy in poor mobilizers: results from the German compassionate use program. Bone Marrow Transplant 48:1045–1052. doi:10.1038/bmt.2010.249
51. Micallef INM, Ansell SM, Buadi F, Dingli D, Dispenzieri A, Gastineau DA, Gertz MA, Hayman SR, Hogan WJ, Inwards DJ, Johnston PB, Kumar S, Lacy MQ, Litzow MR, Porrata LF, Wolf R, Miceli T, Winters JL (2009) A risk adapted approach utilising plerixafor in autologous peripheral blood stem cell mobilization. Blood 114 (ASH Abstract Book): Abstract 3211
52. Micallef IN, Inwards DJ, Dispenzieri A, Gastineau DA, Gertz MA, Hayman S, Hogan WJ, Johnston PB, Kumar S, Lacy M, Litzow MR, Porrata LE, Buadi F, Ansell SM, Dingli D, Wolf R, Miceli T, Winters JL (2010) A risk adapted approach utilizing plerixafor in autologous peripheral blood stem cell mobilization. Biol Blood Marrow Transplant 16(2):S197–S198
53. Abhyankar SH, Aljitawi O, Ganguly S, McGuirk JP, DeJarnette SD, Merkel DA (2010) An Algorithmic approach to evaluate the optimal use of plerixafor (Mozobil®) for autologous hematopoietic Peripheral Blood Stem Cell (PBSC) collections based on peripheral circulating CD34 counts and Day One collection yield in patients with multiple myeloma (MM) and lymphoma (NHL, HD). Biol Blood Marrow Transplant 16(2):S164–S165
54. Horwitz M, Khan T, Long G, Gasparetto C, Sullivan K, Chute J, Rizzieri D, Drago S, Chao N (2010) Plerixafor given "just in time" for Peripheral Blood Stem Cell mobilization of patients with suboptimal response to G-CSF. Biol Blood Marrow Transplant 16(2):S208
55. Costa LJ, Alexander ET, Hogan KR, Schaub C, Fouts TV, Stuart RK (2011) Development and validation of a decision-making algorithm to guide the use of plerixafor for autologous hematopoietic stem cell mobilization. Bone Marrow Transplant 46:64–69
56. Duarte RF, Martin-Henao G, D'Addio A, Gayoso J, Shaw BE, Russell NH, Lemoli R, Worel N (2010) Predictability of stem cell mobilisation following GCSF ± plerixafor based on Day 4 CD34+ cell levels: basis for a preemptive model of plerixafor use in patients with lymphoma and myeloma who mobilise poorly. Bone Marrow Transplant 42(Suppl 2):Abstract 1022
57. Douglas K, Sinclair JE, McQuaker IG, Clark A, Copland M, Soutar R, Singer I, Morrison AE, Hung A, Clarke P, Parker AN (2011) A pro-active approach to plerixafor use and subsequent apheresis can reduce failed autologous PBSC mobilization rates to virtually zero after two mobilization attempts: a single-centre series of 40 consecutive PBSC mobilization episodes using plerixafor in 37 patients. Bone Marrow Transplant 46(Suppl 2):Abstract 1149
58. Shaughnessy P, Islas-Ohlmayer M, Murphy J et al (2010) Plerixafor plus G-CSF resulted in similar cost but more predictable days of apheresis compared to chemotherapy plus G-CSF for mobilization of autologous hematopoietic stem cells. Biol Blood Marrow Transplant 16(2):S203
59. Campen CJ, Armstrong EP, Christian JA, Hadeed S, Yeager AM (2010) Comparative cost-effectiveness of plerixafor plus G-CSF versus cyclophosphamide versus G-CSF for autologous stem cell mobilization in patients with NHL. Biol Blood Marrow Transplant 16(2):S206
60. Pusic I, Kymes SM, Lambert DL, Gregory M, DiPersio JF (2010) Health economic outcome analysis of stem cell mobilization with granulocyte colony-stimulating factor (G-CSF) plus plerixafor versus G-CSF alone in preparation for autologous stem cell transplantation (ASCT) in patients with non-hodgkin's lymphomas (NHL). Biol Blood Marrow Transplant 16(2):S212
61. Douglas KW, Parker AN, Hayden PJ, Rahemtulla A, D'Addio A, Lemoli RM, Rao K, Maris M, Pagliuca A, Uberti, J, Scheid C, Noppeney R, Cook G, Bokhari SW, Worel N, Mikala G,

Masszi T, Taylor R, Treisman J (2011) Plerixafor for PBSC mobilisation in myeloma patients with advanced renal failure: safety and efficacy data in a series of 21 patients from Europe and the U.S.A. Bone Marrow Transplant (Bone marrow Transplant advance, online publication 28 Feburary 2011: doi:10:1038/bmt 2009)

62. Fish JD, Grupp SA (2008) Stem cell transplantation for neuroblastoma (Review). Bone Marrow Transplant 41(2):159–165
63. Li Y, Huang S, Wang X, Zhou D, Huang K, Guo H, Fang J, Chen C, Liu Q (2010) Rituximab combined with autologous peripheral blood stem cell transplantation improve therapeutic effects of chemotherapy in pediatric patients with Burkitt's lymphoma. J Trop Pediatr 56(5): 337–341
64. Termuhlen AM, Klopfenstein K, Olshefski R, Rosselet R, Yeager ND, Soni S, Gross TG (2008) Mobilization of PML-RARA negative blood stem cells and salvage with autologous peripheral blood stem cell transplantation in children with relapsed acute promyelocytic leukemia. Pediatr Blood Cancer 51(4):521–524
65. Sevilla J, Diaz MA, Fernandez-Plaza S, Gonzalez-Vicent M, Madero L (2004) Risks and methods for peripheral blood progenitor cell collection in small children (Review). Transfus Apher Sci 31(3):221–231
66. Cecyn KZ, Seber A, Ginani VC, Goncalves AV, Caram EM, Oguro T, Oliveira OM, Carvalho MM, Bordin JO (2005) Large-volume leukapheresis for peripheral blood progenitor cell collection in low body weight pediatric patients: a single center experience. Transfus Apher Sci 32(3):269–274
67. Aabideen K, Anoop P, Ethell ME, Potter MN (2011) The feasibility of plerixafor as a second-line stem cell mobilizing agent in children. J Pediatr Hematol Oncol 33(1):65–67
68. Bernardo VA, Ng JS, Joyce MJ (2011) Use of plerixafor with Granulocyte Colony-Stimulating Factor for stem cell mobilization in a pediatric patient. Ann Pharmacother 45(2):e12
69. Toledano H, Yahel A, Cohen IJ et al (2010) Successful mobilization, harvest and transplant of peripheral blood stem cells using AMD3100 and G-CSF following high dose craniospinal irradiation for medulloblastoma in a young child. Pediatr Blood Cancer 54:613–615
70. Flatt T, Lewing K, Gonzalez C, Anthony K, Ryan R, Jones R, Gamis A, Dalal J (2010) Successful mobilization with AMD3100 and filgrastim with engraftment of autologous peripheral blood stem cells in a heavily pretreated pediatric patient with recurrent Burkitt lymphoma. Pediatr Hematol Oncol 27(2):138–149
71. Strahlendorf C, Chan G (2007) Successful peripheral blood stem cell mobilisation using AMD3100 in an 8-year-old child (Abstract). J Clin Apher 22(2):60–61
72. Shenoy S, Asselin B, Dalal J, Goyal R, Kaufman JL, Loeb D, McCarty J, Robertson K, Strahlendorf C, Walters MC, Angell J, Huebner D, Shaw PJ (2010) Safety and efficacy of hematopoietic stem cell remobilization with plerixafor (Mozobil®) + G-CSF in pediatric patients with malignant disorders. Blood 116(21) (ASH Abstract Book): Abstract 2245
73. Robertson KA, Pradhan K, Goebel S et al (2006) Mobilization of peripheral blood CD34 stem cells in a heavily pre-treated pediatric medulloblastoma patient using AMD3100 and G-CSF. Biol Blood Marrow Transplant 12(2 Suppl 1):75–76, Abstract 216
74. Stephen K, Montgomery K, Bateman C et al (2006) Successful mobilisation, harvest and transplant of stem cells following AMD3100 in 3 pediatric patients: the Australian experience. Biol Blood Marrow Transplant 12(2 Suppl 1):157, Abstract 457
75. Kořístek Z, Sterba J, Kepák T, Douglas K, Sastry J, Duarte R & Mohty M, European Consortium on Stem Cell Mobilisation (ECOSM) (2011). European pediatric experience with plerixafor for autologous PBSC mobilization from children failing to mobilize PBSC by conventional means: an initial series of 6 patients from 2 centres. Bone Marrow Transplant 46(Suppl 2): Abstract 1157
76. Chen N, Aleksa K, Woodland C, Rieder M, Koren G (2006) Ontogeny of drug elimination by the human kidney. Pediatr Nephrol 21:160–168
77. Knudsen LM, Nielsen B, Gimsing P, Geisler C (2005) Autologous stem cell transplantation in multiple myeloma: outcome in patients with renal failure. Eur J Haematol 75(1):27–33

Chapter 9
Influence of Different Stem Cell Mobilization Strategies on Graft Composition and Outcome of Autologous or Allogeneic Transplantation

Stefan Fruehauf and Guido Tricot

Abstract Autologous and allogeneic hematopoietic stem cell (HSC) transplantation are considered the standard of care for many malignancies including lymphoma, myeloma, and some leukemias. In many cases, mobilized peripheral blood has become the preferred source for HSCs. The efficacy of different mobilization regimens and transplant outcomes based on cell doses has been well studied. However, the characteristics of the stem cell graft may be of equal importance with respect to patient outcomes following autologous or allogeneic transplant. This review summarizes available preclinical and clinical data for bone marrow and mobilized peripheral blood HSC graft characteristics, defined as the cell types found in the graft as well as their gene expression profiles. This manuscript also explores how graft characteristics can impact bone marrow homing, engraftment, immune reconstitution, and other posttransplant outcomes in both the allogeneic and autologous settings.

Keywords Autologous transplant • Allogeneic transplant • Plerixafor • Chemomobilization • Graft characteristics

S. Fruehauf (✉)
Center for Tumor Diagnostics and Therapy, Paracelsus Klinik,
Am Natruper Holz 69, Osnabrück, 49076, Germany
e-mail: prof.stefan.fruehauf@pk-mx.de

G. Tricot
Department of Medicine, Utah Blood and Marrow Transplant and Myeloma Program,
University of Utah School of Medicine, Salt Lake City, UT, USA

S. Fruehauf et al. (eds.), *Novel Developments in Stem Cell Mobilization: Focus on CXCR4*, DOI 10.1007/978-1-4614-1960-0_9,

Introduction

Hematopoietic stem cell transplantation (HSCT) as a treatment modality for disease dates back to studies performed in the late 1930s and early 1940s [1–5]. An important breakthrough occurred in the 1970s with the detection of the human leukocyte antigen (HLA) system, which allowed allogeneic transplants without potentially fatal complications, such as rejection and severe graft-vs.-host disease (GVHD) [6, 7]. A second important breakthrough occurred in the mid-1980s, when several groups showed that it was possible to collect hematopoietic stem cells (HSCs) from the peripheral blood by apheresis after administration of chemotherapy [8–11] or growth factors, such as granulocyte colony-stimulating factor (G-CSF) [filgrastim (Neupogen®; Amgen, Thousand Oaks, CA, USA)] and granulocyte–macrophage colony-stimulating factor (GM-CSF) [sargramostim (Leukine®; Genzyme Corporation, Cambridge, MA, USA)] [12, 13].

To date, peripheral blood remains the most common source of HSCs, and several agents are available or under investigation for HSC mobilization. Chemotherapeutic agents such as cyclophosphamide and other cytostatic drugs have been used in conjunction with growth factors to mobilize stem cells into the peripheral blood [14–16]. In addition, disease-specific regimens, including ICE (ifosfamide, carboplatin, and etoposide), RICE (rituximab + ICE), IVE (ifosfamide, vincristine, and etoposide), DHAP (cisplatin, cytarabine, and dexamethasone), and D-PACE (dexamethasone, cisplatin, adriamycin, cyclophosphamide, and etoposide), have been used in combination with cytokines for HSC mobilization into the peripheral blood [17–20]. Cytokines alone [e.g., G-CSF, GM-CSF, and stem cell factor (SCF) (Stemgen®; Biovitrum, Stockholm, Sweden)] have been extensively studied and are known to effectively mobilize HSCs, but typically result in lower $CD34^+$ cell numbers [21]. Plerixafor (Mozobil®; Genzyme, Cambridge, MA, USA), a new small molecule, has been approved by the United States Food and Drug Administration and European Medicines Agency for use in HSC mobilization for autologous transplant for patients with lymphoma and multiple myeloma.

Agents that are being explored for use in HSC mobilization, but not currently approved by regulatory authorities, include Cdc42 activity-specific inhibitor and natalizumab [22–24]. Cdc42 activity-specific inhibitor is a small molecule that inhibits the activity of Cdc42—a Rho GTPase shown to facilitate HSC interactions with the bone marrow microenvironment [25]. Natalizumab is an α-VLA-4/CD49d monoclonal antibody against $\beta 1$ integrin and thereby interferes with VLA-4 ($\alpha 4,\beta 1$) interactions with the bone marrow [22, 23]. Small molecule inhibitors of VLA-4 are currently being studied in experimental settings in combination with plerixafor, and the finding of their synergistic effect on mobilization warrants further exploration of their clinical use [26].

This review summarizes available preclinical and clinical literature focusing on graft characteristics, defined as the cell types found in the graft (e.g., $CD34^+$ or $CD3^+$; see Table 9.1 for hematopoietic cell marker definitions) [27] and the gene expression profiles of those cells. Specifically, this chapter discusses how graft characteristics can affect bone marrow homing, engraftment, immune reconstitution, and outcomes after autologous or allogeneic transplant.

Table 9.1 Hematopoietic cell markers [27]

CD antigen	Cell type	Functions
CD3	Thymocytes and T cells	Associated with the TCR and required for cell surface expression of and signal transduction by the TCR
CD4	Thymocyte subsets and T cells	Co-receptor for MHC class II molecules and receptor for HIV-1 and HIV-2 gp120; binds Lck on cytoplasmic face of membrane
CD8	Thymocyte subsets and cytotoxic T cells	Co-receptor for MHC class I molecules; binds Lck on cytoplasmic face of membrane
CD11a (LFA-1)	Lymphocytes, granulocytes, monocytes, and macrophages	αL subunit of integrin LFA-1 (associated with CD18); binds to CD54 (ICAM-1), CD102 (ICAM-2), and CD50 (ICAM-3)
CD25	Activated T cells, B cells, and monocytes	IL-2 receptor α chain
CD31 (PECAM-1)	Monocytes, platelets, granulocytes, T cell subsets, and endothelial cells	Adhesion molecule; mediates both leukocyte-endothelial and endothelial-endothelial interactions
CD33	Myeloid progenitor cells and monocytes	Binds sialoconjugates
CD34	Hematopoietic precursors and capillary endothelium	Ligand for CD62L
CD38	Early B and T cells, activated T cells, germinal center B cells, and plasma cells	NAD glycohydrolase; augments B-cell proliferation
CD45RA	B cells, T cell subsets (naïve T cells), and monocytes	Tyrosine phosphatase; augments signaling through antigen receptor of B and T cells
CD48	Leukocytes	Putative ligand for CD244
CD49d (VLA-4)	Broad distribution includes B cells, thymocytes, monocytes, granulocytes, and dendritic cells	α4 integrin; associates with CD29 and binds fibronectin, MAdCAM-1, and VCAM-1

(continued)

Table 9.1 (continued)

CD antigen	Cell type	Functions
CD49e (VLA-5)	Broad distribution includes memory T cells, monocytes, platelets	α5 integrin; associates with CD29 and binds fibronectin; invasion
CD54 (ICAM-1)	Hematopoietic and nonhematopoietic cells	Binds CD11a/CD18 integrin (LFA-1) and CD11b/CD18 integrin (Mac-1) receptor
CD58 (LFA-3)	Hematopoietic and nonhematopoietic cells	Adhesion molecule; binds CD2
CD62L (L-selectin)	B cells, T cells, monocytes, and NK cells	Leukocyte adhesion molecule; binds CD34 and GlyCAM and mediates rolling interactions with endothelium
CD90 (Thy-1)	$CD34^+$ prothymocytes	Unknown
CD106 (VCAM-1)	Endothelial cells	Adhesion molecule, ligand for VLA-4
CD110	Platelets	MPL (TPO) receptor
CD133	Stem/progenitor cells	Unknown
CD150	Thymocytes and activated lymphocytes	Unknown
CD184 (CXCR4)	Preferentially expressed in the more immature $CD34^+$ hematopoietic stem cells	Binds to SDF-1; acts as a cofactor for fusion and entry of T-cell line

CXCR chemokine receptor, *GlyCAM* glycosylation-dependent cell adhesion molecule, *HIV* human immunodeficiency virus, *LFA* leukocyte function antigen, *MAdCAM* mucosal addressin cell adhesion molecule, *MPL* myeloproliferative leukemia virus oncogene, *NAD* nicotinamide adenine dinucleotide, *NK* natural killer, *PECAM* platelet endothelial cell adhesion molecule, *SDF* stromal cell-derived factor, *TPO* thrombopoietin, *VLA* very late antigen

Mechanisms of HSC Mobilization

Hematopoietic stem cells exist at a very low (0.04%) frequency in steady-state peripheral blood [28, 29]. Most HSCs remain tethered to the bone marrow through adhesion molecule/receptor interactions with bone marrow stromal cells, osteoblasts, and osteoclasts [30]. Several protein–protein interactions help anchor HSCs within the bone marrow, including the chemokine receptor CXC motif receptor 4 (CXCR4) and its cognate ligand stromal cell-derived factor-1 (SDF-1 or CXCL12), CD44—hyaluronic acid, c-kit—kit ligand, very late antigen-4 (VLA-4)—VCAM-1 or fibronectin, and CD62—CD62L or L-selectin [31–34].

Current mobilization regimens increase HSCs in the peripheral blood above steady-state levels by disrupting the normal bone marrow microenvironment through several mechanisms (Fig. 9.1). After chemotherapy administration, CD34⁺ cells in peripheral blood increase as the patient's white blood cell count starts to recover [35]. Although the exact mechanism remains poorly characterized, neutrophil proteases

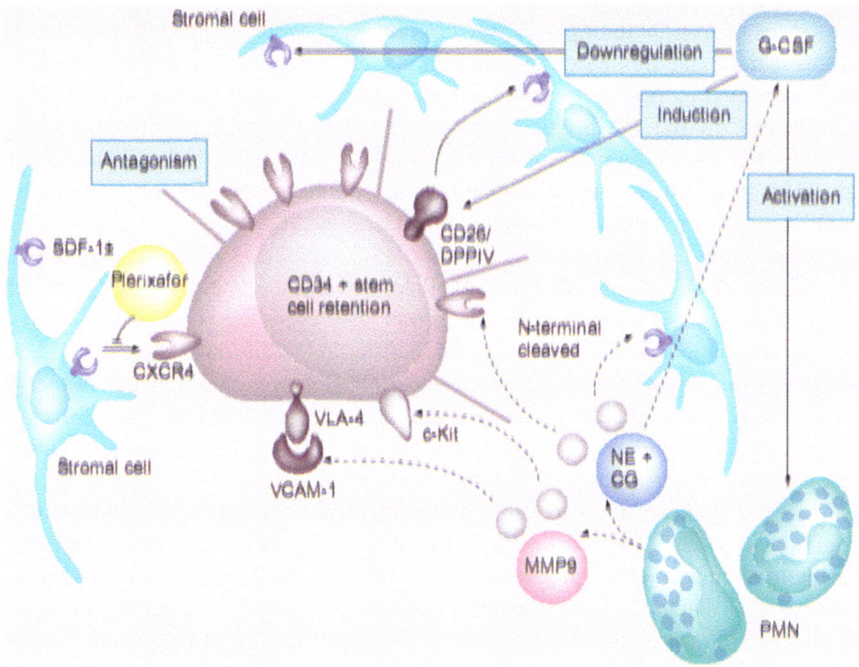

Fig. 9.1 Mechanisms of stem cell mobilization. Granulocyte colony-stimulating factor (G-CSF) mobilizes CD34⁺ cells via downregulation of stromal cell-derived factor-1 (SDF-1) expression and induction of CD26/dipeptidyl peptidase IV (DPPIV) cleavage of cell surface SDF-1. In addition, G-CSF stimulates polymorphonuclear (PMN) leukocyte cell release of the proteases neutrophil elastase (NE), cathepsin G (CG), and matrix metalloproteinase-9 (MMP9), which cleave VCAM-1, c-kit, and SDF-1, releasing stem cells from the bone marrow into the peripheral blood. Plerixafor mobilizes stem cells through direct antagonism of CXC motif receptor 4 (CXCR4), which inhibits the interaction of SDF-1 with CXCR4. VLA, very late antigen. Adapted from *Future Oncol.* (2005) 1(3), 375–383 with permission of Future Medicine Ltd

capable of adhesion molecule cleavage (e.g., neutrophil elastase and cathepsin G) accumulate in the bone marrow and likely contribute to HSC release from the bone marrow into the peripheral blood [36]. It is thought that G-CSF catalyzes HSC mobilization by downregulating mRNA and protein levels of the chemokine SDF-1 and by promoting accumulation of matrix metalloproteinase-9, neutrophil elastase, and cathepsin G, which can cleave kit ligand and SDF-1 in addition to VCAM-1 [36–40]. By contrast, plerixafor is a direct CXCR4 antagonist, which reversibly inhibits the CXCR4–SDF-1 interaction, releasing HSCs from the bone marrow into the peripheral blood [41–46].

Recent studies show that the CXCR4–CXCL12 axis is downstream of CD26 and downstream of the G-CSF receptor so that plerixafor can be used as a single agent to mobilize hematopoietic stem and progenitor cells in normal donors or patients that have an intrinsic defect in their response to G-CSF treatment [47].

Impact of Novel Mobilization Regimens on Poor Mobilizers

Numerous factors, including age, previous rounds of chemotherapy, prior radiation, exposure to lenalidomide or alkylating agents, and bone marrow involvement have been identified as risk factors for poor mobilization in lymphoma and myeloma patients [15, 48–61]. Plerixafor, in combination with G-CSF, has shown the ability to overcome many poor prognostic factors including age [62], previous chemotherapy [63], prior treatment with lenalidomide or fludarabine [64, 65], failed first mobilization attempt [66, 67], and low platelet counts [62–68].

Out of scope for this review is whether HSCs mobilized by novel regimens in predicted poor mobilizers and failed mobilizers are of the same quality as those collected from patients without such risk factors. Cell cycle status, activation, and ex vivo expansion kinetics have been shown to differ in G-CSF-mobilized $CD34^+$ cells collected from “good” and “poor” mobilizers [69]. However, the clinical relevance of these observations remains to be elucidated. Recent clinical data have emerged regarding patients with non-Hodgkin’s lymphoma (NHL) who failed a first mobilization attempt and were successfully remobilized using plerixafor in combination with G-CSF [67]. Median times to neutrophil and platelet engraftment were similar in remobilized patients and those who collected successfully on the first attempt [67]. Furthermore, all patients maintained durable grafts at the 12-month follow-up [67]. This suggests that the cells mobilized by plerixafor in patients who failed prior mobilization are of at least the same quality as those collected from patients during the first mobilization attempt.

Tumor Cell Mobilization

Tumor cells can be detected in the peripheral blood of patients with myeloma and NHL prior to and following mobilization [70–73]. However, the potential impact of tumor cell reinfusion on patient outcomes following autologous transplant remains controversial. Small studies have reported that patients receiving grafts with lower tumor burden demonstrated improved survival outcomes [74–77]. However, in randomized phase III trials, CD34$^+$ cell selection resulted in a 2–3 log reduction in graft tumor cell contamination but did not impact engraftment, median overall survival, disease-free survival, and relapse rate [78, 79]. In addition, a recent study demonstrated no difference in progression-free survival (PFS) or overall survival (OS) for MM and NHL patients receiving autografts with or without detectable tumor cells [80].

Autograft tumor contamination has been shown to vary by HSC source and apheresis day. Several studies have shown that peripheral blood HSC collections are less likely to contain tumor cells compared with bone marrow [81–86]. In particular, two studies compared premobilization bone marrow harvests with mobilized peripheral blood autografts from the same patients and found that bone marrow harvests were contaminated at higher frequencies and with a greater number of tumor cells [81, 86]. However, these findings are not universal, as additional studies reported that peripheral blood collections were at least as likely to be contaminated by tumor cells as bone marrow harvests [87, 88]. Interestingly, tumor cell contamination may also vary by apheresis day. While some groups have observed no increase in tumor cell load, others demonstrated that grafts collected on apheresis days 5 or 6 were more likely to be contaminated by tumor cells [81, 89–91]. It remains an open question whether reducing the number of days required to collect HSCs would reduce tumor burden.

Whether graft tumor contamination varies by mobilization regimen is an important consideration. Autografts collected following either chemomobilization or cytokine-alone mobilization have been shown to contain tumor cells [92–94]. The impact of the novel agent plerixafor on tumor cell contamination has recently been investigated by several groups. In clinical studies of patients with NHL and multiple myeloma, increased mobilization of tumor cells over what was detected following administration of G-CSF alone was not observed following the addition of plerixafor [95–97].

Graft Content Studies in Preclinical Models, Autologous Transplant Patients, and Allogeneic Transplant Donors

Graft Cell Types

Cell types in grafts collected from unmobilized or G-CSF-mobilized bone marrow, typically collected by surgical bone marrow harvest, or in mobilized peripheral blood collected by apheresis differ with regard to primitive hematopoietic progenitors, total T cells, dendritic cells (DCs), and T regulatory cells (Tregs). In turn, the abundance of these cell types can affect transplant outcomes. Primitive progenitors are present in high numbers/frequency in mobilized peripheral blood, are highly clonogenic, and have been shown to improve early neutrophil and platelet engraftment and long-term progenitor cell recovery after autologous HSCT (aHSCT) [98–102].

Dendritic cells are antigen-presenting cells that prime naïve T cells to new antigens, and there are two major types: myeloid DCs (DC1) and lymphoid DCs (DC2) [103]. Myeloid DCs typically drive T-cell differentiation toward Th 1 cells that promote cytotoxic T lymphocytes, which can contribute to GVHD and to a graft-vs.-leukemia effect in allogeneic transplant patients [104–106]. Lymphoid DCs can drive T-cell differentiation toward Th 2 cells, which primarily stimulate B cells [104, 105]. Infusion of greater total lymphocyte doses has been shown to benefit immune reconstitution, OS, and PFS in autologous transplant patients [107–109]. In allogeneic graft recipients, increased graft Tregs and DC2 can help reduce GVHD [110–112]. Studies of graft content in preclinical models, autologous transplant patients, and allogeneic transplant donors have identified differences in graft content depending on the source and/or mobilization regimen.

Graft Content in Preclinical Models

Preclinical work in mice has shown that mobilization with G-CSF or chemotherapy+G-CSF resulted in the collection of cells with superior clonogenicity [as judged by the presence of colony forming unit-culture (CFU-C) and colony forming unit-spleen (CFU-S)] compared with unmobilized peripheral blood capable of short- and long-term engraftment and repopulation [113–116]. One study determined that the clonogenicity of chemomobilized cells was greater than that of G-CSF-mobilized cells [114]. Regarding immune cell phenotypes, mobilization with G-CSF has been shown to induce polarization toward DC2 in mice [117].

Preclinical studies in mice have compared the mobilization of primitive hematopoietic precursors by several mobilization agents [46, 118, 119]. Threefold more Sca-1$^+$ c-kit$^+$ lineage (SKL) cells, which contain long-term multipotent progenitor cells, were collected per milliliter of blood when mice were mobilized by plerixafor+G-CSF than when mice were mobilized by G-CSF [46, 120, 121]. In addition, recent studies in mice have examined the use of the CXCR2 agonist GROβ (CXCL2), either alone or in conjunction with G-CSF or plerixafor, for the mobilization of primitive hematopoietic precursors [118, 119]. The combination of plerixafor and GROβ mobilized approximately twice as many CD150$^+$CD48$^-$ SKL cells, which are involved in T-cell development [122–124], and markers of long-term repopulating cells than did G-CSF, plerixafor, or GROβ alone [119]. In addition, SKL cells mobilized by plerixafor+GROβ expressed higher levels of the adhesion receptors CD11a (LFA-1), CD49e (VLA-5), and CD49d than did those mobilized by plerixafor or GROβ alone, which may contribute to improved bone marrow homing [119]. Annexin V staining of mobilized cells showed that G-CSF (6.4±1.5%), plerixafor (10.4±2.6%), and GROβ (4.5±1.2%) alone each mobilized a greater percentage of apoptotic cells than did the combination of plerixafor+GROβ (2.9±0.4%) [119]. Although not compared directly with chemomobilization in these studies, novel combinations of mobilization agents have the potential to mobilize more primitive HSCs, which have a greater repopulation capacity.

Graft Content in Autologous Transplant Patients

Current regimens mobilize grafts with varying clonogenicity. Although the use of G-CSF has been shown to stimulate the release of cells with high clonogenic potential, several studies suggest that chemomobilized grafts may have greater clonogenic potential, as evidenced by the collection of two- to fourfold more burst-forming unit erythrocytes and two- to sixfold more GM-CFUs per nucleated cell than that after cytokine-only mobilization (see Table 9.2 for a summary of autologous graft content) [98, 125–138]. Long-term culture-initiating cells (LTC-ICs) were also found at 12-fold higher levels in chemomobilized grafts than in grafts mobilized by G-CSF alone [125]. After 4 days of G-CSF administration, plerixafor administration was shown to increase the frequency of LTC-ICs by a further 1.6-fold [129].

Mobilization with G-CSF, chemotherapy + G-CSF, or plerixafor + G-CSF has been shown to mobilize primitive hematopoietic precursors, including $CD34^+CD33^-$, $CD34^+CD38^-$, $CD34^+CD133^+$, $CD34^+Thy1^+$, and $CD34^+HLADR^-$ cells [126, 129, 140–142]. The presence of primitive precursors, such as $CD34^+CD33^-$ cells, has been predictive of platelet engraftment after aHSCT [101, 143]. The effects of cyclophosphamide on $CD34^+CD33^-$ cell collection have been mixed. For example, one study reported a higher percentage of these cells in patients mobilized by cyclophosphamide + G-CSF than in patients mobilized by G-CSF alone, whereas $CD34^+CD38^-$, $CD34^+Thy1^+$, and $CD34^+HLADR^-$ subsets remained unchanged [126]. However, a second study showed that mobilization with cyclophosphamide + G-CSF decreased the number of immature $CD34^+$ cells [141]. In a third study, the proportion of primitive $CD34^+CD38^-$ progenitors (as a percentage of total $CD34^+$ cells) was higher in patients mobilized by G-CSF than in patients mobilized by chemotherapy + G-CSF; however, this difference was offset by a higher total collected cell number in the chemotherapy + G-CSF group, which resulted in higher $CD34^+CD38^-$ cell counts in the apheresis product [98]. Plerixafor administration resulted in a nearly threefold greater proportion and an eightfold higher number of primitive $CD34^+CD38^-$ precursors in the peripheral blood compared with 4 days of G-CSF mobilization [129]. Although not compared directly, chemotherapy, cytokines, and plerixafor each preferentially mobilize different primitive progenitor subsets.

Specific immunomodulating graft cell subsets, including DCs, are altered after mobilization with different regimens. In one study, G-CSF administration increased DC1 by 2.6-fold and DC2 by 5.9-fold in the peripheral blood in one study [130] while in a second study, total DCs increased twofold after G-CSF mobilization [131]. The effects of chemomobilization on graft DC content and polarization have been mixed [131–134]. Regarding polarization, one group showed that chemomobilization polarized DCs toward DC2, with the DC1:DC2 ratio decreasing tenfold in apheresis collections [134]. Similarly, another study demonstrated that mobilization with chemotherapy + G-CSF yielded a higher proportion of DC2 in the graft and a lower DC1:DC2 ratio than did chemotherapy + G-CSF + GM-CSF [135]. In contrast, Gazitt et al. showed that there was no DC polarization after chemomobilization with cyclophosphamide in combination with G-CSF, GM-CSF, or

Table 9.2 Cell types mobilized by G-CSF, chemotherapy, or plerixafor in autologous transplant patients [98, 125–138]

Cell type	G-CSF mobilization	Chemomobilization	Plerixafor mobilization
Clonogenic		Greater numbers of clonogenic cells and LTC-IC than G-CSF mobilization [125–128]	Higher frequency of LTC-IC compared with G-CSF mobilization [129]
Primitive hematopoietic precursors	Higher proportion of $CD34^+CD38^-$ cells compared to chemomobilization [98]	Higher proportion of $CD34^+CD33^-$ cells compared to G-CSF mobilization [126] Higher absolute number of $CD34^+CD38^-$ cells compared to G-CSF mobilization [98]	Greater proportion and number of $CD34^+CD38^-$ cells [129] and higher proportion of CD34-AlDH-bright cells [139] compared to G-CSF mobilization
Dendritic Cell	Total cells increased compared to BM [130, 131] DC2 preferentially mobilized [130, 131]	Polarization results are mixed [131–135]	No further polarization when administered following 4 days of G-CSF observed [136]
T regulatory cells	Proportion of $CD25^+$ cells increased [137]		
$CD3^+$ T cells			Increased compared to G-CSF mobilization [138]
$CD4^+$ T cells			Increased compared to G-CSF mobilization [138]
$CD8^+$ T cells			Increased compared to G-CSF mobilization [138]
Natural killer cells			Increased compared to G-CSF mobilization [138]

DC2 dendritic cell type 2, *G-CSF* granulocyte colony-stimulating factor, *LTC-ICs* long-term culture-initiating cells

G-CSF+GM-CSF [132]. However, a greater number of total DCs were mobilized by cyclophosphamide+GM-CSF than by cyclophosphamide+G-CSF; cyclophosphamide+G-CSF+GM-CSF mobilized an intermediate number of DCs [133]. Plerixafor administration after 4 days of G-CSF resulted in a greater than twofold further increase in both DC1 and DC2, with no additional DC polarization [136]. Because increased pretransplant and posttransplant total DC levels have been shown to correlate with longer OS, it is of interest to examine whether elevated graft DC levels directly correlate to improved aHSCT outcomes [144].

Other cell types, including immunosuppressant Tregs, cytotoxic T cells, and natural killer (NK) cells, are also collected from patients. After G-CSF mobilization, Tregs were found to be nearly threefold higher in the peripheral blood of patients with NHL and multiple myeloma [130]. Cyclophosphamide mobilization has been shown to decrease T-cell counts threefold compared with baseline. By the time of collection, most chemomobilized patients will recover only one-third of their T-cell levels. Although the relative ratios of most T cells ($CD4^+$ central memory, effector memory, late effector, and $CD8^+$ cells) did not change from precyclophosphamide measurements, the proportion of $CD25^+$ cells (including Tregs) increased two- to threefold [137]. Because cyclophosphamide has been shown to be toxic to Tregs, their presence in chemomobilized autografts may be attributable to G-CSF administration [145, 146]. A recent study demonstrated that autologous grafts mobilized by plerixafor+G-CSF had a significantly higher Treg content than did chemomobilized grafts (median: 11.3% compared with 7.5%; $P=0.04$) [147]. Consistent with their function as immunomodulators, Tregs have been shown to inhibit the cytotoxicity of autologous $CD8^+$ T cells in vitro and thus may suppress anticancer immune responses in patients [148–153]. Whether infused Treg levels correlate with immunosuppression and anticancer immune activity in patients remains to be elucidated. Regarding immune cell graft content, $CD3^+$, $CD4^+$, and $CD8^+$ T cells and NK cells increased 4-, 5-, 2.5-, and 3-fold more, respectively, in collections from patients mobilized by plerixafor+G-CSF than in patients mobilized by G-CSF alone [138]. Interestingly, immune cell subsets were shown to vary by mobilization day (1 vs. 2) and disease (NHL vs. multiple myeloma). Specifically, greater $CD3^+$, $CD4^+$, and $CD8^+$ cells were collected on apheresis day 1 compared to day 2. When comparing disease state, NHL patients collected less $CD4^+$, $CD19^+$, and $CD56^+$ cells than myeloma patients [154]. Infusion of greater lymphocyte and NK cell doses has been shown to improve immune reconstitution and correlated with better OS and PFS [107–109].

Allogeneic Graft Content

The cell content of allogeneic grafts isolated from healthy donor bone marrow and/or mobilized peripheral blood has been analyzed, with a focus on primitive progenitors, clonogenic potential, and total T cell, Treg, and DC populations (see Table 9.3 for the summary of allogeneic graft content) [105, 134, 140, 141, 147, 155–161]. Although grafts mobilized by G-CSF contain fewer primitive hematopoietic precursors, they

Table 9.3 Cell types mobilized by G-CSF or plerixafor in allogeneic transplant donors [105, 134, 140, 141, 147, 155–161]

Cell type	G-CSF mobilization	Plerixafor mobilization
Clonogenic	Similar composition to bone marrow [141]	
Primitive hematopoietic precursors	Fewer primitive precursors than bone marrow [155]	Similar levels compared to G-CSF mobilization [140] Higher levels of primitive $CD34^{dim}$ population [156]
Dendritic Cell	DC2 preferentially mobilized [105, 134]	
T regulatory cells	Little change in levels compared with bone marrow [147, 157]	
$CD3^+$ T cells	Increased compared with bone marrow [158, 159]	Increased compared with G-CSF mobilization [160, 161]
$CD4^+$ T cells	Increased compared with bone marrow [158, 159]	Increased compared with G-CSF mobilization [161]
$CD8^+$ T cells	Increased compared with bone marrow [158, 159]	

DC2 dendritic cell type 2, *G-CSF* granulocyte colony-stimulating factor

have been shown to be as clonogenic as bone marrow, as measured by LTC-IC frequency [141, 155]. The proportion of myelomonocytic-committed cells was significantly higher in peripheral blood than in bone marrow, but the proportion of erythroid progenitors in peripheral blood was not significantly different from that in bone marrow [141]. The utility of plerixafor as a mobilization agent in allogeneic donors has also been explored. Regarding clonogenic potential, plerixafor was shown to mobilize GM-CFUs and burst-forming unit erythrocytes [46]. A pair-wise comparison of the proportion of primitive progenitors present in apheresis products from individuals who received plerixafor and then G-CSF, with a 10-day washout period between treatments, showed no significant differences in the $CD34^+$ subtypes: $CD34^+CD133^-$, $CD34^+CD133^+$, $CD34^+CD38^-$, and $CD34^+CD38^+$ [140]. Interestingly, a new population of $CD34^+$ cells was recently identified after plerixafor treatment. Flow cytometric analysis of $CD34^+$ cell subsets mobilized by either plerixafor or G-CSF in healthy donors identified a $CD34^{dim}CD45RA^+$ cell population that is unique to plerixafor-mobilized donors (60%; six of ten donors analyzed) [156]. Up to 20% of $CD34^+$ cells in plerixafor-mobilized grafts were $CD34^{dim}CD45RA^+$ cells compared with <2% of G-CSF-mobilized $CD34^+$ cells [156]. Extensive FACS and functional analyses demonstrated that these cells are plasmacytoid progenitors of DC2 cells. These $CD34^{dim}CD45RA^+$ cells express high levels of the proliferation marker Ki-67 [162]. To which extent these highly proliferative cells survive the freeze–thaw process that is applied routinely in the autologous setting is currently unclear and needs further study. In summary, plerixafor may mobilize more primitive and different additional precursors than other agents.

Dendritic cells are important immunomodulatory cells, and an increased dose of DC2 has been correlated with a decreased incidence of GVHD in allogeneic transplant recipients [112]. Arpinati et al. [105] showed that G-CSF treatment induced DC polarization toward DC2 in healthy donors, and approximately five times more DC2 were found in peripheral blood than in bone marrow. Similarly, another study showed that although G-CSF mobilization did not alter the proportion of total DCs in the collected graft, the DC1:DC2 ratio decreased eightfold, which suggests that DC2 are preferentially mobilized [134].

The T-cell content can have a profound effect on allogeneic transplant outcomes. For example, increased $CD3^+$ T-cell doses have been shown to be associated with an increased incidence of acute GVHD (aGVHD) [163, 164]. G-CSF mobilization results in at least fourfold more T cells in peripheral blood than in unmobilized bone marrow [158, 159] while effector memory and naïve T cells decreased during G-CSF mobilization [157]. Grafts mobilized by plerixafor alone or in combination with G-CSF had an even higher T-cell content than did those mobilized by G-CSF [160]. Devine et al. [161] similarly showed that $CD3^+$ and $CD4^+$ T cells were higher in grafts collected after mobilization with single-agent plerixafor than after mobilization with G-CSF. Although plerixafor-mobilized grafts have a higher T-cell content than bone marrow, the allogeneic transplant of these cells in a small cohort of patients does not appear to increase aGVHD rates higher than historical controls. However, these results require further validation in a larger trial. This suggests that either plerixafor-mobilized T cells or other graft characteristics may contribute to greater host tolerance [158, 161].

Regulatory T cells have shown the ability to combat GVHD, and their presence in allogeneic grafts has been shown to correlate with a reduction in GVHD and improved OS [110]. Regulatory T-cell levels have been shown to vary little in allogeneic donors receiving different mobilization regimens. Studies have shown no difference in Treg levels when comparing unmobilized bone marrow or peripheral blood and G-CSF-mobilized peripheral blood [147]. When compared with multiple myeloma or NHL patients, healthy donors mobilized fewer Tregs [147]. However, 3 weeks after the completion of G-CSF treatment, Tregs have been measured at a twofold higher level in the peripheral blood than in unmobilized peripheral blood [157]. In contrast, $CD3^+CD4^-CD8^-$ Tregs were preferentially mobilized by G-CSF and were found in higher numbers in mobilized peripheral blood than in unmobilized bone marrow [165]. The Treg content of plerixafor-mobilized donors has not yet been evaluated. Although not shown to be mobilized to a great extent by G-CSF, given their ability to modulate GVHD, Treg graft content may be of great importance to allogeneic transplantation.

Depending on the regimen used (G-CSF, plerixafor, or a combination of the two), the first day of collection with respect to donor mobilization initiation varied. For example, individuals who received single-agent plerixafor in the studies by Liles et al. [114] and Devine et al. [115] underwent apheresis on the same day that mobilization started (day 1) or on day 5 of mobilization with G-CSF or plerixafor + G-CSF. In these studies, plerixafor-treated donors, in whom mobilization and collection occurred on the same day, exhibited higher T-cell levels in their grafts than did those mobilized by G-CSF alone [160, 161]. When plerixafor was combined with G-CSF, the number of T cells collected was lower than the number collected after plerixafor alone, but was still significantly higher than the number collected after G-CSF alone

[160]. Thus, it is possible that different mobilization regimens and administration schedules result in differential mobilization kinetics of various cell subsets, which, in turn, could affect the graft content.

Cell Cycle Status

Although there is little functional effect of cell cycle on hematopoietic engraftment based on in vitro tests and transplant studies, cell cycle status may become important when considering ex vivo graft manipulations. For example, when considering the use of a purging agent to eliminate cancer cells from autografts, an understanding of the cell cycle of normal HSCs is critical. A cell cycle-dependent purging technique may better spare normal HSCs collected from the peripheral blood while targeting cancer cells undergoing division. However, some cancerous cells are also noncycling. Differences in the cell cycle status of bone marrow and mobilized peripheral blood have been demonstrated.

Mobilized peripheral blood HSCs have shown a markedly different cell cycle profile than that of bone marrow HSCs. Data from preclinical models and from individuals undergoing mobilization for an autologous or allogeneic transplant suggest that G-CSF mobilization results in a lower proportion of cells in $S/G_2/M$ in mobilized peripheral blood than in unmobilized bone marrow [142, 166, 167]. This cell cycle profile correlates with a gene expression profile showing increased expression of cell cycle inhibitory genes in G-CSF-mobilized peripheral blood [168]. The effect of chemomobilization on cell cycle status has been investigated in preclinical models and autologous transplant patients and is similar to that observed with G-CSF [116, 142, 166]. Finally, although plerixafor-mobilized peripheral blood HSCs appear to have a cell cycle profile more closely related to bone marrow HSCs than to those mobilized using other regimens, most of the mobilized $CD34^+$ cells are not in the $S/G_2/M$ phase.

Gene Expression Analysis

Given that mobilization regimens vary with respect to mechanism of action, it is not unexpected that gene expression profiles differ between the same cell types mobilized by different methods. Altered gene expression could lead to phenotypic changes that dictate HSC viability, homing capability, and engraftment potential.

Preclinical Gene Expression Data

Global gene (17,500 cDNA probes) microarray analysis of $CD34^+$ cells isolated from macaques that received either G-CSF, plerixafor, G-CSF+plerixafor, or

Table 9.4 Gene expression changes following mobilization in preclinical models [46, 169–171]

Gene/ gene category	Mobilization regimen	Expression change
CXCR4	Plerixafor	Increased compared to G-CSF mobilization [169, 170]
VLA-4	Plerixafor	Increased compared to G-CSF mobilization [170]
VLA-5	Plerixafor	Increased compared to G-CSF mobilization [46]
CD62L (L-selectin)	G-CSF	Increased compared to plerixafor mobilization [46]
Adhesion molecules	Plerixafor or G-CSF	Lower compared to unmobilized bone marrow [171]
T-cell related	Plerixafor	Increased compared to G-CSF mobilization [169]
B-cell related	Plerixafor	Increased compared to G-CSF mobilization [169]
Mast cell related	Plerixafor	Increased compared to G-CSF mobilization [169]
Neutrophil related	G-CSF	Increased compared to plerixafor mobilization [169]
Macrophage related	G-CSF	Increased compared to plerixafor mobilization [169]

CXCR4 CXC motif receptor 4, *G-CSF* granulocyte colony-stimulating factor, *VLA-4* very late antigen-4, VLA-5, very late antigen-5

plerixafor alone yielded three distinct clusters [169]. Genes expressed by T cells, B cells, and mast cells were enriched in plerixafor-mobilized cells, whereas genes expressed by neutrophils and macrophages were enriched in G-CSF-mobilized cells (Table 9.4) [46, 169–171]. Genes expressed by B cells were enriched in plerixafor+G-CSF mobilized cells to a greater degree than in cells mobilized by either agent alone [169]. This suggests that the phenotypes of cells mobilized by plerixafor+G-CSF may vary considerably from those mobilized with either agent alone.

Individual genes postulated to be involved in bone marrow homing and engraftment have been shown to vary with different mobilization regimens. One study in macaques showed that a significantly higher proportion of plerixafor-mobilized CD34$^+$ cells expressed CXCR4 both on the cell surface (53 ± 23% compared with 11 ± 9%; $P = 0.02$) and intracellularly compared with G-CSF [170]. Similarly, gene expression of CXCR4 was also found to be significantly upregulated in plerixafor-mobilized cells [169]. The adhesion molecule VLA-4 was also expressed at a significantly higher proportion in plerixafor-mobilized CD34$^+$ cells than in G-CSF-mobilized CD34$^+$ cells (71 ± 13% compared with 41 ± 23%; $P = 0.03$). These cell surface proteins may have contributed to the superior in vitro migration toward SDF-1 and repopulating ability of plerixafor-mobilized cells in this study relative to cells mobilized by G-CSF alone [170]. Cell surface expression of either protein was not significantly different between plerixafor-mobilized peripheral blood and bone marrow [170]. CD34$^+$ cells mobilized by plerixafor+G-CSF expressed significantly higher levels of the adhesion protein very late antigen-5 (VLA-5), whereas G-CSF-mobilized CD34$^+$ cells expressed significantly higher CD62L levels and included a greater proportion of cells expressing CD62L [46]. In mice, cell surface expression of several adhesion molecules, but not of CXCR4, was higher in bone marrow cells than in plerixafor- or G-CSF-mobilized cells, which suggests that hypoadhesion may be a prerequisite for bone marrow egress [171].

Table 9.5 Gene expression changes following mobilization in autologous patients and allogeneic donors [129, 168, 172–175]

Gene/gene category	Mobilization regimen	Expression change
CXCR4	Chemomobilization	Decreased compared to premobilization levels [172]
CXCR4	G-CSF	Increased compared to unmobilized bone marrow [173]
CXCR4	Plerixafor	Unchanged compared to premobilization levels [173]
CXCR4	Plerixafor + G-CSF	Increased compared to G-CSF mobilization [129, 174]
Cell cycle progression	G-CSF	Decreased compared to bone marrow [168] Decreased compared to plerixafor + G-CSF mobilization [174]
DNA synthesis	G-CSF	Decreased compared to bone marrow [168]
Antiapoptosis	Plerixafor + G-CSF	Increased compared to G-CSF mobilization [174]
Cell adhesion	Plerixafor + G-CSF	Increased compared to G-CSF mobilization [174]
Cell motility	Plerixafor + G-CSF	Increased compared to G-CSF mobilization [174]
Pro-apoptosis	G-CSF	Increased compared to plerixafor + G-CSF mobilization [174]
Hematopoiesis-associated miRNAs	G-CSF, plerixafor, or plerixafor + G-CSF	Increased compared to unmobilized peripheral blood [175]

CXCR4 CXC motif receptor 4, *G-CSF* granulocyte colony-stimulating factor, *miRNA* microribonucleic acid

Gene Expression Studies in Autologous and Allogeneic Grafts

Because of its central role in HSC mobilization and engraftment, CXCR4 expression has been monitored in several studies, and its expression differs based on mobilization regimen (Table 9.5) [129, 168, 172–175]. CD34^{+} cells isolated from the peripheral blood of NHL patients mobilized by cyclophosphamide + G-CSF, GM-CSF, or G-CSF followed by GM-CSF all exhibited a lower CXCR4 expression than did premobilized peripheral blood CD34^{+} cells [172]. Mobilization with G-CSF resulted in a higher expression of CXCR4 in allogeneic grafts than in bone marrow [168, 176]. Cell surface CXCR4 expression was shown to decrease after plerixafor administration; however, expression rebounded to pre-plerixafor levels in the apheresis product [173]. Two additional studies reported higher CXCR4 expression in peripheral blood CD34^{+} cells after plerixafor administration in combination with G-CSF compared with G-CSF alone [129, 174]. CXCR4 expression may impact bone marrow homing [40] and unlike cytokine or plerixafor mobilization, its expression may be negatively impacted by cyclophosphamide. Increased adhesion molecule expression may benefit bone marrow homing, but may be detrimental to HSC mobilization. Interestingly, decreased CXCR4 expression has been shown to correlate with improved HSC mobilization [176]. Conversely, lower CD34^{+} cell harvests from the bone marrow have been shown to correlate with decreased CXCR4 expression [176].

The expression of several gene types that might contribute to transplanted cell survival and engraftment is altered when comparing bone marrow and mobilized peripheral blood. CD34^{+} cell expression of cell cycle progression and DNA synthesis genes was greater for bone marrow than for G-CSF-mobilized peripheral blood while expression of cell cycle inhibition and apoptosis genes (including caspases 3, 4, and 8) was greater in G-CSF-mobilized peripheral blood compared with bone marrow [168]. The cell cycle gene expression profile correlates with the fact that more bone marrow HSCs than peripheral blood HSCs are cycling [167]. Interestingly, long-term changes in gene expression have been documented in donors mobilized by G-CSF, with 53 cell growth, proliferation, and communication genes upregulated and 69 downregulated up to 9 months after mobilization [177]. Compared to G-CSF alone, CD34⁺ cells mobilized by plerixafor plus G-CSF had higher expression of antiapoptosis, cell cycle promotion, cell adhesion, and cell motility genes and lower expression of pro-apoptotic genes [174]. Expression of the adhesion molecules LFA-1, CD62L, CD44, VLA-4, or platelet endothelial cell adhesion molecule was not significantly different before or after plerixafor administration after 4 days of G-CSF [173]. Taken together, plerixafor-mobilized cells exhibit a gene expression profile that is favorable to survival and bone marrow homing.

Many genes associated with Tregs were upregulated in T cells isolated from G-CSF-treated donor peripheral blood, but not in unmobilized peripheral blood; many of these genes remained upregulated 3 weeks after G-CSF administration [157]. In addition, the expression of genes associated with Th 1 cells decreased, whereas those associated with Th 2 cells increased, which provided further evidence of the Th 2 polarization of G-CSF-mobilized donors [157]. Importantly, genes associated with antigen processing and GVHD were downregulated after G-CSF administration [157]. Taken together, T cells mobilized by G-CSF had a gene expression profile that suggested greater tolerance toward host cells. This may partially explain why allogeneic transplant of G-CSF-mobilized grafts (with a greater T-cell content than bone marrow) did not cause significantly elevated aGVHD rates [178]. However, over the long-term, chronic GVHD (cGVHD) rates are higher in patients who receive mobilized peripheral blood than in those who receive bone marrow, which suggests the involvement of other factors [178].

RNA profiling can provide global assessments of gene expression changes. The RNA profiles of healthy donor CD34⁺ cells isolated from bone marrow clustered with plerixafor-mobilized HSCs more closely than with G-CSF-mobilized HSCs [156]. This finding suggests that global gene expression is altered to a lesser extent when cells are mobilized by plerixafor than when mobilized by G-CSF. Thus, plerixafor-mobilized cells may be more akin to bone marrow than G-CSF-mobilized cells [156]. Interestingly, genes upregulated by a combination of G-CSF and plerixafor included many not upregulated by either agent alone [156]. This finding is consistent with the concept of synergy between the two agents and suggests that the manner in which CD34⁺ cells are mobilized by the combination of G-CSF and plerixafor may not simply be a function of two exclusive mechanisms of action. In addition, microRNA (miRNA) profiling demonstrated that expression of hematopoiesis-associated miRNAs was higher in mobilized HSCs (regardless of regimen) compared to unmobilized peripheral blood, suggesting greater repopulation capacity for HSCs [175]. Interestingly, mobilization with plerixafor alone or in conjunction with G-CSF resulted in a distinct miRNA profile compared with G-CSF-mobilized cells [175].

Clinical Implications of Graft Content

The ultimate goal of mobilization for autologous stem cell transplantation is to obtain cells that result in durable engraftment and rapid and sustained hematopoietic recovery, which in turn affects long-term outcomes such as OS and PFS. Similarly, for allogeneic transplantation, it is important to collect a graft that will allow durable engraftment, rapid hematopoietic recovery, and minimal incidence of aGVHD and cGVHD. These goals are affected by both the cell types present in the graft and the intrinsic qualities of these cells.

Effect of Graft Content in Preclinical Models

Bone Marrow Homing

Bone marrow homing is a complex cellular activity dependent on the coordination of intracellular gene expression and the response to extracellular stimuli. Using mouse models, Bonig et al. [179] identified increased cell motility as a factor that contributes to improved bone marrow homing. In general, mobilized CD34$^+$ cells (irrespective of the mobilization regimen used) display increased homing potential compared to unprimed bone marrow [171, 179]. It appears that homing is dependent not only on CXCR4, but also on adhesion molecules and intrinsic cell motility capacity [118, 119, 170, 179].

Bone Marrow Repopulation

Homing capability can estimate the ability of cells to migrate toward the bone marrow, but whether cells actually engraft and repopulate once in the marrow space is of great importance. Much of the recent published data have focused on novel mobilization agents such as plerixafor and GROβ, with comparisons frequently made with G-CSF. Competitive repopulation assays in mice showed that cells mobilized by plerixafor + G-CSF were more successful at repopulation than those mobilized by either agent alone [46]. Importantly, cells mobilized by plerixafor or plerixafor + G-CSF showed a great capacity for self-renewal, as transplanted cells isolated from a first recipient repopulated a second lethally irradiated mouse [46].

The effects of cell cycle on repopulation remain largely uncharacterized. Ex vivo cell cycle activation of CD34$^+$ cells has resulted in more rapid short-term granulocyte recovery, but has not correlated with short- or long-term engraftment in a nonhuman primate model of aHSCT [180].

Plerixafor-mobilized long-term repopulating rhesus macaque cells as determined by gene marking and competitive repopulation assays [170]. Twenty-four months posttransplant, plerixafor-mobilized peripheral blood mononuclear cells and granulocytes were still detectable, whereas G-CSF-mobilized cells were not

[170]. Lentiviral marking studies showed an accelerated lymphocyte reconstitution and long-term multilineage recovery after transplantation of lentiviral-transduced rhesus $CD34^+$ cells mobilized by G-CSF and plerixafor compared to a graft mobilized with G-CSF and SCF [181]. One year after transplantation, all animals had 2–10% transgene expression in all blood cell lineages.

Similarly, work in a canine model system showed that plerixafor-mobilized peripheral blood mononuclear cells supported autologous and allogeneic transplants for over 1 year [182]. In another study, plerixafor + GROβ mobilized threefold more marrow repopulating units than did G-CSF, plerixafor, or GROβ alone. Furthermore, the engraftment capacity of cells mobilized by plerixafor + GROβ was superior to that of cells mobilized by any agent alone as determined by chimerism analyses 6 months after competitive transplant [119]. These preclinical studies suggest that novel agents and combination regimens may mobilize cells with improved repopulation capacity.

Clinical Effect of Autologous Graft Content

Bone Marrow Homing

With respect to clinical outcomes, better spontaneous and SDF-1-induced $CD34^+$ cell migration has been shown to correlate with faster neutrophil engraftment after transplant, independent of cell dose [183]. However, individual gene contributions to bone marrow homing remain unclear. For example, when examined in isolation, CXCR4 expression did not correlate with either spontaneous or SDF-1-induced migration in cells mobilized by chemotherapy + G-CSF [183]. Interestingly, the transplant of $CD34^+$L-selectin$^+$ cells correlated significantly better with rapid platelet engraftment than absolute $CD34^+$ cell dose, suggesting that adhesion molecule expression benefits homing [184]. Thus, cell migration is a more complex process than solely the ability to receive SDF-1 signals and adhere. General cell motility, the result of a wide variety of genes, contributes strongly to migration. Plerixafor-mobilized grafts have exhibited increased expression of genes that may facilitate migration and engraftment, including those involved in antiapoptosis, cell cycle promotion, and cell motility [174]. It remains to be seen whether elevated expression of these gene types correlates with improved engraftment.

Engraftment

Hematopoietic engraftment can be divided into short-term recovery (neutrophils, platelets, and RBCs) and long-term engraftment (primitive progenitor cells). The dose of infused $CD34^+$ cells remains the most important determining factor of neutrophil and platelet engraftment [185–187]. However, the presence of other graft cell subtypes has also been shown to affect hematologic recovery. For example,

$CD34^+CD33^-$ cell dose ($>1.38\times10^6$ $CD34^+$ cells/kg) was shown to better predict platelet recovery than $CD34^+$ cell dose [101]. In addition, higher $CD34^+CD33^-$ cell doses have correlated with rapid neutrophil recovery [100, 143]. An increased dose of $CD34^+CD110^+$ (CD110 is the thrombopoietin receptor, which is essential for platelet production [188, 189]) cells has been shown to be highly predictive of platelet transfusion independence within 21 days posttransplant [190]. Threshold values of 5×10^5 total CFUs and 2.5×10^4 CFU-megakaryocytes have also been shown to predict rapid platelet recovery [191]. It has been suggested that colony forming cells and colony forming cells-megakaryocytes be used when infused doses are near or below 2×10^6 $CD34^+$ cells/kg to predict platelet recovery [191]. Taken together, the contributions of a wide variety of cell types can both predict and influence timely engraftment.

Recently, human $CD8^+CD3^+TCR^-$ cells were shown to facilitate hematopoietic engraftment of suboptimal cell doses in nonobese diabetic/severe combined immunodeficiency (NOD/SCID) mice [192]. When $CD34^+$ cells were co-cultured with $CD8^+CD3^+TCR^-$ cells in vitro, hematopoietic colony formation was increased and shown to be a direct effect of $CD8^+CD3^+TCR^-$ cells. Interestingly, these cells have been shown to be present at levels two- to fivefold higher in G-CSF-mobilized peripheral blood than in bone marrow, cord blood, and normal peripheral blood and may help facilitate engraftment of peripheral blood HSCs in patients, especially for those receiving lower $CD34^+$ cell doses [192].

Because primitive progenitor cells have excellent repopulation and proliferation capacities [193, 194], increasing their number in the graft might improve long-term engraftment outcomes. In fact, LTC-IC number, not $CD34^+$ cell dose or GM-CFU number, in mobilized peripheral blood correlated with 1-year marrow progenitor cell recovery after aHSCT [102]. Conversely, the number of LTC-ICs autografted from bone marrow or peripheral blood (mobilized or steady state) did not correlate with short-term neutrophil, platelet, or RBC recovery [195, 196]. In a recent study, nearly all patients (91%) transplanted with G-CSF + plerixafor-mobilized peripheral blood progenitor cells reached the target of full and sustained platelet reconstitution (>150/nL) within 30 days [129]. In a previous study of chemomobilized patients, the threshold of 150 platelets/nL was reached within 180 days in only 63% of aHSCT recipients [197]. Similarly, 65% of patients who received $2–7\times10^6$ $CD34^+$ cells/kg required 1–7 months to reach the same platelet threshold [198]. These data support the notion that G-CSF + plerixafor-mobilized grafts contain more primitive hematopoietic cells with superior long-term engraftment potential [129].

Immune Reconstitution

Immune reconstitution after aHSCT is vital to stave off infection and promote early survival. The use of $CD34^+$ selected grafts (lymphocyte depleted) has allowed evaluation of accessory cell importance with respect to immune reconstitution and infection. Absolute lymphocyte count (ALC) recovery is an established surrogate marker for immune reconstitution, and improved ALC recovery posttransplant has been predictive of superior OS and PFS [107, 199, 200]. In turn, infusion of greater lymphocyte numbers has correlated with improved OS and PFS [107–109]. Of several cell types examined, only increased NK cell dose correlated with faster ALC recovery [107]. Interestingly, NK cell numbers have been shown to be threefold higher in collections from NHL patients mobilized by plerixafor + G-CSF than in those mobilized by G-CSF alone [138]. Patients receiving plerixafor + G-CSF mobilized cells exhibited higher ALC recovery 15 days posttransplant [138]. In addition, after a median follow-up of 20 months, 0 of 7 patients in the plerixafor + G-CSF group but 15 of 29 (52%) patients in the G-CSF group relapsed [138]. However, a direct causal relationship between better ALC recovery and relapse rate was not examined by this group. The transplant of greater lymphocyte doses (including $CD3^+$, NK, and $CD8^+$ cells) has correlated with faster neutrophil recovery, while increased $CD4^+$ cell doses were associated with decreased infection rates [141].

The contributions other graft cell types can make to aHSCT outcomes should not be ignored. For example, the content of DCs both before and after transplant was shown to correlate with better survival outcomes [144]. Specifically, high DC1 and total DC levels before transplant and high DC1, DC2, and total DC levels after transplant were shown to correlate with improved OS [144]. Although the impact of several cell types on aHSCT has been elucidated, it is likely that others remain to be identified.

Effect of Graft Content on Allogeneic Transplant Outcomes

Bone Marrow Repopulation

Timely bone marrow repopulation and engraftment are the early goals of aHSCT, and mouse models have been useful in assessing bone marrow repopulation of human HSCs mobilized by different regimens. A pair-wise comparison of donors mobilized with plerixafor and then G-CSF demonstrated that bone marrow repopulation was significantly higher in mice transplanted with 2×10^7 plerixafor-mobilized mononuclear cells than in mice transplanted with the same dose of G-CSF-mobilized cells ($P < 0.05$) [140]. Furthermore, NOD/SCID repopulating cells were present at a significantly higher frequency in plerixafor-mobilized cells than in G-CSF-mobilized cells [140]. Similarly, donors mobilized greater than threefold more NOD/SCID repopulating cells when administered plerixafor compared with G-CSF. However, G-CSF + plerixafor mobilized more NOD/SCID repopulating cells than either treatment alone, suggesting synergy between these agents [46].

T-Cell Content and GVHD

The contributions of immune cell types to allogeneic transplant outcomes have been difficult to study in isolation. Increased doses of allogeneic $CD3^+$ cells have been shown to be associated with increased aGVHD, but also with decreased treatment-related mortality, better leukemia-free survival, and improved OS [163, 164]. In addition, Waller et al. [201] showed that high doses of $CD4^{bright}$ T cells were associated with decreased event-free survival (EFS) and cGVHD but increased relapse. Activated ($CD152^+$) T cells and NK cells were negative predictors of cGVHD in a prospective trial of allogeneic transplantation [202]. Furthermore, the ratio of CD4 to CD8 cells was negatively associated with disease-free survival and OS [203]. Thus, several studies have indicated increased T-cell content could contribute to GVHD, however, the characteristics of T cells collected may also impact patient outcomes.

Despite higher T-cell content, G-CSF-mobilized grafts are not necessarily associated with higher aGVHD rates [158, 204–206]. Furthermore, Devine et al. [161] showed in a small cohort that despite higher T-cell content, allogeneic transplant of plerixafor-mobilized grafts did not result in aGVHD or cGVHD rates greater than a historical G-CSF-mobilized control population. However, these results require further validation in a larger trial. These findings suggest that the characteristics of graft T cells are important when discussing transplant outcomes. For example, $CD62L^+$ naïve T cells have been shown to be more alloreactive and thus may contribute more to GVHD than $CD62L^-$ memory T cells [207, 208]. These cell populations were not different in peripheral blood cells before and after plerixafor administration [161]. The mobilizing agent used may also play a role in GVHD protection, because Morris et al. [209] showed lower alloreactivity in donor T cells mobilized by pegylated G-CSF than in those mobilized by standard G-CSF. Gene expression is also likely to influence GVHD, and the profile of G-CSF-mobilized T cells suggests greater host tolerance [157]. Another possible explanation for the low incidence of GVHD was that G-CSF- and plerixafor-mobilized grafts may contain more Tregs, potentially offsetting higher $CD3^+$ cell levels. Thus, absolute levels of different cell types may not sufficiently explain transplant outcomes. Further study into the cellular characteristics of grafts is warranted.

Several studies have shown that transplanting high Treg numbers can prevent GVHD in mice [210–213] and this has been studied in allogeneic transplant patients as well. In a study of 34 patients who received HLA-identical sibling donor cells after standard intensity conditioning, those receiving higher Treg numbers had a 45% lower cumulative incidence of aGVHD than those receiving lower Treg numbers [110]. Multivariate analysis identified low graft Treg content as an independent prognostic factor for aGVHD [110]. Importantly, no difference in relapse rate was observed between these two groups, and OS was improved in those receiving higher Treg doses [110]. Similarly, patients experiencing early (within 30–45 days after transplant) Treg recovery had a lower incidence of aGVHD [111]. Conversely, the proportion of circulating Tregs was lower in patients with GVHD [111]. Treg frequency has been shown to vary by mobilization regimen in autologous transplant patients [147], however, it remains to be vigorously studied in the allogeneic setting.

Effects of Dendritic Cells on GVHD

The effects of DCs are also an important consideration when discussing GVHD. Myeloid DCs typically drive differentiation toward Th 1 cells, which promote cytotoxic T cells (contributors to GVHD), whereas DC2 can drive T-cell differentiation toward Th 2 cells, which promote allergic responses [104, 105]. Larger DC2 numbers correlated with significantly shorter EFS, lower cGVHD incidence, and higher relapse incidence [112]. Because G-CSF treatment induces polarization toward DC2, the higher T-cell content observed in G-CSF-mobilized grafts compared with bone marrow may be tempered by increased DC2 levels [105]. Gene expression analysis of plerixafor-mobilized donor cells has revealed no evidence of T-cell polarization [214]. Thus, DC polarization may help modulate the impact of GVHD in peripheral blood-derived grafts.

Conclusions

This review summarized current preclinical, autologous, and allogeneic data regarding the characteristics of grafts mobilized by different regimens and the effects of cell subsets on homing, engraftment, and transplant outcomes. In aHSCT patients, DC and Treg graft content varies after mobilization with different regimens. Mobilization by G-CSF stimulates the release of DCs, with a polarization toward DC2, whereas chemomobilization results in a similar polarization without an increase in the total DC content [130, 141]. Currently, no evidence suggests DC polarization following mobilization with plerixafor. Total Tregs were shown to increase after G-CSF mobilization, and the proportion of Tregs in the graft increased after chemomobilization [130, 137, 147]. Dendritic cell levels are elevated in allogeneic donors after G-CSF mobilization, and, as in autologous patients, are polarized toward DC2 [105, 134]. Greater numbers of T cells have been found in G-CSF- and plerixafor-mobilized peripheral blood than in unmobilized bone marrow, but this has not been shown to correlate with increased aGVHD rates [158–161, 204].

CD34 remains the most widely surrogate for HSC mobilization and collection efficacy. In fact, baseline peripheral blood $CD34^+$ cell counts measured before mobilization with single-agent G-CSF or chemotherapy + G-CSF can be used to estimate mobilization efficiency and may help identify those at risk for mobilization failure [215, 216]. In addition, postmobilization peripheral blood $CD34^+$ cell counts have been shown to be highly predictive of collection success and can be used to identify poorer mobilizers before collection failure [217]. Some groups use a postmobilization $CD34^+$ cell count of $<10/\mu L$ while others reported a postmobilization of <20 $CD34^+$ cells/μL as trigger for administration of plerixafor to attempt to avoid mobilization failure [218, 219]. Preliminary analysis showed that for collection of the minimum $CD34^+$ cell harvest (2×10^6 $CD34^+$ cells/kg), a blood $CD34^+$ cell count on day 4 of $\geq10/\mu L$ is required, while an optimal harvest (5×10^6 $CD34^+$ cells/kg) requires ≥20 $CD34^+$ cells/μL on day 4 [220]. If blood $CD34^+$ values fall below the threshold, plerixafor should be added according to this algorithm.

Although $CD34^+$ remains the most widely used cell type to predict aHSCT engraftment outcomes, other cell subtypes have proven important as well. G-CSF + plerixafor mobilization has resulted in collection of higher proportions of primitive $CD34^+CD38^-$ cells [129]. Henon et al. suggested an optimal threshold of

5×10^4 $CD34^+CD38^-$ cells/kg body weight for rapid and sustained engraftment (Henon P, Sovalat H, Bourderont D, Ojeda-Uribe M, Arkam Y, Wunder E, et al. Role of the $CD34^+$ 38^- cells in posttransplant hematopoietic recovery. Stem Cells 1998;16(Suppl. 1):113–22). Future studies should re-address the relevance of cell type specific thresholds for $CD34^+$ or $CD34^+CD38^-$ cells, particularly in poor mobilizers.

In the allogeneic transplant setting, total T-cell content, the presence of DCs, and the frequency of Tregs have been shown to modulate GVHD. As our understanding of the underlying mechanisms related to HSCT (e.g., homing, engraftment, GVHD, and immune reconstitution) improves, it may have implications for treatment practices and patient outcomes. Furthermore, grafts can be manipulated more extensively ex vivo to elicit the desired response in patients. For example, $CD34^+$ selection could be applied to donor grafts with the intent of transplanting a higher $CD34^+$ cell dose to ensure higher rates of chimerism.

Great strides have been made recently in our understanding of the biology of HSCT, but much remains to be elucidated. The gene expression studies presented in this review offer a good starting point for the analysis of the differences between cells mobilized by different regimens. A next step is to begin to draw more correlations between the molecular characteristics of collected cells, mobilization efficacy, and transplant outcomes. It will be necessary to continue to evaluate the contributions to patient outcomes of different mobilization regimens and the cell types mobilized by these regimens.

Acknowledgments S.F. received research funding and honoraria from Genzyme Corporation for clinical studies and oral presentation regarding plerixafor. G.T has nothing to disclose. Financial support for medical editorial assistance was provided by Genzyme Corporation. The authors thank Richard Balzer, Ph.D. (MediTech Media) for medical editorial assistance with this manuscript. We gratefully acknowledge Elsevier's permission to reuse material.

References

1. Osgood EE, Riddle MC, Mathews TJ (1939) Aplastic anemia treated with daily transfusions and intravenous marrow. Ann Intern Med 13:357–367
2. Morrison M, Samwick AA (1940) Intramedullary (sternal) transfusion of human bone marrow. JAMA 115:1708–1711
3. Thomas ED, Buckner CD, Banaji M et al (1977) One hundred patients with acute leukemia treated by chemotherapy, total body irradiation, and allogeneic marrow transplantation. Blood 49:511–533
4. Mathe G, Amiel JL, Schwarzenberg L, Cattan A, Schneider M (1965) Adoptive immunotherapy of acute leukemia: experimental and clinical results. Cancer Res 25:1525–1531
5. van Bekkum DW, de Vries MJ (1967) Radiation Chimeras. Academic Press, New York
6. Thomas E, Storb R, Clift RA et al (1975) Bone-marrow transplantation (first of two parts). N Engl J Med 292:832–843
7. Thomas ED, Storb R, Clift RA et al (1975) Bone-marrow transplantation (second of two parts). N Engl J Med 292:895–902
8. Reiffers J, Bernard P, David B et al (1986) Successful autologous transplantation with peripheral blood hemopoietic cells in a patient with acute leukemia. Exp Hematol 14:312–315

9. Korbling M, Dorken B, Ho AD, Pezzutto A, Hunstein W, Fliedner TM (1986) Autologous transplantation of blood-derived hemopoietic stem cells after myeloablative therapy in a patient with Burkitt's lymphoma. Blood 67:529–532
10. Kessinger A, Armitage JO, Landmark JD, Weisenburger DD (1986) Reconstitution of human hematopoietic function with autologous cryopreserved circulating stem cells. Exp Hematol 14:192–196
11. Juttner CA, To LB, Haylock DN, Branford A, Kimber RJ (1985) Circulating autologous stem cells collected in very early remission from acute non-lymphoblastic leukaemia produce prompt but incomplete haemopoietic reconstitution after high dose melphalan or supralethal chemoradiotherapy. Br J Haematol 61:739–745
12. Duhrsen U, Villeval JL, Boyd J, Kannourakis G, Morstyn G, Metcalf D (1988) Effects of recombinant human granulocyte colony-stimulating factor on hematopoietic progenitor cells in cancer patients. Blood 72:2074–2081
13. Socinski MA, Cannistra SA, Elias A, Antman KH, Schnipper L, Griffin JD (1988) Granulocyte–macrophage colony stimulating factor expands the circulating haemopoietic progenitor cell compartment in man. Lancet 1:1194–1198
14. Goldschmidt H, Hegenbart U, Haas R, Hunstein W (1996) Mobilization of peripheral blood progenitor cells with high-dose cyclophosphamide (4 or 7 g/m^2) and granulocyte colony-stimulating factor in patients with multiple myeloma. Bone Marrow Transplant 17:691–697
15. Haas R, Mohle R, Fruhauf S et al (1994) Patient characteristics associated with successful mobilizing and autografting of peripheral blood progenitor cells in malignant lymphoma. Blood 83:3787–3794
16. Seggewiss R, Buss EC, Herrmann D, Goldschmidt H, Ho AD, Fruehauf S (2003) Kinetics of peripheral blood stem cell mobilization following G-CSF-supported chemotherapy. Stem Cells 21:568–574
17. Moskowitz CH, Bertino JR, Glassman JR et al (1999) Ifosfamide, carboplatin, and etoposide: a highly effective cytoreduction and peripheral-blood progenitor-cell mobilization regimen for transplant-eligible patients with non-Hodgkin's lymphoma. J Clin Oncol 17:3776–3785
18. Kewalramani T, Zelenetz AD, Nimer SD et al (2004) Rituximab and ICE as second-line therapy before autologous stem cell transplantation for relapsed or primary refractory diffuse large B-cell lymphoma. Blood 103:3684–3688
19. Bishton MJ, Lush RJ, Byrne JL, Russell NH, Shaw BE, Haynes AP (2007) Ifosphamide, etoposide and epirubicin is an effective combined salvage and peripheral blood stem cell mobilisation regimen for transplant-eligible patients with non-Hodgkin lymphoma and Hodgkin disease. Br J Haematol 136:752–761
20. Pavone V, Gaudio F, Guarini A et al (2002) Mobilization of peripheral blood stem cells with high-dose cyclophosphamide or the DHAP regimen plus G-CSF in non-Hodgkin's lymphoma. Bone Marrow Transplant 29:285–290
21. Fruehauf S, Seggewiss R (2003) It's moving day: factors affecting peripheral blood stem cell mobilization and strategies for improvement [corrected]. Br J Haematol 122:360–375
22. Bonig H, Wundes A, Chang KH, Lucas S, Papayannopoulou T (2008) Increased numbers of circulating hematopoietic stem/progenitor cells are chronically maintained in patients treated with the CD49d blocking antibody natalizumab. Blood 111:3439–3441
23. Zohren F, Toutzaris D, Klarner V, Hartung HP, Kieseier B, Haas R (2008) The monoclonal anti-VLA-4 antibody natalizumab mobilizes CD34+ hematopoietic progenitor cells in humans. Blood 111:3893–3895
24. Liu W, Wang L, Shang X et al (2008) Mobilization of Hematopoitic Stem/Progenitor Cells by a Cdc42 Activity-Specific Inhibitor. Blood 112:32–33
25. Yang L, Wang L, Geiger H, Cancelas JA, Mo J, Zheng Y (2007) Rho GTPase Cdc42 coordinates hematopoietic stem cell quiescence and niche interaction in the bone marrow. Proc Natl Acad Sci USA 104:5091–5096
26. Ramirez PA, Rettig M, Holt M, Ritchey J, DiPersio JF (2008) Rapid mobilization of long term repopulating hematopoietic stem cells (HSC) with AMD15057, a small molecule inhibitor of VLA4; synergism with AMD3100 and G-CSF. Blood 112:229–230

27. Janeway CA, Travers P, Walport M, Shlomchik MJ (eds) (2005) Immunobiology. Garland Science Publishing, New York
28. Fruehauf S, Haas R, Zeller WJ, Hunstein W (1994) CD34 selection for purging in multiple myeloma and analysis of CD34+ B cell precursors. Stem Cells 12:95–102
29. Sutherland DR, Keating A, Nayar R, Anania S, Stewart AK (1994) Sensitive detection and enumeration of CD34+ cells in peripheral and cord blood by flow cytometry. Exp Hematol 22:1003–1010
30. Kollet O, Dar A, Shivtiel S et al (2006) Osteoclasts degrade endosteal components and promote mobilization of hematopoietic progenitor cells. Nat Med 12:657–664
31. Lapidot T, Kollet O (2002) The essential roles of the chemokine SDF-1 and its receptor CXCR4 in human stem cell homing and repopulation of transplanted immune-deficient NOD/SCID and NOD/SCID/B2m(null) mice. Leukemia 16:1992–2003
32. Papayannopoulou T, Priestley GV, Nakamoto B, Zafiropoulos V, Scott LM, Harlan JM (2001) Synergistic mobilization of hemopoietic progenitor cells using concurrent beta1 and beta2 integrin blockade or beta2-deficient mice. Blood 97:1282–1288
33. Avigdor A, Goichberg P, Shivtiel S et al (2004) CD44 and hyaluronic acid cooperate with SDF-1 in the trafficking of human CD34+ stem/progenitor cells to bone marrow. Blood 103:2981–2989
34. Deichmann M, Kronenwett R, Haas R (1997) Expression of the human immunodeficiency virus type-1 coreceptors CXCR-4 (fusin, LESTR) and CKR-5 in CD34+ hematopoietic progenitor cells. Blood 89:3522–3528
35. Richman CM, Weiner RS, Yankee RA (1976) Increase in circulating stem cells following chemotherapy in man. Blood 47:1031–1039
36. Levesque JP, Hendy J, Takamatsu Y, Williams B, Winkler IG, Simmons PJ (2002) Mobilization by either cyclophosphamide or granulocyte colony-stimulating factor transforms the bone marrow into a highly proteolytic environment. Exp Hematol 30:440–449
37. Heissig B, Hattori K, Dias S et al (2002) Recruitment of stem and progenitor cells from the bone marrow niche requires MMP-9 mediated release of kit-ligand. Cell 109:625–637
38. Levesque JP, Takamatsu Y, Nilsson SK, Haylock DN, Simmons PJ (2001) Vascular cell adhesion molecule-1 (CD106) is cleaved by neutrophil proteases in the bone marrow following hematopoietic progenitor cell mobilization by granulocyte colony-stimulating factor. Blood 98:1289–1297
39. Petit I, Szyper-Kravitz M, Nagler A et al (2002) G-CSF induces stem cell mobilization by decreasing bone marrow SDF-1 and up-regulating CXCR4. Nat Immunol 3:687–694
40. Semerad CL, Christopher MJ, Liu F et al (2005) G-CSF potently inhibits osteoblast activity and CXCL12 mRNA expression in the bone marrow. Blood 106:3020–3027
41. Martin C, Burdon PC, Bridger G, Gutierrez-Ramos JC, Williams TJ, Rankin SM (2003) Chemokines acting via CXCR2 and CXCR4 control the release of neutrophils from the bone marrow and their return following senescence. Immunity 19:583–593
42. Martin C, Bridger GJ, Rankin SM (2006) Structural analogues of AMD3100 mobilise haematopoietic progenitor cells from bone marrow in vivo according to their ability to inhibit CXCL12 binding to CXCR4 in vitro. Br J Haematol 134:326–329
43. Hatse S, Princen K, Bridger G, De Clercq E, Schols D (2002) Chemokine receptor inhibition by AMD3100 is strictly confined to CXCR4. FEBS Lett 527:255–262
44. Fricker SP, Anastassov V, Cox J et al (2006) Characterization of the molecular pharmacology of AMD3100: a specific antagonist of the G-protein coupled chemokine receptor, CXCR4. Biochem Pharmacol 72:588–596
45. Gerlach LO, Skerlj RT, Bridger GJ, Schwartz TW (2001) Molecular interactions of cyclam and bicyclam non-peptide antagonists with the CXCR4 chemokine receptor. J Biol Chem 276:14153–14160
46. Broxmeyer HE, Orschell CM, Clapp DW et al (2005) Rapid mobilization of murine and human hematopoietic stem and progenitor cells with AMD3100, a CXCR4 antagonist. J Exp Med 201:1307–1318

47. Paganessi LA, Walker AL, Tan LL, Holmes I, Rich E, Fung HC, Christopherson KW 2nd (2011) Effective mobilization of hematopoietic progenitor cells in G-CSF mobilization defective CD26–/– mice through AMD3100-induced disruption of the CXCL12–CXCR4 axis. Exp Hematol 39(3):384–390
48. Morris CL, Siegel E, Barlogie B et al (2003) Mobilization of CD34+ cells in elderly patients (>/= 70 years) with multiple myeloma: influence of age, prior therapy, platelet count and mobilization regimen. Br J Haematol 120:413–423
49. Hosing C, Saliba R, Ahlawat S et al (2009) Poor hematopoietic stem cell mobilizers: a single institution study of incidence and risk factors in patients with recurrent or relapsed lymphoma. Am J Hematol 84:335–337
50. Bensinger W, Appelbaum F, Rowley S et al (1995) Factors that influence collection and engraftment of autologous peripheral-blood stem cells. J Clin Oncol 13:2547–2555
51. Demirer T, Buckner CD, Gooley T et al (1996) Factors influencing collection of peripheral blood stem cells in patients with multiple myeloma. Bone Marrow Transplant 17:937–941
52. Dreger P, Kloss M, Petersen B et al (1995) Autologous progenitor cell transplantation: prior exposure to stem cell-toxic drugs determines yield and engraftment of peripheral blood progenitor cell but not of bone marrow grafts. Blood 86:3970–3978
53. Lee JL, Kim SB, Lee GW et al (2003) Collection of peripheral blood progenitor cells: analysis of factors predicting the yields. Transfus Apher Sci 29:29–37
54. Moskowitz CH, Stiff P, Gordon MS et al (1997) Recombinant methionyl human stem cell factor and filgrastim for peripheral blood progenitor cell mobilization and transplantation in non-Hodgkin's lymphoma patients–results of a phase I/II trial. Blood 89:3136–3147
55. Sugrue MW, Williams K, Pollock BH et al (2000) Characterization and outcome of "hard to mobilize" lymphoma patients undergoing autologous stem cell transplantation. Leuk Lymphoma 39:509–519
56. Gordan LN, Sugrue MW, Lynch JW et al (2003) Poor mobilization of peripheral blood stem cells is a risk factor for worse outcome in lymphoma patients undergoing autologous stem cell transplantation. Leuk Lymphoma 44:815–820
57. Paripati H, Stewart AK, Cabou S et al (2008) Compromised stem cell mobilization following induction therapy with lenalidomide in myeloma. Leukemia 22:1282–1284
58. Popat U, Saliba R, Thandi R et al (2009) Impairment of filgrastim-induced stem cell mobilization after prior lenalidomide in patients with multiple myeloma. Biol Blood Marrow Transplant 15:718–723
59. Kumar S, Dispenzieri A, Lacy MQ et al (2007) Impact of lenalidomide therapy on stem cell mobilization and engraftment post-peripheral blood stem cell transplantation in patients with newly diagnosed myeloma. Leukemia 21:2035–2042
60. Perea G, Sureda A, Martino R et al (2001) Predictive factors for a successful mobilization of peripheral blood CD34+ cells in multiple myeloma. Ann Hematol 80:592–597
61. Micallef IN, Apostolidis J, Rohatiner AZ et al (2000) Factors which predict unsuccessful mobilisation of peripheral blood progenitor cells following G-CSF alone in patients with non-Hodgkin's lymphoma. Hematol J 1:367–373
62. Micallef IN, DiPersio JF, Nademanee AP et al (2009) Efficacy of plerixafor plus G-CSF compared to G-CSF plus placebo for mobilisation of CD34+ haematopoietic progenitor cells in patients older than 60 years with non-Hodgkin's lymphoma or multiple myeloma. Bone Marrow Transplant 42:105
63. Stiff P, Micallef I, McCarthy P et al (2009) Treatment with plerixafor in non-Hodgkin's lymphoma and multiple myeloma patients to increase the number of peripheral blood stem cells when given a mobilizing regimen of G-CSF: implications for the heavily pretreated patient. Biol Blood Marrow Transplant 15:249–256
64. Micallef INM, Tarantolo SR, McSweeney PA, Klien LM, Calandra GC, Huebner DH (2009) Plerixafor can predictably mobilize hematopoietic stem cells in patients with multiple myeloma previously treated with lenalidomide. Haematologica 94:292
65. Schriber JRS, McCarty JM, McGuirk JM, Spitzer GS, Uberti JPU, Calandra GC (2009) Plerixafor can predictably mobilize hematopoietic stem cells in patients with non-Hodgkin's lymphoma

previously treated with fludarabine and undergoing autologous stem cell transplantation. Haematologica 94:289
66. Calandra G, McCarty J, McGuirk J et al (2008) AMD3100 plus G-CSF can successfully mobilize CD34+ cells from non-Hodgkin's lymphoma, Hodgkin's disease and multiple myeloma patients previously failing mobilization with chemotherapy and/or cytokine treatment: compassionate use data. Bone Marrow Transplant 41:331–338
67. Micallef IN, Stiff PJ, DiPersio JF et al (2009) Successful stem cell remobilization using plerixafor (Mozobil) plus granulocyte colony-stimulating factor in patients with non-hodgkin lymphoma: results from the plerixafor NHL phase 3 study rescue protocol. Biol Blood Marrow Transplant 15:1578–1586
68. Micallef IN, Jacobsen E, Shaughnessy P, Marulkar S, Mody P, van Rhee F (2009) Plerixafor (Mozobil®) plus G-CSF is effective in mobilizing hematopoietic stem cells in patients with concurrent thrombocytopenia undergoing autologous hematopoietic stem cell transplantation. Blood 114:1251
69. Ivanovic Z, Kovacevic-Filipovic M, Jeanne M, et al (2010) CD34+ cells obtained from "good mobilizers" are more activated and exhibit lower ex vivo expansion efficiency than their counterparts from "poor mobilizers". Transfusion 50:120–127.
70. Franklin WA, Glaspy J, Pflaumer SM et al (1999) Incidence of tumor-cell contamination in leukapheresis products of breast cancer patients mobilized with stem cell factor and granulocyte colony-stimulating factor (G-CSF) or with G-CSF alone. Blood 94:340–347
71. Billadeau D, Quam L, Thomas W et al (1992) Detection and quantitation of malignant cells in the peripheral blood of multiple myeloma patients. Blood 80:1818–1824
72. Lemoli RM, Cavo M, Fortuna A (1996) Concomitant mobilization of plasma cells and hematopoietic progenitors into peripheral blood of patients with multiple myeloma. J Hematother 5:339–349
73. Demirkazik A, Kessinger A, Armitage JO et al (2001) Progenitor and lymphoma cells in blood stem cell harvests: impact on survival following transplantation. Bone Marrow Transplant 28:207–212
74. Gribben JG, Neuberg D, Freedman AS et al (1993) Detection by polymerase chain reaction of residual cells with the bcl-2 translocation is associated with increased risk of relapse after autologous bone marrow transplantation for B-cell lymphoma. Blood 81:3449–3457
75. Gertz MA, Witzig TE, Pineda AA, Greipp PR, Kyle RA, Litzow MR (1997) Monoclonal plasma cells in the blood stem cell harvest from patients with multiple myeloma are associated with shortened relapse-free survival after transplantation. Bone Marrow Transplant 19:337–342
76. Kopp HG, Yildirim S, Weisel KC, Kanz L, Vogel W (2009) Contamination of autologous peripheral blood progenitor cell grafts predicts overall survival after high-dose chemotherapy in multiple myeloma. J Cancer Res Clin Oncol 135:637–642
77. Vogel W, Kopp HG, Kanz L, Einsele H (2005) Myeloma cell contamination of peripheral blood stem-cell grafts can predict the outcome in multiple myeloma patients after high-dose chemotherapy and autologous stem-cell transplantation. J Cancer Res Clin Oncol 131:214–218
78. Stewart AK, Vescio R, Schiller G et al (2001) Purging of autologous peripheral-blood stem cells using CD34 selection does not improve overall or progression-free survival after high-dose chemotherapy for multiple myeloma: results of a multicenter randomized controlled trial. J Clin Oncol 19:3771–3779
79. Bourhis JH, Bouko Y, Koscielny S et al (2007) Relapse risk after autologous transplantation in patients with newly diagnosed myeloma is not related with infused tumor cell load and the outcome is not improved by CD34+ cell selection: long term follow-up of an EBMT phase III randomized study. Haematologica 92:1083–1090
80. Ho J, Yang L, Banihashemi B et al (2009) Contaminating tumour cells in autologous PBSC grafts do not influence survival or relapse following transplant for multiple myeloma or B-cell non-Hodgkin's lymphoma. Bone Marrow Transplant 43:223–228
81. Mateo G, Corral M, Almeida J et al (2003) Immunophenotypic analysis of peripheral blood stem cell harvests from patients with multiple myeloma. Haematologica 88:1013–1021

82. Ross AA, Cooper BW, Lazarus HM et al (1993) Detection and viability of tumor cells in peripheral blood stem cell collections from breast cancer patients using immunocytochemical and clonogenic assay techniques. Blood 82:2605–2610
83. Kessinger A, Armitage JO, Smith DM, Landmark JD, Bierman PJ, Weisenburger DD (1989) High-dose therapy and autologous peripheral blood stem cell transplantation for patients with lymphoma. Blood 74:1260–1265
84. Moss TJ, Sanders DG, Lasky LC, Bostrom B (1990) Contamination of peripheral blood stem cell harvests by circulating neuroblastoma cells. Blood 76:1879–1883
85. Vose JM, Sharp G, Chan WC et al (2002) Autologous transplantation for aggressive non-Hodgkin's lymphoma: results of a randomized trial evaluating graft source and minimal residual disease. J Clin Oncol 20:2344–2352
86. Vescio RA, Han EJ, Schiller GJ et al (1996) Quantitative comparison of multiple myeloma tumor contamination in bone marrow harvest and leukapheresis autografts. Bone Marrow Transplant 18:103–110
87. Kanteti R, Miller K, McCann J et al (1999) Randomized trial of peripheral blood progenitor cell vs bone marrow as hematopoietic support for high-dose chemotherapy in patients with non-Hodgkin's lymphoma and Hodgkin's disease: a clinical and molecular analysis. Bone Marrow Transplant 24:473–481
88. Leonard BM, Hetu F, Busque L et al (1998) Lymphoma cell burden in progenitor cell grafts measured by competitive polymerase chain reaction: less than one log difference between bone marrow and peripheral blood sources. Blood 91:331–339
89. Kiel K, Cremer FW, Ehrbrecht E et al (1998) First and second apheresis in patients with multiple myeloma: no differences in tumor load and hematopoietic stem cell yield. Bone Marrow Transplant 21:1109–1115
90. Lincz LF, Crooks RL, Way SL, Granter N, Spencer A (2001) Tumour kinetics in multiple myeloma before, during, and after treatment. Leuk Lymphoma 40:373–384
91. Gazitt Y, Tian E, Barlogie B et al (1996) Differential mobilization of myeloma cells and normal hematopoietic stem cells in multiple myeloma after treatment with cyclophosphamide and granulocyte–macrophage colony-stimulating factor. Blood 87:805–811
92. Cremer FW, Kiel K, Wallmeier M, Haas R, Goldschmidt H, Moos M (1998) Leukapheresis products in multiple myeloma: lower tumor load after mobilization with cyclophosphamide plus granulocyte colony-stimulating factor (G-CSF) compared with G-CSF alone. Exp Hematol 26:969–975
93. Anagnostopoulos A, Aleman A, Yang Y et al (2004) Outcomes of autologous stem cell transplantation in patients with multiple myeloma who received dexamethasone-based nonmyelosuppressive induction therapy. Bone Marrow Transplant 33:623–628
94. Narayanasami U, Kanteti R, Morelli J et al (2001) Randomized trial of filgrastim versus chemotherapy and filgrastim mobilization of hematopoietic progenitor cells for rescue in autologous transplantation. Blood 98:2059–2064
95. Fruehauf S, Ehninger G, Hubel K, et al (2010) Mobilization of peripheral blood stem cells for autologous transplant in non-Hodgkin's lymphoma and multiple myeloma patients by plerixafor and G-CSF and detection of tumor cell mobilization by PCR in multiple myeloma patients. Bone Marrow Transplant 45:269–275.
96. Tricot G, Cottler-Fox M, Calandra G (2010) Safety and efficacy assessment of plerixafor in patients with multiple myeloma proven or predicted to be poor mobilizers, including assessment of tumor cell mobilization. Bone Marrow Transplant 45:63–68.
97. DiPersio JF, Bridger G, Calandra G (2009) Effect of plerixafor (AMD 3100) plus G-CSF on tumor cell mobilization among patients with lymphoma. Biol Blood Marrow Transplant 15:37
98. Mohle R, Pforsich M, Fruehauf S, Witt B, Kramer A, Haas R (1994) Filgrastim post-chemotherapy mobilizes more CD34+ cells with a different antigenic profile compared with use during steady-state hematopoiesis. Bone Marrow Transplant 14:827–832
99. Haas R, Mohle R, Pforsich M et al (1995) Blood-derived autografts collected during granulocyte colony-stimulating factor-enhanced recovery are enriched with early Thy-1+ hematopoietic progenitor cells. Blood 85:1936–1943

100. Dercksen MW, Rodenhuis S, Dirkson MK et al (1995) Subsets of CD34+ cells and rapid hematopoietic recovery after peripheral-blood stem-cell transplantation. J Clin Oncol 13:1922–1932
101. Millar BC, Millar JL, Shepherd V et al (1998) The importance of CD34+/CD33− cells in platelet engraftment after intensive therapy for cancer patients given peripheral blood stem cell rescue. Bone Marrow Transplant 22:469–475
102. Benboubker L, Binet C, Cartron G et al (2002) Frequency and differentiation capacity of circulating LTC-IC mobilized by G-CSF or GM-CSF following chemotherapy: a comparison with steady-state bone marrow and peripheral blood. Exp Hematol 30:74–81
103. Banchereau J, Steinman RM (1998) Dendritic cells and the control of immunity. Nature 392:245–252
104. Rissoan MC, Soumelis V, Kadowaki N et al (1999) Reciprocal control of T helper cell and dendritic cell differentiation. Science 283:1183–1186
105. Arpinati M, Green CL, Heimfeld S, Heuser JE, Anasetti C (2000) Granulocyte-colony stimulating factor mobilizes T helper 2-inducing dendritic cells. Blood 95:2484–2490
106. Xia G, Truitt RL, Johnson BD (2006) Graft-versus-leukemia and graft-versus-host reactions after donor lymphocyte infusion are initiated by host-type antigen-presenting cells and regulated by regulatory T cells in early and long-term chimeras. Biol Blood Marrow Transplant 12:397–407
107. Porrata LF, Gastineau DA, Padley D, Bundy K, Markovic SN (2003) Re-infused autologous graft natural killer cells correlates with absolute lymphocyte count recovery after autologous stem cell transplantation. Leuk Lymphoma 44:997–1000
108. Porrata LF, Gertz MA, Geyer SM et al (2004) The dose of infused lymphocytes in the autograft directly correlates with clinical outcome after autologous peripheral blood hematopoietic stem cell transplantation in multiple myeloma. Leukemia 18:1085–1092
109. Porrata LF, Litzow MR, Inwards DJ et al (2004) Infused peripheral blood autograft absolute lymphocyte count correlates with day 15 absolute lymphocyte count and clinical outcome after autologous peripheral hematopoietic stem cell transplantation in non-Hodgkin's lymphoma. Bone Marrow Transplant 33:291–298
110. Wolf D, Wolf AM, Fong D et al (2007) Regulatory T-cells in the graft and the risk of acute graft-versus-host disease after allogeneic stem cell transplantation. Transplantation 83:1107–1113
111. Rezvani K, Mielke S, Ahmadzadeh M et al (2006) High donor FOXP3-positive regulatory T-cell (Treg) content is associated with a low risk of GVHD following HLA-matched allogeneic SCT. Blood 108:1291–1297
112. Waller EK, Rosenthal H, Sagar L (2002) DC2 effect on survival following allogeneic bone marrow transplantation. Oncology (Williston Park) 16:19–26
113. Wierenga PK, Setroikromo R, Kamps G, Kampinga HH, Vellenga E (2002) Peripheral blood stem cells differ from bone marrow stem cells in cell cycle status, repopulating potential, and sensitivity toward hyperthermic purging in mice mobilized with cyclophosphamide and granulocyte colony-stimulating factor. J Hematother Stem Cell Res 11:523–532
114. Neben S, Marcus K, Mauch P (1993) Mobilization of hematopoietic stem and progenitor cell subpopulations from the marrow to the blood of mice following cyclophosphamide and/or granulocyte colony-stimulating factor. Blood 81:1960–1967
115. Yamamoto Y, Yasumizu R, Amou Y et al (1996) Characterization of peripheral blood stem cells in mice. Blood 88:445–454
116. Morrison SJ, Wright DE, Weissman IL (1997) Cyclophosphamide/granulocyte colony-stimulating factor induces hematopoietic stem cells to proliferate prior to mobilization. Proc Natl Acad Sci USA 94:1908–1913
117. Pan L, Delmonte J Jr, Jalonen CK, Ferrara JL (1995) Pretreatment of donor mice with granulocyte colony-stimulating factor polarizes donor T lymphocytes toward type-2 cytokine production and reduces severity of experimental graft-versus-host disease. Blood 86:4422–4429
118. Fukuda S, Bian H, King AG, Pelus LM (2007) The chemokine GRObeta mobilizes early hematopoietic stem cells characterized by enhanced homing and engraftment. Blood 110:860–869

119. Pelus LM, Singh P (2008) The combination of AMD3100 Plus GRO{beta} rapidly mobilizes hematopoietic stem cells with enhanced homing. Adhesion and survival properties. Blood 112:34
120. Osawa M, Hanada K, Hamada H, Nakauchi H (1996) Long-term lymphohematopoietic reconstitution by a single CD34-low/negative hematopoietic stem cell. Science 273:242–245
121. Matsuzaki Y, Kinjo K, Mulligan RC, Okano H (2004) Unexpectedly efficient homing capacity of purified murine hematopoietic stem cells. Immunity 20:87–93
122. Cocks BG, Chang CC, Carballido JM, Yssel H, de Vries JE, Aversa G (1995) A novel receptor involved in T-cell activation. Nature 376:260–263
123. Killeen N, Stuart SG, Littman DR (1992) Development and function of T cells in mice with a disrupted CD2 gene. EMBO J 11:4329–4336
124. Gonzalez-Cabrero J, Wise CJ, Latchman Y, Freeman GJ, Sharpe AH, Reiser H (1999) CD48-deficient mice have a pronounced defect in CD4(+) T cell activation. Proc Natl Acad Sci USA 96:1019–1023
125. Cesana C, Carlo-Stella C, Regazzi E et al (1998) CD34+ cells mobilized by cyclophosphamide and granulocyte colony-stimulating factor (G-CSF) are functionally different from CD34+ cells mobilized by G-CSF. Bone Marrow Transplant 21:561–568
126. Dazzi C, Cariello A, Rosti G et al (2000) Is there any difference in PBPC mobilization between cyclophosphamide plus G-CSF and G-CSF alone in patients with non-Hodgkin's Lymphoma? Leuk Lymphoma 39:301–310
127. Alegre A, Tomas JF, Martinez-Chamorro C et al (1997) Comparison of peripheral blood progenitor cell mobilization in patients with multiple myeloma: high-dose cyclophosphamide plus GM-CSF vs G-CSF alone. Bone Marrow Transplant 20:211–217
128. Koc ON, Gerson SL, Cooper BW et al (2000) Randomized cross-over trial of progenitor-cell mobilization: high-dose cyclophosphamide plus granulocyte colony-stimulating factor (G-CSF) versus granulocyte–macrophage colony-stimulating factor plus G-CSF. J Clin Oncol 18:1824–1830
129. Fruehauf S, Veldwijk MR, Seeger T, et al (2009) A combination of granulocyte colony-stimulating factor (G-CSF) and AMD3100 (plerixafor) mobilizes more primitive peripheral blood progenitor cells than G-CSF alone: results of a European phase II study. Cytotherapy 11:992–1001.
130. Vela-Ojeda J (2006) Garcia-Ruiz Esparza MA, Reyes-Maldonado E, et al. Peripheral blood mobilization of different lymphocyte and dendritic cell subsets with the use of intermediate doses of G-CSF in patients with non-Hodgkin's lymphoma and multiple myeloma Ann Hematol 85:308–314
131. Morse MA, Vredenburgh JJ, Lyerly HK (1999) A comparative study of the generation of dendritic cells from mobilized peripheral blood progenitor cells of patients undergoing high-dose chemotherapy. J Hematother Stem Cell Res 8:577–584
132. Gazitt Y, Akay C, Thomas C 3rd (2006) No polarization of type 1 or type 2 precursor dendritic cells in peripheral blood stem cell collections of non-hodgkin's lymphoma patients mobilized with cyclophosphamide plus G-CSF, GM-CSF, or GM-CSF followed by G-CSF. Stem Cells Dev 15:269–277
133. Gazitt Y, Shaughnessy P, Devore P (2001) Mobilization of dendritic cells and NK cells in non-Hodgkin's lymphoma patients mobilized with different growth factors. J Hematother Stem Cell Res 10:177–186
134. Ferrari S, Rovati B, Porta C et al (2003) Lack of dendritic cell mobilization into the peripheral blood of cancer patients following standard- or high-dose chemotherapy plus granulocyte-colony stimulating factor. Cancer Immunol Immunother 52:359–366
135. Lonial S, Hicks M, Rosenthal H et al (2004) A randomized trial comparing the combination of granulocyte–macrophage colony-stimulating factor plus granulocyte colony-stimulating factor versus granulocyte colony-stimulating factor for mobilization of dendritic cell subsets in hematopoietic progenitor cell products. Biol Blood Marrow Transplant 10:848–857
136. Gazitt Y, Freytes CO, Akay C, Badel K, Calandra G (2007) Improved mobilization of peripheral blood CD34+ cells and dendritic cells by AMD3100 plus granulocyte-colony-stimulating factor in non-Hodgkin's lymphoma patients. Stem Cells Dev 16:657–666

137. Condomines M, Quittet P, Lu ZY et al (2006) Functional regulatory T cells are collected in stem cell autografts by mobilization with high-dose cyclophosphamide and granulocyte colony-stimulating factor. J Immunol 176:6631–6639
138. Holtan SG, Porrata LF, Micallef IN et al (2007) AMD3100 affects autograft lymphocyte collection and progression-free survival after autologous stem cell transplantation in non-Hodgkin lymphoma. Clin Lymphoma Myeloma 7:315–318
139. Taubert I, Saffrich R, Zepeda-Moreno A, Hellwig I, Eckstein V, Bruckner T, Ho AD, Wuchter P (2011) Characterization of hematopoietic stem cell subsets from patients with multiple myeloma after mobilization with plerixafor. Cytotherapy 13(4):459–466
140. Hess DA, Bonde J, Craft TP et al (2007) Human progenitor cells rapidly mobilized by AMD3100 repopulate NOD/SCID mice with increased frequency in comparison to cells from the same donor mobilized by granulocyte colony stimulating factor. Biol Blood Marrow Transplant 13:398–411
141. Menendez P, Caballero MD, Prosper F et al (2002) The composition of leukapheresis products impacts on the hematopoietic recovery after autologous transplantation independently of the mobilization regimen. Transfusion 42:1159–1172
142. Fruehauf S, Veldwijk MR, Kramer A, Haas R, Zeller WJ (1998) Delineation of cell cycle state and correlation to adhesion molecule expression of human CD34+ cells from steady-state bone marrow and peripheral blood mobilized following G-CSF-supported chemotherapy. Stem Cells 16:271–279
143. Sampol Mayol A, Besalduch Vital J, Galmes Llodra A et al (1998) CD34+ cell dose and CD33– subsets: collection and engraftment kinetics in autologous peripheral blood stem cells transplantation. Haematologica 83:489–495
144. Dean R, Masci P, Pohlman B et al (2005) Dendritic cells in autologous hematopoietic stem cell transplantation for diffuse large B-cell lymphoma: graft content and post transplant recovery predict survival. Bone Marrow Transplant 36:1049–1052
145. Ghiringhelli F, Larmonier N, Schmitt E et al (2004) CD4+CD25+ regulatory T cells suppress tumor immunity but are sensitive to cyclophosphamide which allows immunotherapy of established tumors to be curative. Eur J Immunol 34:336–344
146. Lutsiak ME, Semnani RT, De Pascalis R, Kashmiri SV, Schlom J, Sabzevari H (2005) Inhibition of CD4(+)25+ T regulatory cell function implicated in enhanced immune response by low-dose cyclophosphamide. Blood 105:2862–2868
147. Kao G, Stevenson K, Kim E, Spanjaard E, Kim HT, Ritz J (2008) Autologous Peripheral Blood Stem Cell Products from Patients with Hematologic Malignancies Have Increased Frequency of Regulatory T Cells (CD4+FoxP3+ Treg). Blood 112:806
148. Woo EY, Yeh H, Chu CS et al (2002) Cutting edge: Regulatory T cells from lung cancer patients directly inhibit autologous T cell proliferation. J Immunol 168:4272–4276
149. Liyanage UK, Moore TT, Joo HG et al (2002) Prevalence of regulatory T cells is increased in peripheral blood and tumor microenvironment of patients with pancreas or breast adenocarcinoma. J Immunol 169:2756–2761
150. Marshall NA, Christie LE, Munro LR et al (2004) Immunosuppressive regulatory T cells are abundant in the reactive lymphocytes of Hodgkin lymphoma. Blood 103:1755–1762
151. Curiel TJ, Coukos G, Zou L et al (2004) Specific recruitment of regulatory T cells in ovarian carcinoma fosters immune privilege and predicts reduced survival. Nat Med 10:942–949
152. Viguier M, Lemaitre F, Verola O et al (2004) Foxp3 expressing CD4+CD25(high) regulatory T cells are overrepresented in human metastatic melanoma lymph nodes and inhibit the function of infiltrating T cells. J Immunol 173:1444–1453
153. Mittal S, Marshall NA, Duncan L, Culligan DJ, Barker RN, Vickers MA (2008) Local and systemic induction of CD4+CD25+ regulatory T-cell population by non-Hodgkin lymphoma. Blood 111:5359–5370
154. Elquza E, Spier C, Fiederlein R, Salamon D, Yeager AM (2009) Effects of mobilization with granulocyte colony stimulating factor (G-CSF) and plerixafor On lymphocyte subsets in autologous peripheral bBlood stem cell (PBSC) apheresis products. Blood 114:843–844
155. Lemoli RM, Tafuri A, Fortuna A et al (1998) Biological characterization of CD34+ cells mobilized into peripheral blood. Bone Marrow Transplant 22(Suppl 5):S47–S50

156. Rettig MP, Shannon WD, Ritchey J et al (2008) Characterization of human CD34+ hematopoietic stem cells following administration of G-CSF or plerixafor. Blood 112:1192
157. Toh HC, Sun L, Soe Y et al (2009) G-CSF induces a potentially tolerant gene and immunophenotype profile in T cells in vivo. Clin Immunol 132:83–92
158. Korbling M, Huh YO, Durett A et al (1995) Allogeneic blood stem cell transplantation: peripheralization and yield of donor-derived primitive hematopoietic progenitor cells (CD34+ Thy-1dim) and lymphoid subsets, and possible predictors of engraftment and graft-versus-host disease. Blood 86:2842–2848
159. Dreger P, Haferlach T, Eckstein V et al (1994) G-CSF-mobilized peripheral blood progenitor cells for allogeneic transplantation: safety, kinetics of mobilization, and composition of the graft. Br J Haematol 87:609–613
160. Liles WC, Rodger E, Broxmeyer HE et al (2005) Augmented mobilization and collection of CD34+ hematopoietic cells from normal human volunteers stimulated with granulocyte-colony-stimulating factor by single-dose administration of AMD3100, a CXCR4 antagonist. Transfusion 45:295–300
161. Devine SM, Vij R, Rettig M et al (2008) Rapid mobilization of functional donor hematopoietic cells without G-CSF using AMD3100, an antagonist of the CXCR4/SDF-1 interaction. Blood 112:990–998
162. Rettig MP, McFarland K, Ritchey J et al (2009) Preferential mobilization of CD34+ plasmacytoid dendritic cell precursors by plerixafor. Blood 114:19
163. Urbano-Ispizua A, Rozman C, Pimentel P et al (2002) Risk factors for acute graft-versus-host disease in patients undergoing transplantation with CD34+ selected blood cells from HLA-identical siblings. Blood 100:724–727
164. Dong L, Wu T, Zhang MJ, Gao ZY, Lu DP (2007) CD3+ cell dose and disease status are important factors determining clinical outcomes in patients undergoing unmanipulated haploidentical blood and marrow transplantation after conditioning including antithymocyte globulin. Biol Blood Marrow Transplant 13:1515–1524
165. Tayebi H, Kuttler F, Saas P et al (2001) Effect of granulocyte colony-stimulating factor mobilization on phenotypical and functional properties of immune cells. Exp Hematol 29:458–470
166. Uchida N, He D, Friera AM et al (1997) The unexpected G0/G1 cell cycle status of mobilized hematopoietic stem cells from peripheral blood. Blood 89:465–472
167. Lemoli RM, Tafuri A, Fortuna A et al (1997) Cycling status of CD34+ cells mobilized into peripheral blood of healthy donors by recombinant human granulocyte colony-stimulating factor. Blood 89:1189–1196
168. Steidl U, Kronenwett R, Rohr UP et al (2002) Gene expression profiling identifies significant differences between the molecular phenotypes of bone marrow-derived and circulating human CD34+ hematopoietic stem cells. Blood 99:2037–2044
169. Donahue RE, Jin P, Bonifacino AC et al (2009) Plerixafor (AMD3100) and granulocyte colony stimulating factor (G-CSF) mobilize different CD34+ cell populations based on global gene and microRNA expression signatures. Blood 114:2530–2541
170. Larochelle A, Krouse A, Metzger M et al (2006) AMD3100 mobilizes hematopoietic stem cells with long-term repopulating capacity in nonhuman primates. Blood 107:3772–3778
171. Bonig H, Chudziak D, Priestley G, Papayannopoulou T (2009) Insights into the biology of mobilized hematopoietic stem/progenitor cells through innovative treatment schedules of the CXCR4 antagonist AMD3100. Exp Hematol 37:402e.1–415e.1
172. Gazitt Y, Liu Q (2001) Plasma levels of SDF-1 and expression of SDF-1 receptor on CD34+ cells in mobilized peripheral blood of non-Hodgkin's lymphoma patients. Stem Cells 19:37–45
173. Oelschlaegel U, Bornhauser M, Boxberger S et al (2007) Kinetics of CXCR-4 and adhesion molecule expression during autologous stem cell mobilisation with G-CSF plus AMD3100 in patients with multiple myeloma. Ann Hematol 86:569–573
174. Fruehauf S, Seeger T, Maier P et al (2006) The CXCR4 antagonist AMD3100 releases a subset of G-CSF-primed peripheral blood progenitor cells with specific gene expression characteristics. Exp Hematol 34:1052–1059

175. Jin P, Wang E, Ren J et al (2008) Differentiation of two types of mobilized peripheral blood stem cells by microRNA and cDNA expression analysis. J Transl Med 6:39
176. Dlubek D, Drabczak-Skrzypek D, Lange A (2006) Low CXCR4 membrane expression on CD34(+) cells characterizes cells mobilized to blood. Bone Marrow Transplant 37:19–23
177. Amariglio N, Jacob-Hirsch J, Shimoni A, Leiba M, Rechavi G, Nagler A (2007) Changes in gene expression pattern following granulocyte colony-stimulating factor administration to normal stem cell sibling donors. Acta Haematol 117:68–73
178. Stem Cell Trialists' Collaborative Group (2005) Allogeneic peripheral blood stem-cell compared with bone marrow transplantation in the management of hematologic malignancies: an individual patient data meta-analysis of nine randomized trials. J Clin Oncol 23:5074–5087
179. Bonig H, Priestley GV, Oehler V, Papayannopoulou T (2007) Hematopoietic progenitor cells (HPC) from mobilized peripheral blood display enhanced migration and marrow homing compared to steady-state bone marrow HPC. Exp Hematol 35:326–334
180. Drouet M, Herodin F, Norol F, Mourcin F, Mayol JF (2001) Cell cycle activation of peripheral blood stem and progenitor cells expanded ex vivo with SCF, FLT-3 ligand, TPO, and IL-3 results in accelerated granulocyte recovery in a baboon model of autologous transplantation but G0/G1 and S/G2/M graft cell content does not correlate with transplantability. Stem Cells 19:436–442
181. Uchida N, Bonifacino A, Krouse AE, Metzger ME, Csako G, Lee-Stroka A, Fasano RM, Leitman SF, Mattapallil JJ, Hsieh MM, Tisdale JF, Donahue RE (2011) Accelerated lymphocyte reconstitution and long-term recovery after transplantation of lentiviral-transduced rhesus CD34(+) cells mobilized by G-CSF and plerixafor. Exp Hematol 39:795–805.
182. Burroughs L, Mielcarek M, Little MT et al (2005) Durable engraftment of AMD3100-mobilized autologous and allogeneic peripheral-blood mononuclear cells in a canine transplantation model. Blood 106:4002–4008
183. Voermans C, Kooi ML, Rodenhuis S, van der Lelie H, van der Schoot CE, Gerritsen WR (2001) In vitro migratory capacity of CD34+ cells is related to hematopoietic recovery after autologous stem cell transplantation. Blood 97:799–804
184. Dercksen MW, Gerritsen WR, Rodenhuis S et al (1995) Expression of adhesion molecules on CD34+ cells: CD34+ L-selectin+cells predict a rapid platelet recovery after peripheral blood stem cell transplantation. Blood 85:3313–3319
185. Sola C, Maroto P, Salazar R et al (1999) Bone marrow transplantation: prognostic factors of peripheral blood stem cell mobilization with cyclophosphamide and filgrastim (r-metHuG-CSF): the CD34+ cell dose positively affects the time to hematopoietic recovery and supportive requirements after high-dose chemotherapy. Hematology 4:195–209
186. Weaver CH, Hazelton B, Birch R et al (1995) An analysis of engraftment kinetics as a function of the CD34 content of peripheral blood progenitor cell collections in 692 patients after the administration of myeloablative chemotherapy. Blood 86:3961–3969
187. Limat S, Woronoff-Lemsi MC, Milpied N et al (2000) Effect of cell determinant (CD)34+ cell dose on the cost and consequences of peripheral blood stem cell transplantation for non-Hodgkin's lymphoma patients in front-line therapy. Eur J Cancer 36:2360–2367
188. Ramsfjell V, Borge OJ, Cui L, Jacobsen SE (1997) Thrombopoietin directly and potently stimulates multilineage growth and progenitor cell expansion from primitive (CD34+ CD38–) human bone marrow progenitor cells: distinct and key interactions with the ligands for c-kit and flt3, and inhibitory effects of TGF-beta and TNF-alpha. J Immunol 158:5169–5177
189. Kaushansky K (1995) Thrombopoietin: the primary regulator of megakaryocyte and platelet production. Thromb Haemost 74:521–525
190. Sartor MM, Garvin F, Antonenas V, Bradstock KF, Gottlieb DJ (2007) Failure to achieve a threshold dose of CD34+ CD110+ progenitor cells in the graft predicts delayed platelet engraftment after autologous stem cell transplantation. Bone Marrow Transplant 40:851–857
191. Hogge DE, Lambie K, Sutherland HJ et al (2000) Quantitation of primitive and lineage-committed progenitors in mobilized peripheral blood for prediction of platelet recovery post autologous transplant. Bone Marrow Transplant 25:589–598

192. Bridenbaugh S, Kenins L, Bouliong-Pillai E et al (2008) Clinical stem-cell sources contain CD8+CD3+ T-cell receptor-negative cells that facilitate bone marrow repopulation with hematopoietic stem cells. Blood 111:1735–1738
193. Larochelle A, Vormoor J, Hanenberg H et al (1996) Identification of primitive human hematopoietic cells capable of repopulating NOD/SCID mouse bone marrow: implications for gene therapy. Nat Med 2:1329–1337
194. Terstappen LW, Huang S, Safford M, Lansdorp PM, Loken MR (1991) Sequential generations of hematopoietic colonies derived from single nonlineage-committed CD34+CD38– progenitor cells. Blood 77:1218–1227
195. Dahl E, Burroughs J, DeFor T, Verfaillie C, Weisdorf D (2003) Progenitor content of autologous grafts: mobilized bone marrow vs mobilized blood. Bone Marrow Transplant 32: 575–580
196. Sutherland HJ, Eaves CJ, Lansdorp PM, Phillips GL, Hogge DE (1994) Kinetics of committed and primitive blood progenitor mobilization after chemotherapy and growth factor treatment and their use in autotransplants. Blood 83:3808–3814
197. Klaus J, Herrmann D, Breitkreutz I et al (2007) Effect of CD34 cell dose on hematopoietic reconstitution and outcome in 508 patients with multiple myeloma undergoing autologous peripheral blood stem cell transplantation. Eur J Haematol 78:21–28
198. Haas R, Witt B, Mohle R et al (1995) Sustained long-term hematopoiesis after myeloablative therapy with peripheral blood progenitor cell support. Blood 85:3754–3761
199. Porrata LF, Inwards DJ, Micallef IN, Ansell SM, Geyer SM, Markovic SN (2002) Early lymphocyte recovery post-autologous haematopoietic stem cell transplantation is associated with better survival in Hodgkin's disease. Br J Haematol 117:629–633
200. Gordan LN, Sugrue MW, Lynch JW, Williams KD, Khan SA, Moreb JS (2003) Correlation of early lymphocyte recovery and progression-free survival after autologous stem-cell transplant in patients with Hodgkin's and non-Hodgkin's lymphoma. Bone Marrow Transplant 31: 1009–1013
201. Waller EK, Rosenthal H, Jones TW et al (2001) Larger numbers of CD4(bright) dendritic cells in donor bone marrow are associated with increased relapse after allogeneic bone marrow transplantation. Blood 97:2948–2956
202. Skert C, Damiani D, Michelutti A, et al (2009) Kinetics of Th1/Th2 cytokines and lymphocyte subsets to predict chronic GVHD after Allo-SCT: results of a prospective study. Bone Marrow Transplant 44:729–737
203. Xu LP, Luo XH, Chang YJ, et al (2009) High CD4/CD8 ratio in allografts predicts adverse outcomes in unmanipulated HLA-mismatched/haploidentical hematopoietic stem cell transplantation for chronic myeloid leukemia. Ann Hematol 88:1015–1024
204. Zeng D, Dejbakhsh-Jones S, Strober S (1997) Granulocyte colony-stimulating factor reduces the capacity of blood mononuclear cells to induce graft-versus-host disease: impact on blood progenitor cell transplantation. Blood 90:453–463
205. Bensinger WI, Martin PJ, Storer B et al (2001) Transplantation of bone marrow as compared with peripheral-blood cells from HLA-identical relatives in patients with hematologic cancers. N Engl J Med 344:175–181
206. Powles R, Mehta J, Kulkarni S et al (2000) Allogeneic blood and bone-marrow stem-cell transplantation in haematological malignant diseases: a randomised trial. Lancet 355:1231–1237
207. Chen BJ, Cui X, Sempowski GD, Liu C, Chao NJ (2004) Transfer of allogeneic CD62L– memory T cells without graft-versus-host disease. Blood 103:1534–1541
208. Foster AE, Marangolo M, Sartor MM et al (2004) Human CD62L– memory T cells are less responsive to alloantigen stimulation than CD62L+ naive T cells: potential for adoptive immunotherapy and allodepletion. Blood 104:2403–2409
209. Morris ES, MacDonald KP, Rowe V et al (2004) Donor treatment with pegylated G-CSF augments the generation of IL-10-producing regulatory T cells and promotes transplantation tolerance. Blood 103:3573–3581
210. Hoffmann P, Ermann J, Edinger M, Fathman CG, Strober S (2002) Donor-type CD4(+) CD25(+) regulatory T cells suppress lethal acute graft-versus-host disease after allogeneic bone marrow transplantation. J Exp Med 196:389–399

211. Cohen JL, Trenado A, Vasey D, Klatzmann D, Salomon BL (2002) CD4(+)CD25(+) immunoregulatory T Cells: new therapeutics for graft-versus-host disease. J Exp Med 196:401–406
212. Taylor PA, Lees CJ, Blazar BR (2002) The infusion of ex vivo activated and expanded CD4(+)CD25(+) immune regulatory cells inhibits graft-versus-host disease lethality. Blood 99:3493–3499
213. Ruzek MC, Waire JS, Hopkins D et al (2008) Characterization of in vitro antimurine thymocyte globulin-induced regulatory T cells that inhibit graft-versus-host disease in vivo. Blood 111:1726–1734
214. Smith AL, Jungnam J, Rao S et al (2007) Significant alterations in T-cell TH1 and TH2 cytokine gene profiles associated with G-CSF mobilization do not occur in T-cells mobilized with AMD3100. Blood 110:962a
215. Fruehauf S, Haas R, Conradt C et al (1995) Peripheral blood progenitor cell (PBPC) counts during steady-state hematopoiesis allow to estimate the yield of mobilized PBPC after filgrastim (R-metHuG-CSF)-supported cytotoxic chemotherapy. Blood 85:2619–2626
216. Fruehauf S, Schmitt K, Veldwijk MR et al (1999) Peripheral blood progenitor cell (PBPC) counts during steady-state haemopoiesis enable the estimation of the yield of mobilized PBPC after granulocyte colony-stimulating factor supported cytotoxic chemotherapy: an update on 100 patients. Br J Haematol 105:786–794
217. Sinha S, Gastineau DA, Hogan WJ et al (2009) Predicting poor peripheral blood stem cell mobilization in multiple myeloma (MM) using initial peripheral CD34 counts: developing target-based cut-points for early intervention. Blood 114:1252–1253
218. Micallef I, Ansell SM, Buadi F et al (2009) A risk adapted approach utilizing plerixafor in autologous peripheral blood stem cell mobilization. Blood 114:1244
219. Nademanee AP, Stadtmauer E, Micallef IN et al (2009) Plerixafor (Mozobil®) plus G-CSF is more efective than placebo plus G-CSF in mobilizing CD34+ hematopoietic stem cells in patients with multiple myeloma who have low (<20 cells/mcl) peripheral blood CD34+ cell count. Blood 114:1252
220. Alexander E, Costa LJ, Taylor M et al (2009) Cost-effective use of plerixafor for hematopoietic stem cells mobilization: development and validation of a decision-making algorithm. Blood 114:1246

Chapter 10
Relevance and Clinical Implications of Tumor Cell Mobilization in Autologous Transplantation of Multiple Myeloma and Non-Hodgkin's Lymphoma

Stefan Fruehauf, Anthony D. Ho, Jessie Hanrahan, Frank J. Hsu, and John F. DiPersio

Abstract Autologous transplantation of peripheral blood (PB) hematopoietic stem cells is a widely used strategy for reconstitution of blood cells following high-dose chemotherapy for hematologic malignancies, such as multiple myeloma and non-Hodgkin's lymphoma. Stem cells for transplantation are usually obtained from PB after treatment with chemotherapy with or without cytokine [usually, granulocyte colony-stimulating factor (G-CSF)] or after treatment with cytokine alone (such as G-CSF). The use of autologous peripheral blood stem cells for transplantation is associated with the risk of contamination of the graft with tumor cells and whether this impacts response rates, progression-free survival, and overall survival is still debatable. This review summarizes the controversy around tumor cell mobilization (TCM), complexity of detection of minimal residual diseases, available diagnostic tools, differences in TCM with available mobilization regimens, and the potential effect of TCM on clinical outcome.

Keywords Plerixafor • Tumor cell mobilization • Hematopoeitic stem cell transplantation • Non-Hodgkin's lymphoma • Multiple myeloma • AMD3100

S. Fruehauf (✉)
Center for Tumor Diagnostics and Therapy, Paracelsus Klinik, Am Natruper Holz 69, Osnabrück 49076, Germany
e-mail: prof.stefan.fruehauf@pk-mx.de

A.D. Ho
Department of Internal Medicine V, Heidelberg University Hospital, Heidelberg, Germany

J. Hanrahan • F.J. Hsu
Genzyme Corporation, Cambridge, MA, USA

J.F. DiPersio
Division of Oncology, Siteman Cancer Center, Washington University School of Medicine, St. Louis, MO 63110, USA

S. Fruehauf et al. (eds.), *Novel Developments in Stem Cell Mobilization: Focus on CXCR4*, DOI 10.1007/978-1-4614-1960-0_10,

Introduction

Tumor cells can be detected in the peripheral blood (PB) of patients with various cancer types and can contaminate autologous stem cell products derived from the bone marrow or leukapheresis [9, 35, 66]. Standard cancer treatment, such as chemotherapy or radiation, might by itself induce significant mobilization of tumor cells into the PB and has been reported to be associated with metastases [10]. Similarly, common methods employed to mobilize peripheral blood stem cells (PBSCs), such as chemotherapy and cytokines, might also mobilize tumor cells and lead to significant contamination of the apheresis products [2, 10, 48].

Given the low number of tumor cells compared to normal cells and the heterogeneity of tumor cells, their detection presents a major challenge. Tumor cell detection is further complicated by the fact that very few tumor-specific cellular markers exist and many of the available assays are exploratory in nature. Additionally, the sensitivity and specificity of the detection methods vary enormously and are highly dependent upon the methods employed and the source of the cells analyzed (e.g., bone marrow sample, apheresis sample, PB sample).

It is possible that tumor cells in the reinfused apheresis product could lead to relapse. However, it also may be likely that relapse is due to the regrowth of residual disease following incomplete eradication of tumor cells by high-dose chemotherapy and radiation therapy [40, 80]. This review, with a focus on hematological malignancies like multiple myeloma (MM) and non-Hodgkin's lymphoma (NHL), provides an overview of the methods used for detection of malignant cells in these entities, the levels of tumor cell contamination found following the more common methods of mobilization, including chemotherapy, cytokines, and the newly approved mobilizing agent plerixafor.

Methods of Tumor Cell Detection

Multiple methods have been developed for the detection of tumor cell mobilization (TCM), including immunocytochemistry [43, 51], cell culture [59, 82], flow cytometry, and polymerase chain reaction (PCR; both allele-specific oligonucleotide [ASO] and quantitative real time). The sensitivity of the TCM assays can be increased by analyzing multiple samples, increasing the number of cells tested in the sample, and employing sensitive reverse transcriptase PCR methods (RT-PCR). Flow cytometry is considered a low-sensitivity method capable of detecting 1 tumor cell in about 1,000 peripheral blood mononuclear cells (PBMCs) [55]. Comparatively, quantitative PCR methods are highly sensitive, detecting as few as one tumor cell in a million PBMCs. Ultimately, the applicability of each method is determined by the level of tumor contamination considered to be clinically relevant and the detection limits of each assay.

Flow Cytometry

Malignancies, such as MM, arise from a monoclonal population of B cells, and therefore each tumor cell expresses a unique immunoglobulin (Ig) molecule. In addition, plasma cells from patients with MM generally have an abnormal DNA content (aneuploidy) and an increased RNA content [5, 6, 16].

In this detection method, cells are labeled with anti-Ig light-chain and anti-Ig heavy-chain antibodies conjugated to fluorochromes and the DNA is stained. The cells are then analyzed by flow cytometry which allows for automated cellular analysis [7]. The results of this method can be easily analyzed, profiling normal cells versus tumor cells. The data from this method are presented as the percentage of Ig light-chain cells (kappa and lamda), as a DNA index (ratio of $G_{1/0}$ DNA peaks of tumor and control cells [4]) and/or as an RNA index (ratio of mean RNA content of tumor $G_{1/0}$ cells to control lymphocytes [6]). Detection of Ig light-chain restriction and a DNA index of anything other than 1 are indicatives of tumor cells. Additionally, as mentioned above, MM cells may have increased cytoplasmic immunoglobulin (CIg) which can be detected by flow cytometry [7]. This data is represented as a CIg index (ratio of median CIg fluorescence intensities of aneuploid and diploid G_1 cells from the same patient sample).

Flow cytometry is highly reproducible, relatively inexpensive, and is a quick throughput method [65]. However, flow cytometry may require large sample volumes [65] and the sensitivity of this assay is limited to about 1 tumor cell in 1,000 PBMCs [63]. Since the technique of flow cytometry is to count cells labeled with a fluorochrome, for a low-frequency event such as tumor cell contamination a large number of PBMCs must be counted in order to accurately detect low quantities of tumor cells. Even with modern high-speed machines, there are practical limits to the number of cells that can be analyzed by this method due to the time required to perform these tests and the quantity of cells available. In addition, the specificity of the assay may be impacted by the reagents used and their ability to accurately distinguish tumor cells from normal cells [39, 65]. Immunophenotyping using multiple antibodies can increase the sensitivity of flow cytometry to $1{:}10^5$ [55], allowing for the detection of aberrant plasma cells [54, 55]. However, this can be technically challenging as it requires a large quantity of cells to be analyzed in order to achieve accurate statistics.

Polymerase Chain Reaction Analysis

PCR can be used to detect the presence (or absence) of tumor cells. Tumor cells from a specific cancer type generally have unique DNA sequences, often resulting from gene rearrangements, which are absent in normal cells. The unique DNA sequence can be detected by designing specific PCR primers capable of amplifying the tumor-specific sequences of DNA. PCR has many advantages in that the method requires very little sample and is relatively simple and inexpensive to perform. Disadvantages of the PCR method include false positives and the fact that very few gene sequences have been identified that may be broadly applied to a cancer indication (e.g., *BCL-2* for certain lymphomas, Bcr-Abl for chronic myelogenous leukemia). In many instances, gene rearrangements and mutations are specific to an individual patient's tumor and are not applicable to other patients with the same type of cancer. In these cases, a patient-specific detection test must be developed for each individual. The detection sensitivity of PCR is one tumor cell in 10^5–10^7 PBMCs [65].

PCR to Detect TCM in Multiple Myeloma

In MM, malignant plasma cells arise from a single B-cell clone. During B-cell ontogeny, a functional immunoglobulin heavy-chain gene complex is formed. The formation of the Ig heavy chain results in a unique gene sequence specific to the B-cell clone from which it arose [18, 44]. Mutational events occur at the junctional splice sites and often within the complementarity determining regions (CDRs). The CDRs represent primary contact points for antigen interaction; these "binding sites" are often subject to significant mutational events following antigen exposure. The CDR3 region of the Ig-variable heavy-chain gene spans three different Ig gene segments: VH–D–JH. Because of the enormous genetic diversity of this region, as well as the other CDRs, these Ig-variable heavy-chain gene segments represent true tumor-specific markers. All tumor cells in an individual patient share an identical rearranged Ig gene sequence, resulting from rearrangements of the VH, D, and JH gene segments [18, 44]. B-cell-specific primers, which are patient specific, can be designed to these gene segments and used to detect tumor cells by sensitive PCR techniques.

Real-time quantitative PCR can be performed to amplify the CDR3 region of the clonally rearranged VDJ segments of the Ig heavy-chain gene [53, 61, 87] using allele-specific, and therefore patient-specific, oligonucleotides (ASO-PCR [3, 9, 20]). ASO-PCR can be used to specifically detect these unique DNA sequences and assess the mobilization of MM tumor cells. The quantitative ASO-PCR method determines the frequency of tumor genes with respect to the total DNA content. This result is then used to calculate the tumor cell frequency compared to total PBMCs. Using the total PBMC concentration, the total tumor cell concentration can be calculated. The detection sensitivity of this method is 1:10^4 cells [53] to 1:10^6 cells [19, 65].

To perform this assay, a sample of tumor must be obtained, the Ig VH gene segment must be sequenced, and tumor-specific primers must be designed and tested beforehand. Once the PCR detection assay is established, total genomic DNA is isolated from PB, apheresis product, or other sample. The isolated DNA and the gene-specific primers are then used in a PCR reaction. Quantitative PCR methods can be used to determine the level of contamination within a sample or, in the case of no DNA amplification, indicate the absence of tumor cells at the level of the sensitivity of the assay.

This method is extremely laborious (requiring original patient tumor samples and primers designed for each patient), technically challenging, and expensive. However, ASO-PCR is highly sensitive, tumor specific, and requires a small sample.

PCR to Detect TCM in Non-Hodgkin's Lymphoma

Approximately 80% of patients with NHL with follicular histology have a translocation t(14;18) of the *BCL-2* gene [83], and the presence of this translocation can be exploited through the use of PCR in diagnostic settings [15, 62, 84].

Approximately 60–70% of breakpoints fall within a well-defined area, known as the major breakpoint region (MBR) of the 3′-untranslated part of the *BCL-2* gene. Using primers that flank the most common consensus regions of the MBR and modified to fluoresce when hybridized with complementary DNA, PCR can be used to detect *BCL-2* gene rearrangements [39]. Methods, such as quantitative, real-time PCR, can be used to detect translocations down to 0.002% or 1/50,000 cells.

For this assay, total genomic DNA is isolated from PB, apheresis product, or other sample. The isolated DNA and the gene-specific primers are then used in a quantitative PCR reaction; the amplification of the ß-actin gene is used as a control. Standard curves are calculated for the *BCL-2* rearrangement and ß-actin and used to quantify DNA within each sample. These curves control for PCR efficiency and detection limits. A typical lower limit of detection for this assay is 0.01 ng of tumor DNA in a 1 μg DNA sample per PCR, which correlates to approximately two tumor cells per PCR. If no *BCL-2* amplification is detected in the PCR product, this indicates the absence of the t(14;18) translocation in the MBR of the *BCL-2* gene or that levels are below the limit of detection.

This method is highly sensitive and commercial primers are available that can be used for all patients. However, rearrangements involving other regions, including the minor breakpoint cluster, are not detectable with this assay. Additionally, given that the translocation is not found in all patients with NHL, this method is not applicable to all patients and could lead to false negatives. Another disadvantage of this method is that the t(14;18) translocation is observed with increasing frequency in normal lymphocytes as a function of age [26].

Tumor Cell Contamination of Peripheral Blood Prior to Mobilization

Tumor cells can be found circulating in the peripheral blood in patients with hematological malignancies. One study showed a wide variation prior to treatment (i.e., any chemotherapy) in the frequency/number of circulating tumor cells in PB of patients with MM. Among 14 patients with MM, 13 tested positive for the presence of tumor cells by ASO-PCR with tumor cell frequency varying for 12 patients from

0.001 to 1.0%, and 1 patient with 32% [9, 66]. In another study of 23 patients with MM, all patients had detectable circulating plasma cells with a range of 0.1–1.8% of mononuclear cell (MNC) fraction [52]. Some studies have reported a correlation of tumor burden and stage of disease with the incidence of circulating tumor cells [14, 33, 41, 60, 67]; others, however, have reported that the incidence of tumor cells in PB in certain cancers, such as MM, appeared to be independent of bone marrow tumor burden and stage of disease [22, 66].

Tumor Contamination After Mobilization

Tumor cell contamination of PBSC products routinely occurs and has been reported following the use of all common mobilization methods [28]. A wide variation in the frequency of tumor cell levels, ranging from 0.01% to greater than 10%, has been reported in virtually all mobilized PBSC harvests [34]. The kinetics of tumor cell mobilization, underlying residual tumor burden in the patient, and mobilization method used are important factors that impact the contamination of the apheresis product. Several groups have reported that higher proportions of hematopoietic progenitor cells are observed early during apheresis (first 2 days), whereas peak levels of myeloma cells occur in the later days of apheresis [24, 35]. However, other studies have found no variation in the kinetics of tumor cell and $CD34^+$ stem cell mobilization [46, 47, 54, 62].

Chemomobilization

Prior to the development of cytokines for stem cell mobilization, it was noted that there were transient increases in hematopoietic stem cells (HSCs) in peripheral blood following the administration of myelosuppressive chemotherapy [1, 64]. The earliest protocols to mobilize stem cells used chemotherapy alone [49, 74] and later protocols used chemotherapy followed by daily administration of cytokines (granulocyte colony-stimulating factor, G-CSF, or granulocyte–macrophage colony-stimulating factor [GM-CSF]) [27, 38, 72]. In general, chemotherapeutic agents induce stem cell mobilization by reducing bone marrow reserves and forcing stem cell expansion and hematopoiesis [8].

In MM patients, studies have shown that patients have between 0.1 and 1% clonal B cells in hematopoietic stem cell collections following chemomobilization resulting in the infusion of $0.5–5 \times 10^8$ myeloma cells with each transplant [24, 34, 52, 68]. A recent study by Kopp et al. examined the amount of tumor cell contamination in the stem cell product and the resulting outcome following transplantation. The study reported that 27% of stem cell products from 60 patients with MM were contaminated with large quantities of tumor cells ($>4.5 \times 10^5$ cells/kg) following mobilization with chemotherapy or chemotherapy plus G-CSF, and 73% of stem cell products were contaminated with low levels of tumor cells ($\leq 4.5 \times 10^5$ cells/kg) [48]. A study by Ho et al. of contaminating tumor cells in PBSC and influence on outcomes showed tumor contamination of the PBSC graft in 36% (32/89) of patients with NHL and 25% (17/69) of patients with MM following chemomobilization with varying regimens [42] (Table 10.1).

Mobilization with Cytokines

The use of cytokines (most commonly G-CSF and GM-CSF) began in the late 1980s following the report of the mobilizing effects of cytokines [38, 72] and a later report of long-term hematopoietic reconstitution in patients transplanted with only cytokine-mobilized PBSCs [56]. The most commonly used cytokine, G-CSF, works by granulocyte expansion/activation, protease release, and cleavage of adhesion molecules [8, 29].

Tumor contamination of the peripheral blood apheresis product has also been noted in patients receiving only cytokines for mobilization. In a retrospective study of 61 patients with NHL, PBSC samples were examined from 26 patients who did not receive a mobilizing regimen and 35 patients who had mobilization of stem cells with cytokines (22 with G-CSF and 12 with GM-CSF) [23]. Among patients in the cytokine-mobilized group, 37% had tumor contamination in the apheresis product compared with 19% of the nonmobilized group, but this difference was not statistically significant.

Studies Comparing Mobilization Methods

An early study in eight patients with MM compared the tumor load of the leukapheresis product following mobilization with G-CSF and following G-CSF plus cylophosphamide [21]. This study concluded that mobilization by cyclophosphamide plus G-CSF leads to a lower number of malignant cells per $CD34^+$ cell in the leukapheresis product compared with G-CSF alone. A later study examined response rates and survival of various treatment regimens in 135 patients with MM and reported graft contamination with monoclonal plasma cells following mobilization of stem cells. Of the 102 patients receiving G-CSF alone, 25% had tumor contamination and of the 33 patients receiving chemomobilization 51% had tumor contamination [2]. In a randomized study of 47 patients with lymphoma, PCR tumor cell data were available for 22 patients with NHL; 11 patients received mobilization with G-CSF alone and 10 patients received chemotherapy and G-CSF [57]. A high rate of patients in both groups had tumor contamination of the harvested PBSC product (92 and 90%, respectively) (Table 10.1).

Table 10.1 Mobilization methods and tumor cell contamination of apheresis products

First author (reference)	Mobilization method	Number of patients/ disease type	Method for detection of tumor cells	Percentage of patients with tumor cells detected	Level of contamination
Gazitt [34]	Chemotherapy	10/MM	PCR	100% (10 patients)	$<0.4–8400 \times 10^4$
Ho [42]	Chemotherapy	89/NHL 69/MM	PCR	36% of collections contaminated with NHL tumor cells 25% of collections contaminated with MM tumor cells	Reported as detectable or not detectable according to the method (method sensitive to detect 1:100,000 cells)
Kopp [48]	Chemotherapy and G-CSF	60/MM	FACS caliber flow cytometry	27% of collections contaminated with high levels 73% of collections contaminated with low levels	$\leq 4.5 \times 10^5$ tumor cells/kg $>4.5 \times 10^5$ tumor cells/kg
Lemoli [52]	Chemotherapy and G-CSF	23/MM	FACS	100% (23 patients)	Mean = 0.7% circulating myeloma cells (range 0.2–2.7%)
Schiller [68]	Chemotherapy and G-CSF	37 (14 had tumor contamination measured)/MM	PCR	57% (8/14)	0.23–0.0015%
Demirkazik [23]	Cytokines	26/NHL (not mobilized) 35/NHL (mobilized)	PCR	37% of collections contained tumor contamination in the mobilized group compared with 19% in the nonmobilized group	G-CSF mobilized group: Median GM-CFC $\times 10^4$ kg/L blood = 0.21 (0.017–5.8) Nonmobilized group: Median GM-CFC $\times 10^4$ kg/L blood = 0.0054 (0.00013–0.072)
Anagnostopoulos [2]	G-CSF or chemotherapy	33/MM (G-CSF alone) 102/MM (chemotherapy)	Flow cytometry	25% of collections contaminated with tumor cells (G-CSF alone) 51% of collections contaminated with tumor cells (chemotherapy)	All patients: B-2 microglobulin median = 3.2 (range 0.2–34.1)
Narayanasami [57]	G-CSF or chemotherapy and GCSF	47/lymphoma (TCM data reported on 22 patients with NHL)	PCR	11/12 patients (92%) in G-CSF-alone arm 9/10 patients (90%) in chemotherapy + G-CSF arm	Not reported
Cremer [21]	G-CSF or chemotherapy and G-CSF	8/MM	PCR	All 8 patients had detectable malignant cells in the leukapheresis product	0.0006–0.256%
Fruehauf [31]	Plerixafor plus G-CSF	7/MM	PCR	3/7 had detectable tumor cells 4/7 had no detectable tumor cells	Observed fold change from pre-plerixafor to pre-apheresis: 0.11- to 1.08-fold
DiPersio [25]	Plerixafor plus G-CSF	11/NHL (5 G-CSF only 6 plerixafor plus G-CSF)	PCR	1/5 G-CSF had detectable levels of tumor cells 6/6 had no detectable levels of tumor cells	Not reported

Plerixafor Plus G-CSF

Plerixafor is a newly marketed product approved in the USA for use with G-CSF for stem cell mobilization. Plerixafor is a selective and reversible antagonist of CXCR4 and disrupts its interaction with SDF-1, thereby releasing HSCs in the circulation.

The effect of plerixafor plus G-CSF on tumor cell contamination has been investigated in NHL [25, 36] and MM patients [31, 76]. Samples were collected for evaluation of tumor cell contamination from 11 patients with NHL [25] and 7 patients [31] or 10 patients [76] with MM who were in plerixafor clinical trials. In the samples of 11 patients with NHL, 5 received G-CSF alone and 6 received plerixafor plus G-CSF. Samples were analyzed by quantitative PCR for *BCL-2* translocation [25]. Of these NHL patients, ten had undetectable levels of translocated *BCL-2* in the leukapheresis product and one patient who received G-CSF alone had detectable levels (Table 10.1).

In the seven patients with MM, samples for PCR were obtained at baseline prior to any therapy, following G-CSF and before plerixafor, and then again following plerixafor and prior to apheresis (Fruehauf et al. 2009). After receiving plerixafor, 3/7 patients had slightly increased tumor cells in the peripheral blood compared to G-CSF alone and 4/7 had decreased tumor cells. For all patients, the change in tumor cell level ranged from 0.11–1.08 times the pre-plerixafor level. Tricot et al. analyzed PB samples by flow cytometry in ten patients with MM. A total of nine paired samples were available for analysis pre- and post first and second dose of plerixafor. None of the PB samples showed >1% light-chain-restricted cells, except for the first apheresis product of one patient, which had 2% kappa cells with a DNA index of 1 and 1% lambda cells with a DNA index of 1. Plasma cells with aneuploid DNA content were not observed in any of the samples [76].

Although the total number of patients examined overall was limited, there did not appear to be an increase of tumor cells in the apheresis product following plerixafor above that observed or expected with G-CSF. Thus, contamination of an apheresis product would be expected to be similar to that obtained by standard G-CSF mobilization.

Effect of Tumor Cell Contamination on Clinical Outcomes

Early reports examining the presence of tumor contamination in PBSC products and clinical outcome (response and survival) of patients transplanted with these products have reached different conclusions regarding the clinical implications of this finding [37, 68]. A recent study by Ho et al. examined NHL ($n=89$) and MM ($n=69$) patients undergoing autologous stem cell transplants. The study compared the outcome of patients transplanted with HSCs free of tumor cells to those transplanted with HSCs contaminated with tumor cells [42]. The results of this study demonstrated that the contamination of HSCs with tumor cells had no influence on PFS or OS, even when aggressive or indolent histologies are considered separately. Similarly, another study found that the tumor cell content of PB progenitor cell grafts was not predictive of clinical outcome in patients with diffuse B-cell lymphoma and follicular lymphoma [11]. Finally, another study in 61 NHL patients found that lymphoma contamination of transplanted apheresis products had no apparent impact on event-free and overall survival (OS) [23].

In contrast, other studies have reported poorer clinical outcomes in patients transplanted with HSCs contaminated with tumor cells [13, 53, 69, 78, 79]. A recent study by Kopp et al. described a correlation between tumor contamination and outcome in patients with MM receiving chemomobilized stem cell products [48]. The results of this study suggested that the level of tumor cell contamination correlated with a poorer overall survival. However, the level of tumor cell contamination was large ($>4.5\times10^5$ cell/kg). [If one assumes a patient weight of 85 kg and an apheresis cell concentration of about 100×10^6 PBMC/mL, this roughly correlates to 4 tumor cells in 1,000 PBMCs.] In the study, lower quantities of tumor had no significant impact on progression-free survival (PFS) or OS. This indicates that the level of tumor contamination of the apheresis product needs to be very high in order to affect clinical outcome and that minimal or moderate amounts of tumor cell contamination may not be clinically significant. Of note, the use of chemotherapy for mobilization did not reduce the subsequent collection of tumor cells or the purported impact on outcome.

Tumor cell contamination has driven the development of methods to reduce, or purge, the quantity of tumor cells within the stem cell product. These "purging" methods have included the direct removal of tumor cells by antibodies plus complement, magnetic bead separation, exposure of the stem cell product to chemotherapy in vitro, or selection and use of purified stem cells. Since malignant cells from patients with MM and NHL generally do not express CD34, positive selection of CD34$^+$ cells has been used to separate stem cells from tumor cells. Studies have demonstrated that this method markedly reduces tumor contamination by several logs (median 2–3 logs) [30, 45, 68, 71, 75, 77]. However, despite large reductions of tumor burden, long-term follow-up has not demonstrated that purging leads to clinical benefit [50].

Two phase-III randomized trials comparing patients who received autografts purged of tumor cells (CD34$^+$-selected PBSC) to those with unselected PBSCs were conducted in patients with MM [12, 73]. Both studies used a highly sensitive, tumor-specific PCR technique to identify the Ig heavy-chain sequence of the myeloma clone and determine the level of tumor cell contamination. Both studies achieved a large reduction in tumor burden (~1–6 log tumor load reduction), but no significant differences between the two groups in terms of response, event (progression)-free survival, or OS were observed.

Given these findings, the authors of each of these phase III studies speculated that reinfused myeloma cells may not be a significant cause of relapse, but that failure to eradicate the disease within the patient with high-dose chemotherapy may be a stronger contributor to relapse. Allogeneic (and therefore tumor free) bone marrow transplants for myeloma, where patients showed a high risk of relapse approaching 50% [32], also suggest that improved disease eradication within the patient may be a more important goal than purging tumor cells from the reinfused product. Similar clinical outcomes and results have been reported for patients with NHL who received tumor-purged products in a case-matched comparison study using the EBMT registry [81] (Table 10.2).

Table 10.2 Effect of tumor cell contamination of apheresis products on clinical outcomes

First author (reference)	Mobilization method	Number of patients/disease	Conclusions
Blystad [11]	Chemotherapy plus G-CSF	43/NHL	The level of contamination of the PBPC/CD34⁺ cells ranged from 0 to 8.3%. No relationship could be shown between the total number of tumor cells infused and relapsed. Patients receiving PCR-positive or PCR-negative PBPC grafts had similar progression-free survival (PFS) ($P=0.49$)
Bourhis [12]	Chemotherapy and G-CSF	111/MM	Despite significant tumor cell reduction, CD34⁺ selection does not reduce RR and increases the risk of severe post-transplant infections. There was also no difference in RR between patients in either arm who received grafts with detectable tumor cells and those receiving grafts with no detectable tumor cells, suggesting that reinfused tumor cells may not be the main cause of relapse after autologous transplant in myeloma
Brown [13]	Chemotherapy or chemotherapy and G-CSF	103/NHL	The only predictors of decreased progression-free survival proved to be histologic BM involvement at time of harvest [hazard ratio (HR) 2.27, 95% confidence interval (CI) 1.3–3.9, $P<0.004$] and PCR detectable disease in the BM product after purging (HR 4.18, 95% CI 1.99–8.8, $P=0.0002$). No significant predictors of overall survival (OS) were identified
Ho [42]	Chemotherapy	89/NHL 69/MM	Patients with contaminating tumor cells in autologous peripheral blood stem cells (PBSCs) do not have worsened OS or PFS in MM or NHL. Tumor cells detected by sensitive molecular methods in PBSC collections may be distinct from cells contaminating marrow and appear to have limited utility in identifying patients with MM and B-cell NHL who would benefit from purging strategies
Kopp [48]	Chemotherapy and G-CSF	60/MM	Patients with $>4.5\times10^5$ plasma cells/kg contaminating the PBSC graft received after high-dose chemotherapy have a significantly reduced overall survival. Whether high contamination of grafts with plasma cells might reflect residual in vivo tumor mass prior to stem cell transplantation and a generally more aggressive behavior of malignant myeloma cells in these patients or whether reinfused plasma cells contribute to an unfavorable course of disease remains to be determined
Kornacker [50]	Chemotherapy and G-CSF or G-CSF	241/NHL	Patients with disease recurrence within 1 year from transplant and those who had received autoSCT as second-line treatment had significantly reduced survival by multivariate analysis, whereas Follicular Lymphoma International Prognostic Index score, age, remission status at autoSCT, high-dose regimen, and ex vivo purging had no impact

(continued)

Table 10.2 (continued)

First author (reference)	Mobilization method	Number of patients/disease	Conclusions
Lopez-Perez [53]	G-CSF alone (12 patients) and chemotherapy plus G-CSF (11 patients)	23/MM	Patients with clonally free products were more likely to obtain CR following transplant (64% vs. 17%, $P=0.02$) and a longer progression-free survival (40 months in patients transplanted with polyclonal products vs. 20 with monoclonal ones, $P=0.03$). These results were consistent when the overall survival was considered, since it was better in those patients with negative apheresis than it was in those with positive (83% vs. 36% at 5 years from diagnosis, $P=0.01$). These findings indicate that the presence of clonality rearranged VDJH segments is related to the response and outcome in MM-transplanted patients
Schiller [68]	Chemotherapy plus G-CSF	37/MM	Peripheral blood progenitor cells are an effective form of purified hematopoietic support achieving substantial reduction in myeloma cell contamination. At infused cell doses of greater than 2×10^6 $CD34^+$ cells/kg, this product provides safe, rapid, and sustained hematologic recovery in patients receiving myeloablative chemotherapy. Whether this form of purified stem cell support produces improved progression-free survival in multiple myeloma requires further trials
Stewart [73]	Chemotherapy and G-CSF	190/MM	This phase III trial demonstrated that although CD34 selection significantly reduces myeloma cell contamination in PBPC collections, no improvement in disease-free or overall survival was achieved
Vogel [78]	Chemotherapy and G-CSF	74/MM	Patients with graft contamination of more than 4.5×10^5 plasma cells/kg had a high risk of early disease progression after high-dose chemotherapy
Vose [79]	Chemotherapy or chemotherapy plus G-CSF	93/NHL	Patients with aggressive NHL receiving HSCT randomized to PBSCT demonstrated improved neutrophil engraftment and platelet and RBC transfusion independence. The complete response rate and EFS were not statistically different by randomization arm. Patients whose harvests were positive for minimal residual disease by molecular analysis had poorer EFS
Williams [81]	Not reported	224/NHL	Time to hematologic engraftment, response to ABMT, and number of procedure-related deaths were similar in purged and unpurged patients. The overall survival rate was 54% at 5 years in purged patients and 48.3% in unpurged patients ($P=0.1813$). The PFS rates were 44.3 and 44.6%, respectively ($P=.1961$). Patterns of relapse, including bone marrow relapse, were similar in both groups

Mechanism of Tumor Growth

Tumor cells appear to increase, or are "mobilized," into the PB following treatment with standard chemotherapy and radiation [10]. In preclinical models, Biswas et al. demonstrated that when established tumors are treated with chemotherapy or radiation, an increase in circulating tumor cells could be measured resulting in increased lung metastases. The observed TCM and metastatic effect were blocked by neutralizing antibodies to transforming growth factor beta (TGFβ). TGFβ is known to be a critical inducer of epithelial mesenchymal transition (EMT), which causes a morphologic and physiologic change in the tumor cell, leading to increased migration and metastases. Interestingly, in studies in which putative breast cancer stem cells have been identified, similar effects of TGFβ on the induction of EMT and metastasis have been demonstrated [70]. Therefore, TCM appears to occur following standard cancer treatments, and though other factors may be involved this effect appears to be primarily driven by the pro-metastatic effect of TGFβ.

The tumor microenvironment is now recognized as a key factor in the growth of tumor cells. This symbiotic relationship includes the production of cytokines, such as TGFβ and VEGF, by the tumor that stimulate the production of stroma, blood vessels, and other factors that provide the tumor with a supportive microenvironment in which to grow. Stromal cells produce and express SDF-1 which engages tumor cell CXCR4 receptors and induces antiapoptotic signaling. Several groups have demonstrated that blockade of CXCR4 with plerixafor or similar agents can sensitize tumor cells to chemotherapy, increase their effectiveness, and lead to prolonged survival of animals [17, 58, 85, 86]. These data are the basis for ongoing clinical studies investigating the use of plerixafor in combination with chemotherapy or biologic treatments for AML and CLL. Therefore, even though tumor cells might migrate/mobilize under certain conditions, they may readily undergo apoptosis and their metastatic potential may be diminished.

Conclusion

The detection of tumor cells continues to remain extremely difficult given the low number of tumor cells compared to normal cells and the large variety of potential tumor types. The sensitivity and specificity of the various tumor cell detection methods vary and are highly dependent on the method used and the source of the cells analyzed making it difficult to compare results across studies published in the literature. Despite these limitations, it has long been recognized that tumor cell contamination occurs during the mobilization and collection of stem cells from patients with MM and lymphoma following G-CSF or chemomobilization. Tumor cell contamination following plerixafor administration appears to be similar or less than that following G-CSF mobilization alone when the same number of $CD34^{+}$ stem cells are collected.

Of critical importance is the relevance of TCM on clinical outcome. It is possible that tumor cells in the reinfused apheresis product could be responsible for relapse. However, it is more likely that relapse is due to the regrowth of residual cancer in the patient following incomplete eradication of tumor cells by high-dose chemotherapy and radiation therapy. The later scenario is demonstrated by the significant relapse rate in cancer patients receiving "tumor-free" allogeneic stem cells from healthy donors and the fact that in autologous transplants the most common sites of relapse are prior sites of disease. In addition, phase II and large, randomized phase III studies have demonstrated that even a large reduction of tumor cells in the apheresis product had no impact on clinical outcome as measured by disease-free or overall survival. In studies in which tumor cell contamination was associated with poorer overall survival, the correlation was only significant when the level of tumor contamination was very high ($>4.5 \times 10^5$ cells/kg), as detected by flow cytometry. Finally, the reinfusion with tumor cells during autologous HSC transplantation of MM and NHL patients appears to have no influence on progression-free or overall survival, even when aggressive or indolent histologies are considered separately. Collectively, these data suggest that new treatment paradigms for myeloma and lymphoma should focus on increasing the chemosensitivity of the tumor and eliminating residual disease.

Acknowledgments JDP, SF, and ADH have received research funding and honoraria from Genzyme Corporation. CC, JH, and FJH are employees of Genzyme Corporation.
We gratefully acknowledge Elsevier's permission to reuse material.

References

1. Abrams RA, Johnston-Early A, Kramer C, Minna JD, Cohen MH, Deisseroth AB (1981) Amplification of circulating granulocyte-monocyte stem cell numbers following chemotherapy in patients with extensive small cell carcinoma of the lung. Cancer Res 41:35–41
2. Anagnostopoulos A, Aleman A, Yang Y, Donato M, Weber D, Champlin R, Smith T, Alexanian R, Giralt S (2004) Outcomes of autologous stem cell transplantation in patients with multiple myeloma who received dexamethasone-based nonmyelosuppressive induction therapy. Bone Marrow Transplant 33:623–628
3. Bakkus MH, Bouko Y, Samson D, Apperley JF, Thielemans K, Van Camp B, Benner A, Goldschmidt H, Moos M, Cremer FW (2004) Post-transplantation tumour load in bone marrow, as assessed by quantitative ASO-PCR, is a prognostic parameter in multiple myeloma. Br J Haematol 126:665–674
4. Barlogie B, Gohde W, Johnston DA, Smallwood L, Schumann J, Drewinko B, Freireich EJ (1978) Determination of ploidy and proliferative characteristics of human solid tumors by pulse cytophotometry. Cancer Res 38:3333–3339
5. Barlogie B, Johnston DA, Smallwood L, Raber MN, Maddox AM, Latreille J, Swartzendruber DE, Drewinko B (1982) Prognostic implications of ploidy and proliferative activity in human solid tumors. Cancer Genet Cytogenet 6:17–28
6. Barlogie B, Raber MN, Schumann J, Johnson TS, Drewinko B, Swartzendruber DE, Gohde W, Andreeff M, Freireich EJ (1983) Flow cytometry in clinical cancer research. Cancer Res 43:3982–3997

7. Barlogie B, Alexanian R, Pershouse M, Smallwood L, Smith L (1985) Cytoplasmic immunoglobulin content in multiple myeloma. J Clin Invest 76:765–769
8. Bensinger W, DiPersio JF, McCarty JM (2009) Improving stem cell mobilization strategies: future directions. Bone Marrow Transplant 43:181–195
9. Billadeau D, Quam L, Thomas W, Kay N, Greipp P, Kyle R, Oken MM, Van Ness B (1992) Detection and quantitation of malignant cells in the peripheral blood of multiple myeloma patients. Blood 80:1818–1824
10. Biswas S, Guix M, Rinehart C, Dugger TC, Chytil A, Moses HL, Freeman ML, Arteaga CL (2007) Inhibition of TGF-beta with neutralizing antibodies prevents radiation-induced acceleration of metastatic cancer progression. J Clin Invest 117:1305–1313
11. Blystad AK, Delabie J, Kvaloy S, Holte H, Valerhaugen H, Ikonomou I, Kvalheim G (2004) Infused CD34 cell dose, but not tumour cell content of peripheral blood progenitor cell grafts, predicts clinical outcome in patients with diffuse large B-cell lymphoma and follicular lymphoma grade 3 treated with high-dose therapy. Br J Haematol 125:605–612
12. Bourhis JH, Bouko Y, Koscielny S, Bakkus M, Greinix H, Derigs G, Salles G, Feremans W, Apperley J, Samson D, Bjorkstrand B, Niederwieser D, Gahrton G, Pico JL, Goldschmidt H (2007) Relapse risk after autologous transplantation in patients with newly diagnosed myeloma is not related with infused tumor cell load and the outcome is not improved by CD34+ cell selection: long term follow-up of an EBMT phase III randomized study. Haematologica 92:1083–1090
13. Brown JR, Feng Y, Gribben JG, Neuberg D, Fisher DC, Mauch P, Nadler LM, Freedman AS (2007) Long-term survival after autologous bone marrow transplantation for follicular lymphoma in first remission. Biol Blood Marrow Transplant 13:1057–1065
14. Brugger W, Bross KJ, Glatt M, Weber F, Mertelsmann R, Kanz L (1994) Mobilization of tumor cells and hematopoietic progenitor cells into peripheral blood of patients with solid tumors. Blood 83:636–640
15. Buchonnet G, Lenain P, Ruminy P, Lepretre S, Stamatoullas A, Parmentier F, Jardin F, Duval C, Tilly H, Bastard C (2000) Characterisation of BCL2-JH rearrangements in follicular lymphoma: PCR detection of 3′ BCL2 breakpoints and evidence of a new cluster. Leukemia 14:1563–1569
16. Bunn PA Jr, Krasnow S, Makuch RW, Schlam ML, Schechter GP (1982) Flow cytometric analysis of DNA content of bone marrow cells in patients with plasma cell myeloma: clinical implications. Blood 59:528–535
17. Burger J, Burkle A (2007) The CXCR4 chemokine receptor in acute and chronic leukaemia: a marrow homing receptor and potential therapeutic target. Br J Haematol 137:288–296
18. Cook GP, Tomlinson IM, Walter G, Riethman H, Carter NP, Buluwela L, Winter G, Rabbitts TH (1994) A map of the human immunoglobulin VH locus completed by analysis of the telomeric region of chromosome 14q. Nat Genet 7:162–168
19. Corradini P, Voena C, Tarella C, Astolfi M, Ladetto M, Palumbo A, Van Lint MT, Bacigalupo A, Santoro A, Musso M, Majolino I, Boccadoro M, Pileri A (1999) Molecular and clinical remissions in multiple myeloma: role of autologous and allogeneic transplantation of hematopoietic cells. J Clin Oncol 17:208–215
20. Corradini P, Ladetto M, Zallio F, Astolfi M, Rizzo E, Sametti S, Cuttica A, Rosato R, Farina L, Boccadoro M, Benedetti F, Pileri A, Tarella C (2004) Long-term follow-up of indolent lymphoma patients treated with high-dose sequential chemotherapy and autografting: evidence that durable molecular and clinical remission frequently can be attained only in follicular subtypes. J Clin Oncol 22:1460–1468
21. Cremer FW, Kiel K, Wallmeier M, Haas R, Goldschmidt H, Moos M (1998) Leukapheresis products in multiple myeloma: lower tumor load after mobilization with cyclophosphamide plus granulocyte colony-stimulating factor (G-CSF) compared with G-CSF alone. Exp Hematol 26:969–975
22. Cristofanilli M, Broglio KR, Guarneri V, Jackson S, Fritsche HA, Islam R, Dawood S, Reuben JM, Kau SW, Lara JM, Krishnamurthy S, Ueno NT, Hortobagyi GN, Valero V (2007) Circulating tumor cells in metastatic breast cancer: biologic staging beyond tumor burden. Clin Breast Cancer 7:471–479

23. Demirkazik A, Kessinger A, Armitage JO, Bierman PJ, Lynch J, Vose J, Chan W, Sharp JG (2001) Progenitor and lymphoma cells in blood stem cell harvests: impact on survival following transplantation. Bone Marrow Transplant 28:207–212
24. Desikan K, Barlogie B, Jagannath S, Vesole D, Siegel D, Fassas A, Munshi N, Singhal S, Mehta J, Tindle S, Nelson J, Bracy D, Mattox S, Tricot G (1998) Comparable engraftment kinetics following peripheral-blood stem-cell infusion mobilized with granulocyte colony-stimulating factor with or without cyclophosphamide in multiple myeloma. J Clin Oncol 16:1547–1553
25. DiPersio JF, Bridger G, Calandra G (2009) Effect of plerixafor (AMD 3100) plus G-CSF on tumor cell mobilization among patients with lymphoma. Biol Blood Marrow Transplant 15(2):37
26. Dolken G, Dolken L, Hirt C, Fusch C, Rabkin CS, Schuler F (2008) Age-dependent prevalence and frequency of circulating t(14;18)-positive cells in the peripheral blood of healthy individuals. J Natl Cancer Inst Monogr (39):44–47
27. Duhrsen U, Villeval JL, Boyd J, Kannourakis G, Morstyn G, Metcalf D (1988) Effects of recombinant human granulocyte colony-stimulating factor on hematopoietic progenitor cells in cancer patients. Blood 72:2074–2081
28. Franklin WA, Glaspy J, Pflaumer SM, Jones RB, Hami L, Martinez C, Murphy JR, Shpall EJ (1999) Incidence of tumor-cell contamination in leukapheresis products of breast cancer patients mobilized with stem cell factor and granulocyte colony-stimulating factor (G-CSF) or with G-CSF alone. Blood 94:340–347
29. Fruehauf S, Seggewiss R (2003) It's moving day: factors affecting peripheral blood stem cell mobilization and strategies for improvement [corrected]. Br J Haematol 122:360–375
30. Fruehauf S, Haas R, Zeller WJ, Hunstein W (1994) CD34 selection for purging in multiple myeloma and analysis of CD34$^+$ B cell precursors. Stem Cells 12(1):95–102
31. Fruehauf S, Ehninger G, Hubel K, Topaly J, Goldschmidt H, Ho AD, Muller S, Moos M, Badel K, Calandra G (2010) Mobilization of peripheral blood stem cells for autologous transplant in non-Hodgkin's lymphoma and multiple myeloma patients by plerixafor and G-CSF and detection of tumor cell mobilization by PCR in multiple myeloma patients. Bone Marrow Transplant 45:269–275
32. Gahrton G, Svensson H, Cavo M, Apperly J, Bacigalupo A, Bjorkstrand B, Blade J, Cornelissen J, de Laurenzi A, Facon T, Ljungman P, Michallet M, Niederwieser D, Powles R, Reiffers J, Russell NH, Samson D, Schaefer UW, Schattenberg A, Tura S, Verdonck LF, Vernant JP, Willemze R, Volin L (2001) Progress in allogenic bone marrow and peripheral blood stem cell transplantation for multiple myeloma: a comparison between transplants performed 1983–93 and 1994–8 at European Group for Blood and Marrow Transplantation centres. Br J Haematol 113:209–216
33. Gallagher DJ, Milowsky MI, Ishill N, Trout A, Boyle MG, Riches J, Fleisher M, Bajorin DF (2009) Detection of circulating tumor cells in patients with urothelial cancer. Ann Oncol 20:305–308
34. Gazitt Y, Reading C, Hoffman R, Lee J-H, Barlogie B, Vesole D, Jagannath S, Condono J, Lee B, Wickerma A, Tricot G (1995) Purified CD34+ Lin- Thy+ stem cells do not contain clonal myeloma cells. Blood 86:381–189
35. Gazitt Y, Tian E, Barlogie B, Reading CL, Vesole DH, Jagannath S, Schnell J, Hoffman R, Tricot G (1996) Differential mobilization of myeloma cells and normal hematopoietic stem cells in multiple myeloma after treatment with cyclophosphamide and granulocyte-macrophage colony-stimulating factor. Blood 87:805–811
36. Gazitt Y, Freytes CO, Akay C, Badel K, Calandra G (2007) Improved mobilization of peripheral blood CD34+ cells and dendritic cells by AMD3100 plus granulocyte-colony-stimulating factor in non-Hodgkin's lymphoma patients. Stem Cells Dev 16:657–666
37. Gertz MA, Witzig TE, Pineda AA, Greipp PR, Kyle RA, Litzow MR (1997) Monoclonal plasma cells in the blood stem cell harvest from patients with multiple myeloma are associated with shortened relapse-free survival after transplantation. Bone Marrow Transplant 19:337–342

38. Haas R, Ho A, Bredthauer U, Cayeux S, Egerer G, Knauf W, Hunstein W (1990) Successful autologous transplantation of blood stem cells mobilized with recombinant human granulocyte-macrophage colony-stimulating factor. Exp Hematol 18:94–98
39. Haas R, Moos M, Karcher A, Mohle R, Witt B, Goldschmidt H, Fruehauf S, Flentje M, Wannenmacher M, Hunstein W (1994) Sequential high-dose therapy with peripheral-blood progenitor-cell support in low-grade non-Hodgkin's lymphoma. J Clin Oncol 12:1685–1692
40. Hamlin PA, Zelenetz AD, Kewalramani T, Qin J, Satagopan JM, Verbel D, Noy A, Portlock CS, Straus DJ, Yahalom J, Nimer SD, Moskowitz CH (2003) Age-adjusted International Prognostic Index predicts autologous stem cell transplantation outcome for patients with relapsed or primary refractory diffuse large B-cell lymphoma. Blood 102:1989–1996
41. Hiraiwa K, Takeuchi H, Hasegawa H, Saikawa Y, Suda K, Ando T, Kumagai K, Irino T, Yoshikawa T, Matsuda S, Kitajima M, Kitagawa Y (2008) Clinical significance of circulating tumor cells in blood from patients with gastrointestinal cancers. Ann Surg Oncol 15:3092–3100
42. Ho J, Yang L, Banihashemi B, Martin L, Halpenny M, Atkins H, Sabloff M, McDiarmid SA, Huebsch LB, Bence-Bruckler I, Giulivi A, Allan DS (2009) Contaminating tumour cells in autologous PBSC grafts do not influence survival or relapse following transplant for multiple myeloma or B-cell non-Hodgkin's lymphoma. Bone Marrow Transplant 43:223–228
43. Hsieh HB, Marrinucci D, Bethel K, Curry DN, Humphrey M, Krivacic RT, Kroener J, Kroener L, Ladanyi A, Lazarus N, Kuhn P, Bruce RH, Nieva J (2006) High speed detection of circulating tumor cells. Biosens Bioelectron 21:1893–1899
44. Hsu FJ, Levy R (1995) Preferential use of the VH4 Ig gene family by diffuse large-cell lymphoma. Blood 86:3072–3082
45. Hundsdörfer P, Fruehauf S, Haberkorn M, Höft R, Haas R, Zeller WJ (1999) Comparison of different lymphoma cell purging modalities: An experimental study with K422 lymphoma cells. Acta Haematol 101:185–192
46. Kiel K, Cremer FW, Ehrbrecht E et al (1998) First and second apheresis in patients with multiple myeloma: no differences in tumor load and hematopoietic stem cell yield. Bone Marrow Transplant 21:1109–1115
47. Knudsen LM, Rasmussen T, Nikolaisen K, Johnsen HE (2001) Mobilisation of tumour cells along with CD34+ cells to peripheral blood in multiple myeloma. Eur J Haematol 67:289–295
48. Kopp HG, Yildirim S, Weisel KC, Kanz L, Vogel W (2009) Contamination of autologous peripheral blood progenitor cell grafts predicts overall survival after high-dose chemotherapy in multiple myeloma. J Cancer Res Clin Oncol 135:637–642
49. Körbling M, Dörken B, Ho A, Pezzutto A, Hunstein W, Fliedner T (1986) Autologous transplantation of blood-derived hemopoietic stem cells after myeloablative therapy in a patient with Burkitt's lymphoma. Blood 67:529–532
50. Kornacker M, Stumm J, Pott C, Dietrich S, Sussmilch S, Hensel M, Nickelsen M, Witzens-Harig M, Kneba M, Schmitz N, Ho AD, Dreger P (2009) Characteristics of relapse after autologous stem-cell transplantation for follicular lymphoma: a long-term follow-up. Ann Oncol 20:722–728
51. Krivacic RT, Ladanyi A, Curry DN, Hsieh HB, Kuhn P, Bergsrud DE, Kepros JF, Barbera T, Ho MY, Chen LB, Lerner RA, Bruce RH (2004) A rare-cell detector for cancer. Proc Natl Acad Sci USA 101:10501–10504
52. Lemoli RM, Cavo M, Fortuna A (1996) Concomitant mobilization of plasma cells and hematopoietic progenitors into peripheral blood of patients with multiple myeloma. J Hematother 5:339–349
53. Lopez-Perez R, Garcia-Sanz R, Gonzalez D, Balanzategui A, Chillon MC, Alaejos I, Mateos MV, Caballero MD, Mateo G, Nieto MJ, Gonzalez M, San Miguel JF (2000) The detection of contaminating clonal cells in apheresis products is related to response and outcome in multiple myeloma undergoing autologous peripheral blood stem cell transplantation. Leukemia 14:1493–1499
54. Mateo G, Corral M, Almeida J, Lopez-Berges C, Nieto J, Garcia-Marcos A, Vazquez L, del Canizo C, Orfao A, San Miguel JF (2003) Immunophenotypic analysis of peripheral blood stem cell harvests from patients with multiple myeloma. Haematologica 88:1013–1021

55. Menendez P, Caballero M, Prosper F, Del Canizo M, Perez-Simon J, Mateos M, Nieto M, Corral M, Romero M, Garcia-Conde J, Montalban M, San Miguel J, Orfao A (2002) The composition of leukapheresis products impacts on the hematopoietic recovery after autologous transplantation independently of the mobilization regimen. Transfusion 42:1159–1172
56. Mielcarek M, Torok-Storb B (1997) Phenotype and engraftment potential of cytokine-mobilized peripheral blood mononuclear cells. Curr Opin Hematol 4:176–182
57. Narayanasami U, Kanteti R, Morelli J, Klekar A, Al-Olama A, Keating C, O'Connor C, Berkman E, Erban J, Sprague K, Miller K, Schenkein D (2001) Randomized trial of filgrastim versus chemotherapy and filgrastim mobilization of hematopoietic progenitor cells for rescue in autologous transplantation. Blood 98:2059–2064
58. Nervi B, Ramirez P, Holt M, Rettig M, Ritchey J, Prior J, Piwnica-Worms D, Bridger G, Ley T, DiPersio J (2006) CXCR4/SDF-1 is a key regulator for leukemia migration and homing to the BM: impact of AMD3100 on in vivo response to chemotherapy. Blood 108:171a–172a
59. Pantel K, Brakenhoff RH, Brandt B (2008) Detection, clinical relevance and specific biological properties of disseminating tumour cells. Nat Rev Cancer 8:329–340
60. Pecora AL, Lazarus HM, Jennis AA, Preti RA, Goldberg SL, Rowley SD, Cantwell S, Cooper BW, Copelan EA, Herzig RH, Meagher R, Kennedy MJ, Akard LR, Jansen J, Ross A, Prilutskaya M, Glassco J, Kahn D, Moss TJ (2002) Breast cancer cell contamination of blood stem cell products in patients with metastatic breast cancer: predictors and clinical relevance. Biol Blood Marrow Transplant 8:536–543
61. Pott C, Tiemann M, Linke B, Ott MM, von Hofen M, Bolz I, Hiddemann W, Parwaresch R, Kneba M (1998) Structure of Bcl-1 and IgH-CDR3 rearrangements as clonal markers in mantle cell lymphomas. Leukemia 12:1630–1637
62. Price CG, Meerabux J, Murtagh S, Cotter FE, Rohatiner AZ, Young BD, Lister TA (1991) The significance of circulating cells carrying t(14;18) in long remission from follicular lymphoma. J Clin Oncol 9:1527–1532
63. Radich JP, Mao M, Stepaniants S, Biery M, Castle J, Ward T, Schimmack G, Kobayashi S, Carleton M, Lampe J, Linsley PS (2004) Individual-specific variation of gene expression in peripheral blood leukocytes. Genomics 83:980–988
64. Richman CM, Weiner RS, Yankee RA (1976) Increase in circulating stem cells following chemotherapy in man. Blood 47:1031–1039
65. Ross AA (2000) Detection and significance of minimal residual disease from solid tumor malignancies in stem cell autografts. In: Ho AD, Haas R, Champlin RE editor. Hematopoietic Stem Cell Transplantation. 1st ed. New York: Informa Healthcare. pp. 275–290.
66. Ross AA, Cooper BW, Lazarus HM, Mackay W, Moss TJ, Ciobanu N, Tallman MS, Kennedy MJ, Davidson NE, Sweet D et al (1993) Detection and viability of tumor cells in peripheral blood stem cell collections from breast cancer patients using immunocytochemical and clonogenic assay techniques. Blood 82:2605–2610
67. Sastre J, Maestro ML, Puente J, Veganzones S, Alfonso R, Rafael S, Garcia-Saenz JA, Vidaurreta M, Martin M, Arroyo M, Sanz-Casla MT, Diaz-Rubio E (2008) Circulating tumor cells in colorectal cancer: correlation with clinical and pathological variables. Ann Oncol 19:935–938
68. Schiller G, Vescio R, Freytes C, Spitzer G, Sahebi F, Lee M, Wu CH, Cao J, Lee JC, Hong CH et al (1995) Transplantation of CD34+ peripheral blood progenitor cells after high-dose chemotherapy for patients with advanced multiple myeloma. Blood 86:390–397
69. Sharp JG, Kessinger A, Mann S, Crouse DA, Armitage JO, Bierman P, Weisenburger DD (1996) Outcome of high-dose therapy and autologous transplantation in non-Hodgkin's lymphoma based on the presence of tumor in the marrow or infused hematopoietic harvest. J Clin Oncol 14:214–219
70. Shipitsin M, Campbell LL, Argani P, Weremowicz S, Bloushtain-Qimron N, Yao J, Nikolskaya T, Serebryiskaya T, Beroukhim R, Hu M, Halushka MK, Sukumar S, Parker LM, Anderson KS, Harris LN, Garber JE, Richardson AL, Schnitt SJ, Nikolsky Y, Gelman RS, Polyak K (2007) Molecular definition of breast tumor heterogeneity. Cancer Cell 11:259–273
71. Shpall EJ, Jones RB, Bearman SI, Franklin WA, Archer PG, Curiel T, Bitter M, Claman HN, Stemmer SM, Purdy M et al (1994) Transplantation of enriched CD34-positive autologous marrow into breast cancer patients following high-dose chemotherapy: influence of CD34-positive peripheral-blood progenitors and growth factors on engraftment. J Clin Oncol 12:28–36

72. Socinski MA, Cannistra SA, Elias A, Antman KH, Schnipper L, Griffin JD (1988) Granulocyte-macrophage colony stimulating factor expands the circulating haemopoietic progenitor cell compartment in man. Lancet 1:1194–1198
73. Stewart AK, Vescio R, Schiller G, Ballester O, Noga S, Rugo H, Freytes C, Stadtmauer E, Tarantolo S, Sahebi F, Stiff P, Meharchard J, Schlossman R, Brown R, Tully H, Benyunes M, Jacobs C, Berenson R, White M, DiPersio J, Anderson KC, Berenson J (2001) Purging of autologous peripheral-blood stem cells using CD34 selection does not improve overall or progression-free survival after high-dose chemotherapy for multiple myeloma: results of a multicenter randomized controlled trial. J Clin Oncol 19:3771–3779
74. Stiff PJ, Murgo AJ, Wittes RE, DeRisi MF, Clarkson BD (1983) Quantification of the peripheral blood colony forming unit-culture rise following chemotherapy. Could leukocytaphereses replace bone marrow for autologous transplantation? Transfusion 23:500–503
75. Szczepek AJ, Bergsagel PL, Axelsson L, Brown CB, Belch AR, Pilarski LM (1997) CD34+ cells in the blood of patients with multiple myeloma express CD19 and IgH mRNA and have patient-specific IgH VDJ gene rearrangements. Blood 89:1824–1833
76. Tricot G, Cottler-Fox MH, Calandra G (2010) Safety and efficacy assessment of plerixafor in patients with multiple myeloma proven or predicted to be poor mobilizers, including assessment of tumor cell mobilization. Bone Marrow Transplant 45:63–68
77. Vescio RA, Hong CH, Cao J, Kim A, Schiller GJ, Lichtenstein AK, Berenson RJ, Berenson JR (1994) The hematopoietic stem cell antigen, CD34, is not expressed on the malignant cells in multiple myeloma. Blood 84:3283–3290
78. Vogel W, Kopp HG, Kanz L, Einsele H (2005) Myeloma cell contamination of peripheral blood stem-cell grafts can predict the outcome in multiple myeloma patients after high-dose chemotherapy and autologous stem-cell transplantation. J Cancer Res Clin Oncol 131:214–218
79. Vose JM, Sharp G, Chan WC, Nichols C, Loh K, Inwards D, Rifkin R, Bierman PJ, Lynch JC, Weisenburger DD, Kessinger A, Armitage JO (2002) Autologous transplantation for aggressive non-Hodgkin's lymphoma: results of a randomized trial evaluating graft source and minimal residual disease. J Clin Oncol 20:2344–2352
80. Vose J, Bierman P, Loberiza F, Lynch J, Bociek G, Weisenburger D, Armitage J (2008) Long-term outcomes of autologous stem cell transplantation for follicular non-Hodgkin lymphoma: effect of histological grade and Follicular International Prognostic Index. Biol Blood Marrow Transplant 14:36–42
81. Williams CD, Goldstone AH, Pearce RM, Philip T, Hartmann O, Colombat P, Santini G, Foulard L, Gorin NC (1996) Purging of bone marrow in autologous bone marrow transplantation for non-Hodgkin's lymphoma: a case-matched comparison with unpurged cases by the European Blood and Marrow Transplant Lymphoma Registry. J Clin Oncol 14:2454–2464
82. Wu GQ, Sharp JG, Wu G, Vose J, Greiner TC, Chan WC (1997) The detection of minimal lymphoma by molecular and combined culture-molecular methods. Br J Haematol 99:873–881
83. Yunis JJ, Oken MM, Kaplan ME, Ensrud KM, Howe RR, Theologides A (1982) Distinctive chromosomal abnormalities in histologic subtypes of non-Hodgkin's lymphoma. N Engl J Med 307:1231–1236
84. Zelenetz AD, Chu G, Galili N, Bangs CD, Horning SJ, Donlon TA, Cleary ML, Levy R (1991) Enhanced detection of the t(14;18) translocation in malignant lymphoma using pulsed-field gel electrophoresis. Blood 78:1552–1560
85. Zeng Z, Samudio IJ, Munsell M, An J, Huang Z, Estey E, Andreeff M, Konopleva M (2006) Inhibition of CXCR4 with the novel RCP168 peptide overcomes stroma-mediated chemoresistance in chronic and acute leukemias. Mol Cancer Ther 5:3113–3121
86. Zeng Z, Shi YX, Samudio IJ, Wang RY, Ling X, Frolova O, Levis M, Rubin JB, Negrin RR, Estey EH, Konoplev S, Andreeff M, Konopleva M (2009) Targeting the leukemia microenvironment by CXCR4 inhibition overcomes resistance to kinase inhibitors and chemotherapy in AML. Blood 113:6215–6224
87. Zhou P, Zhang Y, Martinez C, Kalakonda N, Nimer SD, Comenzo RL (2003) Melphalan-mobilized blood stem cell components contain minimal clonotypic myeloma cell contamination. Blood 102:477–479

Chapter 11
Plerixafor: Data from the Compassionate Use Program

Maximilian M. Fresen and Kai Hübel

Introduction

High-dose chemotherapy followed by autologous stem cell transplantation (SCT) represents the standard of care in relapsed or refractory Hodgkin's lymphoma (HD) and non-Hodgkin's lymphoma (NHL). It is also an important therapeutic step in the therapy of multiple myeloma (MM) to improve progression-free survival. Application of high-dose chemotherapy is depending on the collection of a sufficient amount of $CD34^+$ stem cells. Most investigators describe a minimum harvest of 2.0×10^6 $CD34^+$ cells/kg bodyweight (BW) for patients with lymphoma and of 4.0×10^6 cells/kg BW for patients with MM undergoing tandem transplantation. Unfortunately, up to 45% of patients fail to mobilize the minimum amount for this important therapeutic approach, being considered as "poor mobilizers" [1–5]. Factors predisposing poor mobilization are age >60 years, progressive disease, severe bone marrow involvement, previous chemo- and/or radiotherapy, type of chemotherapy, previously failed mobilization attempts, platelet counts $<100 \times 10^9$/L prior to apheresis, and the development of neutropenic fever during mobilization [3, 6–10]. Usually hematopoietic growth factors (HGFs) like granulocyte colony-stimulating factor (G-CSF), granulocyte–macrophage colony-stimulating factor (GM-CSF), or stem cell factor (SCF) alone or combined with various chemotherapy regimens (chemomobilization) are used for mobilization. Application of chemotherapeutic agents alone is also possible to mobilize stem cells into peripheral blood. Although there are many combinations of chemotherapy regimens with or without HGF, as well as HGF alone, the ideal mobilization regimen still needs to be identified. Observation of leukocytosis in HIV-positive patients treated with the CXCR4-inhibitor plerixafor (formerly known as "AMD3100") led to discovery of the anchor mechanism of bone marrow

M.M. Fresen • K. Hübel (✉)
Internal Medicine, University Clinic Köln, Köln 50937, Germany
e-mail: kai.hubel@uni-koeln.de

S. Fruehauf et al. (eds.), *Novel Developments in Stem Cell Mobilization: Focus on CXCR4*, DOI 10.1007/978-1-4614-1960-0_11,

stromal cells expressing stromal cell derived factor 1 alpha (SDF-1α) and its cognate receptor CXCR4 on $CD34^+$ stem cells. Thus, plerixafor represents the first substance of a new class of mobilization agents which offers a chance for patients who failed previous mobilization attempts. In a clinical phase I trial, Liles et al. [11] showed that a single dose of 240 μg/kg BW of plerixafor was more effective than a 5-day treatment with G-CSF. Two large blinded, placebo-controlled, randomized phase III trials included patients who are most reliant on successful mobilization and autologous SCT, i.e. patients with NHL and MM [12, 13]. Both trials showed significant advantages in the plerixafor group compared to the placebo group concerning the primary endpoint of yielding $>5\times10^6$ $CD34^+$ cells/kg body weight (BW) in patients with NHL and $>6\times10^6$ $CD34^+$ cells/kg BW in patients with MM. The percentage of patients who successfully met the primary endpoint was significantly higher in the plerixafor group than in the placebo group: 59 versus 20% in patients with NHL and 71.6 versus 34.4% in patients with MM, respectively. These trials for the novel CXCR4-inhibitor plerixafor excluded patients who failed prior conventional mobilization. However, these transplant candidates were in need of novel mobilization regimens and strategies allowing them to proceed to the life-saving therapeutic approach of autologous SCT.

Before approval by the US Food and Drug Association (FDA) in December 2008 and by the European Medicines Evaluation Agency (EMEA) in July 2009, a named-patient compassionate use program (CUP) opened in Europe in July 2008. The CUP granted access to the drug for patients diagnosed with lymphoma and multiple myeloma who failed to mobilize sufficient numbers of PBSC with conventional mobilization attempts and were not eligible for plerixafor registration trials. In 13 countries, physicians took the opportunity of enrolling the hard-to-mobilize patients into the CUP. Plerixafor (Mozobil®) was contributed by Genzyme, Naarden, The Netherlands after registration of the patients. Beside the mobilization outcome, data from the CUPs were also used to identify side effects.

The Protocol

In the final version of the CUP protocol from July 2008, the inclusion and exclusion criteria as well as the operational sequences for G-CSF and plerixafor administration were as follows:

Inclusion Criteria

1. Age from 18 to 78 years.
2. Eligible to undergo autologous hematopoietic SCT.
3. Patient has failed previous conventional therapies for hematopoietic stem cell collection, or based upon a low peripheral blood $CD34^+$ cell count following

conventional therapy is not considered by the physician to have a reasonable chance of collecting enough cells.

4. Adequate pulmonary, cardiac, and renal functions sufficient to undergo apheresis process and transplantation.
5. Eastern Cooperatice Oncology Group (ECOG) performance status 0 or 1.
6. White blood cell count (WBC) $>2.5 \times 10^9/L$.
7. Absolute neutrophil count (ANC) $>1.5 \times 10^9/L$.
8. Platelet count $>85 \times 10^9/L$.
9. Serum creatinine ≤ 1.5 mg/dL.
10. Serum aspartate aminotransferase (AST/GOT), serum alanine aminotransferase (ALT/GPT), and total bilirubine <2× upper limit of normal (ULN).
11. No active infection of hepatitis B or C.
12. Signed informed consent.
13. Women of child-bearing potential or female partners of male patients agree to use an approved form of contraception.
14. Center carrying out mobilization and apheresis must also store the product and carry out the autologous transplantation.

Exclusion Criteria

1. Diagnosis of any acute or chronic leukemia (including plasma cell leukemia) or myelodysplastic syndrome (the blood of patients with MM had to be microscopically evaluated 24 h prior to the first dose of plerixafor for the presence of blasts or plasma cells).
2. A co-morbid condition which, in the view of the treating physician, renders the patient to a high risk from treatment complications.
3. Vasculitis or autoimmune disease.
4. Brain metastasis or carcinomatous meningitis or any other malignancy unless the patient has been disease-free for at least 5 years following curative intent therapy.
   Exceptions: patients with the following diagnosis will not be excluded.
   - Patients with treated nonmelanoma skin cancer, in situ carcinoma, or cervical intraepithelial neoplasia, regardless of the disease-free duration, if definitive treatment for the condition has been completed.
   - Patients with organ-confined prostate cancer without evidence of recurrent or progressive disease based on prostate-specific antigen (PSA) values if hormonal therapy has been initiated or a radical prostatectomy has been performed.
5. Clinical significant heart disease, e.g., indicated by ECG or other study results suggestive of previously undiagnosed cardiac ischemia or a history of clinically significant rhythm disturbance (arrhythmias), or other conduction abnormality in the last year.

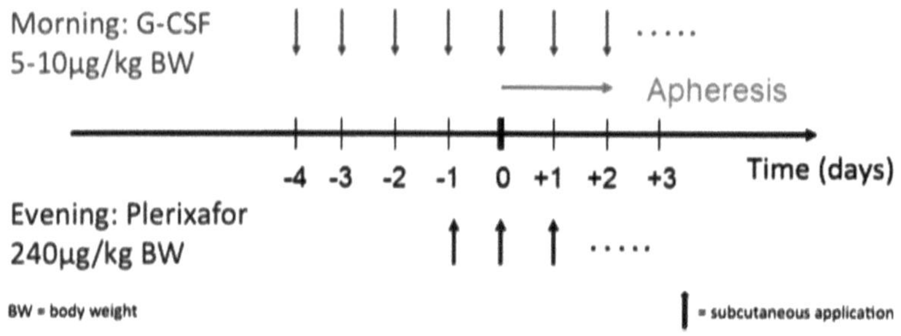

Fig. 11.1 Sequence of G-CSF and plerixafor administration

6. Acute infection and/or fever (temperature >38°C).
7. Hypercalcemia (>1 mg/dL above the ULN).
8. Pregnant or breastfeeding women.
9. Patients of child-bearing potential unwilling to implement adequate birth control.
10. Patients known to be HIV positive.
11. Obese patients exceeding 175% of ideal body weight.
12. Patients receiving experimental treatment during mobilization.

Time Schedule of Mobilization and Treatment Phase

First, patients received a mobilization regimen of nonpegylated G-CSF according to the local practice guidelines. A dosage of 10 μg/kg BW G-CSF had to be administered in the morning for 4 days before a subcutaneous dose of 240 μg/kg BW of plerixafor was given into the abdominal region in the evening of the fourth day 10–11 h prior to apheresis. After administration by a nurse or physician, the patient had to be observed for 60 min for adverse events. At least 1 h before apheresis procedure was started on day 5, another dose of G-CSF was given.

The steps of plerixafor application in the evening and G-CSF application in the morning followed by apheresis were repeated until the required amount of cells was reached (see Fig. 11.1). Processed blood volume was determined according to local practice guidelines.

According to preferences of the transplant center, the combination of G-CSF, chemotherapy, and plerixafor was also feasible.

After patients received high-dose therapy and consecutive autologous SCT, engraftment of neutrophiles and platelets had to be monitored. Patients' relapse, progressive disease, or progression-free survival was also monitored when available.

Results

Patients Collective

Hospitals and health care institutes of 13 European countries took part in Genzyme's Plerixafor CUP. Patients from Austria, Belgium, Croatia, Czech Republic, France, Germany, Hungary, Italy, Poland, Portugal, Slovakia, Spain, and UK were enrolled. The inclusion and exclusion criteria granted access to plerixafor for patients who may benefit from autologous SCT; therefore, patients diagnosed with NHL, MM, Hodgkin's lymphoma (HD) were included as well as patients diagnosed with other malignant and nonmalignant diseases. These patients had seminoma, Ewing sarcoma, germ cell tumors, testicular, and thyroidal cancer. Children with Wiskott–Aldrich syndrome (WAS) and neuroblastoma were enrolled in the German CUP.

A total of 707 patients—389 males and 318 females—were included. Three hundred and twenty-eight patients were diagnosed with NHL, 279 with MM, 70 with HD, and 30 patients were included in the group of other diseases. For patients' characteristics, see Table 11.1.

Patients Diagnosed with Non-Hodgkin's Lymphoma

Three hundred and twenty-eight patients (173 males and 155 females) diagnosed with NHL were enrolled in the European CUPs. The median age was 58 years (range 13–81 years). The median weight was 72.45 kg (range 41.5–130 kg), and patients had received a median of two prior chemotherapy regimens (range 0–10). Although primarily patients who failed a previous conventional mobilization regimen were included, patients were also eligible if they were suspected of being unable to gather a sufficient amount of $CD34^+$ cells in advance. So the median of previous mobilization regimen was 1 with a range from 0 up to a remarkable number of 7 failed mobilization attempts. For conventional mobilization treatment, chemotherapy alone or combined with G-CSF was used as well as G-CSF alone or in combination with SCF.

In a median of two apheresis sessions (range 1–5), patients yielded a median of 2.485×10^6 $CD34^+$ cells/kg BW (range 0–17.37). A total of 197 patients (60%) gathered the defined mininum of 2.0×10^6 $CD34^+$ cells/kg BW and 76 of them (39.6%) needed only a single apheresis session. One hundred and seventy-one patients (52.1%) proceeded to high-dose chemotherapy and underwent autologous SCT. Thirty-three patients (10.1%) reached the primary endpoint of the plerixafor phase III registration trial and yielded more than 5.0×10^6 $CD34^+$ cells/kg BW. There were no differences in stem cell harvest regarding prior mobilization attempts or prior chemotherapeutic regimens.

Table 11.1 Patients' characteristics and results

	NHL	MM	HD	Others	Total
Patients (*n*)	328	279	70	30	707
Age (years)					
Median	58	60	37	26	58
Range (min, max)	(13, 81)	(28, 76)	(19, 76)	(2, 70)	(2, 81)
Sex (*n*)					
Female	155	116	37	10	318
Male	173	163	33	20	389
Weight (kg)					
Median	72.45	75	77	54.5	74
Range (min, max)	(41.5, 130)	(47, 120)	(48, 120)	(14, 92)	(14, 130)
Prior lines of treatment (n)					
Median (range)	2 (0, 10)	2 (0, 10)	3 (0, 5)	2 (0, 12)	2 (0, 12)
Radiation pretreatment (%)	41 (12.5%)	49 (17.6%)	19 (27.1%)	6 (20%)	115 (16.3%)
Previous failed mobilizations (n)					
Median	1	1	1	1	1
Range (min, max)	(0, 7)	(0, 3)	(1, 3)	(1, 2)	(0, 7)
Apheresis sessions (n)					
Median	2	2	2	2	2
Range (min, max)	(1, 5)	(1, 5)	(1, 4)	(1, 4)	(1, 5)
Yield ($\times 10^6$ $CD34^+$ cells/kg BW)					
Median	2.485	3.63	3.04	4.32	3.1
Range (min, max)	(0, 17.37)	(0, 32.6)	(0, 8.62)	(0, 29.32)	(0, 32.6)
$n > 5.0 \times 10^6$ (%)	33 (10.1%)	83 (29.7%)	12 (17.1%)	12 (40%)	140 (19.8%)
$n > 2.0 \times 10^6$ (%)	197 (60.1%)	216 (77.4%)	45 (64.3%)	21 (70%)	479 (67.8%)
Engraftment of platelets (days)					
Median	15	14	14.5	12.5	14
Range (min, max)	(8, 79)	(9, 191)	(2, 36)	(10, 30)	(2, 191)

Patients' platelet counts recovered after a median of 15 days within a range of 8 and 79 days after re-infusion of hematopoietic stem cells.

Patients Diagnosed with Multiple Myeloma

A total of 279 patients diagnosed with MM were enrolled. One hundred and sixty-three men and 116 women with a median age of 60 (range of 28 up to an age of 76 years) received plerixafor. All MM patients had a median weight of 75 kg (range 47–120 kg), had received a median of two prior lines of treatment, and had failed a median of one prior conventional mobilization attempt (range 0–3). As in the group of patients diagnosed with NHL, MM patients without prior mobilization attempts were included. One 59-year-old man had already been treated with ten different chemotherapy regimens. For conventional mobilization treatment, G-CSF with or without chemotherapy was used. No SCF was used.

In the group of MM patients, a median cell count of 3.63×10^6 $CD34^+$ cells/kg BW (range 0–32.6) has been yielded in a median of two apheresis sessions (range 1–5). A total of 216 patients (77.4%) gathered the defined minimum of 2.0×10^6 $CD34^+$ cells/kg BW. Fifty percent of those (108/216) needed only one apheresis session. Eighty-three patients (29.7%) yielded more than 5.0×10^6 $CD34^+$ cells/kg BW.

A total of 210 patients (75.3%) with MM proceeded to high-dose chemotherapy and underwent autologous SCT. Platelet recovery was observed after a median of 14 days (range 9–191 days).

Patients Diagnosed with Hodgkin's Lymphoma

Seventy patients diagnosed with HD were enrolled in the CUP. Thirty-three male and 37 female patients with a median weight of 77 kg (range 48–120) got access to plerixafor. As expected, patients with HD were younger than patients diagnosed with NHL or MM. The median age was 37 years (range 19–76). Although patients diagnosed with HD had a higher median amount of three prior lines of treatment than NHL and HD patients, the maximum of previous chemotherapy regimen was with a value of 5 lower than in the other groups. Like in the other two groups, HD patients had failed a median of one previous conventional mobilization attempt (range 1–3). For conventional mobilization treatment, chemotherapy alone or combined with G-CSF was used as well as G-CSF alone or in combination with SCF.

After receiving the mobilization regimen in the CUP, HD patients yielded a median of 3.04×10^6 $CD34^+$ cells/kg BW (range 0–8.62) in a median of two apheresis sessions (range 1–4).

A total of 45 patients (64.3%) yielded the defined minimum of 2.0×10^6 $CD34^+$ cells/kg BW and 20 of them (44.4%) gathered enough cells even during the first apheresis session. Thirty-nine patients (86.7%) proceeded to high-dose chemotherapy and autologous SCT. Platelet recovery could be observed after a median of 14.5 days (range 2–36) after re-infusion of hematopoietic stem cells.

Patients with Other Malignant and Nonmalignant Diseases

This group of patients is definitely the most heterogeneous because of the many different entities of enrolled diseases. The opening of the CUP for these patients was possible due to the inclusion criteria, allowing plerixafor in patients who failed a conventional mobilization treatment independent of underlying disease. Thus, if the application of high-dose chemotherapy was considered as being a therapeutic approach, but insufficient $CD34^+$ cell yield prevented therapeutic progress, enrollment into the CUP was possible (except for leukemias or MDS). Thirty patients were enrolled, among them patients diagnosed with Ewing sarcoma, germ cell tumors, medulloblastoma and neuroblastoma, composite carcinoma, semoma and nonseminomatous testicular cancer, thyroid and ovarian cancer. In addition, patients with nonmalignant diseases like WAS, systemic amyloidosis and one patient with Evans syndrome—a combination of autoimmune hemolytic anemia and idiopathic thrombocytopenic purpura [14] were included.

Patients in this group had a median age of 26 years with a range from 2 up to 70 years and were even younger than HD patients because of the enrollment of 11 minors—5 diagnosed with WAS, 3 with Ewing sarcoma, 2 with neuroblastoma, and 1 with medulloblastoma. The median weight was 54.5 kg (range 14–92). Patients had received a median of two prior lines of treatment (range 0–12) and failed a median of one previous conventional mobilization regimen (range 1–2). As a matter of course, children with WAS had received no prior chemotherapy. The patient with thyroidal cancer had only received radioiodine therapy. As in the group of MM patients, G-CSF with or without chemotherapy was used. No SCF was used for prior conventional mobilization.

All 30 patients yielded a median of 4.32×10^6 $CD34^+$ cells/kg BW (range 0–29.32) in a median of two apheresis sessions (range 1–4). Although 21 patients (70.0%) gathered the defined minimum of 2.0×10^6 $CD34^+$ cells/kg BW, only 16 patients (53.3%) proceeded to high-dose chemotherapy and autologous SCT. The best mobilization result with the highest yield of 29.32×10^6 $CD34^+$ cells/kg BW was achieved by a 2-year-old boy diagnosed with WAS and a weight of 14 kg.

After transplantation, recovery of platelets could be observed after a median of 12.5 days (range 10–30 days).

Result Overview and Selected Cases

Based on the promising results of phase III trials, the plerixafor CUP was started in 13 European countries, allowing access to plerixafor before approval by the authorities. A total of 707 patients with a median age of 58 (range 2–81) were enrolled yielding a median of 3.1×10^6 $CD34^+$ cells/kg BW (range 0–32.6). In contrast to the phase III trials, patients with HD and other malignant as well as nonmalignant diseases were included. Thus, the CUP provided an insight to mobilization of patients who are in the need of a sufficient cell yield but belong to a group with bad preconditions, resembling the hard-to-mobilize patient. The best yield of 32.6×10^6 $CD34^+$ cells was achieved by a 40-year-old male patient from Portugal diagnosed with multiple myeloma. This patient had received one conventional mobilization regimen with chemotherapy and G-CSF. After two apheresis sessions, he collected 2.6×10^6 $CD34^+$ cells/kg BW, so he had a high risk of failing the desired yield for tandem transplantation. After one boost by plerixafor, the third apheresis added 30×10^6 $CD34^+$ cells/kg BW, allowing both receiving high-dose therapy and a fast engraftment.

Another important insight from the CUP was given by patients who were treated aberrantly from the protocol. In the German CUP, nine patients (four NHL, three MM, one composite lymphoma, and one CLL/NHL) received plerixafor without G-CSF or with G-CSF for less than 4 days. Seven of them (77.8%) gathered more than 2.0×10^6 $CD34^+$ cells/kg BW. The median cell yield was 3.3×10^6 $CD34^+$ cells/kg BW (range 1.6–8.7). The best result in this small group of patients was also achieved by a patient diagnosed with MM. These results underline not only the finding by Liles et al. [11] that a dose of plerixafor is more effective than a 5-day treatment of G-CSF, but also showed the effectiveness of plerixafor as single therapy.

Plerixafor in Children

Some malignant as well as nonmalignant diseases have a higher prevalence in children or young adults. Originally considered to be a glioma, medulloblastoma is known to be of the family of cranial primitive neuroectodermal tumors (PNET) and represents the most common malignant brain tumor in childhood (James G. Gurney, Malcolm A. Smith, Greta R. Bunin, CNS and Miscellaneous Intracranial and Intraspinal Neoplasms, SEER Pediatric Monograph, National Cancer Institute). Although a common genetic locus is responsible for a large percentage of PNET and Ewing sarcoma [15], the diseases are considered of being different. While Ewing sarcomas are most commonly related to bone, PNET are generally not. Ewing sarcomas occur typically in adolescents aged from 15 to 19 years and are often treated with multidrug chemotherapy as well as local disease control with surgery and radiation [16]. Neuroblastoma is the third most common malignant neoplasia in childhood. Like Ewing sarcomas and PNET, high-risk neuroblastoma is usually treated with intensive chemotherapy, surgery, radiation therapy, and hematopoietic SCT [17]. In these different entities, high-dose chemotherapy is frequently indicated; therefore, successful stem cell mobilization and harvest are required.

Due to the fact that clinical trials in pediatric population are hard to perform, only few data concerning plerixafor use in children exist. In the CUP, 11 children and young adults were included (3 Ewing sarcoma, 1 medulloblastoma, 2 neuroblastoma, and 5 WAS). Enrolled patients had a median age of 5 years (range 2–17) and a median weight of 18 kg (range 14–72). Children diagnosed with WAS had never received prior chemotherapy and had only failed one prior steady-state mobilization. Following the protocol's plerixafor administration scheme, seven patients (63.6%) gathered the defined minimum of $CD34^+$ cells and yielded a median of 9.69×10^6 $CD34^+$ cells/kg BW (range 1.49–29.53). Mobilization success was not associated with underlying disease—two patients with Ewing sarcoma, one patient with WAS, and another with neuroblastoma failed to gather enough cells.

Plerixafor in a Patient with Impaired Renal Function

In the German CUP, a 44-year-old female patient diagnosed with IgG lambda MM (Durie and Salmon stage IIIb, first diagnosed in April 2008) was enrolled. The patient developed an impaired renal function with a nephritic syndrome due to Bence-Jones proteinuria requiring dialysis. In medical history, she was also diagnosed with a long-QT syndrome and dilatative cardiomyopathy with global impaired cardiac function. The patient had received three different chemotherapy regimens prior to mobilization: three cycles of vincristine, adriamycin, dexamethasone (VAD) followed by bortezomib, dexamethasone, and lenalidomide, and three cycles of bortezomib and dexamethasone. Due to the diagnosis of dilatative cardiomyopathy in November 2008, steady-state mobilization seems reasonable. Before the start of plerixafor, creatinine was elevated at a level of 4.32 mg/dL (380.16 μM). Following the first shot of plerixafor, it increased to 7.95 mg/dL. Neutrophile granulocytes were elevated at $38.93 \times 10^9/\mu L$ when apheresis procedure was started. On the second day, neutrophiles were elevated at $55.08 \times 10^9/\mu L$. After two apheresis sessions, a total of 5.98×10^6 $CD34^+$ cells/kg BW could be yielded allowing tandem transplantation.

After improvement of the cardiomyopathy, the patient received high-dose chemotherapy with melphalan followed by autologous SCT (2.72×10^6 $CD34^+$ cells/kg BW) in 2009. Neutrophiles recovered after 10 days and thrombocytes after 14 days.

In November 2009, the patient successfully received a donor kidney and was still alive in March 2011.

Plerixafor in Germ Cell Tumor Patients

In the group of other malignant and nonmalignant diseases, six male patients were enrolled in the CUP. Five patients were diagnosed with nonseminomatous germ cell tumors and one had seminoma. The median age was 49 years (range 27–62). All patients had at least stage IIc according to the AJCC classification and had experienced a relapse after a median of 3.5 prior therapies (range 1–6). All patients had received pretreatment with at least one platinum compound, an alkylating agent and etoposide. Prior (failed) mobilization regimens consisted of daily doses of G-CSF combined with chemotherapy. Chemotherapy regimens for mobilization were cisplatinum, ifosphamide, paclitaxel (TIP) in three cases, cisplatinum, etoposide, and ifosphamide (PEI), cisplatinum and ifosphamide (CI), and paclitaxel with ifosphamide (PI). For re-mobilization, five patients received chemomobilization with TIP (three cases), PEI, and PI; one patient attempted steady-state mobilization.

After a median of four apheresis sessions (range 2–6), patients gathered a median of 2.6×10^6 $CD34^+$ cells/kg BW (range 1.9–24.79). Four patients (66.6%) succeeded in yielding a sufficient amount of $CD34^+$ cells to proceed to high-dose chemotherapy. One patient did not reach the threshold by collecting only 1.9×10^6 $CD34^+$ cells/kg BW. In one patient, no apheresis procedure was started due to an insufficient value of $CD34^+$ cells in peripheral blood. No drug related side effects were reported.

Three of four patients with a sufficient amount of $CD34^+$ cells proceeded to high-dose chemotherapy. One patient was not transplanted due to progressive disease before high-dose therapy. After transplantation, recovery of neutrophiles was observed after a median of 10.33 days (range 8–12). Platelet recovery (defined as platelets >20/nL) was monitored after a median of 12.5 days (range 12–13). One patient did not experience platelet recovery.

The data published by Kobold et al. [18] suggest a safe and effective use of plerixafor in germ cell tumor patients. Even in heavily pretreated patients—one had 19 platinum-containing cycles of chemotherapy in medical history—plerixafor was able to allow collection of a sufficient amount of $CD34^+$ cells to undergo high-dose chemotherapy.

Plerixafor in an Elderly Patient

Age >60 years and bone marrow involvement are generally accepted criteria predisposing mobilization failure. As a logical consequence, elderly patients were enrolled in the CUP. Here, we describe the mobilization of a 68-year-old male patient diagnosed with follicular lymphoma (NHL) stage IVb with bone marrow infiltration in July 2006. The patient had received a pre-phase therapy with vincristine and prednisone followed by eight cycles of R-CHOP. He also received radiation with 45 Gy and reached a good partial remission in April 2007. When he was diagnosed with a first relapse, he was treated with six cycles of bendamustine and rituximab (BR). Re-staging CT scans revealed a mixed response in August 2008, so the patient received rituximab monthly. In March 2009, he was diagnosed with a second relapse and R-DHAP was chosen with a mobilization attempt out of the second cycle. Because of hearing impairment, cisplatinum had to be substituted by carboplatinum. From April to May 2009, the second cycle of R-DHAP was given. Plerixafor was administrated on two consecutive days and the patient was able to collect a total of 8.7×10^6 $CD34^+$ cells/kg BW. In August 2009, high-dose therapy with ibritumomab tiuxetan and rituximab followed by carmustine, etoposide, cytarabine, and melphalan (Z-BEAM) was administrated. All collected $CD34^+$ cells were re-infused. Recovery of the WBC was monitored on day 8. On day 12, platelet was recorded. In this case, plerixafor was used for the first mobilization attempt because of two factors predisposing mobilization failure.

Safety Profile of Plerixafor

In the MM registration trial of plerixafor, patients of the study and the control group experienced the same rate of adverse events (AEs): 140 of 147 (95.2%) in the plerixafor group and 140 of 151 (97.2%) in the placebo group had at least one AE. Most of these events were mild to moderate, and the most common AEs considered related to plerixafor administration were GI disorders and injection site reactions. Although during the study 57 of 147 patients (38.8%) in the interventional group and 48 of 151 patients (31.8%) in the placebo group had at least one severe AE, the majority of these events was considered not to be related to study treatment [13].

In the MM patients' registration trial, 95 AEs in 147 patients of the intervention group were registered. The most common was GI disorder, which occurred in 59 patients (40.1%) in the intervention group and 23 patients (15.2%) in the placebo group. Other monitored side effects were general disorders (fatigue) and injection site erythema which occurred in 42 patients (28.6%) in the plerixafor group. Fourteen patients had bone pain (9.5%) and 19 patients suffered from headache or paraesthesia (12.9%).

Similar results were observed in the registration trial in NHL patients. Both groups experienced the same rate of AEs: 146 of 150 (97.3%) patients in the plerixafor group and 138 of 145 (95.2%) patients in the placebo group experienced at least one AE. Most AEs were mild to moderate.

In this registration trial, the most common side effects were also GI disorders and injection site reactions. Three patients were identified, who experienced severe AEs that were related to study medication: in the plerixafor group one patient had hypotension and dizziness after study drug administration and another patient had thrombocytopenia after apheresis. In the placebo group, one patient suffered from nonischemia chest pain.

A total of 98 AEs in 150 patients (65.3%) of the intervention group were registered. As in the MM registration trial, the most common AE was GI disorders. Other occurred AEs included injection erythema and pruritus, bone pain, headache, and paresthesia [12].

Like in the registration trials, all AEs and severe AEs during the CUP were recorded from the time of first plerixafor injection. The severity of AEs and severe AEs were assessed in the categories mild, moderate, and severe, as well as being related or unrelated to plerixafor administration, according to the physician's judgment. All serious related AEs were reported to Genzyme Pharmacovigilance Europe.

Similar to the registration trials, diarrhea, flatulence, and gut discomfort were the most common side effects in the Spanish and British CUP, occurring in 34% of enrolled patients (19/56). Other monitored AEs were injection site reactions in ten patients (18%), bone pain in two patients (4%), hot flushing in two patients (4%), and other toxicities in nine patients (16%). No severe AEs were monitored [19].

In the German CUP with 60 enrolled patients, exhaustion and GI disorders were the most common side effects observed in three cases (5%) each. Dyspnea, balance disorders, hypotension, blood pressure increase, sweating, general pain, and nausea occurred in one case each (1.7%). All observed AEs were mild and manageable [20].

Conclusion

Data from the CUP suggested plerixafor as a valuable additive in patients with NHL, MM, and HD who failed prior mobilization attempts as well as in patients with generally accepted risk factors, who tend to fail a regular mobilization attempt. CUP data also brought first experience of a new drug in children, germ cell tumor patients, as well as in a lot of entities not regarded in former trials. Some patients included in the CUP were treated aberrantly from the protocol and received plerixafor after G-CSF administration for less than 4 days or even without G-CSF. Stem cell collection in those patients was as successful as in patients who received G-CSF for 4 days before plerixafor administration emphasizing the effect of the drug on stem cell mobilization.

Compared to mobilization regimens containing chemotherapy, plerixafor provides an increased predictability of stem cell yield and timing without risks of chemotherapy administration like infectious complications or agent-specific adverse events. In re-mobilization, plerixafor and G-CSF also appear to be superior to other previously described alternative re-mobilization regimens, including higher doses of G-CSF, combinations of G-CSF with other growth factors, as well as a number of chemotherapy regimens combined with growth factors [6, 21–25]. With a favorable safety profile and a remarkable effect on mobilization outcome, plerixafor resembles a valuable additive in patients in the need of high-dose chemotherapy with stem cell salvage. This approach permits saving medical resources by less mobilization attempts and the treatment of their complications.

References

1. Kessinger A, Sharp JG (2003) The whys and hows of hematopoietic progenitor and stem cell mobilization. Bone Marrow Transplant 31(5):319–329
2. Koenigsmann M et al (2004) The role of diagnosis in patients failing peripheral blood progenitor cell mobilization. Transfusion 44(5):777–784
3. Mendrone A Jr et al (2008) Factors affecting hematopoietic progenitor cell mobilization: an analysis of 307 patients. Transfus Apher Sci 39(3):187–192
4. Moog R (2008) Management strategies for poor peripheral blood stem cell mobilization. Transfus Apher Sci 38(3):229–236
5. Pastore D et al (2004) Good and poor CD34+ cells mobilization in acute leukemia: analysis of factors affecting the yield of progenitor cells. Bone Marrow Transplant 33(11):1083–1087
6. Pusic I et al (2008) Impact of mobilization and remobilization strategies on achieving sufficient stem cell yields for autologous transplantation. Biol Blood Marrow Transplant 14(9):1045–1056
7. Kuittinen T et al (2004) Prediction of mobilisation failure in patients with non-Hodgkin's lymphoma. Bone Marrow Transplant 33(9):907–912
8. Pavone V et al (2006) Poor mobilization is an independent prognostic factor in patients with malignant lymphomas treated by peripheral blood stem cell transplantation. Bone Marrow Transplant 37(8):719–724
9. Akhtar S et al (2008) Factors affecting autologous peripheral blood stem cell collection in patients with relapsed or refractory diffuse large cell lymphoma and Hodgkin lymphoma: a single institution result of 168 patients. Leuk Lymphoma 49(4):769–778
10. Wuchter P et al (2010) Poor mobilization of hematopoietic stem cells-definitions, incidence, risk factors, and impact on outcome of autologous transplantation. Biol Blood Marrow Transplant 16(4):490–499
11. Liles WC et al (2005) Augmented mobilization and collection of CD34+ hematopoietic cells from normal human volunteers stimulated with granulocyte-colony-stimulating factor by single-dose administration of AMD3100, a CXCR4 antagonist. Transfusion 45(3):295–300
12. DiPersio JF et al (2009) Phase III prospective randomized double-blind placebo-controlled trial of plerixafor plus granulocyte colony-stimulating factor compared with placebo plus granulocyte colony-stimulating factor for autologous stem-cell mobilization and transplantation for patients with non-Hodgkin's lymphoma. J Clin Oncol 27(28):4767–4773

13. DiPersio JF et al (2009) Plerixafor and G-CSF versus placebo and G-CSF to mobilize hematopoietic stem cells for autologous stem cell transplantation in patients with multiple myeloma. Blood 113(23):5720–5726
14. Evans RS et al (1951) Primary thrombocytopenic purpura and acquired hemolytic anemia; evidence for a common etiology. AMA Arch Intern Med 87(1):48–65
15. Iwamoto Y (2007) Diagnosis and treatment of Ewing's sarcoma. Jpn J Clin Oncol 37(2):79–89
16. Lahl M, Fisher VL, Laschinger K (2008) Ewing's sarcoma family of tumors: an overview from diagnosis to survivorship. Clin J Oncol Nurs 12(1):89–97
17. Fish JD, Grupp SA (2008) Stem cell transplantation for neuroblastoma. Bone Marrow Transplant 41(2):159–165
18. Kobold S et al (2011) Plerixafor is effective and safe for stem cell mobilization in heavily pretreated germ cell tumor patients. Bone Marrow Transplant 46(8):1053–1056
19. Duarte RF et al (2011) Plerixafor plus granulocyte CSF can mobilize hematopoietic stem cells from multiple myeloma and lymphoma patients failing previous mobilization attempts: EU compassionate use data. Bone Marrow Transplant 46(1):52–58
20. Hubel K et al (2011) Plerixafor with and without chemotherapy in poor mobilizers: results from the German compassionate use program. Bone Marrow Transplant 46(8):1045–1052
21. Boeve S et al (2004) Analysis of remobilization success in patients undergoing autologous stem cell transplants who fail an initial mobilization: risk factors, cytokine use and cost. Bone Marrow Transplant 33(10):997–1003
22. Fraipont V et al (2000) Successful mobilization of peripheral blood HPCs with G-CSF alone in patients failing to achieve sufficient numbers of CD34+ cells and/or CFU-GM with chemotherapy and G-CSF. Transfusion 40(3):339–347
23. Goterris R et al (2005) Impact of different strategies of second-line stem cell harvest on the outcome of autologous transplantation in poor peripheral blood stem cell mobilizers. Bone Marrow Transplant 36(10):847–853
24. Weaver CH et al (1998) Second attempts at mobilization of peripheral blood stem cells in patients with initial low CD34+ cell yields. J Hematother 7(3):241–249
25. Lefrere F et al (2004) Successful peripheral blood stem cell harvesting with granulocyte colony-stimulating factor alone after previous mobilization failure. Haematologica 89(12): 1532–1534

Chapter 12
Stem Cell Mobilization with Chemomobilization Plus Plerixafor in Hard-to-Mobilize Patients: The Experience at Kuopio University Hospital, Finland

Esa Jantunen and Tapio Nousiainen

Abstract Mobilization of blood stem cells to support high-dose chemotherapy is difficult in a significant proportion of patients intended for autologous stem cell transplantation (ASCT). Depending on definitions, disease and previous therapy 5–30% of patients can be considered as hard-to-mobilize. Plerixafor is a novel drug mainly studied in combination with G-CSF mobilization although chemotherapy followed by G-CSF (chemomobilization) is still considered standard in many patients. We have evaluated addition of plerixafor to chemomobilization in patients who appear to mobilize poorly. Between 01.08.2009 and 31.12.2010 altogether 20 patients received plerixafor at our department. Two patients with non-Hodgkin's lymphoma (NHL) who had failed a previous chemomobilization were successfully remobilized with chemomobilization plus plerixafor. Eighteen patients (14 NHL, 3 multiple myeloma, 1 Hodgkin's lymphoma) received plerixafor either due to low blood CD34$^+$ (B-CD34$^+$) cell counts (median 3×10^6/L, range <1–12) ($n = 14$) or poor yield of the previous collections ($n = 4$). The median number of plerixafor injections in preemptive use was 1 (1–3). B-CD34$^+$ counts increased a median of fourfold (no change to 16-fold). Stem cell collections were started in 16 patients (89%). The median yield was 2.7×10^6/kg CD34$^+$ cells (1.6–6.4). The minimum collection target ($\geq 2 \times 10^6$/kg CD34$^+$ cells) was achieved in all myeloma patients and in 11/14 (79%) of NHL patients. Out of 20 patients mobilized with chemotherapy plus G-CSF plus plerixafor, 15 have received high-dose therapy with successful engraftment in all but

E. Jantunen (✉)
Department of Medicine, Kuopio University Hospital and University of Eastern Finland/Clinical Medicine, P.O.B. 1777, Kuopio 70211, Finland
e-mail: esa.jantunen@kuh.fi

T. Nousiainen
Department of Medicine, Kuopio University Hospital, P.O.B. 1777, Kuopio 70211, Finland

S. Fruehauf et al. (eds.), *Novel Developments in Stem Cell Mobilization: Focus on CXCR4*, DOI 10.1007/978-1-4614-1960-0_12,

one patient who had delayed platelet engraftment (6 months). Plerixafor added to chemomobilization is safe and efficient in the majority of patients but more studies in regard to optimal timing and dosage are needed.

Keywords Plerixafor • Poor mobilization • Preemptive use • Stem cells • Lymphoma • Myeloma • Apheresis

Introduction

A significant proportion of patients with lymphoid malignancies intended to high-dose therapy with autologous stem cell rescue (ASCT) are hard-to-mobilize with conventional mobilization regimens including chemotherapy followed by granulocyte colony-stimulating factor (G-CSF) (chemomobilization) or with G-CSF alone. Depending on patient characteristics and definitions, about 5–30% of the patients can be considered hard to mobilize [1, 13, 14], in some patient groups like chronic lymphocytic leukemia the proportion may be even higher [15] as well as—at least based on our limited personal experience—in patients with Waldenström's macroglobulinemia (unpublished). In general, myeloma patients are easier to mobilize with about 5% belonging to this category [22] but in patients with non-Hodgkin's lymphoma (NHL) and in patients with Hodgkin's lymphoma (HL), the proportion of hard-to-mobilize patients may be in the order of 20–25% [20, 22]. In a German series including more than 800 patients with MM or NHL, the proportion of patients failing to reach blood CD34⁺ cell counts of 10×10^6/L was 10.8% [25]. Patients who fail blood stem cell mobilization may need remobilization is bone marrow harvest which may delay ASCT with potentially negative patient outcomes and increased costs. In some instances, ASCT should be withheld completely as a treatment option.

Plerixafor is a small molecule that causes reversible and transient disruption of the interaction of chemokine receptor CXCR4 and stroma-derived growth factor 1 causing a rapid release of $CD34^+$ cells from marrow to circulation facilitating stem cell collection [21, 24]. In a phase II study, G-CSF plus plerixafor was superior to G-CSF alone to mobilize blood stem cells in lymphoma and myeloma patients [7]. In a compassionate use study for remobilization, success rate of G-CSF plus plerixafor ranged from 60 to 76% [2]. These studies were followed by two phase III studies in NHL [5] and myeloma patients [4] showing that the combination of G-CSF plus plerixafor was superior to G-CSF alone in terms of blood $CD34^+$ counts, achieving the collection target and resulting in efficient engraftment after high-dose therapy.

Chemomobilization is still a widely used mobilization strategy in both lymphoma and myeloma patients as it allows higher $CD34^+$ cell yields than mobilization with G-CSF alone [1] resulting in fewer apheresis sessions. It has also the additional benefit of antitumour efficacy, the importance of which is dependent on disease and disease status. As we have used chemomobilization in 99% of our patients mobilized at the hematology ward of Department of Medicine, Kuopio University Hospital, it was logical to evaluate the use of plerixafor also in this context when the drug came available for clinical use in 2009 in Europe. In the following we discuss our experiences in preemptive use of plerixafor in chemomobilized patients who have either failed a previous mobilization and more recently in patients who appear to mobilize poorly to avoid collection failure or prolonged collections.

Patients and Methods

Mobilization method employed was cyclophosphamide (2 g/m^2) plus G-CSF (filgrastim 5 μg/kg or single dose pegfilgrastim 6 mg) in myelona patients. In lymphoma patients, disease specific chemotherapy or intermediate-dose cyclophosphamide (4 g/m^2)+G-CSF were used. Myeloma patients were admitted to our ward on day +8–9 and lymphoma patients on day +10–11 from start of chemotherapy (day 0). Blood CD34$^+$ measurements were started when white blood cell (WBC) counts were >1 × 10^9/L and continued daily until completion of aphereses or until realization of mobilization failure. In general, collections were started if B-CD34$^+$ counts measured early in the morning were >20 × 10^6/L but in individual cases also lower counts were accepted to start with collections in hard-to-mobilize patients.

After acceptance by EMEA in July 2009, plerixafor became available for clinical use. Before that time, two patients had received plerixafor for remobilization in compassionate use program. From 1 August 2009 to 31 December 2010, altogether 70 patients with lymphoid malignancies received their first mobilization therapy and were admitted for stem cell collection in the adult hematology ward at Kuopio University Hospital. There were 25 females (36%) and 45 males (64%) with a median age of 57 years (25–70). Thirty-eight patients (54%) had lymphoma (diffuse large B-cell lymphoma 17, mantle cell lymphoma 10, follicular lymphoma 6, peripheral T-cell lymphoma 5), 29 patients (41%) multiple myeloma, and 3 patients (4%) Hodgkin's lymphoma. The mobilization therapy for myeloma patients was low-dose cyclophosphamide (2 g/m^2) (1.5 g/m^2 in one patient) followed by G-CSF (pegfilgrastim 6 mg). In lymphoma patients, the mobilization regiments given were more variable including high-dose cytarabine (n=18), DHAP (n=9), intermediate-dose (4 g/m^2) cyclophosphamide (n=7), ICE (n=4), and CHOP (n=1); as growth factor either filgrastim 5 μg/kg/day or pegfilgrastim (6 or 12 mg) was used.

The patients were admitted to the hematology ward 8 days after CY infusion and 10–11 days after disease-specific chemotherapy. The first measurement of blood CD34$^+$ (B-CD34$^+$) counts were performed early in the next morning (5.30 a.m.) provided that blood leukocyte (WBC) counts were >1 × 10^9/L. B-CD34$^+$ counts were measured by flow cytometry (FACSCanto, Becton Dickinson, San Jose, CA, USA) using ISHAGE protocol with a single platform method (Stem-Kit, Immunotech SAS/Beckman Coulter, France). If B-CD34$^+$ counts were >10 × 10^6/L, collections with a COBE Spectra AutoPBSC™ (Cobe BCT, Lakewood, Colorado, USA) were routinely started after insertion of apheresis catheter. Blood volume processed daily was 2.5 times that of the estimated blood volume during 4–5 h. The minimum collection target was ≥2 × 10^6/kg CD34$^+$ cells, and in younger (<65 years) myeloma patients the minimum target was $\geq 4 \times 10^6$/kg CD34$^+$ cells to facilitate two transplants if feasible. The number of CD34$^+$ cells in the apheresis product was measured using the same method as previously described for B-CD34$^+$ cell counts.

After acceptance of plerixafor for clinical use, addition of this novel drug to chemotherapy plus G-CSF mobilization (chemomobilization) was individually considered in each patient in the following circumstances: (1) low blood B-CD34$^+$ counts ($<10 \times 10^6$/L) at the time of marrow recovery or (2) poor yield of the first apheresis ($<1 \times 10^6$/kg CD34$^+$ cells). Successful collection was defined as $\geq 2 \times 10^6$/kg CD34$^+$ cells collected with maximum of three aphereses.

In patients who started with plerixafor, an extra G-CSF dose (5 μg/kg s.c.) was given to patients who had received pegfilgrastim followed by plerixafor injection (12 mg–24 mg s.c.) at 8–10 p.m. Blood samples for B-CD34$^+$ measurements as well as WBC counts plus differential blood count were taken next morning at 5.30 a.m. Aphereses were started routinely if B-CD34$^+$ counts were $>10 \times 10^6$/L and by individual decision in some patients with B-CD34$^+$ counts between 5 and 10×10^6/L.

Results

Until 31 December 2010, altogether 20 patients with hematological malignancies have received plerixafor added to chemomobilization. There were 7 females and 13 males with a median age of 60 years (27–68). Sixteen patients (80%) had non-Hodgkin lymphoma, three patients (15%) multiple myeloma and one patient Hodgkin lymphoma. Two patients (10%) had failed a chemomobilization attempt and in 18 patients (90%) plerixafor was added preemptively to chemomobilization due to low B-CD34$^+$ counts and/or poor collections. The median number of plerixafor injections was 1 (1–3) and the median dose given per patient was 24 mg (12–72 mg/patient). Eleven patients (55%) received only one plerixafor injection, four patients two injections, and five patients three injections.

In two patients (10%) no collections were started due to low CD34$^+$ counts (1 and 2×10^6/L, respectively). In 18 patients, collections were started, and in 17 patients (85%), a graft containing at least 2×10^6/kg CD34$^+$ cells was collected. The median B-CD34$^+$ count on the days of the first plerixafor dose was 3×10^6/L; it was $<5 \times 10^6$/L in 11 patients (55%), 6–10×10^6/L in 4 patients, and $>10 \times 10^6$/L in 5 patients (decreasing counts in 2 patients). The median WBC count at the time of the first plerixafor dose was 5.2×10^9/L (1.7–35.4). WBC was $<5 \times 10^9$/L in nine patients (45%), 5–10×10^9/L in four patients, and $>10 \times 10^9$/L in seven patients, respectively.

Patients with a Previously Failed Chemomobilization

Both patients with relapsed diffuse large B-cell lymphoma, who had previously failed a chemomobilization attempt, were successfully mobilized with chemomobilization + plerixafor (Table 12.1). The first patient received three plerixafor injections

Table 12.1 Characteristics of patients who had failed a previous chemomobilization and received 2nd mobilization with a chemomobilization plus plerixafor

Gender/ age	Disease/ status	Prior tx	Mobilization regimen	G-CSF	B-CD34⁺ max (×10⁶/L)	Yield (no. aphereses)
M/60	NHL/CR2	R-CHOP × 8 DHAP	DHAP	Pegfilgrastim	1	0 (0)
	II mob		DHAP	Filgrastim	9 (3 plerixafor doses)	2.2 (4)
F/64	NHL/CR2	R-CHOP × 8 R-ICE ×2	ICE	Filgrastim	1	0 (0)
	II mob		AraC	Filgrastim	40 (2 plerixafor doses)	4.0 (2)

Abbreviations: *M* male, *F* female, *NHL* non-Hodgkin's lymphoma, *tx* treatment, *G-CSF* granulocyte colony-stimulating factor, *no.* number, *mob* mobilization, *CR* complete remission, *R* rituximab, *CHOP* cyclophosphamide–doxorubicin–vincristine–prednisolone, *DHAP* dexamethasone-high-dose cytarabine-cisplatinum, *ICE* ifosfamide–carboplatinum–etoposide, *AraC* cytarabine, *B-CD34⁺* blood CD34⁺ count

(72 mg), and collections were started after the second injection (B-CD34$^+$ count 9×10^6/L), thereafter B-CD34$^+$ counts remained stable and started to decrease after the third collection. The other patient received three plerixafor injections (14 mg/day), and collections were started after two injections with B-CD34$^+$ count of 18×10^6/L.

Patients with Preemptive Plerixafor Use

Between 1 August 2009 and 31 December 2010, altogether 18 (26%) out of 70 chemomobilized patients received plerixafor preemptively (Tables 12.2 and 12.3). Altogether, 14/38 NHL patients (37%) received plerixafor compared to only 3/29 (10%) myeloma patients.

Low B-CD34$^+$ counts at the time of marrow recovery (median 3×10^6/L, range <1–12) were the reason for preemptive use in 14 patients (78%), whereas poor yield of the previous apheresis was the reason for plerixafor use in the rest of four patients. In these patients, B-CD34$^+$ counts ranged from 11 to 25×10^6/L.

The median increase of B-CD34$^+$ counts after the first plerixafor dose was four-fold (no change to 16-fold). Stem cell aphereses were started in 16/18 patients (89%). The median yield was 2.7×10^6/kg CD34$^+$ cells (1.6–6.4), and the median number of aphereses was 1 (1–3). The minimum collection target (≥2×10^6/kg CD34$^+$ cells) was achieved in all three MM patients and in 11/14 lymphoma patients (79%). In two patients with NHL, the maximum B-CD34$^+$ counts reached with three plerixafor doses were 1 and 2×10^6/L, respectively and no aphereses were performed.

In general, plerixafor was well tolerated, and no side effects specifically due to this agent could be observed.

Table 12.2 Preemptive use of plerixafor following chemomobilization in patients with non-Hodgkin's lymphoma [17]

Gender/ age	Disease/status	Prior tx	Mobilization regimen	G-CSF	WBCpre ($\times 10^9$/L)	WBCpost ($\times 10^9$/L)	B-CD34$^+$ pre ($\times 10^6$/L CD34$^+$)	B-CD34$^+$ post ($\times 10^6$/L CD34$^+$)	Yield (no. aphereses) ($\times 10^6$/kg CD34$^+$)
M/64	NHL/PR2	CHOP ×6 Fludara ×6 DHAP ×1, RT, IFN	AraC	Pegfilgrastim	13.5	73.2	2	33	3.4 (2)
M/43	NHL/CR2	R-CHOP ×6 R-Benda ×3	AraC	Pegfilgrastim	6.7	9.8	11	48	6.4 (2)
M/68	NHL/CR2	R-CHOP ×6 R-DHAP ×3	CY	Pegfilgrastim	1.7	8.3	<1	<1	0 (0)
M/61	NHL/CR2	CHOEP ×8 R-DHAP ×3	DHAP	Pegfilgrastim	34.6	42.4	3	39	3.2 (1)
M/58	NHL/CR1	R-maxi CHOP ×3 R-AraC ×3	AraC	Pegfilgrastim	13.4	26.4	4	19	2.1 (1)
F/64	NHL/CR2	R-DHAP ×4 R-CHOP ×6	DHAP	Pegfilgrastim	10.5	48.0	7	63	4.2 (1)
F/52	NHL/CR2	R-CHOP ×6 R-DHAP ×1 R-MINE ×2	CY	Pegfilgrastim	2.8	21.5	4	63	3.1 (1)
F/60	NHL/PR1	R-CHOP ×6 R-DHAP ×2	AraC	Filgrastim	35.4	54,9	25 (dec)	49	2.6 (3)
M/51	NHL/PR2	R-CHOP ×8 ICE ×3, RT	ICE	Pegfilgrastim	4.3	17.5	1	11	1.6 (3)

M/51	NHL/CR2	R-COP ×2 R-CHOP ×5 R-AraC ×1	AraC	Filgrastim	26.8	36.7	8	30	2.7 (1)
M/44	NHL/PR1	R-CHOP ×6	CY	Pegfilgrastim	4.0	21.7	12	52	6.1 (3)
M/49	NHL/CR2	R-CHOP ×8 R-Benda ×4	AraC	Filgrastim	4.6	22.8	11	81	6.1 (1)
M/66	NHL/CR2	R-CHOP ×6 R-ICE ×3, RT	ICE	Filgrastim	6.8	37.6	10	41	2.9 (1)
F/65	NHL/PR1	R-CHOP ×2 R-ICE ×3	ICE	Pegfilgrastim	2.3	5.2	<1	<1	0 (0)

Abbreviations: *F* female, *M* male, *tx* treatment, *RT* radiotherapy, *NHL* non-Hodgkin's lymphoma, *CHOP* cyclophosphamide, doxorubicin, vincristine, prednisolone, *fludara* fludarabine, *RT* radiotherapy, *IFN* interferon, *CR* complete remission, *PR* partial remission, *CY* cyclophosphamide, *R* rituximab, *AraC* cytarabine; *DHAP* dexamethasone, high-dose cytarabine, cisplatinum, *Benda* bendamustive, *COP* cyclophosphamide, vincristine, prednisolone, *MINE* methotrexate, ifosfamide, mitoxantrone, etoposide, *ICE* ifosfamide, carboplatinum, etoposide; *WBC* white blood cell count, *pre* on the day of the first plerixafor dose, *post* on the morning after the first plerixafor dose, *dec* decreasing, *no.* number, *B-CD34⁺* blood $CD34^+$ count

Table 12.3 Preemptive use of plerixafor in other patients than NHL [17]

Age/gender	Disease/status	Prior tx.	Mobilization regimen	G-CSF	WBCpre ($\times 10^9$/L)	WBCpost ($\times 10^9$/L)	B-CD34$^+$ pre ($\times 10^6$/L)	B-CD34$^+$ post ($\times 10^6$/L)	Yield (no. aphereses) ($\times 10^6$/kg CD34$^+$)
F/27	HL/CR2	ABVD ×4, DHAP ×3, RT	DHAP	Pegfilgrastim	1.7	12.6	3	21	2.2 (2)
F/56	MM/VGPR	Thal-Dex, Bort-Dex,	CY	Pegfilgrastim	4.4	10.6	7 (dec)	39	2.1 (1)
M/60	MM/VGPR	Thal-Dex, Bort-Dex, RT	CY	Pegfilgrastim	5.5	24.8	16 (dec)	46	2.7 (1)
M/67	MM/PR	Thal-Dex, Len-Dex, RT	CY	Pegfilgrastim	5.2	16.1	2	12	2.1 (2)

Abbreviations: *F* female, *M* male, *tx* therapy, *HL* Hodgkin's lymphoma, *MM* multiple myeloma, *CR* complete remission, *PR* partial remission, *VGPR* very good partial remission, *ABVD* doxorubicin, bleomycin, vinblastine, dacarbazin, *DHAP* dexamethasone, high-dose cytarabine, cisplatinum, *Thal* thalidomide, *Dex* dexamethasone, *Bort* bortezomib, *Len* lenalidomide, *RT* radiotherapy, *CY* cyclophosphamide, *WBC* white blood cell count, *pre* on the day of the first plerixafor dose, *post* on the morning of the first plerixafor dose, *dec* decreasing, *no.* number, *B-CD34$^+$* blood CD34$^+$ count

High-Dose Therapy and Engraftment

Out of 20 patients receiving plerixafor, altogether 15 patients have received high-dose therapy supported by graft collected after chemomobilization plus plerixafor by 31 December 2010. Twelve lymphoma patients have received BEAM (carmustine–etoposide–cytarabine–melphalan) followed by stem cell infusion and pegfilgrastim 6 mg s.c. All patients have engrafted, but one patient had a delayed platelet engraftment (6 months). All three myeloma patients have received high-dose melphalan (200 mg/m^2) followed by stem cell infusion and G-CSF and have engrafted. One patient died due to central nervous system relapse before high-dose therapy, and in two patients high-dose therapy is pending.

Discussion

This series of patients represents the largest single center experience of using plerixafor after chemomobilization in patients who had either failed a previous chemomobilization or who were mobilizing poorly based on B-CD34$^+$ counts and/or low yields of previous collections. This use can be considered as off-label use as the label for the use of plerixafor is in combination with G-CSF in patients with lymphoma or MM and in EU especially in patients mobilizing poorly. Our experience shows that plerixafor used after chemomobilization is safe and effective in the majority of patients allowing efficient collection of stem cell graft to support high-dose therapy. As chemomobilization is widely used especially in Europe, these observations are of considerable interest.

Only one feasibility study combining plerixafor with chemomobilization has previously been published [6]. In that study, 26 MM patients and 14 NHL patients received plerixafor which resulted in an approximately twofold increase in collection yield after plerixafor injection when compared to the collection of the previous day. However, based on B-CD34$^+$ counts and yields, most of the patients in that trial were standard mobilizers or even good mobilizers. Recently, a small series of patients that mobilizes poorly with chemomobilization have received plerixafor have been presented [3, 18], suggesting the efficacy of this strategy. Recently, a German study including 47 chemomobilized patients receiving plerixafor after a previous mobilization failure have been published [11]. These reports as well as the present single center experience suggest that this combination is effective although clearly more data is needed in regard to timing and dosing of plerixafor in this context.

In this series plerixafor was mostly used in patients with NHL which are in general more difficult to mobilize than patients with MM [22]. The need for plerixafor use is also dependent on the mobilization method used as well as the collection target. E.g. if the collection target is high and G-CSF is used alone to mobilize stem cells, only 34% of MM patients mobilized with G-CSF alone achieved collection target of 6×10^6/kg CD34$^+$ cells in a randomized phase III study [4].

In regard to preemptive use, daily monitoring of blood counts and especially B-CD34$^+$ cell counts may be useful to define poor or suboptimal mobilization and to optimize the additive effect of plerixafor. Based on small patients series [3, 16, 18], patients with very low B-CD34$^+$ counts may be difficult to mobilize even with plerixafor. It may be wise to wait until WBC counts are >5–10 × 10^6/L and if at that point B-CD34$^+$ counts are low, adding of plerixafor might be considered [14]. It is possible, however, that stem cell mobilization may improve at least in some patients with time, so in patients with low but rising B-CD34$^+$ counts waiting 1–2 days may be advocated. On the other hand, if B-CD34$^+$ counts are low but do not increase or if they start to decrease, then plerixafor should be added to avoid collection failure. The ability of plerixafor to increase B-CD34$^+$ cell counts within 5–11 h makes this drug suitable to treat patients preemptively if mobilization is considered to be inadequate.

In our series, the majority of the patients were mobilized initially with a combination of chemotherapy and pegfilgrastim. There are no formal studies on combination of pegfilgrastim and plerixafor. Although pegfilgrastim causes higher serum concentrations than filgrastim [19], in general these agents are comparable in regard to mobilization efficiency at least following chemotherapy [23]. It is not known how long the action of pegfilgrastim is continued in a case of high neutrophil counts typically present at recovery phase following chemomobilization. Therefore, we added filgrastim prior to each plerixafor dose in this study. We do not know whether this addition is in fact needed but as it took usually 7–12 days from the pegfilgrastim dosing to apheresis, we have used this approach to ensure maximal mobilization.

In this series of patients the median increase in the amount of B-CD34$^+$ cells after the first plerixafor dose was fourfold with a wide range. One reason for the wide variation might be that some of our patients were "no mobilizers", whereas many others were poor mobilizers and even some late mobilizers. Retrospectively, patients, who received preemptively plerixafor resulting collections of e.g. >4 × 10^6/kg CD34$^+$ cells the next day (four patients in our series), would have been successfully collected without plerixafor with 1–2 additional collections.

Plerixafor added to G-CSF mobilization affects graft composition not only by increasing the number of CD34$^+$ cells collected, but also by increasing the number of CD34$^+$ CD38$^-$ cells [9] as well as the number of T-cells [10]. Whether graft characteristics are important for the long-term outcome of the patients is not known and deserves further studies [8, 12]. There is no published data on mobilization of other cells than CD34$^+$ cells with the triple combination of chemotherapy, G-CSF and plerixafor. Interestingly, there is no data on graft composition either in this context.

Plerixafor is expensive and may add important costs to the stem cell mobilization and collection procedure. On the other hand, collection failure is also expensive and may be associated with adverse patient outcomes. Further studies including economical considerations are needed. Our preemptive strategy may, however, prove to be cost-effective as very few collection failures have been observed since the advent of plerixafor in our unit. There is still more work to be done to better define postmobilization phase patients who may benefit from the preemptive use of plerixafor and to optimize the use of this drug in this context.

To conclude, addition of plerixafor to chemomobilization is effective both in patients who have experienced a collection failure as well as in patients treated preemptively to avoid collection failure or prolonged collections. More studies are needed to optimize timing and dosing of plerixafor in this context as well as to evaluate cost-effectiveness of this approach.

References

1. Bensinger W, DiPersio JF, McCarty JM (2009) Improving stem cell mobilization strategies: future directions. Bone Marrow Transplant 43:181–195
2. Calandra G, McCarty J, McGuirk J et al (2008) AMD3100 plus G-CSF can successfully mobilize CD34+ cells from non-Hodgkin's lymphoma, Hodgkin's disease and multiple myeloma patients previously failing mobilization with chemotherapy and/or cytokine treatment: compassionate use data. Bone Marrow Transplant 41:331–338
3. d'Addio A, Curti A, Worel N et al (2011) The addition of plerixafor is safe and allows adequate PBSC collection in multiple myeloma and lymphoma patients poor mobilizers after chemotherapy and G-CSF. Bone Marrow Transplant 46:356–363
4. DiPersio JF, Stadtmayer EA, Nademanee A et al (2009) Plerixafor and G-CSF versus placebo and G-CSF to mobilize hematopoietic stem cells for autologous stem cell transplantation in patients with multiple myeloma. Blood 113:5720–5726
5. DiPersio JF, Micallef I, Stiff P et al (2009) Phase III prospective randomized double-blind placebo-controlled trial of plerixafor plus granulocyte colony-stimulating factor compared with placebo plus granulocyte colony-stimulating factor for autologous stem-cell mobilization and transplantation for patients with non-Hodgkin's lymphoma. J Clin Oncol 27:4767–4773
6. Dugan MJ, Maziarz RT, Bensinger WI et al (2010) Safety and preliminary efficacy of plerixafor (Mozobil) in combination with chemotherapy and G-CSF: an open-label, multicentre, exploratory trial in patients with multiple myeloma and non-Hodgkin's lymphoma undergoing stem cell mobilization. Bone Marrow Transplant 45:39–47
7. Flomenberg N, Devine S, DiPersio JF et al (2005) The use of AMD3100 plus G-CSF for autologous hematopoietic progenitor cell mobilization is superior to G-CSF alone. Blood 106:1867–1874
8. Fruehauf S, Tricot G (2010) Comparison of unmobilized and mobilized graft characteristics and the implications of cell subsets on autologous and allogeneic transplant outcomes. Biol Blood Marrow Transplant 16:1629–1648
9. Fruehauf S, Veldvijk MTR, Seeger T et al (2009) A combination of granulocyte colony-stimulating factor (G-CSF) and plerixafor mobilizes more primitive peripheral blood progenitor cells than G-CSF alone: results of a European phase II study. Cytotherapy 11:992–1001
10. Holtan SG, Porrata LF, Micallef IN et al (2007) AMD3100 affects autograft lymphocyte collection and progression-free survival in non-Hodgkin lymphoma. Clin Lymphoma Myeloma 7:315–318
11. Hubel K, Fresen MM, Salwander H et al (2011) Plerixafor with and without chemotherapy in poor mobilizers: results from the German compassionate use program. Bone Marrow Transplant 46:1045–1052
12. Jantunen E, Fruehauf S (2011) Importance of blood graft characteristics in autologous stem cell transplantation: implications for optimizing mobilization regimens. Bone Marrow Transplant 46:627–635
13. Jantunen E, Kuittinen T (2008) Blood stem cell mobilization and collection in patients with lymphoproliferative diseases: practical issues. Eur J Haematol 80:287–295
14. Jantunen E, Kvalheim G (2010) Mobilization strategies in hard-to-mobilize patients with lymphoid malignancies. Eur J Haematol 85:463–471

15. Jantunen E, Itälä M, Siitonen T et al (2008) Blood stem cell mobilization and collection in patients with chronic lymphocytic leukaemia: a nationwide analysis. Bone Marrow Transplant 41:239–244
16. Jantunen E, Penttilä K, Pyörälä M et al (2011) Addition of plerixafor to a chemotherapy and G-CSF mobilization in hard-to-mobilize patients. Bone Marrow Transplant 46:308–309
17. Jantunen E, Kuittinen T, Mahlamäki E et al (2011) Efficacy of pre-emptively used plerixafor in patients mobilizing poorly after chemomobilization: a single centre experience. Eur J Haematol 86:299–304
18. Josefsen D, Rechnitzer C, Parto K, Kvalheim G (2010) The use of plerixafor for blood stem cell mobilization reduces the frequency of mobilization failure in patients planned to undergo autologous transplantation. Eur Hematol 4:24–29
19. Kobbe G, Burns I, Fenk R et al (2009) Pegfilgrastim for PBSC mobilization and autologous haematopoietic SCT. Bone Marrow Transplant 43:669–677
20. Kuittinen T, Nousiainen T, Halonen P et al (2004) Prediction of mobilization failure in patients with non-Hodgkin's lymphoma. Bone Marrow Transplant 33:907–912
21. Lemoli RM, d'Addio A (2008) Hematopoietic stem cell mobilization. Haematologica 83:321–324
22. Pusic I, Jiang SY, Landua S et al (2008) Impact of mobilization and remobilization strategies on achieving sufficient stem cell yields for autologous transplantation. Biol Blood Marrow Transplant 14:1045–1056
23. Putkonen M, Rauhala A, Pelliniemi TT, Remes K (2009) Single-dose pegfilgrastim is comparable to daily filgrastim in mobilizing peripheral blood stem cells: a case-matched study in patients with lymphoproliferative malignancies. Ann Hematol 88:673–680
24. Steinberg M, Silva M (2010) Plerixafor: a chemokine receptor 4 antagonist for mobilization of hematopoietic stem cells for transplantation after high-dose chemotherapy for non-Hodgkin's lymphoma. Clin Ther 32:821–843
25. Wuchter P, Ran D, Bruckner T et al (2010) Poor mobilization of hematopoietic stem cells—definitions, incidence, risk factors, and impact on outcome of autologous transplantation. Biol Blood Marrow Transplant 16:490–499

Chapter 13
Blood Stem Cell Mobilization in Solid Tumors: Experience with Plerixafor and Alternative Ways of Hematopoietic Stem Cell Mobilization

Guido Kobbe and Rainer Haas

Abstract High-dose therapy and autologous hematopoietic stem cell transplantation has traditionally been used to treat patients with high-risk hematologic malignancies. In addition, there are some rare solid tumors in children, adolescent, or young adults that may also be treated successfully with high-dose therapy. These include neuroblastoma, medulloblastoma, and Ewing's sarcoma as well as some types of germ cell tumors. In patients suffering from these tumors, blood stem cells have so far been mobilized by G-CSF or GM-CSF alone during steady-state hematopoiesis or in combination with cytotoxic therapy. If treated for recurrent disease, up to 30% of these patients fail traditional mobilization regimens due to extensive pretreatment. Recent evidence suggests that the CXCR4 antagonist Plerixafor may be used to enhance G-CSF mediated mobilization allowing sufficient blood stem cell collections in these so-called "poor mobilizers." This chapter reviews the current literature on the use of Plerixafor in patients with solid tumors and highlights additional experimental agents for blood stem cell mobilization.

Blood Stem Cell Mobilization in Solid Tumors

High-dose therapy and transplantation of peripheral blood stem cells (PBSC) is an accepted therapy for patients with high-risk hematologic malignancies, while its use for patients with solid tumors is relatively rare. According to a report on the transplant activity in Europe, which was published in 2004, between 1991 and 2002,

G. Kobbe (✉) • R. Haas
Department of Hematology, Oncology and Clinical Immunology, University Hospital Düsseldorf, Heinrich Heine University Düsseldorf, Moorenstr. 5, Düsseldorf 40225, Germany
e-mail: Kobbe@med.uni-duesseldorf.de

S. Fruehauf et al. (eds.), *Novel Developments in Stem Cell Mobilization: Focus on CXCR4*, DOI 10.1007/978-1-4614-1960-0_13,

a total of 27,902 patients received high-dose therapy followed by autologous PBSC transplantation for the treatment of a solid tumor [25]. The number of transplantations performed increased from 536 per year in 1991 to 4,154 in 1997, whereas we witnessed a reduction to 1913 in 2002. At least 98% of these high-dose therapies were supported by autologous PBSC transplantations. Since then, there was a further decline in the number as far as solid tumors were concerned. On the other hand, in 2009 we noted an increase in the proportion of allogeneic PBSC transplantations from 2 to 6% out of the 1,454 transplantations performed in that year [5].

This development is a consequence of the discouraging results of high-dose therapy and autologous PBSC transplantation in studies performed in patients with breast cancer as well as in patients with small cell lung cancer. For most of the other solid tumors, data from prospective randomized studies are lacking [21, 22]. Still, adult patients with germ cell tumors and particular types of soft tissue sarcomas as well as children with neuroblastoma, medulloblastoma, and Ewing's sarcoma are candidates for a PBSC-supported high-dose therapy [7, 8, 41, 50, 66].

Blood Stem Cell Mobilization in Patients with Germ Cell Tumors: Early Experience with Plerixafor

The ability to mobilize autologous hematopoietic stem- and progenitor cells, a prerequisite for high-dose chemotherapy, depends on several critical factors that may be viewed as related to particular patient characteristics, disease specific aspects, or effects of the anteceding cytotoxic treatment. When compared with patients who suffer from hematologic malignancies such as multiple myeloma or Non-Hodgkin's lymphoma, the likelihood of harvesting a sufficient number of PBSC for several cycles of high-dose therapy is relatively great in patients with germ cell tumors, since they are mostly young and present without bone marrow involvement.

On the other hand, high-dose therapy is almost exclusively used as a second, third, or fourth line salvage treatment. As a consequence, these patients have received several lines of previous chemotherapy, often combined with radiotherapy at the time when PBSC mobilization is envisaged. Extensive pretreatment with Cisplatin, alkylating agents, and radiotherapy to bone marrow involving sites of active hematopoiesis reduce the so-called "stem cell reserve" and as a consequence hamper the ability to mobilize a sufficient amount of PBSC [23, 24, 27, 37, 61].

Furthermore, high-dose therapy protocols for patients with germ cell tumors are often based on two or more cycles of high-dose therapy. A great amount of $CD34^+$ cells is therefore needed to support each treatment cycle [41, 49]. Although these chemotherapy cycles are not myeloablative, they would be associated with severe, long lasting periods of cytopenia, if not a sufficient number of $CD34^+$ cells was autografted after high-dose therapy. As a result, high-dose sequential therapy in patients with germ cell tumors requires PBSC grafts containing enough $CD34^+$ cells for 3–4 treatment cycles considering also the possibility of a "backup" transplant.

In patients with germ cell tumors, $CD34^+$ cells have traditionally been mobilized during conventional salvage treatment using a combination of intensive, alkylating agents containing chemotherapy in combination with granulocyte-colony stimulating factor (G-CSF) [2, 69].

There are approximately between 30 and 40% of patients, who are unable to mobilize a sufficient number of PBSC mainly because of extensive previous cytotoxic chemotherapy [20, 23, 39]. Before the introduction of the CXCR4 antagonist Plerixafor, strategies to enhance PBSC mobilization and collection in these patients included the introduction of large volume leukaphereses, G-CSF dose escalation, the administration of additional cytokines, or a change of the cytotoxic drugs. The latter approach was taken in the assumption that an intensification by administering Taxanes or high-dose Etoposide would also result in better blood stem cell mobilization as the result of a deeper anteceding nadir [33, 34, 36, 40, 48, 59, 60].

At the time of writing this review, there are several reports on the use of Plerixafor for the mobilization of PBSC in extensively pretreated patients with germ cell tumors. The first patient was reported by Saure from our group in November 2010 [71]. A 26-year-old patient who had received four previous lines of therapy for recurrent testicular cancer was given two doses of Plerixafor during hematopoietic recovery from a cytotoxic mobilization cycle using Paclitaxel and Ifosphamide. Despite of 6 mg Pegfilgrastim and additional boost of conventional G-CSF stimulation at a dose of 10.5 μg/kg twice a day, the maximal concentration of $CD34^+$ cells in the peripheral blood was 4.7 per microliter (4.7×10^6/L) with a white blood count (WBC) of 9,400 per microliter (9.4×10^9/L).

Ten hours after subcutaneous injection of 0.27 mg/kg Plerixafor, the WBC had increased to 50.4×10^9/L and the number of circulating $CD34^+$ cells had risen to 15.5×10^6/L, which enabled a successful apheresis with a harvest containing 2.3×10^6 $CD34^+$ cells per kilogram. As a sufficient number of $CD34^+$ cells for three high-dose cycles was needed additional aphereses were scheduled. On the next day, the peripheral $CD34^+$ cell count had dropped to five $CD34^+$ cells per microliter and only 0.2×10^6/kg $CD34^+$ cells could be collected. In the evening of the same day, the patient received Plerixafor at a dose of 0.27 mg/kg for the second time. In the morning of the following day, the $CD34^+$ cell concentration in the peripheral blood had increased to 23×10^6/L again permitting the collection of 1.8×10^6 $CD34^+$ cells per kilogram. Together with 1.73×10^6 $CD34^+$ cells from an apheresis of a previous mobilization cycle, the patient achieved the amount of PBSC to support three cycles of high-dose therapy consisting of Carboplatin and Etoposide (Fig. 13.1). Within the following months, he completed three cycles of high-dose therapy each time with a timely and stable hematopoietic recovery.

In principle, the case of this young man illustrates two important findings. First, Plerixafor is effective in the mobilization of $CD34^+$ cells in combination with Pegfilgrastim. Second, Plerixafor has to be given on consecutive days because its mobilizing ability of $CD34^+$ cells when combined with G-CSF is time dependent and limited. Therefore, it requires several administrations day by day until the desired yield is achieved.

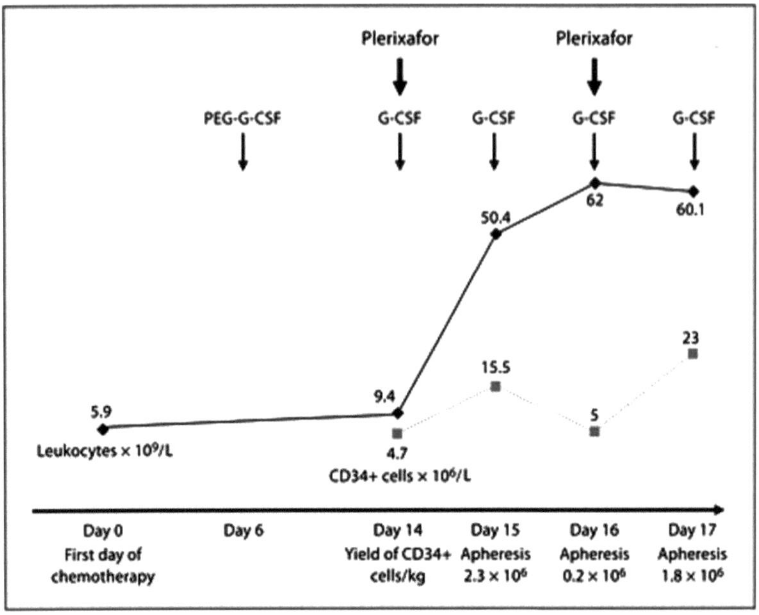

Fig. 13.1 This figure shows peripheral blood CD34+ cell kinetics of an extensively pretreated patient with metastasized testicular germ cell tumor following treatment with Taxol and Ifosphamide, Pegfilgrastim, Filgrastim and Plerixafor. Stimulation with G-CSF alone was insufficient to achieve peripheral blood CD34+ cell counts >10 × 10^6/L and an apheresis yield >2 × 10^6 CD34+/kg. Following treatment with Plerixafor, a sufficient number of CD34+ cells could be collected (taken from [71])

Shortly following this initial report seven additional patients with germ cell tumors who had received Plerixafor to increase the number of circulating CD34+ cells on the occasion of G-CSF supported cytotoxic mobilization therapies were reported. Kobold and colleagues published the cumulative experience from the European Plerixafor compassionate use program [39]. During a 1-year period (11/2008–11/2009) 6 of 17 patients (35%) with relapsed germ cell tumors who were treated in four centers in Germany failed to mobilize. These relapsed patients had underwent a median of 3.5 prior treatment lines (range 1–6) and were envisaged for one or more cycles of high-dose therapy. The G-CSF-based mobilization regimens which had failed included TIP (Cisplatin, Ifosphamide, Paclitaxel, $n=3$), PEI (Cisplatin, Etoposide, Ifosphamide), PI (Cisplatin, Etoposide), or TI (Paclitaxel, Ifosphamide). The patients then received a second round of mobilization using chemotherapy (3× TIP, 1× PEI, 1× PI) with G-CSF or G-CSF during steady state alone ($n=1$) in combination with Plerixafor at a dose of 0.24 mg/kg on the occasion of a median of four aphereses (range 2–6). The addition of Plerixafor permitted in four of the six patients the collection of a sufficient number of CD34+ cells to proceed to high-dose therapy. So far, three patients actually received high-dose Ifosphamide, Carboplatin, and Etoposide or Carboplatin and Etoposide with PBPC support. Two patients showed a prompt and complete hematopoietic recovery, whereas one patient failed to recover a normal platelet count within the follow-up time of six months and still needed platelet transfusions.

Tuffaha and colleagues reported another patient with a recurrent germ cell tumor in third remission who had previously failed two consecutive attempts to mobilize CD34⁺ cells using 2×5 μg/kg/day G-CSF and 2×10 μg/kg/day G-CSF [76]. During a third mobilization attempt with G-CSF (10 μg/kg/day) and Plerixafor at a dose of 0.24 mg/kg, he achieved a total of 5.74×10^6 $CD34^+$ cells per kilogram in two apheresis sessions.

For all patients treated so far, there are no reports on serious adverse effects related to Plerixafor. Similar results were reported by Horwitz and colleagues on the 2010 meeting of the American Society for Clinical Oncology (ASCO) [29]. They presented results of the US Plerixafor compassionate use program in 39 patients with nonhematologic malignancies. Among them were 21 patients with germ cell tumors who had previously failed mobilization attempts with G-CSF alone or in combination with cytotoxic chemotherapy. Following mobilization with G-CSF and Plerixafor 72% of patients achieved PBSC yields greater than 2×10^6 $CD34^+$ cells per kilogram and 64% of patients proceeded to high dose therapy. Eight of the 21 patients with germ cell tumors received tandem high-dose therapy.

In conclusion, a substantial number of patients with recurrent germ cell tumors fail conventional PBSC mobilization using either G-CSF alone or in combination with cytotoxic chemotherapy. Extensive previous therapy is the major cause for mobilization failure. The data presented suggest that Plerixafor successfully enhances $CD34^+$ cell mobilization in a substantial number of these patients. Adequate hematopoietic recovery has been reported in all but one patient who received $CD34^+$ cells that were mobilized by G-CSF ± chemotherapy and Plerixafor. As dose dense chemotherapy is essential for cure of patients with recurrent germ cell tumors, a combination of cytotoxic chemotherapy, G-CSF, and Plerixafor dependent on peripheral blood $CD34^+$ cell levels seems to be a reasonable approach. Decision algorithms for the use of Plerixafor using peripheral blood $CD34^+$ cell concentrations taking into account the number of high-dose cycles envisaged is recommended similar to the algorithm suggested by Costa and colleagues for patients with hematologic malignancies [17].

Experience with Plerixafor for Blood Stem Cell Mobilization in Patients with Solid Malignancies Other than Germ Cell Tumors

Among the 2010 ASCO report of the US Plerixafor compassionate use program there were 18 patients suffering from solid cancers other than germ cell tumors [29]. They included six patients with medulloblastoma, six patients with sarcoma, two with neuroblastoma two with breast cancer, and one each with cervical cancer and chordoma. Seven of these patients were children aged between 8 and 17 years.

In addition to this cumulative report the experience with Plerixafor in a total of 12 children with solid tumors (8 neuroblastoma, 2 medulloblastoma, 1 Wilm's tumor, 1 Ewing's sarcoma) was published in 4 full papers [1, 15, 55, 75]. Similar to the treatment of germ cell tumors in adults, the therapy of these malignancies in children involves combined modality approaches with intensive chemotherapy, surgery, radiotherapy, and serial cycles of high-dose chemotherapy.

If PBSC are mobilized early during first-line chemotherapy collection of adequate numbers to support between 1 and 3 cycles of high-dose is likely for the majority of patients. In contrast, patients who are treated at relapse may have a significantly reduced hematopoietic reserve as a consequence of previous intensive chemoradiotherapy. Nine of the 12 children (75%) that have been reported so far had a successful blood stem cell harvest following the use of Plerixafor in combination with G-CSF. Owing to the small number of patients and the fact that there may be underreporting of unsuccessful mobilization attempts the database for any definite conclusion on this issue is thin. It seems that, similar to the results obtained in adults, a relevant number of poor mobilizers among children with nonhematologic malignancies can successfully mobilize PBSC without any obvious side effects when Plerixafor is added to G-CSF ± chemotherapy.

Alternative Mobilization Strategies

Following the experience in hematopoietic stem cell mobilization made with G-CSF and granulocyte-macrophage colony-stimulating factor GM-CSF, other cytokines such as interleukin 3 (IL-3), IL-8, IL-11, stem cell factor (SCF), flt-3 ligand, and macrophage inflammatory protein-1α (MIP-1α) were considered to be potential candidates for the mobilization of $CD34^{+}$ cells [3, 4, 11, 26, 30, 43, 45, 52]. However, the ability of these cytokines to increase the number of circulating PBSC when given as single agents or in combination was either not superior to that of G-CSF or associated with relevant side effects.

Pegfilgrastim

Still, progress in the field of growth factor mediated mobilization of blood stem cells has been made by the pegylation of Filgrastim [19]. Different from the original, nonpegylated G-CSF, Pegfilgrastim is characterized by a significantly longer half-life because of a substantially reduced renal elimination [58]. In the first clinical mobilization study on this agent, which included patients with multiple myeloma, we could demonstrate safety and efficacy of a single dose of 12 mg Pegfilgrastim in mobilizing PBSC following cytotoxic chemotherapy sufficient for at least one high-dose therapy and subsequent autologous PBSC transplantation [74]. We later showed that the dose of Pegfilgrastim could be lowered to 6 mg without compromising mobilization results (Fig. 13.2) [13].

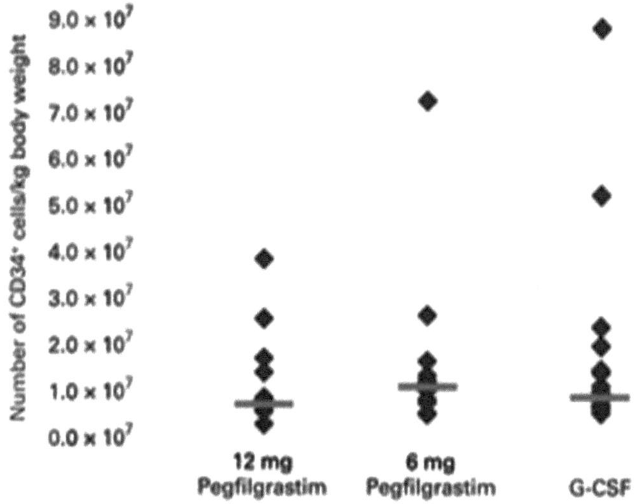

Fig. 13.2 This figure shows a similar mobilization efficacy of 6 and 12 mg Pegfilgrastim in comparison to standard dose G-CSF following high-dose Cyclophosphamide in patients with Multiple Myeloma. Apheresis yields obtained during large volume leukapheresis in a sequential cohort of 35 patients were not significantly different ($p = ns$). Each rhombus represents a patient and the horizontal lines represent medians (taken from [38])

Although clinical results were similar to conventional G-CSF in terms of circulating $CD34^+$ cells and total PBSC yields, it was interesting to note that Pegfilgrastim-exposed $CD34^+$ cells had a subset composition which was different from that of Filgrastim-mobilized $CD34^+$ cells [14]. They included a greater proportion of more primitive $CD34^+$ cells as characterized by lack of CD38 expression. In addition, Pegfilgrastim-mobilized $CD34^+$ cells exhibited a gene expression profile which was significantly different from $CD34^+$ cells mobilized by conventional G-CSF, reflecting the preponderance of a more immature $CD34^+$ cell subset on the transcriptome level (Fig. 13.3). Pegfilgrastim is meanwhile regularly used for PBSC mobilization in patients with hematologic malignancies and solid tumors [38].

Monoclonal Antibodies

To highlight potential alternative mobilization agents in addition to hematopoietic growth factors and the CXCR4 blocking agent Plerixafor, a closer look on the stem cell niche, the bone marrow microenvironment, and the adhesion structures involved in PBSC mobilization and homing is useful (Fig. 13.4).

In addition to osteoblasts, osteoclasts, and endothelial cells, the bone marrow contains different stromal cells including fibroblasts and adipocytes, which provide a highly specialized microarchitecture. The structure of this network of corresponding cells is essential for the differentiation of the various hematopoietic progenitor

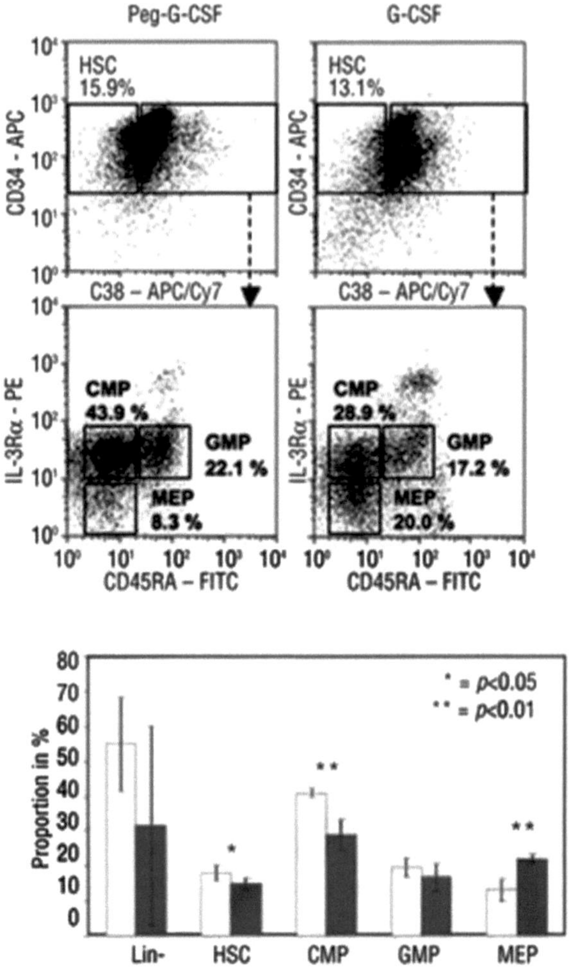

Fig. 13.3 This figure shows different patterns of hematopoietic stem-and progenitor cells in the peripheral blood mobilized with either Pegfilgrastim (*white columns*) or conventional G-CSF (*gray columns*). Pegfilgrastim mobilizes a greater proportion of hematopoietic stem cells and common myeloid progenitors but fewer megakaryocyte-erythrocyte progenitors. The percentage for Lin⁻ cells is related to total CD34⁺ cells while the percentages for hematopoietic stem cells (HSC), common myeloid progenitors (CMP), granulocyte monocyte progenitors (GMP), and megakaryocyte erythrocyte progenitors (MEP) are related to Lin⁻ CD34⁺ cells (taken from [14])

and precursor cells from an early hematopoietic stem cell. Stromal cells produce hematopoietic growth factors and cytokines and mediate adhesive interactions essential for migration, circulation, and proliferation of HSC [67, 77, 79].

Receptors and ligands that are involved in this process include members of the ß1 and ß2 integrin family, selectins, and superimmunoglobulin family. Most of these molecules have been well characterized. Their function has been studied on the progenitor cell level and in mature leukocytes in the context of inflammation and infectious disease [73]. The large majority of their ligands are expressed on endothelial cells, leucocytes, or stromal cells. Binding partners may also represent compounds of the extracellular matrix of the BM microenvironment.

For instance, the ß1 integrins very late antigen 4 ([VLA-4] CD29/CD49d) and VLA-5 (CD29/CD49e) are heterodimers permitting adhesion of hematopoietic progenitor cells to different adhesion structures of the BM stroma. In particular, the

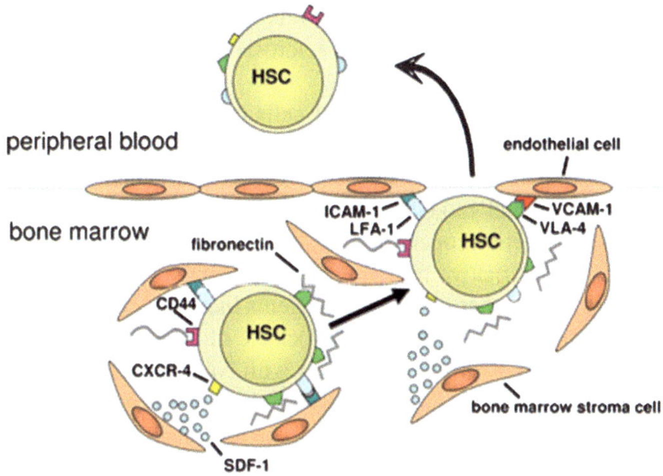

Fig. 13.4 This figure schematically shows the most important adhesion structures for stem cell homing and illustrates the process of hematopoietic stem cell (HSC) mobilization. *ICAM-1* intercellular adhesion molecule 1, *LFA-1* leukocyte function-associated molecule-1, *VCAM-1* vascular cell adhesion molecule 1, *VLA-4* very late antigen 4, *CXCR4* CXC-chemokine receptor type 4

VLA-4-mediated interaction between hematopoietic stem cells and BM stroma is of functional relevance for hematopoiesis as well as for mobilization and homing of CD34⁺ cells [28, 32, 54, 67, 81]. Circulating CD34⁺ cells express VLA-4 at lower levels in comparison to bone marrow CD34⁺ cells, indicating that the release of CD34⁺ cells and their migratory capacity are apparently related to the expression level of VLA-4 [44, 47, 56, 67, 80]. Further evidence elucidating this mechanism is the finding that systemic treatment of primates and mice with monoclonal antibodies directed against VLA-4 resulted in a significant increase of circulating hematopoietic progenitor cells [18, 63, 65, 78].

At the same time, mice treated with an anti-VLA-4 antibody experienced engraftment failure of hematopoietic stem cells [64].

The adhesive properties of CD34⁺ cells not only depend on the magnitude of the expression level but also on the functionality of these integrins. Altered functional state of integrins is known for physiological processes such as platelet aggregation [72], cell migration [31], or embryonic development [51]. Examining the activation state of VLA-4 on CD34⁺ cells from BM and PB during G-CSF-enhanced marrow recovery by flow cytometry, we found a significantly reduced functional activity of the VLA-4 receptor on circulating CD34⁺ cells when compared to steady state bone marrow [47]. In addition the number of circulating CD34⁺ cells during hematopoietic recovery was inversely related to the activation state and not to the expression level of VLA-4. Papayannapoulou and colleagues observed—in accordance to our own results—elevated numbers of circulating CD34⁺ cells in patients with multiple sclerosis who were treated with the humanized recombinant antibody Natalizumab [82]. Following treatment with Natalizumab patients had significantly higher levels of circulating CD34⁺ cells than their baseline levels before antibody treatment and in comparison with patients who had multiple sclerosis but received different kinds of treatments [9, 82].

The increased number of circulating CD34⁺ cells may result from a release of CD34⁺ cells from the VCAM-expressing endothelial niche and/or from prolonged circulation because of impaired homing due to the lack of VLA-4 mediated transendothelial migration. In animal models, the bone marrow repopulating ability of VLA-4 exposed hematopoietic progenitor cells could be demonstrated. Thus, this antibody provides a new alternative for PBSC mobilization, potentially alone or in combination with G-CSF or other mobilization agents like Plerixafor.

Bonig and colleagues studied a combined blockade of α4-integrin and CXCR4 in macaques by sequentially treating the animals with Natalizumab and Plerixafor [10]. While each agent alone had a modest effect on the levels of circulating CD34⁺ cells, they observed a more than additive mobilization of CD34⁺ cells into the peripheral blood by the combination. The same effect was evident in α4-integrin deficient mice. These results suggest that both agents may be used in combination for clinical blood stem cell mobilization.

Similar to VLA-4, the ß2 integrin leukocyte function-associated molecule-1 ([LFA-1], CD18/CD11a) mediates interactions between CD34⁺ hematopoietic progenitor cells and bone marrow stroma. Natural ligands of LFA-1 represent the members of the superimmunoglobulin family intercellular adhesion molecule (ICAM)-1 and ICAM-2. LFA-1 had a lower expression level on circulating CD34⁺ cells when compared to BM-derived CD34⁺ cells. Adhesion and migration of CD34⁺ cells could be inhibited using blocking monoclonal antibodies against LFA-1[56, 57]. This may be of relevance as a humanized monoclonal antibody directed against LFA-1 is available and approved for the treatment of patients with psoriasis.

A relationship has been shown to exist between cell adhesion and signal transduction pathways, which are stimulated by cytokines. Therefore SCF, GM-CSF, or IL-3 are capable of transiently enhancing the adhesiveness of CD34⁺ cells via activation of the integrins VLA-4 and VLA-5 [42, 46].

Additional molecules relevant in the context of blood stem cell mobilization and homing are platelet endothelial cell adhesion molecule-1 (PECAM, CD36) and CD44. CD44 is strongly expressed on CD34⁺ hematopoietic stem and progenitor cells. Osteopontin, hyaluronic acid, and fibronectin are the ligands of CD44 and represent components of the HSC niche and stromal microenvironment. Anti-CD44 directed monoclonal antibodies lower the adhesion of CD34⁺ cells to bone marrow stroma. In addition, they induce mobilization of progenitor cells in mice and prevent hematopoiesis in long-term BM cultures [35, 53, 62, 70].

A major disadvantage of using monoclonal antibodies in the context of blood stem cell mobilization is their prolonged half-life and therefore long lasting effect on stem cell homing an immune cell function. Small molecules targeting for example α4-integrin that are tested in animal models have a short half-life and are therefore better suitable for mobilization purposes [68].

Parathyroid Hormone

Parathyroid hormone (PTH) and the insulin-like growth factors (IGFs) have also been demonstrated to influence the function of the hematopoietic stem cell niches. High endogenous levels or administration of PTH to mice and humans have been shown to expand the number of bone marrow HSCs and increase the number of $CD34^+$ cells in peripheral blood [6, 12, 16]. Our current understanding of the role for PTH and IGF in hematopoietic niches is limited. We therefore believe that both their physiological importance and pharmacological potential warrants further study.

Conclusion

In conclusion, a sufficient harvest of hematopoietic stem and progenitor cells including primitive subsets with high potential for self-renewal is an essential prerequisite for high-dose therapy. The hematopoietic growth factor G-CSF has been used successfully for two decades and has become a valuable cornerstone for the mobilization of PBSC in clinical practice. The introduction of other cytokines such as SCF, IL-11, IL-8, or flt-3 ligand was not better than the two myeloid growth factors G- and GM-CSF but was often associated with significant and untolerable toxicity. New compounds with proven $CD34^+$ cell mobilizing ability include the long lasting compound Pegfilgrastim permitting PBSC mobilization by a single injection as well as the CXCR4 antagonist Plerixafor. Whether $CD34^+$ cells exposed to the monoclonal anti-VLA-4 antibody Natalizumab are suitable for transplantation requires careful animal studies as the engraftment potential has not been evaluated so far. It is interesting to note that both, Plerixafor and Natalizumab, interfere directly with the receptor–ligand cross talk between hematopoietic stem and progenitor cells and their adhesive partners within the stem cell niche. The combination of hematopoietic growth factors and direct inhibition of receptor–ligand interactions provides a principal model to further improve PBSC mobilization. The molecular insight we gain from these studies on normal hematopoietic stem cells may also be helpful in the "mobilization" of leukemic stem cells to render them more susceptible to conventional cytotoxic drugs. This kind of targeted therapy is particularly promising when allogeneic hematopoietic stem cells are available to occupy the stem cell niches disburdened from leukemic cells.

References

1. Aabideen K, Anoop P, Ethell ME, Potter MN (2011) The feasibility of plerixafor as a second-line stem cell mobilizing agent in children. J Pediatr Hematol Oncol 33:65–67
2. Agarwal R, Dvorak CC, Stockerl-Goldstein KE, Johnston L, Srinivas S (2009) High-dose chemotherapy followed by stem cell rescue for high-risk germ cell tumors: the Stanford experience. Bone Marrow Transplant 43:547–552

3. Andrews RG, Bartelmez SH, Knitter GH, Myerson D, Bernstein ID, Appelbaum FR, Zsebo KM (1992) A c-kit ligand, recombinant human stem cell factor, mediates reversible expansion of multiple CD34+ colony-forming cell types in blood and marrow of baboons. Blood 80:920–927
4. Andrews RG, Bensinger WI, Knitter GH, Bartelmez SH, Longin K, Bernstein ID, Appelbaum FR, Zsebo KM (1992) The ligand for c-kit, stem cell factor, stimulates the circulation of cells that engraft lethally irradiated baboons. Blood 80:2715–2720
5. Baldomero H, Gratwohl M, Gratwohl A, Tichelli A, Niederwieser D, Madrigal A, Frauendorfer K (2011) The EBMT activity survey 2009: trends over the past 5 years. Bone Marrow Transplant 46:485–501
6. Ballen KK, Shpall EJ, Avigan D, Yeap BY, Fisher DC, McDermott K, Dey BR, Attar E, McAfee S, Konopleva M, Antin JH, Spitzer TR (2007) Phase I trial of parathyroid hormone to facilitate stem cell mobilization. Biol Blood Marrow Transplant 13:838–843
7. Banna GL, Simonelli M, Santoro A (2007) High-dose chemotherapy followed by autologous hematopoietic stem-cell transplantation for the treatment of solid tumors in adults: a critical review. Curr Stem Cell Res Ther 2:65–82
8. Barrett D, Fish JD, Grupp SA (2010) Autologous and allogeneic cellular therapies for high-risk pediatric solid tumors. Pediatr Clin North Am 57:47–66
9. Bonig H, Wundes A, Chang KH, Lucas S, Papayannopoulou T (2008) Increased numbers of circulating hematopoietic stem/progenitor cells are chronically maintained in patients treated with the CD49d blocking antibody natalizumab. Blood 111:3439–3441
10. Bonig H, Watts KL, Chang KH, Kiem HP, Papayannopoulou T (2009) Concurrent blockade of alpha4-integrin and CXCR4 in hematopoietic stem/progenitor cell mobilization. Stem Cells 27:836–837
11. Brugger W, Bross K, Frisch J, Dern P, Weber B, Mertelsmann R, Kanz L (1992) Mobilization of peripheral blood progenitor cells by sequential administration of interleukin-3 and granulocyte-macrophage colony-stimulating factor following polychemotherapy with etoposide, ifosfamide, and cisplatin. Blood 79:1193–1200
12. Brunner S, Zaruba MM, Huber B, David R, Vallaster M, Assmann G, Mueller-Hoecker J, Franz WM (2008) Parathyroid hormone effectively induces mobilization of progenitor cells without depletion of bone marrow. Exp Hematol 36:1157–1166
13. Bruns I, Steidl U, Kronenwett R, Fenk R, Graef T, Rohr UP, Neumann F, Fischer J, Scheid C, Hubel K, Haas R, Kobbe G (2006) A single dose of 6 or 12 mg of pegfilgrastim for peripheral blood progenitor cell mobilization results in similar yields of CD34+ progenitors in patients with multiple myeloma. Transfusion 46:180–185
14. Bruns I, Steidl U, Fischer JC, Czibere A, Kobbe G, Raschke S, Singh R, Fenk R, Rosskopf M, Pechtel S, von HA, von HA, Wernet P, Tenen DG, Haas R, Kronenwett R (2008) Pegylated granulocyte colony-stimulating factor mobilizes CD34+ cells with different stem and progenitor subsets and distinct functional properties in comparison with unconjugated granulocyte colony-stimulating factor. Haematologica 93:347–355
15. Cardenoux C, Demeocq F, Kanold J, Merlin E, Oudot C, Piguet C, Roussanne MC (2010) Pegfilgrastim plus AMD 3100 for stem-cell mobilization in children. Pediatr Blood Cancer 55:769
16. Coppolino G, Bolignano D, De PL, Giulino C, Mannella A, Riccio M, Mascaro MA, Lombardi G, Fuiano G, Lombardi L, Buemi M (2011) Parathyroid Hormone and Mobilization of Circulating Bone Marrow-Derived Cells in Uremic Patients. J. Investig, Med
17. Costa LJ, Alexander ET, Hogan KR, Schaub C, Fouts TV, Stuart RK (2011) Development and validation of a decision-making algorithm to guide the use of plerixafor for autologous hematopoietic stem cell mobilization. Bone Marrow Transplant 46:64–69
18. Craddock CF, Nakamoto B, Andrews RG, Priestley GV, Papayannopoulou T (1997) Antibodies to VLA4 integrin mobilize long-term repopulating cells and augment cytokine-induced mobilization in primates and mice. Blood 90:4779–4788
19. Curran MP, Goa KL (2002) Pegfilgrastim. Drugs 62:1207–1213

20. Dazzi C, Cariello A, Rosti G, Monti G, Sebastiani L, Argnani M, Nicoletti P, Tienghi A, Leoni M, Fiorentini G, Turci D, Giovanis P, De GU, Marangolo M (1999) Peripheral blood progenitor cell (PBPC) mobilization in heavily pretreated patients with germ cell tumors: a report of 34 cases. Bone Marrow Transplant 23:529–532
21. Farquhar C, Marjoribanks J, Basser R, Hetrick S, Lethaby A (2005a) High dose chemotherapy and autologous bone marrow or stem cell transplantation versus conventional chemotherapy for women with metastatic breast cancer. Cochrane Database Syst Rev CD003142
22. Farquhar C, Marjoribanks J, Basser R, Lethaby A (2005b) High dose chemotherapy and autologous bone marrow or stem cell transplantation versus conventional chemotherapy for women with early poor prognosis breast cancer. Cochrane Database Syst Rev CD003139
23. Ford CD, Green W, Warenski S, Petersen FB (2004) Effect of prior chemotherapy on hematopoietic stem cell mobilization. Bone Marrow Transplant 33:901–905
24. Goldschmidt H, Hegenbart U, Wallmeier M, Hohaus S, Haas R (1997) Factors influencing collection of peripheral blood progenitor cells following high-dose cyclophosphamide and granulocyte colony-stimulating factor in patients with multiple myeloma. Br J Haematol 98:736–744
25. Gratwohl A, Schmid O, Baldomero H, Horisberger B, Urbano-Ispizua A (2004) Haematopoietic stem cell transplantation (HSCT) in Europe 2002. Changes in indication and impact of team density. A report of the EBMT activity survey. Bone Marrow Transplant 34:855–875
26. Haas R, Ehrhardt R, Witt B, Goldschmidt H, Hohaus S, Pforsich M, Ehrlich H, Farber L, Hunstein W (1993) Autografting with peripheral blood stem cells mobilized by sequential interleukin-3/granulocyte-macrophage colony-stimulating factor following high-dose chemotherapy in non-Hodgkin's lymphoma. Bone Marrow Transplant 12:643–649
27. Haas R, Mohle R, Fruhauf S, Goldschmidt H, Witt B, Flentje M, Wannenmacher M, Hunstein W (1994) Patient characteristics associated with successful mobilizing and autografting of peripheral blood progenitor cells in malignant lymphoma. Blood 83:3787–3794
28. Hamamura K, Matsuda H, Takeuchi Y, Habu S, Yagita H, Okumura K (1996) A critical role of VLA-4 in erythropoiesis in vivo. Blood 87:2513–2517
29. Horwitz M, Schriber J, Libby EN, Gorak EJ, Mody P, Marulkar S, Holman PR (2010) Efficacy and safety of hematopoietic stem cell (HSC) remobilization with plerixafor plus G-CSF in patients with non-hematologic malignancies. J Clin Oncol 28(15):e15072
30. Hunter MG, Bawden L, Brotherton D, Craig S, Cribbes S, Czaplewski LG, Dexter TM, Drummond AH, Gearing AH, Heyworth CM, Lord BI, McCourt M, Varley PG, Wood LM, Edwards RM, Lewis PJ (1995) BB-10010: an active variant of human macrophage inflammatory protein-1 alpha with improved pharmaceutical properties. Blood 86:4400–4408
31. Huttenlocher A, Ginsberg MH, Horwitz AF (1996) Modulation of cell migration by integrin-mediated cytoskeletal linkages and ligand-binding affinity. J Cell Biol 134:1551–1562
32. Iikura Y, Sakamoto Y, Imai T, Akai L, Matsuoka T, Sugihara K, Utumi M, Tomikawa M (2001) Dolphin-assisted seawater therapy for severe atopic dermatitis: An immunological and psychological study. Int Arch Allergy Immunol 124:389–390
33. Junghanss C, Leithauser M, Wilhelm S, Kleine HD, Knopp A, Decker S, Alscher A, Casper J, Kohne CH, Freund M (2001) High-dose etoposide phosphate and G-CSF mobilizes peripheral blood stem cells in patients that previously failed to mobilize. Ann Hematol 80:96–102
34. Kanfer EJ, McGuigan D, Samson D, Abboudi Z, Abrahamson G, Apperley JF, Chilcott S, Craddock C, Davis J, MacDonald C, Macdonald D, Olavarria E, Philpott N, Rustin GJ, Seckl MJ, Sekhar M, Stern S, Newlands ES (1998) High-dose etoposide with granulocyte colony-stimulating factor for mobilization of peripheral blood progenitor cells: efficacy and toxicity at three dose levels. Br J Cancer 78:928–932
35. Khaldoyanidi S, Denzel A, Zoller M (1996) Requirement for CD44 in proliferation and homing of hematopoietic precursor cells. J Leukoc Biol 60:579–592
36. Kobbe G, Soehngen D, Heyll A, Fischer J, Thiele KP, Aul C, Wernet P (1997) Large volume leukapheresis maximizes the progenitor cell yield for allogeneic peripheral blood progenitor donation. J Hematother 6:125–131

37. Kobbe G, Sohngen D, Bauser U, Schneider P, Germing U, Thiele KP, Rieth C, Hunerliturkoglu A, Fischer J, Frick M, Wernet P, Aul C, Heyll A (1999) Factors influencing G-CSF-mediated mobilization of hematopoietic progenitor cells during steady-state hematopoiesis in patients with malignant lymphoma and multiple myeloma. Ann Hematol 78:456–462
38. Kobbe G, Bruns I, Fenk R, Czibere A, Haas R (2009) Pegfilgrastim for PBSC mobilization and autologous haematopoietic SCT. Bone Marrow Transplant 43:669–677
39. Kobold S, Isernhagen J, Hubel K, Kilic N, Bogner C, Frickhofen N, Bokemeyer C, Fiedler W (2011) Plerixafor is effective and safe for stem cell mobilization in heavily pretreated germ cell tumor patients. Bone Marrow Transplant 46:1053–1056
40. Kolbe K, Peschel C, Rupilius B, Despres D, Burger K, Sklenar I, Farber L, Huber C, Derigs HG (1997) Peripheral blood stem cell (PBSC) mobilization with chemotherapy followed by sequential IL-3 and G-CSF administration in extensively pretreated patients. Bone Marrow Transplant 20:1027–1032
41. Kollmannsberger C, Beyer J, Bokemeyer C (2009) High-dose chemotherapy in nonseminomatous germ cell cancer. BJU Int 104:1398–1403
42. Kovach NL, Lin N, Yednock T, Harlan JM, Broudy VC (1995) Stem cell factor modulates avidity of alpha 4 beta 1 and alpha 5 beta 1 integrins expressed on hematopoietic cell lines. Blood 85:159–167
43. Laterveer L, Lindley IJ, Heemskerk DP, Camps JA, Pauwels EK, Willemze R, Fibbe WE (1996) Rapid mobilization of hematopoietic progenitor cells in rhesus monkeys by a single intravenous injection of interleukin-8. Blood 87:781–788
44. Leavesley DI, Oliver JM, Swart BW, Berndt MC, Haylock DN, Simmons PJ (1994) Signals from platelet/endothelial cell adhesion molecule enhance the adhesive activity of the very late antigen-4 integrin of human CD34+ hemopoietic progenitor cells. J Immunol 153:4673–4683
45. Lemoli RM, Fogli M, Fortuna A, Motta MR, Rizzi S, Benini C, Tura S (1993) Interleukin-11 stimulates the proliferation of human hematopoietic CD34+ and CD34+CD33-DR- cells and synergizes with stem cell factor, interleukin-3, and granulocyte-macrophage colony-stimulating factor. Exp Hematol 21:1668–1672
46. Levesque JP, Leavesley DI, Niutta S, Vadas M, Simmons PJ (1995) Cytokines increase human hemopoietic cell adhesiveness by activation of very late antigen (VLA)-4 and VLA-5 integrins. J Exp Med 181:1805–1815
47. Lichterfeld M, Martin S, Burkly L, Haas R, Kronenwett R (2000) Mobilization of CD34+ haematopoietic stem cells is associated with a functional inactivation of the integrin very late antigen 4. Br J Haematol 110:71–81
48. Lie AK, Hui CH, Rawling T, Dyson PG, Thorp D, Benic J, Rawling CM, Toogood I, Horvath N, Simmons PJ, To LB (1998) Granulocyte colony-stimulating factor (G-CSF) dose-dependent efficacy in peripheral blood stem cell mobilization in patients who had failed initial mobilization with chemotherapy and G-CSF. Bone Marrow Transplant 22:853–857
49. Lorch A, Kollmannsberger C, Hartmann JT, Metzner B, Schmidt-Wolf IG, Berdel WE, Weissinger F, Schleicher J, Egerer G, Haas A, Schirren R, Beyer J, Bokemeyer C, Rick O (2007) Single versus sequential high-dose chemotherapy in patients with relapsed or refractory germ cell tumors: a prospective randomized multicenter trial of the German Testicular Cancer Study Group. J Clin Oncol 25:2778–2784
50. Lorch A, Bascoul-Mollevi C, Kramar A, Einhorn L, Necchi A, Massard C, De GU, Flechon A, Margolin K, Lotz JP, Germa-Lluch JR, Powles T, Kollmannsberger C, Beyer J (2011) Conventional-dose versus high-dose chemotherapy as first salvage treatment in male patients with metastatic germ cell tumors: evidence from a large international database. J Clin Oncol 29:2178–2184
51. Martin-Bermudo MD, Dunin-Borkowski OM, Brown NH (1998) Modulation of integrin activity is vital for morphogenesis. J Cell Biol 141:1073–1081
52. Mauch P, Lamont C, Neben TY, Quinto C, Goldman SJ, Witsell A (1995) Hematopoietic stem cells in the blood after stem cell factor and interleukin-11 administration: evidence for different mechanisms of mobilization. Blood 86:4674–4680

53. Miyake K, Medina KL, Hayashi S, Ono S, Hamaoka T, Kincade PW (1990) Monoclonal antibodies to Pgp-1/CD44 block lympho-hemopoiesis in long-term bone marrow cultures. J Exp Med 171:477–488
54. Miyake K, Weissman IL, Greenberger JS, Kincade PW (1991) Evidence for a role of the integrin VLA-4 in lympho-hemopoiesis. J Exp Med 173:599–607
55. Modak S, Cheung IY, Kushner BH, Kramer K, Reich L, Cheung NK (2011) Plerixafor plus granulocyte-colony stimulating factor for autologous hematopoietic stem cell mobilization in patients with metastatic neuroblastoma. Pediatr, Blood Cancer
56. Mohle R, Murea S, Kirsch M, Haas R (1995) Differential expression of L-selectin, VLA-4, and LFA-1 on CD34+ progenitor cells from bone marrow and peripheral blood during G-CSF-enhanced recovery. Exp Hematol 23:1535–1542
57. Mohle R, Moore MA, Nachman RL, Rafii S (1997) Transendothelial migration of CD34+ and mature hematopoietic cells: an in vitro study using a human bone marrow endothelial cell line. Blood 89:72–80
58. Molineux G, Kinstler O, Briddell B, Hartley C, McElroy P, Kerzic P, Sutherland W, Stoney G, Kern B, Fletcher FA, Cohen A, Korach E, Ulich T, McNiece I, Lockbaum P, Miller-Messana MA, Gardner S, Hunt T, Schwab G (1999) A new form of Filgrastim with sustained duration in vivo and enhanced ability to mobilize PBPC in both mice and humans. Exp Hematol 27:1724–1734
59. Moncada V, Bolan C, Yau YY, Leitman SF (2003) Analysis of PBPC cell yields during large-volume leukapheresis of subjects with a poor mobilization response to filgrastim. Transfusion 43:495–501
60. Morris T, Ranaghan L, Drake M (1999) Poor stem cell mobilizers–variation in response to G-CSF dose escalation. Bone Marrow Transplant 24:448–449
61. Muramaki M, Miyake H, Hara S, Kamidono S, Hara I (2003) Predicting factors for collection of peripheral blood stem cells in patients with advanced germ cell tumors after cisplatin-based combination chemotherapy. Oncol Rep 10:1545–1549
62. Oostendorp RA, Spitzer E, Brandl M, Eaves CJ, Dormer P (1998) Evidence for differences in the mechanisms by which antibodies against CD44 promote adhesion of erythroid and granulopoietic progenitors to marrow stromal cells. Br J Haematol 101:436–445
63. Papayannopoulou T, Nakamoto B (1993) Peripheralization of hemopoietic progenitors in primates treated with anti-VLA4 integrin. Proc Natl Acad Sci USA 90:9374–9378
64. Papayannopoulou T, Craddock C, Nakamoto B, Priestley GV, Wolf NS (1995) The VLA4/VCAM-1 adhesion pathway defines contrasting mechanisms of lodgement of transplanted murine hemopoietic progenitors between bone marrow and spleen. Proc Natl Acad Sci USA 92:9647–9651
65. Papayannopoulou T, Priestley GV, Nakamoto B (1998) Anti-VLA4/VCAM-1-induced mobilization requires cooperative signaling through the kit/mkit ligand pathway. Blood 91: 2231–2239
66. Peinemann F, Smith LA, Kromp M, Bartel C, Kroger N, Kulig M (2011) Autologous hematopoietic stem cell transplantation following high-dose chemotherapy for non-rhabdomyosarcoma soft tissue sarcomas. Cochrane Database Syst Rev (2): CD008216
67. Prosper F, Stroncek D, McCarthy JB, Verfaillie CM (1998) Mobilization and homing of peripheral blood progenitors is related to reversible downregulation of alpha4 beta1 integrin expression and function. J Clin Invest 101:2456–2467
68. Ramirez P, Rettig MP, Uy GL, Deych E, Holt MS, Ritchey JK, DiPersio JF (2009) BIO5192, a small molecule inhibitor of VLA-4, mobilizes hematopoietic stem and progenitor cells. Blood 114:1340–1343
69. Rick O, Bokemeyer C, Beyer J, Hartmann JT, Schwella N, Kingreen D, Neureither S, Metzner B, Casper J, Wandt H, Hartmann F, Schmoll HJ, Derigs G, Gerl A, Berdel WE, Kanz L, Siegert W (2001) Salvage treatment with paclitaxel, ifosfamide, and cisplatin plus high-dose carboplatin, etoposide, and thiotepa followed by autologous stem-cell rescue in patients with relapsed or refractory germ cell cancer. J Clin Oncol 19:81–88

70. Rosel M, Khaldoyanidi S, Zawadzki V, Zoller M (1999) Involvement of CD44 variant isoform v10 in progenitor cell adhesion and maturation. Exp Hematol 27:698–711
71. Saure C, Weigelt C, Schroeder T, Klarner V, Galonska L, Haas R, Kobbe G (2010) Plerixafor enables successful hematopoietic stem cell collection in an extensively pretreated patient with testicular cancer. Acta Haematol 124:235–238
72. Shattil SJ, Kashiwagi H, Pampori N (1998) Integrin signaling: the platelet paradigm. Blood 91:2645–2657
73. Soligo D, Schiro R, Luksch R, Manara G, Quirici N, Parravicini C, Lambertenghi DG (1990) Expression of integrins in human bone marrow. Br J Haematol 76:323–332
74. Steidl U, Fenk R, Bruns I, Neumann F, Kondakci M, Hoyer B, Graf T, Rohr UP, Bork S, Kronenwett R, Haas R, Kobbe G (2005) Successful transplantation of peripheral blood stem cells mobilized by chemotherapy and a single dose of pegylated G-CSF in patients with multiple myeloma. Bone Marrow Transplant 35:33–36
75. Toledano H, Yahel A, Cohen IJ, Yaniv I, Stein J (2010) Successful mobilization, harvest and transplant of peripheral blood stem cells using AMD3100 and G-CSF following high dose craniospinal irradiation for medulloblastoma in a young child. Pediatr Blood Cancer 54:613–615
76. Tuffaha H, bdel-Rahman FA (2010) Successful stem-cell mobilization and transplantation using plerixafor in a patient with a germ cell tumor. Hematol Oncol Stem Cell Ther 3:203–205
77. Verfaillie CM, Gupta P, Prosper F, Hurley R, Lundell B, Bhatia R (1999) The Hematopoietic Microenvironment: Stromal Extracellular Matrix Components As Growth Regulators For Human Hematopoietic Progenitors. Hematology 4:321–333
78. Vermeulen M, Le PF, Gagnerault MC, Mary JY, Sainteny F, Lepault F (1998) Role of adhesion molecules in the homing and mobilization of murine hematopoietic stem and progenitor cells. Blood 92:894–900
79. Whetton AD, Graham GJ (1999) Homing and mobilization in the stem cell niche. Trends Cell Biol 9:233–238
80. Yamaguchi M, Ikebuchi K, Hirayama F, Sato N, Mogi Y, Ohkawara J, Yoshikawa Y, Sawada K, Koike T, Sekiguchi S (1998) Different adhesive characteristics and VLA-4 expression of CD34(+) progenitors in G0/G1 versus S+G2/M phases of the cell cycle. Blood 92:842–848
81. Yanai N, Sekine C, Yagita H, Obinata M (1994) Roles for integrin very late activation antigen-4 in stroma-dependent erythropoiesis. Blood 83:2844–2850
82. Zohren F, Toutzaris D, Klarner V, Hartung HP, Kieseier B, Haas R (2008) The monoclonal anti-VLA-4 antibody natalizumab mobilizes $CD34^+$ hematopoietic progenitor cells in humans. Blood 111:3893–3895

Chapter 14
Mobilization with Chemotherapy + G-CSF + Plerixafor in Europe: The Italian Experience

Roberto M. Lemoli and Alessandra D' Addio

Abstract The standard mobilization strategy in the majority of the European Transplant Centers involves the combination of disease-specific chemotherapy with granulocyte colony-stimulating factor (G-CSF) (chemomobilization) to obtain both the reduction of tumor burden and the mobilization of peripheral blood stem cells (PBSCs). However, a significant proportion of patients with lymphoid malignancies fail to mobilize enough PBSCs to proceed to autotransplantation. In this regard, chemomobilization does not prevent poor mobilization. Plerixafor (previously known as AMD 3100) has been shown to rapidly increase the number of circulating $CD34^+$ stem/progenitor cells from marrow niches to the circulation when administered alone or in combination with G-CSF. There is limited experience on combining plerixafor with chemotherapy plus G-CSF in patients who mobilize poorly although current evidence suggests that the addition of plerixafor is safe and effective in the large majority of patients with low blood $CD34^+$ cell counts after mobilization and/or poor yield after the first collection(s) (poor mobilizers). Therefore, the mechanism of action of plerixafor inducing the rapid release of $CD34^+$ cells from the bone marrow to the peripheral blood makes this molecule suitable for its "preemptive" use in patients who are hard to mobilize.

Keywords Chemomobilization • Proven poor mobilizer • Predicted poor mobilizer

---

R.M. Lemoli (✉)
Department of Hematology and Oncological Sciences "L. & A. Seràgnoli",
Istitute of Hematology, University of Bologna, Via Massarenti, Bologna 9 40138, Italy
e-mail: roberto.lemoli@unibo.it

A. D' Addio
Hematology Unit, Azienda Istituti Ospitalieri, Cremona, Italy

S. Fruehauf et al. (eds.), *Novel Developments in Stem Cell Mobilization: Focus on CXCR4*, DOI 10.1007/978-1-4614-1960-0_14,

Abbreviations

AHP	Analytic hierarchy process
ASCT	Autologous stem cell transplantation
BM	Bone marrow
G-CSF	Granulocyte colony-stimulating factor
GITMO	Italian Group for stem cell transplantation
GM-CSF	Granulocyte–macrophage colony-stimulating factor
HL	Hodgkin's lymphoma
LVL	Large volume leukapheresis
MM	Multiple myeloma
NHL	Non-Hodgkin's lymphoma
PB	Peripheral blood
PBSCs	Peripheral blood stem cells
WBC	White blood cell

Chemomobilization: The Rationale

High-dose chemotherapy with peripheral blood stem cell (PBSC) support is considered the best therapeutic option for resistant/relapsed non-Hodgkin's lymphoma (NHL), Hodgkin's lymphoma (HL) patients and multiple myeloma (MM) patients [1]. Several studies have conclusively demonstrated that the successful engraftment of PBSCs relies mostly on $CD34^+$ stem/progenitor cell dose, thus making effective PBSC mobilization a critical step for the entire procedure [2].

The minimum dose of $CD34^+$ cells to provide a high likelihood of successful PBSC engraftment is widely considered to be greater than 2×10^6 cells/kg recipient body weight [3–6], whereas the "optimal" number is considered to be $4–6 \times 10^6$ $CD34^+$ cells/kg. As higher numbers of reinfused $CD34^+$ cells have been shown to result in earlier hematopoietic recovery after transplantation and may correlate with longer disease-free and overall survival than lower cell doses [7–9], most centers attempt to collect the optimal PBSC number (target cell dose) rather than the minimum one.

Most mobilization regimens currently used, especially in Europe, in patients with MM and lymphoma combine the administration of granulocyte colony-stimulating factor (G-CSF) with the delivery of a disease-specific chemotherapy or cyclophosphamide to achieve higher $CD34^+$ cell yields than treatment with G-CSF alone [10]. Although failure rates with chemomobilization seem to be as high as with G-CSF alone [3–8], potential clinical benefits of chemomobilization regimens include fewer number of required apheresis sessions compared to G-CSF alone and, most important, second line salvage chemomobilizing regimens, particularly in lymphoma patients, have the main objective to reduce the tumor load and tumor cell contamination in the apheresis product. As for MM patients, there is no convincing evidence that cyclophosphamide has the same role for disease control [10]. When mobilization with chemotherapy plus G-CSF and G-CSF alone have been compared

[1, 11], the addition of chemotherapy resulted in higher infectious morbidity and mucositis incidence, longer duration of neutropenia, need of additional red cell and platelets transfusions, and prolonged hospitalization compared to mobilization with growth factors alone. Furthermore, G-CSF alone allows the easier scheduling of PBSC collection avoiding weekend sessions. Overall, regardless of the addition of chemotherapy, the failure rate with current mobilizing strategies varies between 5 and 40% [1, 10, 12] leading often to suboptimal grafts associated with delayed hematopoietic recovery, need for remobilization or marrow harvest and, sometimes, to treatments other than autologous stem cell transplantation (ASCT) [13–15].

The ideal mobilization regimen would mobilize the optimal number of CD34$^+$ cells in as few apheresis sessions as possible, would increase the proportion of patients proceeding to transplantation, followed by prompt and durable engraftment and high survival rates, with minimal toxicity.

Plerixafor: Mechanism of Action and Rapid Peak Time

Plerixafor (formerly AMD3100) is a CXCR4 chemokine antagonist that has been shown to increase the number of circulating CD34$^+$ cells in healthy volunteers and cancer patients alone or with G-CSF [16]. The key feature of this chemokine receptor–ligand interaction is the rapidity of the mobilization process and stands in clear contrast with G-CSF-based mobilization where up to 4 days of treatment is required before the significant increase of circulating CD34$^+$ cells is observed [17]. Consistent with its antagonistic activity on the CXCR4 receptor, plerixafor also increases the number of circulating white blood cells (WBCs). There are two distinct phases of stem cell mobilization according to different routes of administration: the peak occurs approximately 4 h after intravenous injection, while 10–12 h are required for stem cell release from the bone marrow (BM) after subcutaneous administration. By 24 h, the mobilizing effect of plerixafor is returned to baseline or close to baseline [18]. Therefore, the rapid biological activity of plerixafor allows its administration "on demand" without planning the timing of administration in advance.

Factors Influencing Chemomobilization During and Postmobilization

While the extensive review of the predictive factors affecting PBSC mobilization is beyond the scope of this chapter, few concepts should be discussed concerning the potential negative role of chemotherapy.

During- and postmobilization factors have poorly been exploited due to the lack, so far, of rescue strategies. It is well known that febrile neutropenia is one major complication after administration of mobilizing chemotherapy. The release of proinflammatory cytokines negatively affects stem cell proliferation and mobilization. Need for supportive care such as antibiotics for febrile neutropenia and blood product support is associated with mobilization failure in patients with NHL [10]. Moreover, in patients receiving mobilization with a combination of chemotherapy and G-CSF, slow leukocyte and platelet recovery as well as anemia indicate poor marrow function. However, type and dose of chemotherapy may influence the risk of mobilization failure as severe thrombocytopenia induced by alkylating agents administered during mobilization can be a risk factor for mobilization failure while high-dose cytarabine mobilization regimen often induces severe thrombocytopenia and neutropenia without negatively affect stem cell mobilization [12].

Other factors predicting mobilization failure are: delayed or anticipated timing of apheresis (due to insufficient circulating stem cells monitoring), small volume of processed blood, technical or clinical problems occurring during leukapheresis that may affect PBSC collection even in patients showing a satisfactory peak of $CD34^+$ cells in the peripheral blood (PB).

Nevertheless, the most important factor predicting PBSC harvest failure is the number of circulating $CD34^+$ cells. PB $CD34^+$ cell counts have been shown to correlate with apheresis collections and are widely used as the main parameter to start apheresis session [2]. During the chemomobilization procedure, prior to apheresis, useful markers for successful mobilization have been considered the kinetics of recovery of circulating WBC and the rapid increase of $CD34^+$ cells [11]. Generally, a peak value >20 $CD34^+$ cells/μL in the PB is considered a reliable indicator of good mobilization ability although many transplant centers use 10 cells/μL as the minimum threshold to commence leukapheresis [17]. Conversely, slow increase of PB $CD34^+$ counts at the time of marrow recovery may be indicative of hard-to-mobilize patients. Reviewing the database of the Cell Processing Laboratory of the Institute "Seràgnoli" we found that, after chemomobilization, the combination of low PB $CD34^+$ counts (e.g., <10/μL) and high WBC (e.g., $>5\text{–}10 \times 10^9$/L) predicts for poor, or none, PBSC collection (i.e., $<2 \times 10^6$ $CD34^+$ cells/kg) to proceed to ASCT.

While peak mobilization after G-CSF alone usually occurs 4–5 days after initiation of G-CSF [19], peak mobilization following chemotherapy-based regimens is more variable and generally occurs 10–18 days after last dose of chemotherapy according to different regimens and disease. Thus, daily monitoring of PB $CD34^+$ cells is necessary at the time of hematopoietic recovery during chemomobilization to identify the peak mobilization and to predict poor mobilization. Early identification of poor mobilizers during chemomobilization, regardless of upfront potential predictive risk factors, allows early intervention with plerixafor or other novel drugs.

Who Are the "Proven Poor Mobilizer"?

The definition of "poor" mobilization varies, due to different parameters proposed by different transplant centers to evaluate the extent of mobilization: peak of circulating $CD34^+$ cells, kinetics of increase of PB $CD34^+$ cells, cumulative apheresis yield, the percent of candidate patients undergoing ASCT. Thus, literature data are difficult to analyze and to compare to each other. For these reasons, a GITMO (Italian Group for Stem Cell Transplantation) working group has recently applied the analytic hierarchy process (AHP), a decision making method which was developed to establish priorities and to make the best decision when both quantitative and qualitative aspects of a problem have to be considered and poor information is available [20], to propose the definition of "poor mobilizer" for lymphoproliferative disease. A uniform definition would be important for assessment of PBSC mobilization in clinical trials and as a decision criterion for developing mobilization strategies in clinical practice. Two different definitions were given: "proven poor mobilizer" and "predicted poor mobilizer" [20].

The "proven poor mobilizer" was defined as a patient receiving adequate mobilization (G-CSF dose ≥10 μg/kg if used alone or ≥5 μg/kg after chemotherapy) showing: peak $CD34^+$ circulating cell count <20/μL on day 4–6 after start of mobilization with G-CSF alone or up to 20 days after chemotherapy and G-CSF *or* a patient with less than 2.0×10^6 harvested $CD34^+$ cells/kg (i.e., minimum safe dose for each planned ASCT).

According to this definition, daily monitoring of PB $CD34^+$ cell counts showing suboptimal mobilization (i.e., <20 $CD34^+$ cells/μL) becomes very important. Looking at plerixafor rapid biological activity, the selective preemptive addition of plerixafor can be considered to avoid poor mobilization.

Who Are the "Predicted Poor Mobilizer"?

The "predicted poor mobilizer" was defined as a patient who holds at least one major criterion or at least two minor criteria:

Major Criteria

- Failed previous mobilization attempt not otherwise specified.
- Prior extensive radiotherapy to marrow bearing tissue.
- Full courses of previous therapy including melphalan, fludarabine or other therapies potentially affecting stem cell mobilization.

Minor Criteria

- Advanced phase disease, i.e., at least two prior cytotoxic lines.
- Refractory disease.
- Extensive BM involvement at mobilization.
- BM cellularity <30% at mobilization.
- Age >65 years.

In this category of patients, it may be important that novel mobilization strategies could be used upfront (i.e., with the first mobilization attempt), so that the patient can proceed earlier to high-dose chemotherapy without the need of remobilization.

Therapeutic Options for Poor Mobilizers After Chemomobilization

A variety of strategies have been proposed to increase the CD34⁺ cells yield both in patients who are at risk for poor mobilization, as well as in patients who had failed the first mobilization attempt. These strategies include large volume leukapheresis (LVL), which can be defined as the processing of 3–6 blood volumes, off-label use of high-doses of G-CSF (i.e., 16–32 μg/kg subcutaneously daily to 12–16 μg/kg subcutaneously twice daily), G-CSF sequentially or concurrently combined with GM-CSF (granulocyte–monocyte colony-stimulating factor) (G-CSF, 5–10 μg/kg; GM-CSF, 5 μg/kg or 250 $\mu g/m^2$) with or without chemotherapeutic agents, regimens combining high-dose chemotherapy or novel chemotherapeutic agents with G-CSF, G-CSF-primed BM harvest [21–24].

Published data demonstrate that over 80–90% of all ASCT world-wide are performed using either cytokine-based mobilization or chemomobilization [25]. As discussed above, chemomobilization has been shown in various settings to be more effective than growth factors alone in terms of stem cell number and fewer apheresis sessions, although chemotherapy-related toxicity makes this combination problematic if the chemotherapy is used only for mobilization and not to treat the underlying disease.

Remobilization strategies, including high-dose G-CSF, G-CSF plus GM-CSF, and G-CSF plus chemotherapy, produce success rates of 23–65%, depending on the definition of failure and on whether or not the subsequent mobilization products were pooled.

In a recent single center series using predominantly G-CSF for mobilization (>90% of cases on a total of over 1,000 patients with lymphoproliferative disorders), the failure rates of the first mobilization attempt, defined as the collection of less than 2×10^6 $CD34^+$ cells/kg, were 18.8 and 18.6% for chemomobilization and G-CSF alone, respectively. Mobilized, preapheresis, PB $CD34^+$ count correlated with first day apheresis yield and 20 cells/μL was the minimum threshold needed for a successful day 1 collection. A total of 269 patients underwent subsequent remobilization using chemomobilization, G-CSF, and/or GM-CSF, and G-CSF plus plerixafor. Only 23% of remobilized patients achieved $\geq 2 \times 10^6$ $CD34^+$ cells/kg [13]. In particular, failure rates were 73.5% in patients remobilized with chemotherapy + G-CSF, 81.6% in patients remobilized with growth factors alone but only 27.8% in patients mobilized with G-CSF plus plerixafor. Therefore, this study underlines the concept that patients who fail initial mobilization, either chemomobilization or G-CSF alone, are more likely to fail remobilization unless novel molecules are used. Furthermore, in a compassionate use study of 115 patients who had failed a previous mobilization, the success rate (i.e., $>2 \times 10^6$ $CD34^+$ cells collected/kg) of G-CSF plus plerixafor was 60.3% for NHL, 71.4% for MM and 76.5% for HL, respectively [25] with no difference between patients treated upfront with G-CSF alone or chemomobilization. Similarly, in a European compassionate use series, combination of G-CSF and plerixafor gave successful collections in 71% of patients who had failed a previous mobilization, mostly chemotherapy + G-CSF [26].

The rate of successful remobilization with plerixafor plus G-CSF following failed mobilization has proved to be superior to most remobilization attempts including G-CSF, other cytokines, chemotherapy, and other investigational agents. However, even if successful, remobilization often results in the delay of the delivery of high-dose chemotherapy and ASCT and the substantial use of financial resources.

Plerixafor in Combination with Chemomobilization

Very few data are available on the safety and efficacy of administration of plerixafor added to G-CSF after chemotherapy to mobilize PBSCs. The rationale to use plerixafor in combination with chemobilization is to improve stem cell mobilization and overcome the risk of mobilization failure based on plerixafor rapid mechanism of action and daily monitoring of PB CD34^{+} cells.

In a pilot study conducted by Dugan et al. [27], the safety of plerixafor administration in combination with chemotherapy plus G-CSF was explored. MM and lymphoma patients, who received chemotherapy plus G-CSF mobilization regimen to collect PBSCs prior ASCT, were included in the study. To understand the effects of plerixafor after mobilization with chemotherapy and G-CSF, the study was conducted in four different cohorts. The main goals of the four cohorts were: to evaluate the capacity and the relative contribution of plerixafor to enhance CD34^{+} cell collection in combination of chemotherapy plus G-CSF (cohorts A and B), to evaluate the safety and efficacy of plerixafor as a rescue regimen for patients who failed mobilization with chemotherapy and G-CSF (cohort C) and to explore the potential role of plerixafor to accelerate the time to PBSC collection after WBC recovery from chemotherapy and G-CSF mobilization (cohort D). All patients received plerixafor 0.24 mg/kg/day subcutaneously for up to 5 days. In this study, 40/44 (26 MM and 14 NHL) patients were treated with plerixafor. Plerixafor was well tolerated and its addition to a chemomobilization regimen resulted in an increased mobilization of PBSCs. The mean rate of increase of PB CD34^{+} cells was 2.8 cells/μL/h pre- and 13.3 cells/μL/h post plerixafor administration. Engraftment results after myeloablative chemotherapy and reinfusion of plerixafor-mobilized PBSCs were comparable to those obtained with PBSCs mobilized without plerixafor in historical patients. The data obtained from the analysis of the cohorts suggest that plerixafor can safely be added to chemotherapy-based mobilization regimens and may accelerate the rate of increase in CD34^{+} cells.

In our study [28], we analyzed the mobilization kinetics of 13 MM and lymphoma patients, potential candidates for ASCT, who were failing PBSC mobilization after disease-specific chemotherapy plus G-CSF. To prevent mobilization failure, plerixafor 0.24 mg/kg was added to chemomobilization for up to three injections. MM patients (three) received different induction therapies, but none of them had been treated with lenalidomide or local radiotherapy, and none was in complete remission at the time of mobilization. All lymphoma patients (ten) were heavily pretreated before mobilization and one of them had received fludarabine as induction therapy. Mobilization regimens combining chemotherapy and G-CSF were selected

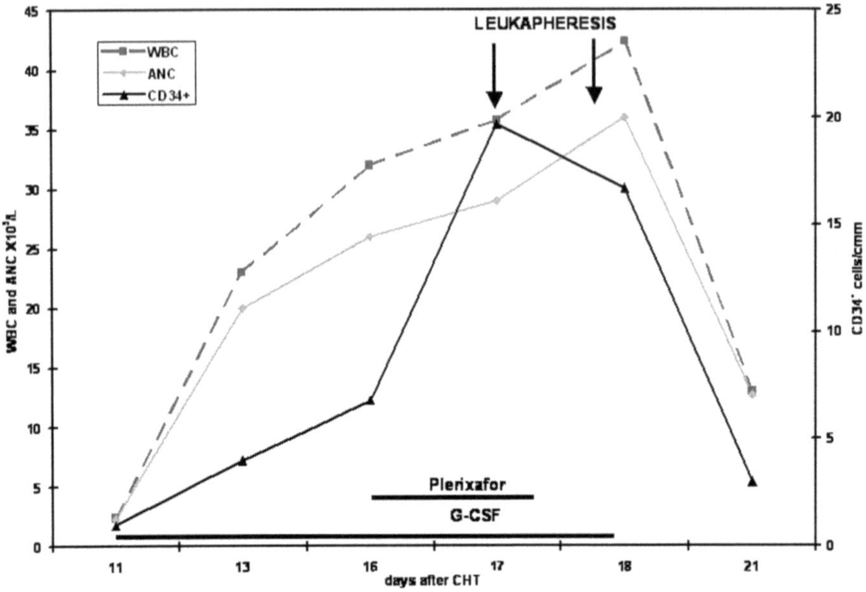

Fig. 14.1 A representative example of the boost of PB CD34⁺ cells observed after plerixafor administration following chemomobilization

following institutional guidelines. In MM patients, plerixafor was administered in two patients because PB CD34⁺ cell concentration dropped down to <10/μL after the initial PBSC collections which were felt to be inadequate considering the poor-prognosis disease, the young age, and the planned double ASCT. The third patient, undergoing dialysis and showing resistant disease, was considered poor mobilizer because of the low concentration of PB CD34⁺ cells (<10 μL) after mobilization chemotherapy. In our study, all MM patients were able to yield an adequate number of CD34⁺ cells to perform the planned ASCT with 1–3 leukaphereses.

All but one lymphoma patients were considered poor mobilizers based on the low concentration of circulating CD34⁺ cells (<10/μL) observed at time of hematological recovery after mobilizing chemotherapy. Plerixafor was administered for a median of two injections (range 1–3) allowing the collection, in all patients, of a sufficient number of CD34⁺ cells to proceed to ASCT. Engraftment after plerixafor-mobilized PBSCs was adequate and no documented infectious complications occurred. We observed a 4.7 median fold-increase in the number of circulating CD34⁺ cells after plerixafor as compared with baseline [from a median of 6.2 (range 1–12) to 21.5 (range 9–88) cells/μL].

In our patients, the preemptive use of plerixafor to G-CSF after chemotherapy seemed to be safe and allowed the rescue of MM and lymphoma patients, who need autologous transplantation but were failing PBSC mobilization. A representative example of the boost of PB CD34⁺ cells observed after plerixafor application is shown in Fig. 14.1.

Furthermore, Attolico et al. [29] investigated the safety and the efficacy of plerixafor added to chemomobilization in 37 Italian MM and lymphoma patients defined as "proven poor mobilizers" according to GITMO panel [20]. Twenty-five/37 patients had a history of previous mobilization failure, combined with other adverse factors for mobilization. Plerixafor (0.24 mg/kg) was added to G-CSF after chemotherapy mobilizing regimen for up to 3 days (median of two plerixafor administrations) being administered the evening before the planned apheresis. The addition of plerixafor allowed the successful collection in 73% of patients with 25/37 patients being able to collect $\geq 2 \times 10^6$ $CD34^+$ cells/kg in 1–3 leukaphereses. Twenty four patients have already been transplanted, showing a rapid and durable hematological recovery [23].

These results confirm the safety and the efficacy of plerixafor added to G-CSF after disease-oriented chemomobilization in patients proven to be poor mobilizers, thus preventing more apheresis procedures and/or more mobilization procedures.

Preemptive use of Plerixafor: Conclusions

Plerixafor is an effective and generally well-tolerated novel drug for PBSC mobilization from the BM to the PB, their collection and subsequent autologous transplantation in adult patients with lymphomas and MM who are planned for high-dose chemotherapy. While it mobilizes $CD34^+$ cells on its own, plerixafor significantly improves the mobilization capacity of G-CSF when the two drugs are used in combination.

Although the experience of adding plerixafor to chemomobilization in hard-to-mobilize patients is limited, early results have shown that this combination is feasible and safe and is able to improve stem cell mobilization by several fold to facilitate timely collection and subsequent stem cell transplantation. The vast majority of the patients reported in eight evaluable patient series (Table 14.1 [27–34]) published so far and reviewed in this chapter achieved the minimum collection target and could proceed to ASCT. Of note, according to the proposed definition of "poor mobilizers" [20] most of these patients may be included in this patient group. At present, there is no available prospective data on chemomobilization and plerixafor in "predicted poor mobilizers".

However, one of the main issues in this setting remains patient selection and timing of plerixafor administration. Available evidence based on small case numbers [27–30] suggests that the beneficial effect of plerixafor after chemomobilization may not be seen with very low blood leukocyte counts although no clear algorithms can be presented due to scanty information available. Conversely, based on available data, plerixafor may be added to patients with low PB $CD34^+$ cell counts (e.g., $<10 \times 10^6$/L) at the time of hematopoietic recovery after chemotherapy (e.g., blood leukocytes $>5 \times 10^9$/L and platelets $>20 \times 10^9$/L) or to patients with poor first collection yield (e.g., $<1 \times 10^6$ $CD34^+$ cells/kg) (proven poor mobilizers). In our own experience, we cannot rule out that some of our patients may have mobilized satisfactory with the continuation of G-CSF alone. However, it is promising that the highest

Table 14.1 Published trials where plerixafor has been added to chemomobilization

Author	Pts (no.)	Diagnosis	Mobilization regimen	Plerixafor injections median (range)	Aphereses median (range)	CD34⁺ cells collected (10^6/kg) median (range)	Success rate[a]
Dugan	40	NHL 14	Per Insitut. preference	1 (1–3)	2 (1–3)	NS	39/40
		MM 26	Based on the disease				
Segel	9	NHL 7	AraC/DHAP 6	2 (1–4)	2 (0–3)	3.3 (0–4.4)	5/9
		HD 2	CHOP2, CY1				
D'Addio	13	NHL 9	CY 4, DHAP 3	2 (1–3)	2 (1–3)	3.7 (2.5–6.6)	13/13
		MM 3	ICE 3, IEV 1				
		HD 1	ESHAP 1, ABVD 1				
Jantunen	7	NHL6	AraC 5, CY2	1 (1–3)	1 (0–4)	2.2 (0–4.2)	6/7
		MM 1					
Josefsen	5	NHL 5	CY 2, MIME 2	1 (1–2)	1 (1–2)	2.6 (0–9.6)	3/7
			ARA-C1				
Basak	10	NS	ICE 4, CY2	NS	NS	NS	NS
			BEACOPP 2, CED				
			Mega-CHOP 1				
Hubel	47[b]	NHL 24	NS	NS	2 (0–3)	2.3 (0–8.8)	15/24
		MM 14	NS	NS	2 (0–5)	4.9 (0–11)	12/14
		HD 2	NS	NS	2	2.4	2/2
		Other 7	NS	NS	2 (1–4)	2.6 (0.9–24.8)	5/7
Olivieri	37	NHL 20	DHAP	2 (1–3)	2 (1–3)	5.4 (2–15.2)	27/37
		MM 17	CTX				

NS not stated, *NHL* non-Hodgkin's lymphoma, *MM* multiple myeloma, *HD* Hodgkin's disease, *AraC* cytarabine, *CY* cyclophosphamide, *DHAP* dexamethasone–cytarabine–cisplatinum, *ICE* ifosfamide–carboplatin–etoposide, *IEV* ifosfamide–epirubicin–etoposide, *ESHAP* etoposide–methylprednisolone–cytarabine–cisplatinum, *ABVD* doxorubicin, bleomycin–vinblastine–dacarbazine, *CHOP* cyclophosphamide–doxorubicin–vincristine–prednisone, *MIME* methyl-GAG-ifosfamide–methotrexate–etoposide, *CED* cyclophosphamide–etoposide–dexamethasone, *BEACOPP* carmustine–etoposide–doxorubicin–cyclophosphamide–vincristine–procarbazine–prednisone, *CTX* cytoxan

[a] At least 2×10^6/kg CD34⁺ cells collected after the first mobilization attempt

[b] All failed at least one mobilization

fold-increase was observed in those patients with <5 circulating CD34⁺ cells/μL, suggesting the role of plerixafor in this "hard-to-mobilize" patient population.

On this basis, the preemptive use of plerixafor may be the most cost-effective way to use this new drug by preventing mobilization failure and need for remobilization or marrow harvest and, perhaps, resulting in a higher number of lymphoma and MM patients submitted to ASCT.

Overall, the decision to add plerixafor to chemotherapy should be based on clinical parameters taking into account predictive criteria (e.g., age, disease status, prior lines of chemotherapy, and prior radiation therapy) as well as "actual" criteria such as the absolute PB $CD34^+$ cell and WBC counts 1 day prior or on the day of PBSC collection and the overall therapeutic goal (e.g., sufficient $CD34^+$ cells for single or double transplantation). In this view, the patient-adapted use of plerixafor in adjunct to G-CSF, based on PB $CD34^+$ count and target cell dose, has been recently proposed by Costa et al. [35] and resulted in a safer and more efficient collection of PBSCs when compared to cyclophosphamide and G-CSF [36].

Noteworthy, in all reviewed studies the administration of plerixafor during chemomobilization was shown to be safe. In particular, we did not observe any clinical adverse events or any variation in laboratory values even in three patients older than 60 years and in one patient undergoing dialysis during mobilization [28]. In this last patient, the dose of plerixafor was not reduced according to renal failure supporting recent data which indicate that plerixafor may be safely used at full dosage to mobilize PBSCs in patients with advanced renal failure [37]. Chemomobilization is widely used in clinical practice and poor mobilization remains a critical problem, therefore studies addressing the optimal use of plerixafor in poor mobilizers after chemotherapy should be pursued. To this end, we have planned a prospective phase II study on the addition of plerixafor to Cy and G-CSF chemomobilization for MM patients intended for double ASCT.

Acknowledgments This work was supported in part by Regione Emilia-Romagna (Progetti di Ricerca Università-Regione Emilia Romagna, Progetto Medicina Rigenerativa, 2007). MIUR (PRIN 2006 and 2008).

References

1. Gertz MA (2010) Current status of stem cell mobilization. Br J Haematol 450:647–62
2. Sinha S, Gastineau D, Micallef I, Hogan W, Ansell S, Buadi F, Dingli D, Dispenzieri A, Gertz M, Greiner C, Hayman S, Inwards D, Johnston P, Lacy M, Litzow M, Porrata L, Winters J L, Kumar S (2011) Predicting PBSC harvest failure using circulating CD34 levels: developing target-based cutoff points for early intervention. Bone Marrow Transplant 46:343–49
3. Bender JG, To LB, Williams S, Schwartzberg LS (1992) Defining a therapeutic dose of peripheral blood stem cells. J Hematother 1:329–41
4. Gazitt Y, Freytes CO, Callander N et al (1999) Successful PBSC mobilization with high-dose G-CSF for patients failing a first round of mobilization. J Hematother 8:173–83
5. Stiff P, Gingrich R, Luger S et al (2000) A randomized phase 2 study of PBPC mobilization by stem cell factor and filgrastim in heavily pretreated patients with Hodgkin's disease or non-Hodgkin's lymphoma. Bone Marrow Transplant 26(5):471–81

6. Tricot G, Jagannath S, Vesole D et al (1995) Peripheral blood stem cell transplants for multiple myeloma: identification of favorable variables for rapid engraftment in 225 patients. Blood 85:588–96
7. Blystad AK, Delabie J, Kvaloy S et al (2004) Infused CD34 cell dose, but not tumour cell content of peripheral blood progenitor cell grafts, predicts clinical outcome in patients with diffuse large B-cell lymphoma and follicular lymphoma grade 3 treated with high-dose therapy. Br J Haematol 125:605–12
8. Shpall EJ, Champlin R, Glaspy JA (1998) Effect of CD34+ peripheral blood progenitor cell dose on hematopoietic recovery. Biol Blood Marrow Transplant 4:84–92
9. Toor AA, Ayers J, Strupeck J et al (2004) Favourable results with a single autologous stem cell transplant following conditioning with busulphan and cyclophosphamide in patients with multiple myeloma. Br J Haematol 124:769–76
10. Bensinger W, DiPersio JF, MacCarty JM (2009) Improving stem cell mobilization strategies: future directions. Bone Marrow Transplant 43:181–95
11. Watanabe H, Watanabe T, Suzuya H, Wakata Y, Kaneko M, Onishi T, Okamoto Y, Abe T, Kawano T, Kagami S, Takaue Y (2006) Peripheral blood stem cell mobilization by granulocyte colony-stimulating factor alone and engraftment kinetics following autologous transplantation in children and adolescents with solid tumor. Bone Marrow Transplant 37(7):661–68
12. Jantunen E, Kvalheim G (2010) Mobilization strategies in hard-to-mobilize patients with lymphoid malignancies. Eur J Haematol 85(6):463–71
13. Pusic I, Jiang SY, Landua S, Uy GL, Rettig MP, Cashen AF, Westervelt P, Vij R, Abboud CN, Stockerl-Goldstein KE, Sempek DS, Smith A, DiPersio JF (2008) Impact of mobilization and remobilizaton strategies on achieving sufficient stem cell yields for autologous transplantation. Biol Blood Marrow Transplant 14:1045–56
14. Hosing C, Rima M, Ahlawat S, Korbling M, Kebriaei P, Alousi A, De Lima M, Okoroji J-G, McMannis J, Qazilbash M, Anderlini P, Giralt S, Champin RE, Khouri I, Popat U (2009) Poor hematopoietic stem cell mobilizers: a single institution study of incidence and risk factors in patients with recurrent or relapsed lymphoma. Am J Hematol 84(6):335–37
15. Wuchter P, Ran D, Bruckner T, Schmitt T, Witzens-Harig M, Neben K, Goldschmodt H, Ho AD (2010) Poor mobilization of hematopoietic stem cells-definitions, incidence, risk factors, and impact on outcome of autologous transplantation. Biol Blood Marrow Transplant 16(4): 490–99
16. Hübel K, Liles WC, Broxmeyer HE, Rodger E, Wood B, Cooper S, Hangoc G, Macfarland R, Bridger GJ, Henson GW, Calandra G, Dale DC (2004) Leucocytosis and mobilization of CD34+ hematopoietic progenitor cells by AMD3100, a CXCR4 antagonist. Support Cancer Ther 1(3):165–72
17. To LB, Haylock DN, Simmons PJ, Juttner CA (1997) The biology and clinical uses of blood stem cells. Blood 89(7):2233–58. Review. No abstract available.
18. Devine SM, Flomenberg N, Vesole DH, Liesveld J, Weisdorf D, Badel K, Calandra G, DiPersio JF (2004) Rapid mobilization of CD34+ cells following administration of the CXCR4 antagonist AMD3100 to patients with multiple myeloma and non-Hodgkin's lymphoma. J Clin Oncol 22(6):1095–102
19. Körbling M (2004) Mobilization regimens for harvesting autologous and allogeneic peripheral blood stem cells. In: Atkinson K, Fibbe WE, Champlin R, Ljungman P, Ritz J, Brenner MK (eds) Clinical Bone Marrow and Blood Stem Cell Transplantation, 3rd edn. Cambridge University Presspp, Cambridge, UK, pp 383–403
20. Olivieri A, Marchetti M, Lemoli RM, Tarella C, Iacone A, Lanza F, Rambaldi A, Bosi A, on behalf of the Italian Group for Stem Cell Transplantation (GITMO) (2011) Proposed definition of "poor mobilizer" in lymphoma and multiple myeloma: an analytic hierarchy process by an ad-hoc Working Group Gruppo ItalianoTrapianto di Midollo Osseo (GITMO) (Bone Marrow Transplant May 30) [E-pub ahead of print]
21. Cassens U, Momkvist PH, Zuehlsdorf M et al (2001) Kinetics of standardized large volume leukapheresis (LVL) in patients do not show a recruitment phenomenon of peripheral blood progenitor cells (PBPC). Bone Marrow Transplant 28:13–20

22. Fu S, Liesveld J (2000) Mobilization of hematopoietic stem cells. Blood Rev 14:205–218
23. Höglund M, Smedmyr B, Simonsson B, Tötterman T, Bengtsson M (1996) Dose-dependent mobilisation of haematopoietic progenitor cells in healthy volunteers receiving glycosylated rHuG-CSF. Bone Marrow Transplant 18:19–27
24. Lemoli RM, de Vivo A, Damiani D, Isidori A, Tani M, Bonini A, Cellini C, Curti A, Gugliotta L, Visani G, Fanin R, Baccarani M (2003) Autologous transplantation of granulocyte colony-stimulating factor-primed bone marrow is effective to support myeloablative chemotherapy in patients with hematological malignancies and poor peripheral blood stem cell mobilization. Blood 102:1595–1600
25. Calandra G, McCarty J, McGuirk J, Tricot G, Crocker SA, Badel K, Grove B, Dye A, Bridger G (2008) AMD3100 plus G-CSF can successfully mobilize CD34+ cells from nonHodgkin's lymphoma, Hodgkin's disease and multiple myeloma patients previously failing mobilization with chemotherapy and/or cytokine treatment: compassionate use data. Bone Marrow Transplant 41:331–338
26. Duarte RF, Shaw BE, Marín P, Kottaridis P, Ortiz M, Morante C, Delgado J, Gayoso J, Goterriz R, Martínez-Chamorro C, Mateos-Mazón JJ, Ramírez C, de la Rubia J, Achtereekte H, Gandhi PJ, Douglas KW, Russell NH (2011) Plerixafor plus granulocyte CSF can mobilize hematopoietic stem cells from multiple myeloma and lymphoma patients failing previous mobilization attempts: EU compassionate use data. Bone Marrow Transplant 46:52–8
27. Dugan MJ, Maziarz RT, Bensinger WI, Nademanee A, Liesveld J, Badel K, Dehner C, Gibney C, Bridger G, Calandra G (2010) Safety and preliminary efficacy of plerixafor (Mozobil) in combination with chemotherapy and G-CSF: an open-label, multicenter, exploratory trial in patients with multiple myeloma and non-Hodgkin's lymphoma undergoing stem cell mobilization. Bone Marrow Transplant 45:39–47
28. D'Addio A, Curti A, Worel N, Douglas K, Motta MR, Rizzi S, Dan E, Taioli S, Giudice V, Agis H, Kopetzky G, Soutar R, Casadei B, Baccarani M, Lemoli RM (2011) The addition of plerixafor is safe and allows adequate PBSC collection in multiple myeloma and lymphoma patients poor mobilizers after chemotherapy and G-CSF. Bone Marrow Transplant 46:356–63
29. Attolico I, Pavone V, Ostun A, Rossini B, Musso M, Cresci Manno A, Martino, M, Iacopino P, Milone G, Tedeschi P, Coluzzi S, Nuccorini R, Pascale S, Di Naroo E, Olivieri A (2011) Plerixafor added to Cheno Therapy plus 6-CSF S, Safe and allows adequate PBSC collection in Predicted poor Mobilizer patients with multiple myeloma or Cymphora Biol Blood Marrow Transplant. Jul 23, [E-Pub ahead of print]
30. Basak GW, Knopinska-Posluszny W, Matuszak M, Kisiel E, Hawrylecka D, Szmigielka-Kaplon A, Urbaniak-Kujda D, Dybko J, Zielinska P, Dabrovska-Iwanicka A, Werkun J, Rzepecki P, Wroblewska W, Wiktor-Jedrzejzak W (2011) Hematopoietic stem cell mobilization with the reversible CXCR4 receptor antagonist plerixafor (AMD3100) – Polish compassionate use experience. Ann Hemato 90:557–68
31. Hubel K, Fresen MM, Salwender H, Basara N, Beier R, Theurich S, Christopeit M, Bogner C, Galm O, Hartwig R, Heits F, Lordick F, Rösler W, Wehler D, Zander AR, Albert MH, Dressler S, Ebinger M, Frickhofen N, Hertenstein B, Kiehl M, Liebler S, von Lilienfeld-Toal M, weidmann E, Weigelt C, Lange F, Kröger N (2011) Plerixafor with and without chemotherapy in poor mobilizers: results from the German compassionate use program. Bone Marrow Transplant 46:1045–52
32. Jantunen E, Penttilä K, Pyörälä M, Mahlamäki E, Kuittinen T, Nousiainen T (2011) Addition of plerixafor to a chemotherapy and G-CSF mobilization in hard-to-mobilize patients. Bone Marrow Transplant [E-pub ahead of print 46:308–9]
33. Josefsen D, Rechnitzer C, Parto K, Kvalheim G (2011) The use of plerixafor for blood stem mobilization reduces the frequency of mobilization failure in patients planned to undergo autologous stem cell transplantation. Eur Haematol 4:24–29
34. Segel E, Sorensen B, d'Amore F, Hokland P (2011) Successful peripheral blood stem cell harvest in mobilization-refractory lymphoma patients. Bone Marrow Transplant 45(suppl. 2): S258 (abstract)

35. Costa LJ, Alexander ET, Hogan KR, Schaub C, Fouts TV, Stuart RK (2011) Development and validation of a decision-making algorithm to guide the use of plerixafor for autologous hematopoietic stem cell mobilization. Bone Marrow Transplant 46:64–9
36. Costa LJ, Milles AN, Alexander ET, Hogan KR, Shabbir M, Schaub C, Stuart RK (2011) Growth factor and patient-adapted use of plerixafor is superior to CY and growth factor for autologous hematopoietic stem cell mobilization. Bone Marrow Transplant 46:523–28
37. Douglas K, Hayden P, Rahemtulla A, D'Addio A, Rao K, Maris M, et al (2011) Plerixafor for PBSC mobilization in myeloma patients with advanced renal failure: safety and efficacy data in a series of 12 patients from the US or European Compassionate Use Programmes and from the US post-licensing. Bone Marrow Transplant 45(Suppl. 2):S3–S23

Chapter 15
Experience with Plerixafor in Poor Mobilizers

Catherine H. Roberts and John M. McCarty

Abstract Using traditional growth factor or chemotherapy-based stem cell mobilization methods, the ability to obtain a stem cell dose that meets the minimum criteria for safety, much less the optimal dose, which increases patients' tolerance and salutary long-term outcome may be ineffective in up to one third of patients. The FDA approval of plerixafor, an antagonist of the α-chemokine receptor CXCR4 for use with G-CSF, was based on its proven ability to enhance peripheral blood and apheresis collection $CD34^+$ cell content. The current body of experience for this agent provides a toolkit of varied strategies by which patients already proven to be unable to collect or those predicted unlikely to mobilize may yet obtain sufficient cells to receive high dose therapy as planned. This chapter will review the currently available clinical data that illustrates the potential benefit of plerixafor in poorly mobilizing patients and will explore the international experience of this drug in combination with G-CSF or chemotherapy-based mobilization and remobilization treatment protocols.

Definitions and Characteristics of Hard-to-Mobilize Patients

Successful outcomes in autologous peripheral blood stem cell transplantation (autoSCT) are critically dependent on the $CD34^+$ stem cell dose infused following myeloablative preparative regimens. A minimum dose of 2×10^6 cells/kg is widely accepted to ensure adequate platelet engraftment and to reduce the incidence of post-transplant MDS, toxicity and relapse [1–3]. While a dose of $4–6 \times 10^6$ cells/kg is commonly considered an optimum target to improve post-transplant engraftment [4],

C.H. Roberts, PhD • J.M. McCarty, MD (✉)
Bone Marrow Transplant Program, Massey Cancer Center, VCU Medical Center, Richmond, VA 23298-0157, USA
e-mail: jmccarty@mcvh-vcu.edu

S. Fruehauf et al. (eds.), *Novel Developments in Stem Cell Mobilization: Focus on CXCR4*, DOI 10.1007/978-1-4614-1960-0_15,

Table 15.1 Risk factors for mobilization failure

Older age [5–7]
Prior failure of mobilization [8]
Prior exposure to stem cell toxic agents
Alkylators [9, 10]
Melphalan [7, 11, 12]
BCNU [12–15]
Lenalidomide [16, 17]
Fludarabine [18, 19]
Platinum compounds [9]
Interferon [20]
Hyper-CVAD [21]
DHAP [22]
More prior chemotherapy [7, 12, 21, 22]
Marrow involvement by disease [15, 23]
Prior marrow radiation [24, 25]
Thrombocytopenia at mobilization [5, 20]
Low steady state PB CD34$^+$ cells [26]
Iron overload [27]
Marrow hypocellularity [5]
Lymphoma diagnosis [8]
FUO/infection [20, 26]

the ideal cell dose has not been established for standardization of practice. With the increasing potential for tandem transplantation in myeloma, higher target stem cell collections remain important for long-term disease management. Patients may be characterized as failing to collect, using the threshold targets described above, or as failing to mobilize as measured by the peripheral blood CD34$^+$ content (PB CD34$^+$) being at least 10 cells/μL on the expected day of first apheresis.

Many factors have been cited as contributing to the difficulty in mobilizing adequate CD34$^+$ cells in patients requiring autoSCT. These include older age, prior mobilization failure, prior exposure to stem cell toxic agents and intensive regimens, a longer pre-mobilization treatment course, marrow involvement by disease, prior marrow radiation exposure, thrombocytopenia at mobilization, iron overload, low steady state PB CD34$^+$ count, marrow hypocellularity, non-Hodgkin's lymphoma (NHL) diagnosis, and infection or sepsis during mobilization attempt (Table 15.1). Despite an extensive body of literature identifying risk factors predicting mobilization failure, a practical predictive scoring system has not been widely successful. Even with such forewarning, the failure rate to collect has been reported from 5% to more than 30% [8, 12, 28, 29]. Even with more sophisticated real-time dynamic predictive measures based on first day PB 34$^+$ cell content and apheresis collection [30], an effective, flexible, and easily implemented intervention for these difficult-to-mobilize patients must be made available. With the advent and approval of the CXCR4 antagonist plerixafor, a new and effective agent has been added to address this difficult clinical problem. A number of different strategies have been devised and reported using plerixafor in the difficult-to-mobilize patient population, and these will be reviewed here.

During its development, testing and approval phase, plerixafor has been known as AMD3100, and is marketed as Mozobil. For the purposes of this chapter, plerixafor will be used to identify this agent regardless of its appellation at the time of publication. Unless otherwise stipulated in this chapter, administration of plerixafor is assumed to be scheduled according to the labeling indication recommending G-CSF daily for 4 days prior to plerixafor administration. Plerixafor is given as a daily dose of 0.24 mg/kg body weight s.c. 10–11 h prior to apheresis attempt, and may be continued for up to 4 days of daily therapy [31].

Traditional Plerixafor Salvage Approaches and Studies

A phase II trial implementing a crossover design compared the activity of G-CSF with and without the combination of plerixafor using a sequential mobilization strategy in multiple myeloma (MM) or NHL was designed to show the feasibility and benefit of the adding plerixafor to G-CSF [32]. The study reported that all mobilization attempts receiving plerixafor plus G-CSF resulted in higher PB CD34$^+$ cells than attempts with G-CSF alone. In nine patients, the minimum 2×10^6 cells/kg target was not reached using G-CSF alone, but all were successfully mobilized with the subsequent planned plerixafor plus G-CSF attempt. This suggested a beneficial role of the plerixafor plus G-CSF combination in the salvage of prior mobilization failure with G-CSF alone. The plerixafor plus G-CSF group experienced fewer apheresis procedures and were more likely to collect 5×10^6 cells/kg.

The plerixafor plus G-CSF mobilization strategy was retrospectively analyzed for its benefit as a salvage approach using a database of patients enrolled in the Compassionate Use Protocol (CUP; Table 15.2) [33]. These patients were a subset of 115 data-audited patients out of a total of more than 200 accepted into the CUP. The majority of the patients analyzed had failed to mobilize with more than 75% measuring a PB CD34$^+$ of <10 cells/μL, having received a median of two prior mobilization attempts before entry into CUP. Plerixafor plus G-CSF was administered as described above, but the endpoint for stopping apheresis attempts was left to the

Table 15.2 Outcomes of MCC single institution CUP trial

	Median	Range
PB CD34/μL day 5 am	24.2	0.96–102.8
Days apheresis	4	1–7
Total collected	3.58	0.36–10.05
Days apheresis ≥2	2	1–7
ANC	10	7–24
PLT	17	10–25
# TX	61	
Collected ≥2	60	
Collected ≥5	18	
Total # collections	70	Four had two AMD collections

discretion of the local investigator. Using a goal of collecting $\geq 2 \times 10^6$ cells/kg, the target collection was met in 60.3% of NHL patients, 71.4% of MM patients and 76.5% of patients with Hodgkin's disease (HD). An insignificant difference was seen when these groups were sub-analyzed for their prior mobilization attempts. For NHL patients, target cell collection was met in 55.9% of patients failing prior G-CSF versus 65.5% of those failing prior chemotherapy mobilization regimens. In Hodgkin's disease (HD), goal was met in 77.8% (G-CSF) versus 75% (Chemotherapy). In MM, 2×10^6 cells/kg were collected in 63.6% of patients failing prior G-CSF versus 75% failing prior chemotherapy. More than 75% of the total CUP population was able to proceed to transplant. In all patients, engraftment occurred on day +11 for neutrophils and day +18 for platelets. Engraftment was durable up to 1 year in all but one poorly mobilized patient transplanted with multiple prior pooled stem cell products and another experiencing a fatal disease relapse before 1 year.

The VCU Massey Cancer Center experience in 66 data audited compassionate use protocol or expanded access program patients with NHL, HD, MM, and AML represents a large single institutional experience. In all, 49/66 failed to mobilize, 16 failed collection, and one considered excessively high risk due to prior radiation. The proportion of patients failing prior chemotherapy-based regimens to G-CSF only was 36:28. These patients were identified early and were initially mobilized with G-CSF plus plerixafor. After a significant post-plerixafor administration increase in PB $CD34^+$ cell concentration to a median of 24.2/μL, the median $CD34^+$ product collected was 3.58 in a median of 4 days apheresis. More than 90% (60/66) achieved a collection of $>2 \times 10^6$ cells/kg and 30% collected $>5 \times 10^6$ cells/kg. AutoSCT was performed in 92.4% of the group with engraftment comparable to the overall population (neutrophil day +10, platelets day +17). Despite similar demographics, these single institution results exceeded those reported for the CUP, and may be due to the earlier intervention with plerixafor salvage. Compared to the CUP data, patients enrolled in our institutional protocol after only one prior mobilization attempt, with the median interval between first attempt and plerixafor plus G-CSF salvage was 2 weeks versus more than a month for the CUP. There may have also been a target bias in the local cohort, in that our policy continued to apheresis patients who could potentially collect the optimal 5×10^6 cells/kg dose. However, it is important to stress that our analysis demonstrated little benefit in prolonging apheresis beyond 5 days continuous collection with plerixafor as the daily apheresis collection dramatically decreased beyond that time point. The results of the first 33 patients in this group was previously reported [34].

The group at Oregon Health and Sciences University similarly reported significant single institutional results from their experience enrolling patients into the CUP [35]. Twenty patients with NHL, HD, MM, and AILD had failed prior G-CSF or chemotherapy-based mobilization regimens. Following the plerixafor salvage regimen with plerixafor plus G-CSF previously outlined, 18 of the 20 patients collected at least 2×10^6 cells/kg and proceeded to autoSCT. A median of 4×10^6 cells/kg were collected in a median of 2 days in patients failing prior chemotherapy-based mobilization, and 3.7×10^6 cells/kg were collected in 2 days in the prior

G-CSF mobilized group. One of these patients required two plerixafor plus G-CSF mobilization attempts and two patients failed to collect a minimum required cell dose to proceed to autoSCT. Neutrophil and platelet engraftment was comparable to transplant to the overall OHSU autoSCT population in the 16 patients undergoing plerixafor salvage.

A large Phase III randomized double-blinded placebo control trial of 298 patients with NHL compared the benefit of adding plerixafor to G-CSF as a first mobilization strategy [36]. This trial included a rescue protocol allowing patients in either study arm to receive open label plerixafor plus G-CSF if they failed to collect $<0.8 \times 10^6$ cells/kg in two apheresis collections or $<2 \times 10^6$ cells/kg in four apheresis collections [37]. Sixty-eight patients were eligible for the rescue protocol with 11 having received the plerixafor plus G-CSF combination and 57 G-CSF plus placebo. Sixty-two patients received open-label plerixafor plus G-CSF (ten with prior plerixafor, 52 G-CSF plus placebo). Forty percentage of the prior plerixafor mobilized patients and 63% of the prior G-CSF alone patients collected $\geq 2 \times 10^6$ cells/kg and were eligible to proceed to autoSCT. Engraftment characteristics in these patients were comparable to those not requiring a rescue mobilization. These data show that plerixafor rescue may be a consideration even in patients failing to collect a sufficient stem cell dose with previous plerixafor plus G-CSF mobilization attempts.

Since its approval by the FDA in December of 2008, the results of a number of other rescue protocols have been published. Tricot [38] reported the use of plerixafor plus G-CSF in MM patients failing a previous mobilization in which $<2 \times 10^6$ cells/kg were collected. Use of the plerixafor plus G-CSF rescue strategy resulted in 7/10 patients collecting $>2 \times 10^6$ cells/kg adequate for subsequent transplant. No myeloma cell tumor contamination was detected in the collected apheresis products. All patients experienced timely and durable engraftment of neutrophils and platelets out to a 6-month follow-up. A subsequent cohort was treated with the addition of plerixafor in a preemptive strategy, which will be described below.

The European Union reported their experience with plerixafor in patients previously failing mobilization. Fifty-six patients with MM or NHL from 15 centers in Spain and the United Kingdom were included in this European compassionate use trial of plerixafor plus G-CSF. The 56-patient panel underwent a total of 76 previous mobilization attempts including G-CSF in 28, chemotherapy plus G-CSF in 43, and G-CSF plus SCF in two. In all, 42/56 (75%) collected $\geq 2 \times 10^6$ cells/kg with plerixafor plus G-CSF on this rescue protocol. On day 5 after plerixafor administration, 71% of patients measured a PB $CD34^+$ of >10 cells/μL and experienced a median 7.6-fold expansion of peripheral blood $CD34^+$ from day 4 G-CSF administration baseline. The regimen was well tolerated with expected engraftment metrics. The EU experience compares favorably with the CUP data previously reported [33].

The Austrian plerixafor salvage experience was reported from a named patient program of patients mobilizing insufficient $CD34^+$ cells to undergo autoSCT [39]. A total of 27 patients treated at eight centers in Austria were given the plerixafor plus G-CSF regimen described previously. Twenty of the 27 patients collected 2×10^6 cells/kg or more with 13 subsequently proceeding on to transplant. PB $CD34^+$ exceeded 10 cells/μL in 74% of patients so treated. Of the initial group, 48% of the patients proceeded on to autoSCT. With a median cell dose delivered of 2.93×10^6 cells/kg, patients engrafted neutrophils at a median of day +12 and platelets by day +14. It is noted that even in patients showing a PB CD34⁺ count of less than 10 cells/μL, harvest resulted in a median of 0.71×10^6 cells/kg with a range of 0.08–2.51×10^6 cells/kg. The authors conclude that patients should proceed to stem cell collection after plerixafor administration even if the PB $CD34^+$ count is below the optimal mobilization target as some of these patients may still benefit.

With the success of plerixafor well documented by the outcomes of these traditional salvage strategies, investigators began to explore additional strategic approaches to the use of plerixafor to reduce mobilization failure rates and to increase the stem cell yield in patients for whom the optimal $\geq 5 \times 10^6$ cells/kg rather than the minimum target was preferred. These included the use of plerixafor with the initial mobilization attempt, combining it with chemotherapy-based mobilization, and incorporating plerixafor earlier in the mobilization process for patients deemed unlikely to meet target collection goals.

Up-Front Plerixafor Mobilization Strategies

With the success of plerixafor in salvage of prior failed stem cell mobilization or collection, several studies determined the feasibility and efficacy of planned up-front administration of plerixafor in all standard and high-risk patients. The potential advantages of this strategy would be to reduce the uncertainty of current predictive methods to identify those unlikely to mobilize, to increase the stem cell yield in the shortest time in collection, and to more certainly predict when patients would be ready for effective stem cell apheresis.

Cashen and the group at Washington University in St. Louis reported the first large phase II study of plerixafor plus G-CSF as an initial mobilization strategy in 19 patients with relapsed or refractory HD [40]. Patients received G-CSF at 10 μg/kg/day and plerixafor at 240 μg/kg s.c. 11 h prior to apheresis procedures after at least 4 days of G-CSF. This approach yielded a higher percentage of optimal stem cell numbers collected compared with the institutional historical G-CSF mobilized control population previously reported [8]. In addition to a higher initial day 1+2 total $CD34^+$ cell collection and a median 3.2-fold higher pre-apheresis PB $CD34^+$ cell count, 63% of the plerixafor plus G-CSF group collected $\geq 5 \times 10^6$ cells/kg compared to only 15% in the historical cohort. The vast majority (95%) of patients collected the minimum $\geq 2 \times 10^6$ cells/kg necessary to proceed to transplant. Accordingly, the proportion of patients not able to proceed to transplant due to insufficient stem cell collection was more favorable in the plerixafor plus G-CSF group, comprising 5 versus 22% in the historical G-CSF alone group. The plerixafor plus G-CSF combination was efficient, with a median 2 apheresis sessions per patient, as was seen in the historical G-CSF alone group.

A second phase II multicenter trial investigated this approach in patients with MM and NHL [41]. As with previously described protocols, G-CSF was given daily for up to 9 days, with plerixafor given on the evening of day 4, 10–11 h prior to the apheresis procedure for up to a maximum of five apheresis sessions. Patients were continued on apheresis until $\geq 5 \times 10^6$ cells/kg were collected and were considered transplant eligible if $\geq 2 \times 10^6$ cells/kg could be collected. Of this group of 23 patients with NHL and 26 with MM, a median of 5.9×10^6 cells/kg were collected in a median of 2 aphereses. In all, 47 of the 49 patients treated (96%) proceeded on to autoSCT. All transplanted patients demonstrated adequate and expected engraftment kinetics. Of the more than half (57%) of the cohort who were deemed heavily pretreated, similar results were seen in fold PB 34^+ counts measured, total collection and number of apheresis sessions required to meet the minimum transplantable stem cell target dose.

The reports of two Phase III multicenter randomized placebo-controlled studies of plerixafor plus G-CSF as first mobilization approach in patients with NHL (Study 3101) and multiple myeloma (Study 3102) were also favorable [36, 42]. All patients in both studies received G-CSF at 10 μg/kg s.c. daily for 4 days. On the evening of day 4, patients received either placebo or plerixafor (240 μg/kg s.c.). As with the previous studies, patients underwent apheresis on day 5 and continued to receive an evening dose of either placebo or plerixafor followed by the morning dose of G-CSF for up to a total of four apheresis sessions or until $\geq 5 \times 10^6$ $CD34^+$ cells/kg were collected. In Study 3102, which examined mobilization with plerixafor in patients with MM, the percentage of patients from whom $\geq 6 \times 10^6$ $CD34^+$ cells/kg were collected in ≥2 days of apheresis served as the primary end point to reflect the potential for tandem transplantation in this disease. As described above, patients unable to obtain the minimum $\geq 2 \times 10^6$ $CD34^+$ cells/kg in either study were eligible for open label use of plerixafor plus G-CSF as a salvage regimen independent of their initial treatment arm. In Study 3101, which evaluated plerixafor for mobilization in patients with NHL, the percentage of patients from whom $\geq 5 \times 10^6$ $CD34^+$ cells/kg were collected in ≥4 days of apheresis was fixed as the primary end point. The 3102 MM study reported that $\geq 6 \times 10^6$ $CD34^+$ cells/kg were collected from 71.6% of patients in the plerixafor group in ≥2 days of apheresis, whereas only 34.4% of patients in the placebo group had reached this goal, a statistically significant difference ($P < 0.0001$). Of note, 54% of the plerixafor group reached target collection in one apheresis session, where 56% of the placebo group required 4 days to reach this same goal. Median PB $CD34^+$ counts were increased 4.8-fold after plerixafor administration, compared to 1.7-fold following placebo comparing values from days 4 and 5 of the protocol. The 3101 NHL study reported that the target yield of $\geq 5 \times 10^6$ $CD34^+$ cells/kg collected in ≤4 apheresis days was reached by 59.3% of patients in the plerixafor group but by only 19.6% of patients in the placebo group, also a statistically significant difference ($P < 0.0001$). While the median PB $CD34^+$ count was similar in both groups on day 4, the plerixafor-treated group had a higher median PB $CD34^+$ (36 vs. 13 cells/μL) and fold increase PB $CD34^+$ cells (5.0 vs. 1.4). A greater portion of the patients receiving plerixafor met the secondary endpoint of collecting $\geq 2 \times 10^6$ $CD34^+$ cells/kg in 4 days or less than controls (86.7 vs. 47.3%). As with the primary endpoint, the time to meet this goal was significantly shorter in the plerixafor-treated group. For both the groups meeting either the primary and secondary endpoints, a similar percentage of patients in the plerixafor group met the collection goal in one apheresis session, where the same proportion was not reached in the control population until four apheresis sessions were completed. More patients proceeded to transplantation in the plerixafor group (90%) than in the placebo group (55%). Transplant engraftment kinetics were not different between the two groups. Graft durability was similar except for platelet counts from day 100 to 6 months post-transplant in NHL patients transplanted with the plerixafor mobilized stem cell products, reflecting the higher $CD34^+$ dose delivered compared to control patients transplanted with G-CSF alone mobilized stem cell products [43]. Lymphoma patients also required fewer red blood cell transfusion requirements. In general, treatment with plerixafor and G-CSF was associated with side effects similar to those seen with treatment with G-CSF alone with most treatment-related mild and transient. The most common AEs were gastrointestinal tract effects, such as diarrhea, nausea and vomiting, and injection-site reactions, such as erythema or edema as previously reported in Phase II and compassionate use protocols. In addition to a significant greater number of plerixafor patients collecting an optimal number of $CD34^+$ cells, this was accomplished in both studies with fewer collection days, indicating that this up-front plerixafor approach could result in a more predictable and efficient use of apheresis resources without decreasing patients' tolerance or undue side effects.

Plerixafor Salvage with Chemotherapy-Based Mobilization

In addition to mobilization strategies employing G-CSF, a significant number of transplant centers prefer the use of a chemotherapy-based mobilization regimen. This practice is even more prevalent in Europe than in the US due in part to transplant funding mechanisms. The decision to utilize a chemotherapy mobilization regimen is often based on disease characteristics, and is often used to enhance continued cytoreduction as much as improving stem cell collection yields. Regimens commonly employed include cytoxan in doses ranging from 1.5 to 4 g/m^2 [44, 45], ICE (ifosfamide, carboplatin, and etoposide) [46], IVE (ifosfamide, epirubicin, and etoposide) [47], DHAP (cytarabine, cisplatin, and dexamethasone), [22] or ESHAP (etoposide, methylprednisolone, cytarabine, and cisplatin) [48].

The limitations to chemo-mobilization include a higher incidence of dose dependent morbidity due to infection, sepsis, hospitalization for drug administration or febrile neutropenia, and drug-specific toxicity when compared to growth factor alone mobilization strategies [45, 49]. In addition, cytoxan-mobilized patients were noted to have a higher probability of post-transplant staph bacteremia [49], slower engraftment kinetics [49], and a higher risk of infection and delayed immune reconstitution due to lymphocytopenia [50]. One problematic issue is the difficulty in predicting the optimal time to initiate stem cell collection in chemo-mobilized patients due to variability in the peak concentration of PB $CD34^+$ cells [46, 51–54]. While not studied as thoroughly as plerixafor plus G-CSF, there are reports of using plerixafor with chemotherapy plus G-CSF in an effort to reduce the variability of peak PB CD34+ cell timing and to increase the proportion of patients meeting intended CD34+ collection goals [55].

Dugan reported the efficacy and safety of adding plerixafor to patients undergoing chemotherapy-based mobilization regimens [56]. In this open label multicenter phase II trial in patients with MM ($n=26$) and NHL ($n=14$), plerixafor was administered to patients receiving a variety of chemotherapy regimens determined by the local institutional disease standard. The local mobilization practice was not altered except for the addition of plerixafor. Three different cohorts were examined in this study. In the first (Cohort A, $n=19$), plerixafor was administered after the first apheresis session to determine if its addition would enhance subsequent CD34+ collection. In Cohort B ($n=15$), plerixafor administration was delayed until the morning of the second apheresis day, 6 h prior to that day's collection attempt. A third Cohort C ($n=1$) served as a rescue strategy for patients in Cohorts A and B who failed to mobilize a PB CD34+ above 20 cells/μL. A fourth cohort D ($n=5$) included patients at one institution that received booster doses of plerixafor immediately proximate to chemotherapy to determine its role in hastening counts recovery. In all, the addition of plerixafor to these disparate chemotherapy regimens was well tolerated, with the expected frequency and severity of adverse events and side effects. Peripheral blood CD34+ counts were raised a median 1.7-fold for all patients in cohorts A and B. Comparing the apheresis yields from pre- and post-plerixafor administration, the mean fold increase in CD34+ cell count/kg collected after plerixafor injection was 2.06-fold over chemotherapy plus G-CSF alone. The different timing of plerixafor administration between these groups showed some differences in this value (1.85× in Cohort A vs. 2.32× in Cohort B) but limited numbers do not allow strict conclusions to be drawn about the relative value of alternative dose timing. The mean fold increase in cell dose collected between patients with MM (2.00×) and NHL (2.15×) was similar. The single patient who did not reach the threshold PB CD34+ cell count after chemotherapy plus G-CSF alone collected a total of 5.23×10^6 CD34+/kg in two apheresis sessions after plerixafor boost. All 40 patients underwent transplantation and exhibited the expected engraftment kinetics. Long-term follow-up of graft durability was assessed in 35 of these 40 and deemed successful in all patients to 1 year post-transplant. Platelet counts were sustained $>100 \times 10^9$/L at 12 months in 75% of NHL patients and 95.4% of MM patients. This study was the first systematic report of the feasibility of adding plerixafor to chemotherapy-based stem cell mobilization.

Some patients treated with plerixafor through European compassionate use protocols were salvaged from failed or failing chemotherapy-based mobilization regimens. Basak reported a small case series of five patients with MM and NHL who failed to mobilize above the threshold PB CD34+ content to predict an adequate collection [57]. After administration of plerixafor, all five demonstrated a significant increase in PB CD34+ cells/μL (range 2.6- to 16-fold) and all collected above the $\geq 2 \times 10^6$ CD34+ cells/kg threshold required to proceed to transplant. All patients tolerated the salvage intervention well.

The German multicenter compassionate use program previously discussed above also included 47 patients in whom plerixafor plus G-CSF was added to chemotherapy [55]. Patients deemed unlikely to have a successful collection, either due to a previously failed attempt or a PB CD34⁺ cell count below 10/μL were enrolled. The group consisted of 24 patients with NHL, 14 patients with MM, and two patients with HD. The NHL patients collected a median of 2.29×10^6 CD34⁺ cells/kg and the MM patients a median of 4.94×10^6 CD34⁺ cells/kg. Collections were accomplished in a median of two apheresis sessions. Overall, the side effect profile was mild to moderate, and transplant engraftment was consistent with overall institutional expectations.

Additional reports of adding plerixafor to patients using more recent preemptive intervention strategies have also supported the feasibility of using plerixafor with a variety of different chemotherapy regimens. These will be discussed in more detail in the next section.

Preemptive Plerixafor Strategies

Given the effectiveness of plerixafor-based salvage strategies in patients proven to be high risk for collection failure by prior failed attempts, alternative strategies to implement plerixafor in a preemptive fashion have become more prevalent and are being more systematically studied. Relegating plerixafor use to a strictly salvage role would identify hard-to-mobilize patients with high certainty, but increases the unpredictability of pharmacy, apheresis, clinic and stem cell laboratory resource use, and extends both time and cost of the stem cell mobilization process when the historically required washout period is implemented between initial and salvage attempts. This is illustrated in Figure 15.1 below, where the peripheral blood CD34⁺ plot of two traditional plerixafor salvage patients from the VCU Massey Cancer Center is plotted (Salvages 1 and 2). These patients with high-risk MM required a target cell dose of $8–10 \times 10^6$ CD34⁺ cells/kg to support planned tandem transplantation, but collected an inadequate cell dose after G-CSF-based mobilization. As seen, the minimally required 7-day washout period not only added additional days of waiting time before effective treatment could begin but also represents another course of G-CSF, laboratory and clinic costs, and additional apheresis and stem cell processing time and costs. From a logistics standpoint, prediction of patient scheduling the apheresis unit and transplant bed resources becomes chaotic in that the unpredictable failure of a patient means apheresis chair slots are underutilized in the planned week and over-scheduled during the next salvage week. When apheresis, stem cell lab, flow cytometry lab, and transplant center staffing is difficult to predict, increased overtime and scheduling conflicts add unnecessary complications and cost to the BMT program. Even if combined with products obtained with the earlier apheresis attempt to reduce the time required for salvage, the additional daily products processed need to be stored, requiring more capital expenditures in freezer storage capacity and stem cell laboratory needs.

With the impressive outcomes described above in the phase II and Phase III frontline plerixafor mobilization approaches, another potential strategy to optimize the predictability of stem cell mobilization and collection would be to use plerixafor in all patients with NHL and MM regardless of risk. The logistics of obtaining sufficient

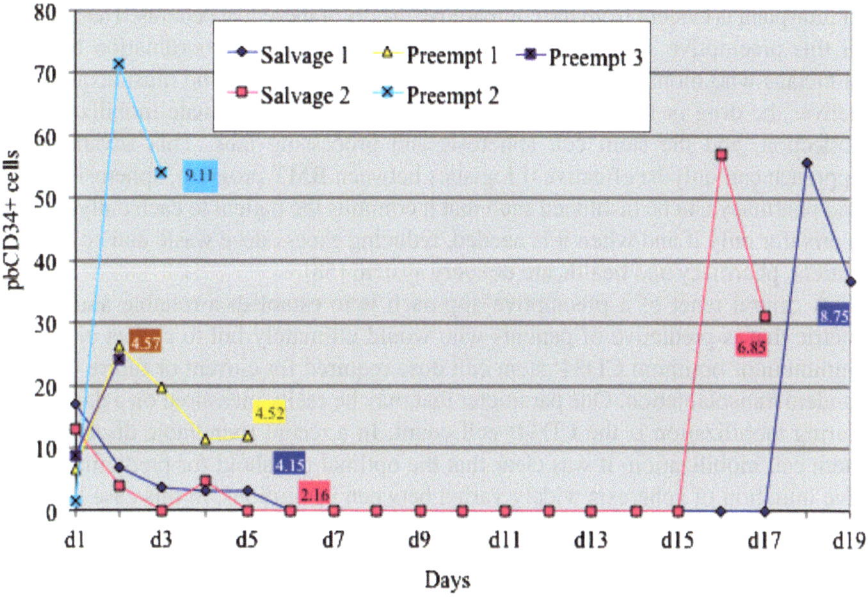

Fig. 15.1 Kinetics of traditional and preemptive plerixafor salvage collection

plerixafor means that in accordance with the FDA-approved administration methods, the drug would have to be available for each patient, either through patient pharmacy insurance benefit requiring advance authorization and ordering, or through pre-positioned patient stocks available in the outpatient transplant clinic. Using this strategy, 23% of lymphoma patients would be expected to save up to 3 days of apheresis in an attempt to collect an optimal cell dose; 35% of patients could expect to save up to 2 days apheresis. Over 37% of myeloma patients would save up to 3 days and 43% up to 2 days of apheresis with up-front use of plerixafor. However, blanket use of this agent would also mean that a significant number of patients would have purchased more plerixafor than required for obtaining an optimal or minimal stem cell dose, unnecessarily raising both transplant center and societal healthcare costs, and resulting in a significant co-pay burden on the part of the patient.

Preemptive salvage strategies administer plerixafor immediately proximate to more individualized objective data suggesting a patient's failure to mobilize or collect. The kinetics of such a strategy is illustrated by the three "Preempt" patients treated at the VCU Massey Cancer Center illustrated in Figure 15.1. In this approach, plerixafor is used to boost a flagging PB $CD34^+$ cell peak, a failing stem cell mobilization or inadequate daily $CD34^+$ stem cell collection attempt while it is underway, without a G-CSF washout period prior to the mobilization reattempt as stipulated in the plerixafor salvage and up-front use study protocols. This approach has merit in that only patients who objectively demonstrate mobilization or collection failure will receive plerixafor, and allows patients to avoid an intervening wait for the salvage attempt. The evidence for a more rapid conclusion of the stem cell collection phase of transplant is evident from the comparative results of these five patients. The logistics of this preemptive salvage method, however, require close coordination between clinicians who monitor the patient's progress, the pharmacy who must acquire and deliver the drug in less than 12 h of demonstration of inadequate mobilization or collection, and the stem cell apheresis and processing labs. This advantageous approach can only be effective if logistics between BMT program, apheresis center and pharmacy can be fashioned such that it commits the patient to each daily dose of plerixafor only if and when it is needed, reducing excess dose waste and cost to the patient, pharmacy and healthcare delivery system [58].

A central tenet of a preemptive approach is to establish a reliable and timely metric that is predictive of patients who would ultimately fail to collect either the minimum or optimum $CD34^+$ stem cell dose required for current or future planned tandem transplantation. One parameter that may be easily measured on a daily basis during mobilization is the $CD34^+$ cell count. In a recent roundtable discussion of stem cell mobilization, it was clear that the optimal threshold for predicting effective initiation of apheresis widely varied between institutions, in this case between 7 and 20 $CD34^+$ cells/μL [59]. The group at Ohio State has devised an algorithm to identify patients likely to require an additional mobilization strategy [59, 60]. Other groups have determined from their local mobilization experience that a level of at least 20 $CD34^+$ cells/μL was highly predictive of collecting at least 2×10^6 $CD34^+$ cells/kg in a single apheresis session [8, 61]. The group at Cleveland Clinic performed a retrospective analysis of 172 patients undergoing G-CSF or G-CSF plus chemotherapy-based stem cell mobilization using recursive partition analysis (RPA) to identify the optimal cutoff values for first day apheresis $CD34^+$ collection yield for patients likely or unlikely to sufficiently collect [30]. In this group, 23 patients failed to collect 2×10^6 $CD34^+$ cells/kg in 5 days of apheresis. Specifically, 22/23 patients who collected $\leq 0.7\times10^6$ $CD34^+$ cells/kg on the first day but only 1/143 who collected more than this amount. When the cumulative first 2 days apheresis collection was considered, 23/30 who collected $\leq 1.54\times10^6$ $CD34^+$ cells/kg failed to collect sufficiently, but none of those collecting more that this threshold. While the precise threshold values predicting minimal and optimal collection for PB $CD34^+$ and apheresis day collections may vary between institutions, this provides a starting point for wider implementation of a preemptive strategy. Thus, it becomes relevant to discriminate between the definition of two patterns of failure, those who fail to mobilize, meaning those whose PB $CD34^+$ cell count fails to rise above or subsequently fall below the target 10–20 $CD34^+$ cells/μL prior to apheresis, and those who fail to collect, referring to those whose daily post-apheresis $CD34^+$ stem cell yield is inadequate to result in a 5-day collection of the targeted minimum or optimal stem cell dose.

The effectiveness and feasibility of this preemptive strategy has been reported both in primary investigations and as subset analyses of overall plerixafor salvage strategies. Some of the retrospective compassionate use G-CSF and chemotherapy plus G-CSF salvage reports described earlier in this chapter included patients who received plerixafor at the time of insufficient measured PB or daily apheresis collection

CD34+ content. In these reports, the earlier application of plerixafor to a G-CSF or chemotherapy-based mobilization regimen increased the PB CD34+ cell content and subsequently improved the likelihood of sufficient and optimal stem cell yields. For example, a retrospective review of 61 patients treated through the Polish compassionate use experience with plerixafor comprised 51 patients who had failed at least one prior mobilization attempt, and ten who had either failed to mobilize ≥20 PB CD34+ cells/μL or who in the local investigators opinion was unlikely to collect a minimum transplant cell dose of 2.0×10^6 CD34+ cells/kg [62]. Overall, 85.2% of this group proceeded to cell collection, and with a median of two aphereses performed, the minimum target collection was obtained from 65.6%, with a median of 2.67×10^6 CD34+ cells/kg. No graft failure was noted for patients in this cohort.

The article by Tricot et al. related their experience in MM patients receiving plerixafor in an open-label phase II study of 20 patients [38]. Ten patients who had been considered proven poor mobilizers were previously discussed and treated according to the traditional plerixafor after washout protocol. An additional ten patients were considered predictably poor mobilizers if after leukocyte recovery from chemotherapy measured PB CD34+ cells were 5–12/μL or in heavily chemotherapy treated patients with a pre-mobilization platelet count of 100,000–150,000/μL. These patients were allowed at least 4 weeks' time for hematologic recovery before G-CSF administration, and were allowed up to 7 days plerixafor administration after a minimum of 7 days G-CSF prior to apheresis. Patients underwent apheresis until ≥5 but $<15 \times 10^6$ CD34+ cells/kg were collected. The PB CD34+ count rose a median of threefold following plerixafor administration, resulting in 80% of the cohort to collect the minimum, and 50% collected more than 5×10^6 CD34+ cells/kg. All patients proceeded to transplant and 6/10 successfully underwent a second autoSCT. All patients engrafted as expected, and graft durability was documented through long-term follow-up.

Four additional author's publications describe larger experiences with planned preemptive or "just-in-time" plerixafor mobilization algorithms. Jantunen analyzed this approach in 63 NHL, HD and MM patients undergoing chemotherapy for stem cell mobilization. Over this 15-month period, 16 patients required plerixafor after the first mobilization due to PB CD34+ counts <10/μL or a first apheresis collection of $<1 \times 10^6$ CD34+ cells/kg. Patients responded to plerixafor with a median fivefold increase in PB CD34+ cells to 39/μL. Apheresis was attempted in 14/16 patients and a median of 2.9×10^6 CD34+ cells/kg was collected in one session. All but one of these patients proceeded to transplant and exhibited normal engraftment. The authors caution that given the high incidence of slow and late CD34+ mobilization in chemotherapy-based strategies, patients may be best served by waiting for WBC recovery to exceed 20×10^6/mL with rising PB CD34+ counts. If at that point, PB CD34+ counts are <10/μL for minimum or <20/μL for optimum cell dose targets, then plerixafor may be introduced. Clearly, clinical situations in which the PB CD34+ count remains low or declines with successive days could be rendered more likely successful from this preemptive plerixafor approach. This same group also reported similar salutary outcomes in a more recent case series of seven patients with NHL and MM in which 6/7 successfully collected $>2\times10^6$ $CD34^+$ cells/kg in one apheresis session following poor $CD34^+$ cell mobilization following chemotherapy [63].

D'Addio also reported a benefit to early introduction of plerixafor in 13 patients with NHL or MM with poor mobilization following chemotherapy plus G-CSF or were thought unlikely to collect sufficiently due to clinical high-risk factors [64]. These patients were continued on G-CSF and plerixafor was administered 10–11 h before the planned apheresis. Compared to baseline, a 4.7-fold increase was seen in the circulating $CD34^+$ cell concentration. All 13 patients collected at least 2×10^6 $CD34^+$ cells/kg and five of the 13 had undergone transplantation at the time of publication. No significant adverse events were recorded with this mobilization approach.

The group at Emory reported a retrospective analysis comparing a preemptive "just in time" plerixafor administration institutional protocol with a cohort of patients who were treated in the year prior to plerixafor approval by the FDA [65]. In this study, of G-CSF mobilized patients, 64 of 188 patients were considered high risk due to pre-existing poor mobilization risk factors ($n=23$) or from insufficient PB $CD34^+$ cell mobilization (<15/μL) after 5 days of G-CSF ($n=41$). The benefit of additional plerixafor was amply demonstrated when compared against 36 similarly high-risk patients mobilized with G-CSF alone with 93 versus 72% collecting the transplant minimum and 42 versus 22% collecting the optimal targets for NHL ($>5\times10^6$ $CD34^+$ cells/kg) and MM ($>10\times10^6$ $CD34^+$ cells/kg). The proportion of patients in the overall study population successfully collecting a transplant dose was higher in patients receiving plerixafor (98%) than in the period where plerixafor was not institutionally available (93% $p=0.04$). An analysis of the costs associated with this just-in-time strategy showed that it increased overall charges by $2,468 per patient, or 17% over G-CSF alone. This increased cost was felt to be easily offset by the higher proportion of high-risk patients able to proceed to transplant.

The MUSC group developed and validated a cost-based decision making algorithm based on the intended target $CD34^+$ transplant cell dose and the PB $CD34^+$ cell count on the fourth day of G-CSF to determine if plerixafor should be added to the G-CSF only mobilization regimen (the MUSC Algorithm, MA, USA) [66, 67]. Comparing 50 patients treated under this algorithm versus 81 mobilized with Cytoxan 2 g/m^2 plus G-CSF, the MA resulted in only 2% of patients failing to meet transplant dose target (3×10^6 $CD34^+$ cells/kg per planned transplant) versus 22% in the Cytoxan cohort. The MA strategy also required fewer days of hospitalization for neutropenic infection, and a shorter interval between initiation of mobilization and transplant admission.

We recently presented a preliminary analysis of the VCU Massey Cancer Center experience of efficacy and economic impact of the initial with plerixafor salvage stem cell mobilization strategies employed from 2004 through April 2010 [68]. Patients with NHL, HD or MM were initially mobilized with either chemotherapy plus G-CSF ($n=97$), G-CSF alone ($n=155$) or with front-line G-CSF plus Plerixafor on the phase III NHL and MM trials discussed above. The mobilization algorithm for these three groups allowed patients to access salvage plerixafor after at least 4 days prior G-CSF through the CUP, Phase III study salvage or Expanded Access Programs after at minimum 7 day washout of G-CSF. A fourth cohort introduced plerixafor in a preemptive pattern if the PB $CD34^+$ cell count was <10/μL after at least 4 days of G-CSF or if a daily collection was less than 0.5×10^6 $CD34^+$ cells/kg. Up to 4 days of plerixafor was administered 11 h prior to apheresis. Using a stringent target of collecting at least 5×10^6 $CD34^+$ cells/kg in 4 days of apheresis, the failure rate was highest in the G-CSF alone and front-line plerixafor group, but lowest in the preemptive plerixafor cohort. In all groups, the total costs accrued from initial mobilization day to the day of transplant admission (including necessary salvage mobilization) was higher in patients failing to meet target $CD34^+$ goal, but with an insignificant difference in the preemptive cohort, suggesting that early plerixafor intervention could moderate costs associated with mobilization or collection failure. Comparing expected costs, a probabilistic weighted average of success and failure costs, the highest expected costs were seen in the blanket up-front use of plerixafor in all patients. Further, the differences in the cost of successful and failed stem cell collection was virtually nil in the preemptive plerixafor strategy. This early intervention strategy was clinically successful with all patients proceeding to transplant with at least a minimum cell dose, and the majority (76.2%) collecting 5×10^6 $CD34^+$ cells/kg in the 4 days of apheresis allowed. This approach also eliminated the need for weekend apheresis due to improved predictability of the mobilization kinetics. Only one patient required apheresis rescheduling due to remobilization. Disease-specific data, along with that from an additional 70 preemptive patients accrued are continuing to be analyzed and will be reported fully in the near future.

These disparate reports support the efficacy, feasibility and safety of a preemptive plerixafor administrative approach. In addition to allowing the administration of this agent to patients who clearly demonstrate its need, this approach allows for more efficient use of transplant, clinical, and apheresis resources and diminishes the lost opportunity time for patients as they await this critical component of the autoSCT process.

Special Consideration Groups: The Plerixafor Experience

Subset reporting of several studies already reviewed above as well as a few case reports comprise the experience of plerixafor use in patients with unique diseases, treatment characteristics that are either not defined by FDA-approved indications or that are recognized as clinical situations in which patients have been found difficult to mobilize sufficiently or optimally.

Patients with MM having prior therapy with lenalidomide have been reported to have excess risk of mobilization failure, ranging from 7 to 77% in some publications [16, 17, 69, 70]. Analyzing a database of 60 patients treated with plerixafor through compassionate use salvage protocols or with initial mobilization attempts through expanded access use programs or the up-front phase III MM trial, Micallef retrospectively examined its impact on patients previously treated with lenalidomide [71]. This patient panel consisted of 20 patients receiving front-line plerixafor and 40 for remobilization. The median number of collected $CD34^+$

cells was 5.6×10^6 CD34$^+$ cells/kg, with the minimum 2×10^6 CD34$^+$ cells/kg collected after one apheresis session in 100% of the initial mobilization and 80% of the salvage mobilization groups. More than 47% of the remobilization cohort collected $\geq 5 \times 10^6$ CD34$^+$ cells/kg. In all, 90% of the entire group proceeded to transplant including one patient transplanted with 1.9×10^6 CD34$^+$ cells/kg, and another transplanted with pooled products. All patients exhibited timely and durable engraftment post-transplant. The International Myeloma Working Group recently cited plerixafor as a strategy to overcome the impaired stem cell mobilization seen in lenalidomide treated patients, reflecting the benefit illustrated in the Micallef study [72].

Multiple myeloma patients who have previously undergone autoSCT without residual stem cell product stored may require remobilization when further transplantation is indicated for disease recurrence. The Central and Eastern European Leukemia Group reported their experience in 76 patients using plerixafor in support of stem cell mobilization including 30 patients with prior autoSCT [73]. The prior autoSCT group were patients either proven to be poor mobilizers after having failed prior attempts ($n = 13$) or those thought unlikely to meet collection target to support subsequent transplantation ($n = 15$). These patients were all heavily pretreated, with 100% having previously been exposed to high dose melphalan, 24.1% to lenalidomide, and 86.2% to velcade-a median of 17 cycles of six different regimens for this group. Additionally, 60% or more of these patients exhibited leukopenia or thrombocytopenia prior to mobilization. These adverse risk features were less prevalent in the group of patients who had not undergone prior autoSCT. The success of plerixafor plus G-CSF for the entire compassionate use cohort was reported as more than 94% mobilizing enough CD34$^+$ cells in the peripheral blood to proceed to apheresis, collecting a median 3.6×10^6 CD34$^+$ cells/kg in two sessions. 44.4% collected $\geq 4 \times 10^6$ CD34$^+$ cells/kg, and 77.6% collected $\geq 2 \times 10^6$ CD34$^+$ cells/kg. In contrast, results in the previously transplanted group proved that this remains a high-risk mobilization group of patients. The first post-plerixafor PB CD34$^+$ cell measurements were lower in the prior transplant group than in those note previously transplanted, (19.5 vs. 30/μL) and the proportion of those with a PB CD34$^+$ cell $\geq$20/μL was also inferior (46.2 vs. 73%). The median total stem cell dose collected was 2.8×10^6 CD34$^+$ cells/kg, compared to 4.2×10^6 CD34$^+$ cells/kg, and only 70% were able to collected more than the minimum threshold stem cell dose for transplant compared to 82% in the non-transplanted group, a statistical trend to significance only. Despite these differences, there was no disparity in the likelihood or timing of engraftment.

Prior treatment of NHL with fludarabine has been reported as a risk factor for patients experiencing inadequate stem cell mobilization and collection [18, 52, 74]. Schriber examined the efficacy of mobilization with plerixafor + G-CSF among NHL patients previously treated with fludarabine through a retrospective analysis of patients with NHL who participated in the compassionate use program [75]. Those patients who received plerixafor + G-CSF and had complete data on the number of cycles of fludarabine and total CD34$^+$ cells collected were included in the analysis. Of the 401 NHL patients in the CUP database, 48 (12%) had documented prior therapy with fludarabine. Complete data on number of cycles of fludarabine and total CD34+ cells collected was available for 33 of these patients. The median number of fludarabine cycles prior to HSC mobilization was five (range 1–50). Among the patients that received prior fludarabine, administration of plerixafor+G-CSF resulted in a median collection of 2.8×10^6 CD34+ cells/kg. A total of 21/33 (63.6%) of the patients collected $\geq 2 \times 10^6$ CD34+ cells/kg necessary to proceed to autoSCT in a median of two apheresis sessions (range 1–6). Overall, 27/33 (81.8%) of the patients proceeded to autoSCT. Median time to neutrophil and platelet engraftment was 12 and 22 days, respectively. The overall collection parameters, and engraftment kinetics were not different from the group of NHL patients without prior fludarabine exposure. This suggests that the majority of patients with NHL pretreated with fludarabine who have failed a previous mobilization regimen can successfully and predictably mobilize CD34+ HSC with plerixafor+G-CSF, and that this approach can overcome the adverse risk impact that fludarabine may have on optimal and effective stem cell collection.

There is a small encouraging reported experience for the use of plerixafor in support of stem cell mobilization of patients with heavily pretreated testicular and germ cell tumors. As these patients are often extensively pretreated, and may be offered tandem transplantation or dose intensive therapy requiring stem cell support for recurrent or refractory disease, successful collection of sufficient cells to support adequate treatment may require plerixafor intervention. Two reports from Germany have been published documenting the experience of plerixafor in support of stem cell mobilization in germ cell tumor patients. The first is a single patient case report of patient with seminoma undergoing scheduled to undergo dose intensive chemotherapy with stem cell support for treatment of a second relapse of disease [76]. The patient was mobilized with G-CSF and PEG-CSF following paclitaxel and ifosfamide chemotherapy. While 1.73×10^6 CD34+ cells/kg were collected in 2 days of apheresis, measurement of the PB CD34+ cells in circulation was 4/μL, and declined further the next day, precluding the likelihood of collecting sufficient stem cells (6×10^6 CD34+ cells/kg) to support three subsequent cycles of carboplatin and etoposide. Plerixafor was administered 10 h prior to apheresis. In the next 2 days, the PB CD34+ cell content had increased by more than three- and nearly fivefold. The final collection total was 4.3×10^6 CD34+ cells/kg in 3 days of collection, and the regimen target was reached by pooling this with the pre-plerixafor collection. When a second mobilization attempt was made to obtain a backup product, the addition of plerixafor to carboplatin/etoposide plus PEG-G-CSF resulted in the collection of 2.6×10^6 CD34+ cells/kg in a single apheresis session. Recovery of neutrophils and platelets were similar across all three stem cell transplantations. A small case series of six heavily pretreated patients (median 3.5 prior lines of therapy) with germ cell tumor was reported [77]. Out of a larger cohort of 17 patients with germ cell tumor undergoing stem cell mobilization, these patients were entered into a plerixafor compassionate use program for having failed a prior chemotherapy plus G-CSF mobilization attempt. The median PB CD34+ cell count increased from 10 to 20 following plerixafor administration, resulting in a 4 day collection of 2.6×10^6 CD34+ cells/kg. Four of the six patients reached the minimum cell dose threshold for autoSCT. Of these, one experienced disease progression prior to high dose chemotherapy, leaving three to proceed to transplant. While these reports constitute a limited dataset for plerixafor use in this disease, given the myelotoxic and stem cell compartment depleting nature of the chemotherapy agents commonly used in the initial treatment and salvage of germ cell tumors, this represents a patient population that may benefit from plerixafor supported stem cell mobilization strategies.

The report of the German compassionate use protocol included 13 patients with "other" diagnoses than NHL, HD or MM, including testicular/germ cell tumor, composite lymphoma, thyroid carcinoma, CLL, Wiskott Aldrich Syndrome, and neuroblastoma [55]. Seven of these patients were mobilized using a varied menu of chemotherapy regimens with G-CSF and plerixafor and six patients mobilized with plerixafor plus G-CSF. The "other" group mobilized with chemotherapy, G-CSF and plerixafor yielded a median of 4.94×10^6 $CD34^+$ cells/kg and the plerixafor plus G-CSF group 16.2×10^6 $CD34^+$ cells/kg. The overall success rate for collection of the minimum acceptable stem cell dose was 76.9% for the entire "Other" composite category.

This publication also reported on plerixafor use in seven pediatric patients with five receiving a non-chemotherapy-based plerixafor plus G-CSF and two with chemotherapy [55]. The non-chemotherapy group collected a median of 17×10^6 $CD34^+$ cells/kg with the chemotherapy cohort yielding a median of 6×10^6 $CD34^+$ cells/kg. All of these groups collected with a median of two apheresis days.

A handful of other brief reports comprise the remainder of the published pediatric experience with plerixafor mobilization. The original US compassionate use program included six pediatric patients, ranging in age from 10 to 18 years. While the mobilization outcomes of this subgroup of patients have not been formally analyzed, they comprise the majority (6/10) of patients in the "other" diagnostic category with documented clinical data in which 80% achieved a collection of at least 2×10^6 $CD34^+$ cells/kg [78]. Most recently, investigators at the Royal Marsden Hospital reported a success rate of 60% in the collection of transplantable stem cell products in five heavily pretreated pediatric patients [79]. Another single case report recounted the successful mobilization, collection and transplantation of a heavily pretreated 13-year old with recurrent Burkitt's lymphoma and concurrent invasive aspergillosis [80]. Toledano reported the use of plerixafor in a 7 year old with metastatic medulloblastoma previously treated with craniospinal irradiation to 36 Gy [81]. An initial attempt was made to collect stem cells using G-CSF alone, but the patient collected a total of 0.3×10^6 $CD34^+$ cells/kg. A single cycle of carboplatin and etoposide was given, and at hematologic recovery the patient was administered G-CSF (10 μg/kg) for 4 days and a single dose of plerixafor 10 h prior to the apheresis attempt. A single apheresis session of 5 h duration collected 11.8×10^6 $CD34^+$ cells/kg. The cells were successfully infused after each of the successive dose intensive chemotherapy cycles, with neutrophil and platelet engraftment occurring within 10–13 days. At the time of publication, the patient remained in clinical and pathologic remission of her disease. While this reported body of evidence remains too small to draw meaningful conclusions, these successful and well-tolerated interventions are encouraging for further studies of plerixafor in the pediatric population.

Ongoing efforts include larger studies and a more systematic retrospective review of the international experience of plerixafor mobilization in young patients.

Conclusions

The development of plerixafor has brought an additional potent tool in the compendium of therapies to support effective stem cell collection for autoSCT. A variety of approaches including remobilization salvage, blanket frontline administration and preemptive dosing of plerixafor have shown efficacy in allowing standard and high-risk patients to obtain not just an acceptable stem cell dose, but a more optimal stem cell dose allowing better long-term outcomes after transplantation. Each of these approaches has differing requirements on the resources of patients and transplantation programs, necessitating careful consideration of the impact of each approach for each institution. The emergence of preemptive plerixafor interventions as a more widely implemented strategy requires careful planning and coordination of clinician, pharmacy, clinical laboratory, apheresis center and stem cell processing laboratory to take full advantage of this effective and increasingly efficient approach to stem cell mobilization salvage. Future studies should focus on the optimal predictive methods of mobilization failure to refine this promising approach to collection of peripheral blood stem cells.

References

1. Desikan KR, Barlogie B, Jagannath S, Vesole DH, Siegel D, Fassas A, Munshi N, Singhal S, Mehta J, Tindle S, Nelson J, Bracy D, Mattox S, Tricot G (1998) Comparable engraftment kinetics following peripheral-blood stem-cell infusion mobilized with granulocyte colony-stimulating factor with or without cyclophosphamide in multiple myeloma. J Clin Oncol 16:1547–1553
2. Weaver CH, Schwartzberg LS, Hainsworth J, Greco FA, Li W, Buckner CD, West WH (1997) Treatment-related mortality in 1000 consecutive patients receiving high-dose chemotherapy and peripheral blood progenitor cell transplantation in community cancer centers. Bone Marrow Transplant 19:671–678. doi:10.1038/sj.bmt.1700713
3. Kalaycio M, Rybicki L, Pohlman B, Sobecks R, Andresen S, Kuczkowski E, Bolwell B (2006) Risk factors before autologous stem-cell transplantation for lymphoma predict for secondary myelodysplasia and acute myelogenous leukemia. J Clin Oncol 24:3604–3610. doi:10.1200/JCO.2006.06.0673
4. Stiff PJ, Micallef I, Nademanee AP, Stadtmauer EA, Maziarz RT, Bolwell BJ, Bridger G, Marulkar S, Hsu FJ, Dipersio JF (2010) Transplanted $CD34^+$ cell dose is associated with long-term platelet count recovery following autologous peripheral blood stem cell transplant in patients with non-Hodgkin lymphoma or multiple myeloma. Biol Blood Marrow Transplant. doi:10.1016/j.bbmt.2010.11.021
5. Hosing C, Saliba RM, Ahlawat S, Korbling M, Kebriaei P, Alousi A, De Lima M, Okoroji JG, Mcmannis J, Qazilbash M, Anderlini P, Giralt S, Champlin RE, Khouri I, Popat U (2009) Poor hematopoietic stem cell mobilizers: a single institution study of incidence and risk factors in

patients with recurrent or relapsed lymphoma. Am J Hematol 84:335–337. doi:10.1002/ajh.21400

6. Morris CL, Siegel E, Barlogie B, Cottler-Fox M, Lin P, Fassas A, Zangari M, Anaissie E, Tricot G (2003) Mobilization of CD34+ cells in elderly patients (>/= 70 years) with multiple myeloma: influence of age, prior therapy, platelet count and mobilization regimen. Br J Haematol 120:413–423
7. Wuchter P, Ran D, Bruckner T, Schmitt T, Witzens-Harig M, Neben K, Goldschmidt H, Ho AD (2010) Poor mobilization of hematopoietic stem cells-definitions, incidence, risk factors, and impact on outcome of autologous transplantation. Biol Blood Marrow Transplant 16:490–499. doi:10.1016/j.bbmt.2009.11.012
8. Pusic I, Jiang SY, Landua S, Uy GL, Rettig MP, Cashen AF, Westervelt P, Vij R, Abboud CN, Stockerl-Goldstein KE, Sempek DS, Smith AL, Dipersio JF (2008) Impact of mobilization and remobilization strategies on achieving sufficient stem cell yields for autologous transplantation. Biol Blood Marrow Transplant 14:1045–1056. doi:10.1016/j.bbmt.2008.07.004
9. Ford CD, Green W, Warenski S, Petersen FB (2004) Effect of prior chemotherapy on hematopoietic stem cell mobilization. Bone Marrow Transplant 33:901–905. doi:10.1038/sj.bmt.1704455
10. Nickenig C, Dreyling M, Hoster E, Ludwig WD, Dorken B, Freund M, Huber C, Ganser A, Trumper L, Forstpointner R, Unterhalt M, Hiddemann W (2007) Initial chemotherapy with mitoxantrone, chlorambucil, prednisone impairs the collection of stem cells in patients with indolent lymphomas—results of a randomized comparison by the German Low-Grade Lymphoma Study Group. Ann Oncol 18:136–142. doi:10.1093/annonc/mdl348
11. Boccadoro M, Palumbo A, Bringhen S, Merletti F, Ciccone G, Richiardi L, Rus C, Bertola A, Giaccone L, Omede P, Musto P (2002) Oral melphalan at diagnosis hampers adequate collection of peripheral blood progenitor cells in multiple myeloma. Haematologica 87:846–850
12. Dreger P, Kloss M, Petersen B, Haferlach T, Loffler H, Loeffler M, Schmitz N (1995) Autologous progenitor cell transplantation: prior exposure to stem cell-toxic drugs determines yield and engraftment of peripheral blood progenitor cell but not of bone marrow grafts. Blood 86:3970–3978
13. Canales MA, Fernandez-Jimenez MC, Martin A, Arrieta R, Caballero MD, Diez J, Quevedo E, Garcia-Bustos J, San Miguel JF, Hernandez-Navarro F (2001) Identification of factors associated with poor peripheral blood progenitor cell mobilization in Hodgkin's disease. Haematologica 86:494–498
14. Clark RE, Brammer CG (1998) Previous treatment predicts the efficiency of blood progenitor cell mobilisation: validation of a chemotherapy scoring system. Bone Marrow Transplant 22:859–863. doi:10.1038/sj.bmt.1701461
15. Drake M, Ranaghan L, Morris TC, Nolan L, Desai ZR, Irvine AE, Jordan A, Magill K, Price S (1997) Analysis of the effect of prior therapy on progenitor cell yield: use of a chemotherapy scoring system. Br J Haematol 98:745–749
16. Paripati H, Stewart AK, Cabou S, Dueck A, Zepeda VJ, Pirooz N, Ehlenbeck C, Reeder C, Slack J, Leis JF, Boesiger J, Torloni AS, Fonseca R, Bergsagel PL (2008) Compromised stem cell mobilization following induction therapy with lenalidomide in myeloma. Leukemia 22:1282–1284. doi:10.1038/sj.leu.2405100
17. Popat U, Saliba R, Thandi R, Hosing C, Qazilbash M, Anderlini P, Shpall E, Mcmannis J, Korbling M, Alousi A, Andersson B, Nieto Y, Kebriaei P, Khouri I, De Lima M, Weber D, Thomas S, Wang M, Jones R, Champlin R, Giralt S (2009) Impairment of filgrastim-induced stem cell mobilization after prior lenalidomide in patients with multiple myeloma. Biol Blood Marrow Transplant 15:718–723. doi:10.1016/j.bbmt.2009.02.011
18. Laszlo D, Galieni P, Raspadori D, Tozzi M, Lauria F, Martinelli G (2004) Fludarabine combination regimen severely affected peripheral blood stem cell mobilization. Acta Haematol 111:228–229. doi:10.1159/000077572
19. Tournilhac O, Cazin B, Lepretre S, Divine M, Maloum K, Delmer A, Grosbois B, Feugier P, Maloisel F, Villard F, Villemagne B, Bastit D, Belhadj K, Azar N, Michallet M, Manhes G, Travade P (2004) Impact of frontline fludarabine and cyclophosphamide combined treatment

on peripheral blood stem cell mobilization in B-cell chronic lymphocytic leukemia. Blood 103:363–365. doi:10.1182/blood-2003-05-1449
20. Putkonen M, Rauhala A, Pelliniemi TT, Remes K (2007) Sepsis, low platelet nadir at mobilization and previous IFN use predict stem cell mobilization failure in patients with multiple myeloma. Cytotherapy 9:548–554. doi:10.1080/14653240701508429
21. Keane C, Gibbs S, Seymour JF, Mills AK, Grimmett K, Van Kuilenberg R, Saal R, Gill D, Prince HM, Marlton P, Mollee P (2006) The Hyper-CVAD chemotherapy regimen has an adverse long-term impact on the ability to mobilize peripheral blood stem cells, which can be readily circumvented by using the early cycles for mobilization. Hematol Oncol 24:159–163. doi:10.1002/hon.784
22. Olivieri A, Brunori M, Capelli D, Montanari M, Massidda D, Gini G, Lucesole M, Poloni A, Offidani M, Candela M, Centurioni R, Leoni P (2004) Salvage therapy with an outpatient DHAP schedule followed by PBSC transplantation in 79 lymphoma patients: an intention to mobilize and transplant analysis. Eur J Haematol 72:10–17. doi:10.1046/j.0902-4441.2004.00171.x
23. Kuittinen T, Nousiainen T, Halonen P, Mahlamaki E, Jantunen E (2004) Prediction of mobilisation failure in patients with non-Hodgkin's lymphoma. Bone Marrow Transplant 33:907–912. doi:10.1038/sj.bmt.1704466
24. Bensinger W, Appelbaum F, Rowley S, Storb R, Sanders J, Lilleby K, Gooley T, Demirer T, Schiffman K, Weaver C et al (1995) Factors that influence collection and engraftment of autologous peripheral-blood stem cells. J Clin Oncol 13:2547–2555
25. Demirer T, Buckner CD, Gooley T, Appelbaum FR, Rowley S, Chauncey T, Lilleby K, Storb R, Bensinger WI (1996) Factors influencing collection of peripheral blood stem cells in patients with multiple myeloma. Bone Marrow Transplant 17:937–941
26. Pastore D, Specchia G, Mestice A, Liso A, Pannunzio A, Carluccio P, Buquicchio C, Greco G, Ciuffreda L, Pietrantuono G, Liso V (2004) Good and poor CD34+ cells mobilization in acute leukemia: analysis of factors affecting the yield of progenitor cells. Bone Marrow Transplant 33:1083–1087. doi:10.1038/sj.bmt.1704437
27. Park IH, Kim Y, Kim JS, Cheong JW, Song JW, Min YH (2008) Transfusion-associated iron overload as a predictive factor for poor stem cell mobilization in patients with haematological malignancies. Transfus Med 18:97–103. doi:10.1111/j.1365-3148.2008.00849.x
28. Weaver CH, Hazelton B, Birch R, Palmer P, Allen C, Schwartzberg L, West W (1995) An analysis of engraftment kinetics as a function of the CD34 content of peripheral blood progenitor cell collections in 692 patients after the administration of myeloablative chemotherapy. Blood 86:3961–3969
29. Tarella C, Di Nicola M, Caracciolo D, Zallio F, Cuttica A, Omede P, Bondesan P, Magni M, Matteucci P, Gallamini A, Pileri A, Gianni AM (2002) High-dose ara-C with autologous peripheral blood progenitor cell support induces a marked progenitor cell mobilization: an indication for patients at risk for low mobilization. Bone Marrow Transplant 30:725–732. doi:10.1038/sj.bmt.1703729
30. Duong HK, Bolwell BJ, Rybicki L, Koo A, Hsi ED, Figueroa P, Dean R, Pohlman B, Kalaycio M, Andresen S, Sobecks R, Copelan E (2011) Predicting hematopoietic stem cell mobilization failure in patients with multiple myeloma: a simple method using day 1 CD34+ cell yield. J Clin Apher. doi:10.1002/jca.20278
31. Genzyme Corporation (2008) Mozobil® (plerixafor injection) package insert. Cambridge, MA
32. Flomenberg N, Devine SM, Dipersio JF, Liesveld JL, Mccarty JM, Rowley SD, Vesole DH, Badel K, Calandra G (2005) The use of AMD3100 plus G-CSF for autologous hematopoietic progenitor cell mobilization is superior to G-CSF alone. Blood 106:1867–1874. doi:10.1182/blood-2005-02-0468
33. Calandra G, Mccarty J, Mcguirk J, Tricot G, Crocker SA, Badel K, Grove B, Dye A, Bridger G (2008) AMD3100 plus G-CSF can successfully mobilize CD34+ cells from non-Hodgkin's lymphoma, Hodgkin's disease and multiple myeloma patients previously failing mobilization with chemotherapy and/or cytokine treatment: compassionate use data. Bone Marrow Transplant 41:331–338. doi:10.1038/sj.bmt.1705908

34. Roberts Ch CH, Candler Ks, Calandra G, Badel K, Mccarty Jm (2007) Single-center experience with the early use of AMD3100 plus G-CSF for mobilization of hematopoietic progenitor cells in patients classified as poor mobilizers ASBMT Tandem Transplant Meeting Keystone, CO 99a
35. Fowler CJ, Dunn A, Hayes-Lattin B, Hansen K, Hansen L, Lanier K, Nelson V, Kovacsovics T, Leis J, Calandra G, Maziarz RT (2009) Rescue from failed growth factor and/or chemotherapy HSC mobilization with G-CSF and plerixafor (AMD3100): an institutional experience. Bone Marrow Transplant 43:909–917. doi:10.1038/bmt.2008.409
36. Dipersio JF, Micallef IN, Stiff PJ, Bolwell BJ, Maziarz RT, Jacobsen E, Nademanee A, Mccarty J, Bridger G, Calandra G (2009) Phase III prospective randomized double-blind placebo-controlled trial of plerixafor plus granulocyte colony-stimulating factor compared with placebo plus granulocyte colony-stimulating factor for autologous stem-cell mobilization and transplantation for patients with non-Hodgkin's lymphoma. J Clin Oncol 27:4767–4773. doi:10.1200/JCO.2008.20.7209
37. Micallef IN, Stiff PJ, Dipersio JF, Maziarz RT, Mccarty JM, Bridger G, Calandra G (2009) Successful stem cell remobilization using plerixafor (mozobil) plus granulocyte colony-stimulating factor in patients with non-hodgkin lymphoma: results from the plerixafor NHL phase 3 study rescue protocol. Biol Blood Marrow Transplant 15:1578–1586. doi:10.1016/j.bbmt.2009.08.005
38. Tricot G, Cottler-Fox MH, Calandra G (2010) Safety and efficacy assessment of plerixafor in patients with multiple myeloma proven or predicted to be poor mobilizers, including assessment of tumor cell mobilization. Bone Marrow Transplant 45:63–68. doi:10.1038/bmt.2009.130
39. Worel N, Rosskopf K, Neumeister P, Kasparu H, Nachbaur D, Russ G, Namberger K, Witt V, Schloegl E, Zojer N, Linkesch W, Kalhs P, Greinix HT (2011) Plerixafor and granulocyte-colony-stimulating factor (G-CSF) in patients with lymphoma and multiple myeloma previously failing mobilization with G-CSF with or without chemotherapy for autologous hematopoietic stem cell mobilization: the Austrian experience on a named patient program. Transfusion 51:968–975. doi:10.1111/j.1537-2995.2010.02896.x
40. Cashen A, Lopez S, Gao F, Calandra G, Macfarland R, Badel K, Dipersio J (2008) A phase II study of plerixafor (AMD3100) plus G-CSF for autologous hematopoietic progenitor cell mobilization in patients with Hodgkin lymphoma. Biol Blood Marrow Transplant 14:1253–1261. doi:10.1016/j.bbmt.2008.08.011
41. Stiff P, Micallef I, Mccarthy P, Magalhaes-Silverman M, Weisdorf D, Territo M, Badel K, Calandra G (2009) Treatment with plerixafor in non-Hodgkin's lymphoma and multiple myeloma patients to increase the number of peripheral blood stem cells when given a mobilizing regimen of G-CSF: implications for the heavily pretreated patient. Biol Blood Marrow Transplant 15:249–256. doi:10.1016/j.bbmt.2008.11.028
42. Dipersio JF, Stadtmauer EA, Nademanee A, Micallef IN, Stiff PJ, Kaufman JL, Maziarz RT, Hosing C, Fruehauf S, Horwitz M, Cooper D, Bridger G, Calandra G (2009) Plerixafor and G-CSF versus placebo and G-CSF to mobilize hematopoietic stem cells for autologous stem cell transplantation in patients with multiple myeloma. Blood 113:5720–5726. doi:10.1182/blood-2008-08–174946
43. Stiff PJ, Micallef I, Nademanee AP, Stadtmauer EA, Maziarz RT, Bolwell BJ, Bridger G, Marulkar S, Hsu FJ, Dipersio JF (2011) Transplanted CD34+ cell dose is associated with long-term platelet count recovery following autologous peripheral blood stem cell transplant in patients with non-Hodgkin lymphoma or multiple myeloma. Biol Blood Marrow Transplant 17:1146–1153
44. Callera F, De Cavenaghi L, Melo CM (2009) Peripheral blood progenitor cell collection without close monitoring of peripheral blood CD34+ cells: a feasible strategy for multiple myeloma or pre-treated non-Hodgkin's lymphoma patients mobilized with low-dose cyclophosphamide plus G-CSF. Transfus Apher Sci 40:91–95. doi:10.1016/j.transci.2009.01.015
45. Jantunen E, Putkonen M, Nousiainen T, Pelliniemi TT, Mahlamaki E, Remes K (2003) Low-dose or intermediate-dose cyclophosphamide plus granulocyte colony-stimulating factor for progenitor cell mobilisation in patients with multiple myeloma. Bone Marrow Transplant 31:347–351. doi:10.1038/sj.bmt.1703840
46. Moskowitz CH, Bertino JR, Glassman JR, Hedrick EE, Hunte S, Coady-Lyons N, Agus DB, Goy A, Jurcic J, Noy A, O'brien J, Portlock CS, Straus DS, Childs B, Frank R, Yahalom J,

Filippa D, Louie D, Nimer SD, Zelenetz AD (1999) Ifosfamide, carboplatin, and etoposide: a highly effective cytoreduction and peripheral-blood progenitor-cell mobilization regimen for transplant-eligible patients with non-Hodgkin's lymphoma. J Clin Oncol 17:3776–3785
47. Fox CP, Mcmillan AK, Bishton MJ, Haynes AP, Russell NH (2008) IVE (ifosfamide, epirubicin and etoposide) is a more effective stem cell mobilisation regimen than ICE (ifosphamide, carboplatin and etoposide) in the context of salvage therapy for lymphoma. Br J Haematol 141:244–248. doi:10.1111/j.1365-2141.2008.07068.x
48. Akhtar S, Tbakhi A, Humaidan H, El Weshi A, Rahal M, Maghfoor I (2006) ESHAP + fixed dose G-CSF as autologous peripheral blood stem cell mobilization regimen in patients with relapsed or refractory diffuse large cell and Hodgkin's lymphoma: a single institution result of 127 patients. Bone Marrow Transplant 37:277–282. doi:10.1038/sj.bmt.1705239
49. Gertz MA, Kumar SK, Lacy MQ, Dispenzieri A, Hayman SR, Buadi FK, Dingli D, Gastineau DA, Winters JL, Litzow MR (2009) Comparison of high-dose CY and growth factor with growth factor alone for mobilization of stem cells for transplantation in patients with multiple myeloma. Bone Marrow Transplant 43:619–625. doi:10.1038/bmt.2008.369
50. Menendez P, Caballero MD, Prosper F, Del Canizo MC, Perez-Simon JA, Mateos MV, Nieto MJ, Corral M, Romero M, Garcia-Conde J, Montalban MA, San Miguel JF, Orfao A (2002) The composition of leukapheresis products impacts on the hematopoietic recovery after autologous transplantation independently of the mobilization regimen. Transfusion 42:1159–1172
51. Arland M, Leuner S, Lange S, Bartsch R, Kahl C, Florschutz A, Franke A, Hoffkes HG (2001) Ifosamide, epirubicin and granulocyte colony-stimulating factor: a regimen for successful mobilization of peripheral blood progenitor cells in patients with multiple myeloma. Hematol Oncol 19:59–66
52. Watts MJ, Ings SJ, Leverett D, Macmillan A, Devereux S, Goldstone AH, Linch DC (2000) ESHAP and G-CSF is a superior blood stem cell mobilizing regimen compared to cyclophosphamide 1.5 g m(−2) and G-CSF for pre-treated lymphoma patients: a matched pairs analysis of 78 patients. Br J Cancer 82:278–282. doi:10.1054/bjoc.1999.0915
53. D'sa S, Yong K, Kyriakou C, Bhattacharya S, Peggs KS, Foulkes B, Watts MJ, Ings SJ, Ardeshna KM, Goldstone AH, Williams CD (2004) Etoposide, methylprednisolone, cytarabine and cisplatin successfully cytoreduces resistant myeloma patients and mobilizes them for transplant without adverse effects. Br J Haematol 125:756–765. doi:10.1111/j.1365-2141.2004.04981.x
54. Shaughnessy P, Islas-Ohlmayer M, Murphy J, Hougham M, Macpherson J, Winkler K, Silva M, Steinberg M, Matous J, Selvey S, Maris M, Mcsweeney PA (2011) Cost and clinical analysis of autologous hematopoietic stem cell mobilization with G-CSF and plerixafor compared to G-CSF and cyclophosphamide. Biol Blood Marrow Transplant 17:729–736. doi:10.1016/j.bbmt.2010.08.018
55. Hubel K, Fresen MM, Salwender H, Basara N, Beier R, Theurich S, Christopeit M, Bogner C, Galm O, Hartwig R, Heits F, Lordick F, Rosler W, Wehler D, Zander AR, Albert MH, Dressler S, Ebinger M, Frickhofen N, Hertenstein B, Kiehl M, Liebler S, Von Lilienfeld-Toal M, Weidmann E, Weigelt C, Lange F, Kroger N (2010) Plerixafor with and without chemotherapy in poor mobilizers: results from the German compassionate use program. Bone Marrow Transplant. doi:10.1038/bmt.2010.249
56. Dugan MJ, Maziarz RT, Bensinger WI, Nademanee A, Liesveld J, Badel K, Dehner C, Gibney C, Bridger G, Calandra G (2010) Safety and preliminary efficacy of plerixafor (Mozobil) in combination with chemotherapy and G-CSF: an open-label, multicenter, exploratory trial in patients with multiple myeloma and non-Hodgkin's lymphoma undergoing stem cell mobilization. Bone Marrow Transplant 45:39–47. doi:10.1038/bmt.2009.119
57. Basak GW, Urbanowska E, Boguradzki P, Torosian T, Halaburda K, Wiktor-Jedrzejczak W (2010) Booster of plerixafor can be successfully used in addition to chemotherapy-based regimen to rescue stem cell mobilization failure. Ann Transplant 15:61–67
58. Dr KMGMK (2010) Plerixafor: a peripheral blood stem cell mobilizer. Pharmacotherapy 30:485–492
59. Giralt S, Alsina MCR, Chao Nj, Devine Sm, Horwitz Me, Jagasia M, Kumar S, Mccarty Jm, Mehta J, Moreb Js, Peterson Fb, Shuster Mw, Schriber Jr, Soiffer Rj, Van Beisen K, Waller Ek

(2009) Challenging the current concepts of stem cell mobilization. Educational Concepts Group. http://web.educationalconcepts.net/monograph/mth029ae2/index.html
60. Devine SHL, Mccarty Jm, Mcsweeney Pa, Micallef I, Schriber Jr (2010) Improving stem cell mobilization results: a CaseBook™ approach educational concepts LLC. http://web.educationalconcepts.net/Monograph/MTH033AE1/index.html
61. Bensinger W, Dipersio JF, Mccarty JM (2009) Improving stem cell mobilization strategies: future directions. Bone Marrow Transplant 43:181–195. doi:10.1038/bmt.2008.410
62. Basak GW, Knopinska-Posluszny W, Matuszak M, Kisiel E, Hawrylecka D, Szmigielska-Kaplon A, Urbaniak-Kujda D, Dybko J, Zielinska P, Dabrowska-Iwanicka A, Werkun J, Rzepecki P, Wroblewska W, Wiktor-Jedrzejczak W (2011) Hematopoietic stem cell mobilization with the reversible CXCR4 receptor inhibitor plerixafor (AMD3100)-Polish compassionate use experience. Ann Hematol 90:557–568. doi:10.1007/s00277-010-1098-7
63. Jantunen E, Penttila K, Pyorala M, Mahlamaki E, Kuittinen T, Nousiainen T (2011) Addition of plerixafor to a chemotherapy plus G-CSF mobilization in hard-to-mobilize patients. Bone Marrow Transplant 46:308–309. doi:10.1038/bmt.2010.93
64. D'Addio A, Curti A, Worel N, Douglas K, Motta MR, Rizzi S, Dan E, Taioli S, Giudice V, Agis H, Kopetzky G, Soutar R, Casadei B, Baccarani M, Lemoli RM (2011) The addition of plerixafor is safe and allows adequate PBSC collection in multiple myeloma and lymphoma patients poor mobilizers after chemotherapy and G-CSF. Bone Marrow Transplant 46:356–363. doi:10.1038/bmt.2010.128
65. Li J, Hamilton E, Vaughn L, Graiser M, Renfroe H, Lechowicz MJ, Langston A, Prichard JM, Anderson D, Gleason C, Lonial S, Flowers CR, Kaufman JL, Waller EK (2011) Effectiveness and cost analysis of "just-in-time" salvage plerixafor administration in autologous transplant patients with poor stem cell mobilization kinetics. Transfusion. 10.1111/j.1537-2995.2011.03136.x
66. Costa LJ, Alexander ET, Hogan KR, Schaub C, Fouts TV, Stuart RK (2011) Development and validation of a decision-making algorithm to guide the use of plerixafor for autologous hematopoietic stem cell mobilization. Bone Marrow Transplant 46:64–69. doi:10.1038/bmt.2010.78
67. Costa LJ, Miller AN, Alexander ET, Hogan KR, Shabbir M, Schaub C, Stuart RK (2011) Growth factor and patient-adapted use of plerixafor is superior to CY and growth factor for autologous hematopoietic stem cells mobilization. Bone Marrow Transplant 46:523–528. doi:10.1038/bmt.2010.170
68. Roberts Ch SR, Edwards R, Anderson J, Mccarty Bw, Scott M, Mccarty Jm (2011) Cost-effective stem cell mobilization: a novel early plerixafor salvage strategy is optimally resource-effective compared to chemotherapy, G-CSF or initial plerixafor strategies. 37th annual meeting of the European Group for blood and marrow transplantation, Paris, France
69. Kumar S, Dispenzieri A, Lacy MQ, Hayman SR, Buadi FK, Gastineau DA, Litzow MR, Fonseca R, Roy V, Rajkumar SV, Gertz MA (2007) Impact of lenalidomide therapy on stem cell mobilization and engraftment post-peripheral blood stem cell transplantation in patients with newly diagnosed myeloma. Leukemia 21:2035–2042. doi:10.1038/sj.leu.2404801
70. Mazumder A, Kaufman J, Niesvizky R, Lonial S, Vesole D, Jagannath S (2008) Effect of lenalidomide therapy on mobilization of peripheral blood stem cells in previously untreated multiple myeloma patients. Leukemia 22:1280–1281. doi:10.1038/sj.leu.2405035 (author reply 1281–1282)
71. Micallef IN, Ho AD, Klein LM, Marulkar S, Gandhi PJ, Mcsweeney PA (2011) Plerixafor (Mozobil) for stem cell mobilization in patients with multiple myeloma previously treated with lenalidomide. Bone Marrow Transplant 46:350–355. doi:10.1038/bmt.2010.118
72. Giralt S, Stadtmauer EA, Harousseau JL, Palumbo A, Bensinger W, Comenzo RL, Kumar S, Munshi NC, Dispenzieri A, Kyle R, Merlini G, San Miguel J, Ludwig H, Hajek R, Jagannath S, Blade J, Lonial S, Dimopoulos MA, Einsele H, Barlogie B, Anderson KC, Gertz M, Attal M, Tosi P, Sonneveld P, Boccadoro M, Morgan G, Sezer O, Mateos MV, Cavo M, Joshua D, Turesson I, Chen W, Shimizu K, Powles R, Richardson PG, Niesvizky R, Rajkumar SV, Durie BG (2009) International myeloma working group (IMWG) consensus statement and guide-

lines regarding the current status of stem cell collection and high-dose therapy for multiple myeloma and the role of plerixafor (AMD 3100). Leukemia 23:1904–1912. doi:10.1038/leu.2009.127
73. Basak GW, Jaksic O, Koristek Z, Mikala G, Basic-Kinda S, Mayer J, Masszi T, Giebel S, Labar B, Wiktor-Jedrzejczak W (2011) Haematopoietic stem cell mobilization with plerixafor and G-CSF in patients with multiple myeloma transplanted with autologous stem cells. Eur J Haematol 86:488–495. doi:10.1111/j.1600-0609.2011.01605.x
74. Eve HE, Seymour JF, Rule SA (2009) Impairment of peripheral blood stem-cell mobilisation in patients with mantle-cell lymphoma following primary treatment with fludarabine and cyclophosphamide +/– rituximab. Leuk Lymphoma 50:463–465. doi:10.1080/10428190802641979
75. Schriber Jr MJ, Mcguirk J, Spitzer G, Uberti Jp, G C (2009) Plerixafor can predictably mobilize hematopoietic stem cells in patients with non-Hodgkin's lymphoma previously treated with fludarabine and undergoing autologous stem cell transplantation 35th annual meeting of the European Group for blood and marrow transplantation Berlin, Germany (abs 0710)
76. Saure C, Weigelt C, Schroeder T, Klarner V, Galonska L, Haas R, Kobbe G (2010) Plerixafor enables successful hematopoietic stem cell collection in an extensively pretreated patient with testicular cancer. Acta Haematol 124:235–238. doi:10.1159/000321509
77. Kobold S, Isernhagen J, Hubel K, Kilic N, Bogner C, Frickhofen N, Bokemeyer C, Fiedler W (2010) Plerixafor is effective and safe for stem cell mobilization in heavily pretreated germ cell tumor patients. Bone Marrow Transplant. doi:10.1038/bmt.2010.264
78. Mccarty JM, J, Grove B, Badel K, Olsen H, Bridger G, Calandra G (2006) AMD3100 Plus G-CSF use in 100 proven poor mobilizers in a compassionate use protocol (CUP). 32nd annual meeting of the European Group for blood and marrow transplantation. Hamburg, Germany
79. Aabideen K, Anoop P, Ethell ME, Potter MN (2011) The feasibility of plerixafor as a second-line stem cell mobilizing agent in children. J Pediatr Hematol Oncol 33:65–67. doi:10.1097/MPH.0b013e3181e9e4c2
80. Flatt T, Lewing K, Gonzalez C, Anthony K, Ryan R, Jones R, Gamis A, Dalal J (2010) Successful mobilization with AMD3100 and filgrastim with engraftment of autologous peripheral blood stem cells in a heavily pretreated pediatric patient with recurrent Burkitt lymphoma. Pediatr Hematol Oncol 27:138–149. doi:10.3109/08880010903447367
81. Toledano H, Yahel A, Cohen IJ, Yaniv I, Stein J (2010) Successful mobilization, harvest and transplant of peripheral blood stem cells using AMD3100 and G-CSF following high dose craniospinal irradiation for medulloblastoma in a young child. Pediatr Blood Cancer 54:613–615. doi:10.1002/pbc.22370

Chapter 16
CXCR4 Antagonists

Klaus Dembowsky, Barbara Romagnoli, Johann Zimmermann, Eric Chevalier, Christian Ludin, and Daniel Obrecht

Introduction

All major pharmaceutical and several Biotech companies have invested over many years significant resources into the field of modulation of chemokines and their receptors for discovery and development novel drugs. Despite these efforts, the outcome has not fulfilled up to now the expectations. Only two compounds have been approved by regulatory authorities and are being marketed: the CCR5 antagonist maraviroc (Celsentri®) acting as HIV entry inhibitor was approved in 2007, followed shortly afterward by the CXCR4 antagonist plerixafor or AMD3100 (Mozobil®): plerixafor was approved in December 2008 by the FDA for subcutaneous injection in combination with granulocyte colony-stimulating factor (G-CSF) to mobilize hematopoietic stem cells (HSCs) to the peripheral blood for collection and subsequent autologous transplantation in patients with non-Hodgkin's lymphoma (NHL) and multiple myeloma (MM). EMA approval followed in August 2009 for Europe to enhance mobilization of stem cells to the bloodstream (in combination with G-CSF) for collection and subsequent autologous transplantation in patients with lymphoma and multiple myeloma whose cells mobilize poorly.

Originally intended to treat HIV infections (similar to the CCR5 antagonist maraviroc), it was noted during clinical development that plerixafor mobilizes HSCs from the bone marrow into the peripheral blood which finally led to marketing of this drug. However, CXCR4 is also expressed by many other cell types and together with its natural ligand SDF-1 (stromal cell-derived factor 1), the axis CXCR4/SDF-1 probably plays an important role in many other different indications as well. Thus, plerixafor (and other CXCR4 antagonists) has and still serves as a prototype drug for exploring many different additional indications.

K. Dembowsky (✉) • B. Romagnoli • J. Zimmermann • E. Chevalier • C. Ludin • D. Obrecht
Polyphor Ltd, Hegenheimermattweg 125, CH-4123, Allschwil, Switzerland
e-mail: klaus.dembowsky@polyphor.com

S. Fruehauf et al. (eds.), *Novel Developments in Stem Cell Mobilization: Focus on CXCR4*, DOI 10.1007/978-1-4614-1960-0_16,

In drug discovery, the chemokine receptor CXCR4 has been targeted by different approaches: by small peptides derived from its ligand SDF-1 and other natural products, by traditional small molecular weight molecules, and more recently also by antibodies. All three approaches have yielded drug-like molecules for preclinical in vitro and in vivo studies, but only a few of these have entered clinical development. The most advanced compounds are POL6326 (Polyphor) and TG-0054 (Taigen) which are currently in Phase II clinical studies for autologous stem cell transplantation.

In the past 10–15 years, stem cell based research and derived cell therapies have seen major progress with harvesting, purification, selection, and optional expansion of human stem cells which are then injected as therapeutic agents for treatment of various diseases with the goal of tissue repair and regeneration and providing alternative therapies. Legislative actions in the EU recently have classified these stem cell based therapies as drugs which need to be manufactured under GMP conditions and regulations. Blockade of CXCR4 mobilizes not only HSCs, but also various other types of stem cells from the bone marrow into the peripheral blood. It is therefore conceivable that such circulating stem or progenitor cells exert similar effects in disease as cell-based therapies. This chapter, therefore, describes also disease areas and indications in which stem cell based research and clinical trials have been conducted or are ongoing and discusses the role of endogenously mobilized stem cells by CXCR4 antagonists.

Physiology of the CXCR4 Receptor

The CXCR4 receptor is a class A G-protein coupled receptor (GPCR) and belongs to the chemokine receptor superfamily, which comprises 19 receptors and at least 46 ligands [1, 2]. The ligand for CXCR4 is stromal cell-derived factor 1 (SDF-1 or CXCL12), a 67-amino acid protein belonging to the ELF-homeostatic and angiostatic chemokines [2] and is produced in the bone marrow (BM) by stromal cells like osteoblasts and endothelial cells. Binding of SDF-1 to CXCR4 activates the Gαi-protein-mediated downstream signaling events which result in calcium efflux, and protein kinase C (PKC) and PI3K/Akt pathway activation [3]. These pathway activations by the CXCR4-SDF-1 axis have pronounced effects on cell migration, chemotaxis of stem cells, cell proliferation, and cell survival [3]. In addition, activation of the CXCR4-SDF axis and AKT-signaling also leads to upregulation of the key angiogenic factor VEGF. Conversely, blockage of CXCR4 suppresses VEGF-promoted tumor angiogenesis and growth [4]. CXCR4 desensitization occurs as a consequence of the phosphorylation of the intracellular C terminus by PKC and GPCR kinases, followed by the interaction with β-arrestin which ultimately leads to receptor internalization. In addition to the roles on receptor desensitization, β-arrestin recruitment has also been associated with regulation of CXCR4 signaling. In particular, it has been shown that β-arrestin 2 enhances the SDF-1-induced chemotaxis which is mediated by MAPK pathway activation [5, 6]. Recently, it was found that SDF-1 also binds to CXCR7 (RDC-1) [7, 8] which was initially considered to be mainly a decoy receptor acting as a SDF-1 scavenger and recently found to activate MAP kinases through β-arrestin, but not G-protein activation [9, 10]. In addition, CXCR7 can signal via formation of heterodimeric receptors with CXCR4. It has also been shown that CXCR7 induces conformational rearrangements within preassembled CXCR4/Gαi protein complexes that impair CXCR4-promoted Gαi protein activation and calcium responses [11].

During embryogenesis, CXCR4 plays a crucial role as knockout of CXCR4 in mice was lethal [12]. A critical function of CXCR4 in the adult life is demonstrated by the existence of two pathologies which are associated with altered function of the CXCR4/SDF-1 axis, namely, the WHIM syndrome [13] and primary myelofibrosis [14].

Functional CXCR4 is detected in a diverse range of cells including peripheral blood lymphocytes (PBL) and monocytes, as well as pre-B cells, mast cells, $CD34^+$ bone marrow progenitor cells, endothelial cells, intestinal and alveolar epithelial cells, astrocytes, microglia, and neurons [15]. Furthermore, CXCR4 is strongly upregulated in over 25 different tumor cells including cancers of epithelial, mesenchymal, and hematopoetic origin [16–18]. Finally, T-tropic HIV uses CXCR4 as a co-receptor (with CCR5) for cell fusion and entry [19, 20].

Crystal structures of a CXCR4 construct bound to two CXCR4 antagonists have recently been described [21]. Notably, one of the ligands was a close analogue of the PEM CXCR4 antagonist POL3026 [22], which served as an early precursor for the discovery and development of POL6326 which is currently in clinical development (see below).

Thus, the CXCR4-SDF-1 axis has fundamental functions in normal and pathologic physiology. It is involved in several crucial disease processes, including HIV infection, cancer cell metastasis, leukemia cell progression, rheumatoid arthritis, asthma, pulmonary fibrosis, and tissue repair.

CXCR4 Antagonists and Antibodies

Since the discovery of CXCR4 and its role in 1996 as main co-receptor for the entry of T-cell line tropic HIV [20], the interest in this receptor has markedly raised. The initial research on CXCR4 was mainly focused on its role in HIV infection. Subsequently, abundant studies were published describing additional roles of the CXCR4/SDF-1 axis in different physiological and pathological processes such as in stem cell mobilization and homing, cancer growth, and metastasis as well as in inflammation.

As a consequence, the potential therapeutic opportunities linked to CXCR4 became more and more apparent and the search for agents targeting and modulating the CXCR4/SDF-1 axis more and more appealing. CXCR4 targeting drugs described so far can be divided into three categories: (1) peptide-like molecules of varying sizes; (2) small molecules; and (3) antibodies.

The first CXCR4 antagonists described belong to the first group of peptide-like molecules and are two unrelated peptides, ALX40-4C and T22 which were discovered as anti-HIV agents even before recognizing that this activity was CXCR4

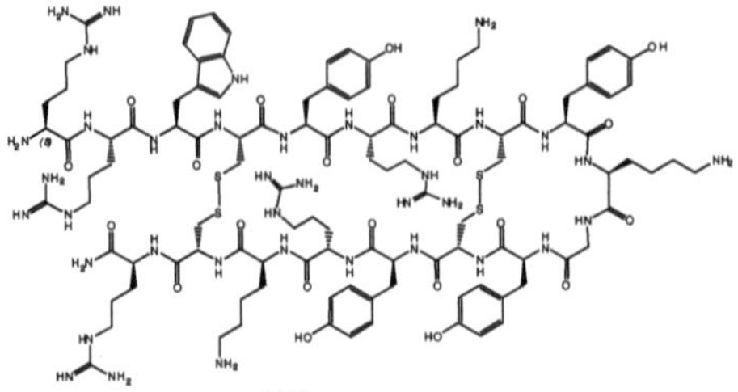

T22

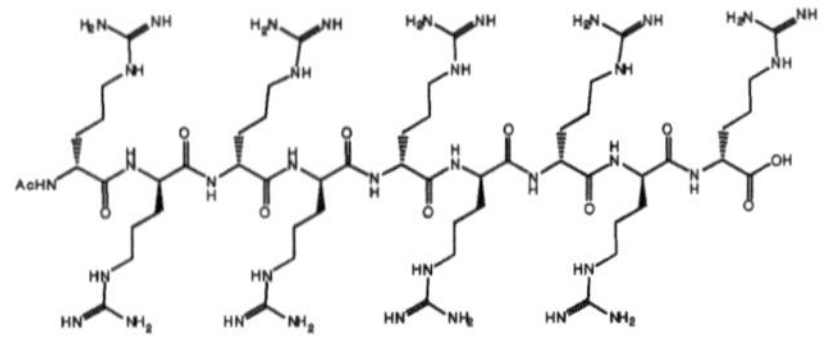

ALX40-4C

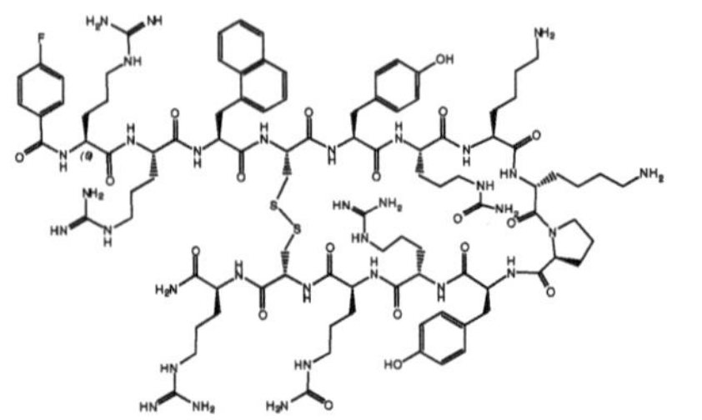

4-F-benzoyl-TN14003

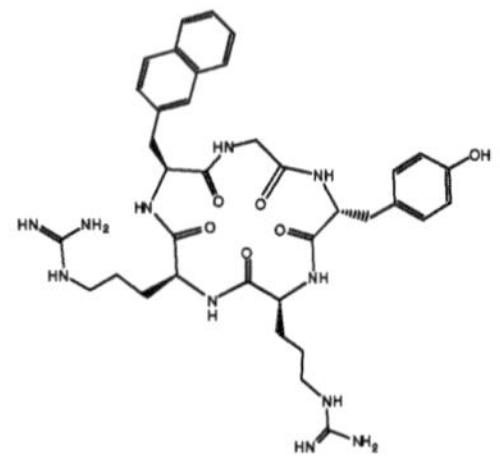

FC-131

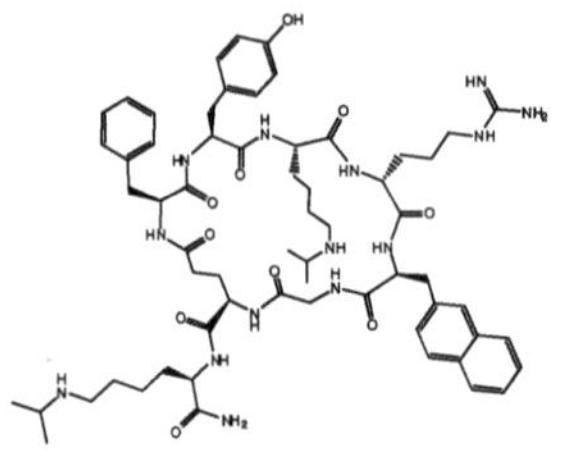

Ly-2510924

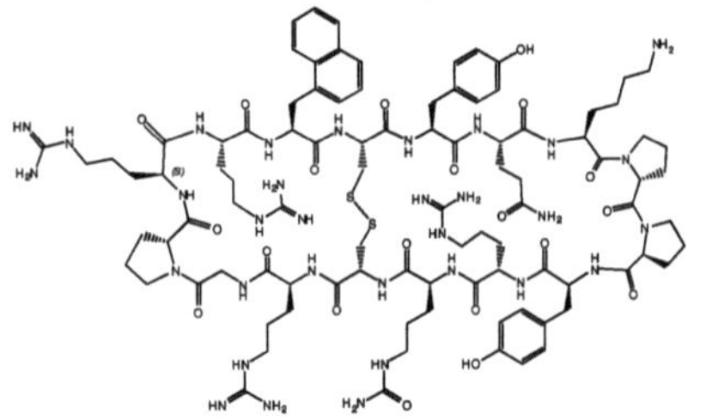

POL3026

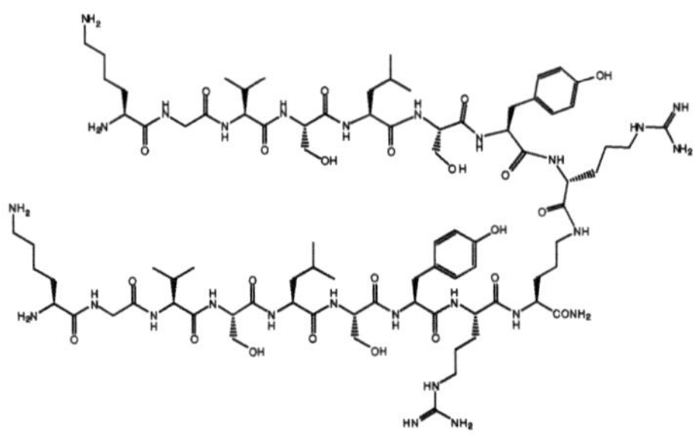

CTCE-9908

Fig. 16.1 Structure of peptide-like CXCR4 antagonists

mediated. ALX40-4C is a *N*-α-acetyl-nona-D-arginine amide developed by Allelix (now NPS Allelix) as anti-HIV agent up to Phase I/II in which the compound was shown to be safe, but also had no significant effect on reducing the viral load [23, 24]. The 18mer peptide T22 with two disulfide bridges (Fig. 16.1) is an analogue of polyphemusin II isolated from the American horseshoe crab and has been synthesized and profiled by Tamamura and Fujii from Kyoto University [25–27]. This peptide was found to be a potent in vitro CXCR4 antagonist (IC_{50} = 10–40 nM depending on the assay) and HIV-inhibitor (IC_{50} = 4–40 nM depending on HIV strains and cell lines). The analysis of the structural motifs responsible for the antagonistic activity has led to the synthesis of several smaller analogues with increased potency and stability [28–30]. In particular, one analogue identified by the same group is 4F-benzoyl-TN14003 (Fig. 16.1), a 14-mer T22 analogue with only one disulfide bridge, which was sufficient to maintain the indispensable β-sheet structure for the CXCR4 antagonist activity [31]. The pharmacological activity of 4F-benzoyl-TN14003 and its parent compounds has been extensively investigated. Interestingly, this peptide was originally claimed to be a CXCR4 antagonist, but then it was observed that a close precursor (T140) behaved as inverse agonist when tested in a cell line expressing a constitutively active mutant receptor [32]. Finally, in a recent patent application, T140 analogues have been reported to have super-agonistic activity causing apoptosis of multiple myeloma and leukemia cells. 4F-Benzoyl-TN14003 is in clinical development by Biokine Therapeutics under the code of BKT140 and a Phase I/II for autologous HSC transplantation in multiple myeloma patients has been successfully completed in 2010.

A further reduction of the size of T140 has led to the cyclopentapeptide FC-131 (Fig. 16.1), in which only the key pharmacophore residues from the larger peptide are conserved [33]. The compound maintains the CXCR4 antagonistic activity of T140 (IC_{50} = 7 nM in a binding assay), but no further development has been reported.

Ely-Lilly has also identified a small peptide (LY-2510924) targeting CXCR4 for treatment of cancer, which in September 2011 has entered into clinical Phase II studies for advanced renal cell carcinoma and lung cancer. One structure from the relevant patent application WO2008/150689A1 is shown in Fig. 16.1.

POL3026 is another T22 analogue with reduced size and is the first compound of a series of potent CXCR4 antagonists developed by Polyphor employing the proprietary Protein Epitope Mimetics (PEM) Technology. POL3026 is a bicyclic 16mer peptide (Fig. 16.1) potently antagonizing CXCR4 antagonist (IC_{50} = 1–2 nM in different in vitro assays) and blocking in vitro HIV-infection with a large panel of HIV strains comprising also some strains resistant to clinically used drugs such as azathymidine (AZT), nevirapine, and the entry inhibitor enfurtivide [34, 35]. Interestingly, the co-crystal structure of CXCR4 with a very close analogue of POL3026 has recently been solved [36] and has further elucidated the binding mode of this compound to the receptor. Further optimization of POL3026 has led to POL6326 with comparable activity, but improved ADMET properties. POL6326 is in clinical development (Phase II) for autologous HSC transplantation in multiple myeloma patients by Polyphor in which efficacy, safety, and excellent tolerability have been demonstrated.

Chemokine Therapeutics has developed CTCE-9908 (Fig. 16.1 from WO2001/85196A2), a CXCR4 antagonist derived from dimerization of two truncated N termini of SDF-1 [37]. This peptide inhibits cancer growth and metastasis in a variety of animal models (e.g., skin, prostate, breast cancer) [38]. Data from Phase I/II

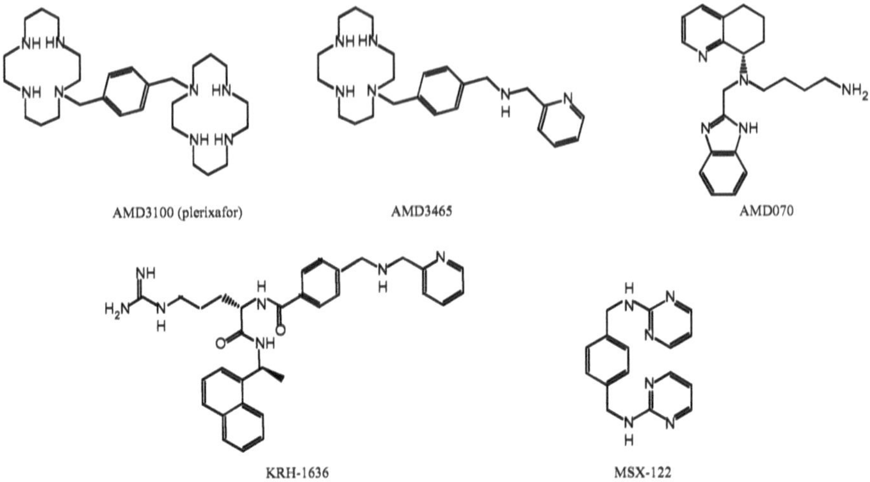

Fig. 16.2 Structure of small molecule CXCR4 antagonists

studies had revealed promising results in cancer patients, but no further development has been reported since then. The development of CTCE9908 is now pursued by British Canadian Biosciences, and a Phase II has been approved in 2010 in several countries for the treatment of cancer diseases.

Whereas all peptides described so far interact with the extracellular domain of CXCR4 (mainly the N terminal and ECL2 portion), the pepducin ATI-2341 is a lipopeptide comprising a peptidic moiety (mimicking the intracellular loop of CXCR4) and a lipid tether allowing the peptide to penetrate the cell membrane and to activate the receptor at the intracellular protein interface [39]. Although displaying agonistic activity in vitro, ATI-2341 behaves in vivo as a CXCR4 antagonist and induces effective peripheral mononuclear cells and HSC mobilization (comparable to plerixafor) in both mice and cynomolgus monkeys.

In parallel to peptide-like CXCR4 antagonists, a large number of nonpeptidic molecules have been described in discovery and preclinical research with only a few of them having reached the clinical stage. The first reported small molecule CXCR4 antagonist is represented by the polycationic bicyclam AMD3100 (plerixafor) (Fig. 16.2). Plerixafor was originally developed by AnorMed (then acquired by Genzyme which is now part of Sanofi Aventis) as HIV entry inhibitor by intravenous application, but this indication was discontinued, maybe because of low efficacy and the observation of adverse cardiac events [40, 41]. During a clinical trial of plerixafor, an increase in white blood cells (WBC) and in particular in HSCs was observed suggesting the potential use of this compound (and CXCR4 antagonists in general) for the mobilization of HSCs. Although plerixafor showed also efficacy in other disease models, such as rheumatoid arthritis, cancer models, and myocardial infarction, no clinical development has been reported for these indications. Plerixafor (Mozobil®) is approved in the USA and Europe for autologous stem cell transplantation in patients with NHL and multiple myeloma in combination with G-CSF. Additional CXCR4 antagonists such as AMD070 and AMD3465 (Fig. 16.2) have been described by AnorMed. The former is a benzimidazole analogue with oral bioavailability and was developed up to Phase II as an anti-HIV agent [42], whereas the later is a monocyclam for which efficacy in disease models of breast cancer and acute myeloid leukemia have been reported for both compounds, but no further development [43].

Another class of orally bioavailable CXCR4 antagonists has been identified by Kureha as anti-HIV agents. Interestingly, the first described prototype KRH-1636 (Fig. 16.2) contains the same pharmacophore that has been identified in the peptidic class of CXCR4 antagonists as indispensable for activity, e.g., a basic group (in particular, guanidine) adjacent to an aromatic moiety [44]. Two optimized analogues, KRH-2731 and KRH-3955, show a more than 1,000-fold increase in potency as CXCR4 antagonists (IC_{50}=5–10 nM) compared to KRH-1636 and inhibit HIV replication in a mouse model after oral administration. However, none of these compounds, although known since 2005, has progressed into clinical development.

MSX-122 is a small molecule (Fig. 16.2) with some similarity to plerixafor, but with two pyrimidine rather than cyclam moieties. This compound has been originally identified by Metastatyx (now Altiris Therapeutics) as an oral anticancer agent for solid tumors, but after completion of Phase I no further development has been reported.

The only other nonpeptide like CXCR4 antagonist in clinical development is TG-0054 by Taigen. After successful completion of a Phase I study, a Phase II for HSC transplantation in NHL and multiple myeloma is ongoing. Additional therapeutic areas under investigation include among others age-related macular degeneration and myocardial infarction.

Other CXCR4 antagonists have been reported which are closely related to AMD070 and comprise a benzimidazole-like and quinolamine moiety separated by a basic group as a spacer. This is the case for CXCR4 antagonists described by GSK and LEO Pharma and they have been investigated mainly as potential therapeutic agents for HIV infections [45]. Other classes of CXCR4 antagonists have been disclosed by ONO Pharmaceuticals, Novartis, and Chemocentryx mainly at the level of patent applications with limited information available on research activities and development status.

Antibodies are the last group of CXCR4 antagonists. Northwest Biotherapeutics has developed two monoclonal antibodies (mAbs) for CXCR4, CX-02, and CX-05, for the treatment of cancers such as leukemia, lymphoma, and solid tumors. The mAbs 517H7 under investigation by Pierre Fabre SA, MDX-1338/BMS-936564 by Bristol-Myers Squibb. The most advanced molecule in terms of clinical development is MDX-1338/BMS-936564 which is in clinical Phase II studies for multiple myeloma.

Another way to modulate the CXCR4/SDF-1 axis consists in the blockade of its natural ligand. This mode of action is represented by PA-517, a therapeutic protein by ProtAffin Biotechnology based on the technology of glycan binding decoy proteins. PA-517 competes with endogenous SDF-1 for the binding to membrane glycosaminoglycans (GAG) which play a key role in the biology of the CXCR4/SDF-1 axis [46, 47]. No further development has been described for this agent after in vivo proof of concept in a metastatic breast cancer model. A RNA-derived inhibitor (Spiegelmer technology) of SDF-1 bound to a PEG-polymer is being developed by Noxxon and is the most advanced molecule in this class of SDF-1 antagonists. After completion of a, first-in-human study Phase I, phase II study is currently ongoing for HSC transplantation alone and in combination with filgrastim (recombinant G-CSF).

In summary, many structurally diverse molecules have been identified and have entered the drug discovery and development pipeline of mostly smaller Biotech companies. The approval of plerixafor for HSCs mobilization and transplantation in combination with G-CSF and the implication of the CXCR4/SDF-1 axis in many different diseases have triggered the entry of different companies into this field which has become competitive.

Stem Cell Mobilization by CXCR4 Antagonists and Transplantation

Transplantation of autologous or allogeneic stem cells has become a standard procedure for treatment of hematological malignancies. In the early times of transplantation, the bone marrow was used as a source for stem cells, but today the infusion of stem cells harvested from the peripheral blood by apheresis has become the standard. Since only small numbers of stem cells are present in peripheral blood, they need to be mobilized from the BM by pharmacological agents. The administration of G-CSF has become the standard for this mobilization and a minimum of two million $CD34^+$ stem cells/kg body weight are required to be collected during aphereses for stem cell transplantation [48]. Recently, exhaustive reviews have been published on the use of CXCR4 antagonists for stem cell mobilization and transplantation [49, 50].

For mobilization of HSCs, G-CSF is routinely given as daily subcutaneous injections over 4–5 days. Although in general G-CSF is well tolerated, skeletal pain and nausea are frequently reported side effects. Despite the routine use of G-CSF, it is not a universally effective mobilizing agent with failure rates of between 5% and 30% [51]. For autologous stem cell transplantation in patients with hematological malignancies, G-CSF is given in the USA as stand-alone therapy, whereas in the EU it is generally given in conjunction with mostly cyclophosphamide-based chemotherapy [52]. The combination of G-CSF requires less apheresis procedures, but also somewhat longer treatment schedules [53, 54]. Notably, in healthy donors who are treated by G-CSF for mobilization and subsequent allogeneic stem cell transplantation the concomitant use of chemotherapy is not indicated. Despite the extensive use of G-CSF for mobilization and stem cell transplantation, there is a need for improved treatment regimens with higher success rates and less adverse events.

HSCs are kept in niches of the BM by the tight, high affinity interaction between receptors and ligands on HSCs and stromal cells. Whereas HSCs express on their surface CXCR4, VLA-4, Kit, CD62L, and CD44, and the corresponding interacting molecules SDF-1, VCAM-1, Kit ligand, CD62, and hyaluronic acid are expressed on cells of the BM stroma, respectively [50, 51]. The interaction between each of these pairs contributes to the retention of stem cells in the BM and blocking the interaction between one or more of them releases HSCs into the peripheral blood.

The relevance of the CXCR4/SDF-1 and VLA-4/VCAM-1 axis in the mobilization of HSCs has been demonstrated in numerous preclinical animal studies, but importantly also in clinical studies. The humanized monoclonal antibody natalizumab (Tysabri®) targeting VLA-4 (CD49d/CD29) which is approved for treatment of relapse multiple sclerosis and more recently for Crohn's disease also releases HSCs into the peripheral blood. Natalizumab results in a five- to seven-fold increase in HSCs which is chronically maintained during therapy. The rather low increase in HSCs results in lower yields of $CD34^+$ cells during apheresis; the accompanying lymphocytosis and the risk of developing progressive multifocal leukoencephalopathy (PML, a demyelinating disease of the central nervous system) preclude the routine use of natalizumab for stem cell mobilization and transplantation [50, 55, 56].

The administration of CXCR4 blocking agents (see section on "CXCR4 Antagonists and Antibodies") results in the mobilization of HSCs. In healthy volunteers in a Phase I study with plerixafor, a dose-dependent mobilization of $CD34^+$ stem cells has been demonstrated [57]. In patients with multiple myeloma and non-Hodgkin's lymphoma, such a dose-dependent effect is less conspicuous or even absent [58]. However, the number of mobilized stem cells after administration of a CXCR4 antagonist, e.g., plerixafor, does not represent the maximal numbers that can be mobilized; this notion is supported by data from CXCR4 conditional knockout animals [59]. Rather, the mobilization of the maximal number of stem cells can only be achieved by blocking several interactions (e.g., VLA-4) and with the combination of G-CSF [51, 56] arguing that the different mechanisms for mobilization act independent of each other. It remains to be shown whether other CXCR4 antagonists behave the same way as plerixafor and result in a limited degree of stem cell mobilization. Preliminary data with analogues of POL6326 show that this type of CXCR4 antagonists may result in a superior mobilization (unpublished data).

From data of a recent clinical trial with autologous stem cell transplantation in multiple myeloma patients it has been concluded that plerixafor given as standalone therapy is insufficient to generate enough HSCs for transplantation [60]. In agreement with these observations, plerixafor has been approved in the USA and EU only in combination with G-CSF for autologous stem cell transplantation in patients with multiple myeloma and NHL. The combination of plerixafor and G-CSF resulted in an increase in the number of stem cells collected in up to four apheresis procedures and/or the need for less numbers of apheresis in patients with these two diseases when compared to the application of G-CSF alone [53, 54]. The recommended dose of plerixafor is 0.24 mg/kg/day by subcutaneous application; however, doses as high as 0.48 mg/kg have been tested with intravenous infusions (see below). Further dose escalation is limited by side effects of plerixafor that include diarrhea and cardiovascular reactions like vasovagal syncopes. It is conceivable that higher degrees of stem cell mobilization may be achieved with a CXCR4 antagonist that can be dosed higher.

Plerixafor has not been approved for use in healthy donors and allogeneic transplantation, but clinical studies with subcutaneous and intravenous administrations have demonstrated that irrespective of the application regimen at the highest dose 25–30% of the donors failed to collect with one apheresis procedure the required number of $CD34^+$ cells (two million cells/kg) to proceed with transplantation. With two apheresis procedure, nearly 100% of donors achieved the required cell numbers [50]. This observation precludes the routine use of plerixafor as stand-alone therapy for stem cell mobilization and collection for allogeneic transplantation in healthy donors.

The approved administration of plerixafor is by the subcutaneous route to patients the night before apheresis is to take place which makes its use inconvenient. It is unclear whether pharmacokinetic properties are the sole reason for this behavior. The use of another CXCR4 antagonist, POL6326, has been reported to result after short 1–2 h intravenous infusions in a rapid mobilization of stem cells so that drug administration and apheresis can be conveniently performed on a single day with drug infusion in the morning followed shortly thereafter by apheresis [61].

The subpopulations of HSCs mobilized by G-CSF and plerixafor have systematically been analyzed by DiPersio and colleagues (for review see 50): $CD34^+$ cells mobilized by plerixafor contain a subset with the phenotype $CD34^{dim}CD45RA^+CD123^{hi}$. This cell type represents progenitors of pre-dendritic cell type 2, but the role they play in homing and engraftment after transplantation awaits further studies. In contrast, $CD34^+$ cells mobilized by G-CSF are enriched with $CD34^+CD45RA^-CD123^{+/-}$ cells (myeloid progenitors and more primitive HSCs). Taubert et al. [62] recently reported that plerixafor mobilizes a subset of a rare and primitive subpopulation of $CD34^+$ HSCs which are $CD38^-$ and stain positively for aldehyde dehydrogenase (ADH^+) (bright) or (high). Although not fully understood yet, the mobilization of these primitive HSCs may have an impact on the engraftment of HSCs mobilized by plerixafor. It would be of great interest to compare the profile of the subpopulations of HSC mobilized by the other CXCR4 antagonists (POL6326 and TG-0054) with that of plerixafor.

Two CXCR4 antagonists are currently in Phase II trials for autologous stem cell transplantation: POL6326 (Polyphor) and TG-0054 (Taigen). Data from a Phase I trial with TG-0054 in healthy volunteers indicate that doses between 1.12 and 4.4 mg/kg are tolerated and result in a 3–14-fold increase in circulating $CD34^+$ cells. Observed side effects were abdominal pain, diarrhea, and nausea and resemble those of plerixafor [63]. Interim data from the ongoing Phase II trial with POL6326 in multiple myeloma patients and autologous stem cell transplantation indicate the compound to be efficacious, very safe, and well tolerated. The optimization of the dosing regimen is so far not limited by side effects and is ongoing to achieve optimal yields in $CD34^+$ cells [62]. In this study, it was also noted that when compared to mobilization with chemotherapy and G-CSF, no or less myeloma tumor cells were detected in the peripheral blood and the apheresis product by POL6326.

Although the debate about clinical and outcome consequences of contamination of the apheresis product by tumor cells in autologous stem cell transplantation is not concluded yet, this could provide a benefit over existing treatments [64].

CXCR4 antagonists are not only able to mobilize HSCs from the BM to the peripheral blood, but may also mobilize tumor cells from either primary hematological (e.g., AML) or solid tumors or metastases, especially in the bone marrow. When CXCR4 antagonists are combined in a timely manner with administration of cytotoxic chemotherapy, the mobilized tumor cells may be killed because the tumor cells loose the protective environment. The combined action of mobilization and cytotoxic agents may result in a reduction of the tumor/metastases and eventually reduce relapses. This principle of chemosensitation has been demonstrated in animal studies for AML [65, 66] and holds promise for clinical trials. Preliminary data from a Phase I/II study in patients with relapsed or refractory AML and plerixafor have reported an increase of the complete remission rate [67].

Stem Cell Mobilization and Tissue Repair

There is more and more evidence that CXCR4$^+$ HSCs can be mobilized from their stores (e.g., the BM) into the peripheral blood during and after tissue or organ injury to initiate repair and regeneratione at these sites. After homing and engraftment of the HSCs at the site of injury, these CXCR4$^+$ cells support the intrinsic mechanisms to limit the damage and possibly also to restore function. The mechanism of action is not yet fully understood, but may include trans-differentiation into the cell types of the injured organ and/or secretion of paracrine factors by the recruited CXCR4$^+$ cells after their homing. Notably, in many organs, the tissue levels of SDF-1 increase after injury and provide a source for chemotaxis of CXCR4$^+$ cells along this SDF-1 concentration gradient

The therapeutic potential of HSCs for tissue repair has been increasingly recognized by large Pharma companies; however, especially Biotech companies and academia have launched several preclinical and clinical research activities to use collected stem cells for different indications. The injection of HSCs is actively being studied in many indications, e.g., myocardial infarction, bone fracture, pancreatic, intestinal, and lung injury to name only a few. The processing of stem cells involves their harvesting, purification, and expansion and finally their injection into the patient. After recent changes in legislation, these processes must be performed under GMP conditions and are not yet possible on a larger scale.

Disruption of the CXCR4/SDF-1 axis during pharmacological treatment with G-CSF or a CXCR4 antagonist also mobilizes HSCs to the peripheral blood [68]. This latter approach holds medical promise with some advanced data demonstrating its therapeutic benefit and therefore represents an alternative to traditional therapies with small molecule drugs or recombinant proteins as discussed below. Pharmacological mobilization of HSCs into the peripheral blood followed by homing and engraftment may indeed serve the same purpose as stem cell therapies in tissue and organ repair and regeneration. In many studies, the CXCR4 antagonist plerixafor (or related molecules) has served as a prototype drug to explore the potential use in tissue or organ repair and regeneration.

In this section, we focus on diseases for which an improvement by the administration or involvement of stem cells has been demonstrated or is highly likely. In the subsequent sections, the focus is on diseases involving the mobilization and migration of inflammatory cells. However, there is often an overlap between these two mechanisms of diseases and a clear separation is not always possible.

Heart and Myocardial Infarction

In a murine model of acute myocardial infarction (AMI), ischemia enhanced the expression of hypoxia inducible factor (HIF-1α) in response to a local hypoxia (after coronary artery occlusion) and subsequently resulted in the expression of SDF-1 in the heart for several days. Increased SDF-1 levels after AMI attract CXCR4-expressing bone marrow derived stem cells to the site of injury via an SDF-1 gradient. In this model, the size of the myocardial infarction was strongly reduced by the application of a CXCR4 antagonist, suggesting that the benefits of hypoxic preconditioning during angina pectoris attacks which often precede a myocardial infarction may be mediated by the CXCR4/SDF-1 axis. Therefore, therapeutic approaches targeting this axis may enhance cardiac progenitor cell based regenerative therapy [69]. Moreover, some CXCR4$^+$ cells that are recruited to the heart in this condition may also act as vascular stem/progenitor cells (including endothelial progenitor cells, EPCs) and promote angiogenesis after AMI [70].

Vascular System: Restenosis After Stent Implantation

In vascular injury (e.g., after stent implantation), SDF-1 expression is increased in smooth muscle cells (SMCs) and accompanied by a transient rise in SDF-1 plasma levels. The SDF-1 gradient recruits CXCR4$^+$ smooth muscle progenitor cell to the site of stent implantation, thus contributing to the maladaptive tissue response that results in thickening of the media (neointima proliferation). The implication of the CXCR4/SDF-1 axis in this neointimal hyperplasia in a murine model of stent implantation (wire injury) has been demonstrated in hyperlipidemic ApoE$^{-/-}$ mice. Chronic pharmacological blockade of CXCR4 using the small molecule antagonist AMD3465 reduces the neointima size by 59%. However, after long-term CXCR4 antagonist treatment, aggravated atherosclerosis was observed, probably due to an increased neutrophil content in the plaque resulting from an increased neutrophil mobilization into the PB [71]. CXCR4 antagonism may therefore be a conceivable and novel approach to limit restenosis after percutaneous interventions through systemic (short term) or local (via drug-eluting stents) application [72].

Bone and Fractures

Bone fractures in the increasingly aging society is one of the major clinical and health economic problems, especially in patients with rheumatoid arthritis (RA) who tend to have lower bone mineral density. Osteoporotic hip fractures are associated with higher mortality. Autologous bone grafts which contain mesenchymal stem cells (MSCs) are currently used for reconstructive bone surgery. Alternatively, stem cell therapy could eventually become a promising and maybe more convenient novel approach for the treatment of bone diseases. In an experimental model of bone fracture, mobilized MSCs were shown to participate in endochondral bone repair. In contrast, a continuous blockade of the CXCR4/SDF-1 axis in mice (SDF-$1^{+/-}$, CXCR$4^{+/-}$, anti–SDF-1 antibody or continuous infusion of the CXCR4 antagonist TF14016) was not effective [73].

The concept of CXCR4^{+} MSCs mobilization and homing suggest that an intermittent administration of a CXCR4 antagonist should be more beneficial than a continuous infusion. After injection MSCs migrated in an exclusively CXCR4-dependent manner to the fracture site, thus supporting this hypothesis. There MSCs improved the fracture healing by improving the biomechanical properties and mineralization of the callus. This improvement correlated well with an increase in cartilage [74].

Pancreas and Type 1 Diabetes

Type 1 insulin-dependent diabetes mellitus (IDDM) is an autoimmune disease resulting from the destruction of the insulin producing pancreatic β-cells. The only real cure is replacement of the β-cell mass, for example through ecto-pancreatic transplantation and islet implantation. These procedures suffer from a chronic shortage of available donor tissue in comparison to the number of potential recipients. One promising alternative approach is the regulated in vivo differentiation of pancreatic islet stem/progenitor cells to produce large numbers of mature, functional islets. In non-obese diabetic (NOD) mice that have a susceptibility to spontaneous development of autoimmune, IDDM, the CXCR4 antagonist plerixafor inhibited the development of disease in prediabetic mice [75]. In another study, islets from BALB/c mice were transplanted to the kidney capsule of hyperglycemic C57BL/6 mice and subsequent treatment of recipients with a CXCR4 antagonist resulted in mobilization of HSCs and in prolongation of islet graft survival [76].

Diseases of the Lung

In several murine models of pulmonary diseases in which the CXCR4/SDF-1 axis was described to be involved in a similar manner as in human airway diseases, adult human MSCs and other stem cells have been used as novel therapeutic approaches.

Instillation of MSCs resulted in improvements of lung function by initiating and supporting regenerative processes.

On the other hand, fibrocytes migrate to damaged lung areas where they interact with local cells, express collagen and thus contribute to fibrosis. Similar to EPCs and the microvasculature, fibrocytes likely contribute to small airway wall thickening in chronic obstructive pulmonary disease (COPD). The potential therapeutic use of stem cells in lung regenerative medicine may thus be a two-edged sword: beneficial effects of MSCs on tissue regeneration, but increase in fibrocytes with potentially worsening the disease. The balance between these two effects depends on the type and composition of cells used for injection and the respective timing [77].

Idiopathic pulmonary fibrosis (*IPF*) is an interstitial inflammatory disease characterized by scarring and fibrosis of the lungs ultimately resulting in terminal respiratory insufficiency. In the rodent bleomycin model, which is frequently used to mimic IPF, SDF-1 levels are increased in serum and bronchial alveolar lavage fluid. These changes are associated with an increase in $CXCR4^+$ cells in the lung and a decrease of $CXCR4^+$ cells in the bone marrow. Administration of MSCs immediately after bleomycin exposure significantly reduces inflammation and collagen deposition. This effect was attributed to secretion of growth factors and cytokines by the instilled MSCs (paracrine effect) that ultimately stimulate tissue repair and regeneration. An alternative mechanism suggests that MSCs home to the lung in response to injury and may exert their beneficial effect by ultimately adopting a lung epithelium-like phenotype [78].

Inhibition of the interaction between CXCR4 and SDF-1 by plerixafor pretreatment in the bleomycin murine model resulted in a decrease of fibrocytes in the lung tissue. These observations provide evidence that CXCR4 antagonists or other specific blockers of the CXCR4/SDF-1 axis may be useful in the prevention (and hopefully treatment) of pulmonary fibrosis by inhibiting the recruitment of $CD45^+CXCR4^+collagenI^+$fibrocytes originating from the BM to the lungs [79].

Acute lung injury (*ALI*) is defined as an acute onset of pulmonary exudates and cellular infiltrates associated with severe hypoxemia. It represents a significant source of morbidity and mortality in patients in intensive care settings. The pathogenesis of ALI has been associated with injury to vascular endothelium and alveolar epithelium as well as sensitivity to endotoxin. In a mouse model of ALI, *Escherichia coli* endotoxin (lipopolysaccharide, LPS) was instilled into the alveoli of the lung followed by intrapulmonary administration of MSCs several hours later. Mice treated with MSCs had reduced lung edema, alveolar capillary permeability, and mortality. In a novel ALI model using ex vivo perfused human lung preparations, allogeneic human MSCs improved alveolar fluid clearance following endotoxin-induced lung injury. These ex vivo human and in vivo murine studies suggest the use of adult MSCs in the treatment of ALI and the closely associated adult respiratory distress syndrome (ARDS) [78].

COPD is a lung disease with both chronic bronchitis and increased mucus secretion eventually resulting in extensive destruction of the alveoli and small airways, e.g., emphysema. COPD is one of the leading causes of death and disability resulting predominantly from cigarette smoking. Pilot clinical studies with the use of allogeneic

MSCs were initiated for the treatment of steroid-resistant COPD; however, the functional outcomes were disappointing (no increase in pulmonary function as measured by forced expiratory volume (FEV1)). The absence of response to the administration of allogeneic MSCs might have been related to the dosage, route of administration, number of infusions, disease stage of COPD, and/or actual composition of the MSC preparation. New clinical trials are being designed to better capture patient response and accurate recording. More recently, compelling studies show that hematopoietic, non-EPC mononuclear cells attracted by VEGF and then kept in place by SDF-1 are critical to support the growth of local vascular cells during angiogenesis. Thus, local vascular progenitors regulate normal vascular homeostasis and remodeling events that are undoubtedly important in the development and progression of COPD [77]. In addition, a recent study showed that a single intratracheal transplantation of bone marrow-derived EPCs could reduce chronic cigarette smoke induced emphysema in mice as assessed by improvement of lung function and histology scores. These findings emphasize the contribution of endothelial cells and the microvasculature in this disease [80].

Cystic fibrosis (*CF*) is a rare hereditary disease which affects mucus clearance, infection resolution, and nutrition. The mutations in the cystic fibrosis transmembrane conductance regulator (CFTR) protein impact the entire body, causing progressive decrease in quality of life and premature death. Although CF is a whole body epithelial disorder, the main cause of morbidity and mortality is respiratory insufficiency due to deficient mucociliary clearance, and chronic infections with *Pseudomonas aeruginosa*. Bone marrow transplantation from healthy mice into $CFTR^{-/-}$ animals significantly improved the response of mice chronically infected with *P. aeruginosa*, ultimately improving clinical scores and lung pathology. Furthermore, preliminary observations show that administration of adult MSCs improved outcome measures and decreased inflammation in the same chronic model of infection and inflammation. These studies underscore the potential of stem cell based therapy in CF [81].

Asthma is an allergic disease associated with airway hyperresponsiveness and inflammation eventually resulting in lung injury due to restricted air flow. Administration of MSCs in the ovalbumin model of asthma significantly decreased airway reactivity and eosinophilia in the bronchoalveolar lavage fluid. The MSCs also had an effect on the direction of the T-cell response shifting the trend of the T cell phenotype away from Th2 helper cell cytokines. This effect was independent from the source of bone marrow derived murine MSCs. In addition, the administration of MSCs resulted in a reduction of inflammation, in epithelial hyperplasia and in extracellular matrix deposition [81].

In models of *pulmonary arterial hypertension* (*PAH*), a CXCR4 antagonist significantly decreased hypoxia-induced pulmonary hypertension and vascular remodeling in rats and mice [82]. Most importantly, rats which were transplanted with bone marrow, cells in which CXCR4 was silenced with siRNA after electroporation, had significantly lower mean pulmonary pressure and wall thickness of pulmonary artery. Thus, selective CXCR4 antagonism may provide novel therapies by decreasing the recruitment of bone marrow derived stem cells to the lung during hypoxia [83].

Kidney Diseases

Focal segment glomerulosclerosis (FSGS) is a common cause of the nephrotic syndrome, associated with kidney CXCR4 overexpression, which often leads to terminal kidney failure. Therapy with steroids and immunosuppressive drugs are the only treatment options, so there is high medical need for a new therapy. Systemically administered human $CD34^+$ HSCs (1 day after ischemia/reperfusion injury) were selectively recruited to sites of injury in immunodeficient mice. These HSCs then promoted kidney repair and regeneration (kidney microvasculature, tubular epithelial cells), enhanced functional recovery, and increased survival. Engraftment of human endothelial cells into the mouse capillary wall was an extremely rare event, indicating that human stem cells mediated renal repair may be due to paracrine mechanisms. These studies highlight human HSCs as a promising therapeutic strategy for promoting renal repair after injury. Blockade of CXCR4 induces mobilization of bone marrow stem cells into the peripheral blood and may have similar effects as administration of HSCs [84].

Neuroscience

Transplantation of bone marrow stem cells has been suggested as a potential therapeutic approach to treat neurodegenerative diseases, however, remains problematic due to issues of engraftment, potential toxicities, and other factors. An alternative strategy is pharmacological-induced recruitment of endogenous stem cells from the bone marrow to a site of injury. SDF-1 is an effective agent for inducing migration of endogenous BM-derived HSCs into the brain shown in a murine Alzheimer's disease (AD) model. This approach warrants further investigations as a potential therapeutic option for the treatment of AD patients in the future [85].

Ophthalmology

Retinal pigment epithelium (RPE) dysfunction has been linked to many devastating eye disorders, including age-related macular degeneration. Damaged RPE are associated with increased SDF-1 release and bone marrow-derived $CXCR4^+$ stem cell migration to the eye. RPE transplantation in humans has rescued photoreceptors and even promoted visual improvements. Some reports demonstrated the clinical feasibility of intravitreal administration of autologous bone marrow-derived mononuclear cells in patients with advanced degenerative retinopathies [86].

Endothelial precursor cells (EPCs) derived from HSCs contribute to choroidal neovascularization (CNV) by signaling through the CXCR4/SDF-1 axis. Hence, CXCR4 antagonism may be useful in preventing neovascularization as observed in the prevention of the laser CNV model by reducing choroidal leakage and angiogenesis [87].

CXCR4 plays a critical role in antigen-induced ocular inflammation (uveitis) by facilitating leukocyte infiltration, which provides a good rationale to target CXCR4 as an anti-inflammatory strategy to treat uveitis [88].

SDF-1 and CXCR4 are increased in hypoxic retina with SDF-1 being localized in glial cells primarily near the surface of the retina and CXCR4 localized in bone marrow derived cells. Antagonists of CXCR4 reduce the migration of HSCs into ischemic retina and strongly suppress VEGF-induced subretinal and CNV [89].

Lupus Erythematosus

In multiple murine models of lupus erythematosus, CXCR4 is significantly upregulated on monocytes, neutrophils, $CD4^+$ T cells, subsets of B, and plasma cells, and is associated with functional consequences including increased cellular migration. The upregulation of SDF-1 has been postulated to promote mobilization and recruitment of $CD34^+$ progenitor cells to sites of damage as a mechanism of repair and repopulation [90]. A total of 15 patients with persistently active refractory systemic lupus erythematosus (SLE) underwent allogeneic MSC transplantation. All patients clinically improved following MSC transplantation with a marked decrease in the SLE disease activity index (SLEDAI) score for up to 1 year. MSC transplantation appears to result in amelioration of disease activity, improvement in serological markers, and stabilization of renal function [91].

Inflammatory Bowel Disease (Crohn's Disease)

Current therapies of inflammatory bowel disease (IBD) do not produce responses in all patients, and nonresponding patients are frequently forced to pursue a surgical option although surgical intervention still will not resolve the disease. Because there are currently no curative options, stem cell based therapeutic approaches could drive major changes in disease management and treatment, as observed in initial promising clinical trials. Patients with Crohn's disease (CD) which undergo allogeneic transplantation for hematological malignancies have been analyzed: among these CD patients 4/5 patients remained free of disease for at least 15 years without any immunosuppressive therapy. Recently, complete normalization of the CD Activity Index (CDAI) was reported after HSC transplantation in two patients with severe, nonresponsive, infliximab-resistant CD. A Phase I clinical trial involving refractory CD patients showed clear evidence of recovery after autologous HSC transplantation. In another clinical trial investigating safety and efficacy of HSC transplantation using autologous, adipose tissue derived stem cells, resulted in complete healing of fistulas in 6/8 patients. Furthermore, it has been shown that allogeneic transplantation of either HSCs or MSCs could also populate the injured regions of the colon in a TNBS-induced experimental colitis rat model resulting in improved gross morphological scores [92].

Rheumatoid Arthritis

Rheumatoid arthritis (RA) is an autoimmune disease of the small joints which can be treated with mAbs against cytokines, notably against tumor necrosis factor α (TNFα) in about 50–60% of affected patients. Curative therapy does currently not exist. Autologous HSC transplantation in RA patients resulted in a clinically positive short-term outcome with low treatment related toxicity. However, most patients relapsed because of residual lesional effector cells. MSCs derived from bone marrow are currently being tested as tissue regenerative and immunomodulating stem cell therapies not only in RA, but also in many other autoimmune diseases after positive data from animal models [93]. Systemic infusion of human adipose tissue-derived MSCs significantly reduced the incidence and severity of collagen-induced arthritis (CIA) in mice by down-regulating the Th1 helper cells driven autoimmune and inflammatory responses. Human adipose tissue-derived MSCs also induced de novo generation of antigen-specific $CD4^{+}CD25^{+}FoxP3^{+}$Treg cells with the capacity to suppress self-reactive T-effector cell responses. Human adipose tissue-derived MSCs emerge as key regulators of immune tolerance by inducing the generation/activation of Treg cells and are thus attractive candidates for a cell-based therapy for RA and other autoimmune diseases [94].

CXCR4 Receptor, Inflammatory Cells, and Inflammatory Diseases

Chemokines were originally identified as potent chemo-attractants of leukocytes, such as neutrophils and monocytes, and therefore, were generally regarded as mediators of acute and chronic inflammation. Several chemokines were subsequently found to be constitutively expressed in lymphoid tissues. Moreover, leukocytes also express specific chemokines and their receptors. Accumulating evidence suggests that in addition to inflammation, chemokines are important regulators in development, homeostasis, and pathophysiological processes associated with osteoporosis, obesity and insulin resistance, viral infections, immune responses, and mobilization of progenitors [95].

The results of many clinical trials with molecules targeting chemokines and chemokine receptors for inflammatory diseases have largely been disappointing. These failures have often been attributed to suboptimal dosing, receptor occupancy, and/or redundancy in the chemokine and their receptor(s) with respect to their physiological and pathophysiological effects [96].

However, two small molecular weight drugs were recently approved by the FDA: maraviroc, an antagonist of CCR5 for the prevention of HIV infection, and plerixafor, a CXCR4 antagonist for HSC mobilization [97]. Preliminary results of a Phase III trial with an orally active CCR9 antagonist for CD are promising (CCX282-B) and the target CCR1 is currently revisited with new molecules. These efforts could lead to the first success for a chemokine receptor antagonist as an anti-inflammatory therapeutic drug and would confirm the importance of chemokine receptors as a target class for inflammatory diseases.

The local invasion by inflammatory cells is a complex process, which is temporally and tightly orchestrated by many immune mediators and cellular effectors. First, patrolling leukocytes are signaled and attracted to the target tissue. To prepare the stage for leukocyte extravasation, the expression of selectins on the surface causes cell rolling (or slowing down) along the endothelial vascular surface. Next, chemokines, integrins, and other adhesive molecules participate in the facilitation of cell activation, firm adhesion, and eventually transmigration into the tissue. This multi-step cascade is indispensable for the exit of the inflammatory cells from the systemic circulation into the tissue. Increasing evidence suggests that CXCR4 and its ligand SDF-1 play an important role in the inflammatory cell trafficking [88].

In this section, we focus on diseases and indications for which an involvement of CXCR4 and its ligand on inflammatory mediators and cells has been demonstrated or is highly likely. From these disease processes, CXCR4 antagonists might thus be introduced into the therapy of inflammatory disorders.

Neutrophils

CXCR4 is also expressed at low levels on the cell surface of mature neutrophils. The interaction between CXCR4 and SDF-1 retains neutrophils within the bone marrow environment as demonstrated by the rare autosomal dominant disorder WHIM (warts, hypogammaglobulinaemia, infections, and myelokathexis). WHIM patients are profoundly neutropenic despite having increased numbers of neutrophils in the bone marrow. These patients have a mutation in CXCR4 which is proposed to be responsible for impaired neutrophil release from the bone marrow by enhancing receptor sensitivity to SDF-1 and thus promoting retention. The role of the CXCR4/SDF-1 interaction in regulating neutrophil egress from the bone marrow is further supported by the finding that CXCR4 deletion in murine myeloid cells results in increased neutrophil release. In addition, treatment with a CXCR4 antagonist or blocking antibody leads to rapid mobilization of neutrophils from bone marrow both in human and mouse [98]. Stress and systemic inflammation are associated with neutrophilia and require the coordination of multiple inflammatory mediators for this acute mobilization of neutrophils from the bone marrow.

Inflammatory Bowel Disease (Ulcerative Colitis)

Recent studies demonstrated that SDF-1 and CXCR4 are constitutively expressed on intestinal epithelial cells, lamina propria T cells, and circulating T cells, but the level of expression is increased in patients with ulcerative colitis (UC). Blockade of

CXCR4 significantly ameliorates dextran sodium sulfate (DSS)-induced colitis in mice, indicating a possible role of the CXCR4/SDF-1 axis in the intestinal inflammatory response [99]. In addition, the number of infiltrated lymphocytes and degree of lymphocyte aggregation was significantly decreased when treated with a CXCR4 antagonist [100].

Lupus Erythematosus

In the immune system, SDF-1 plays a major role in determining differential leukocyte output from the bone marrow. Treatment with a CXCR4 antagonist significantly improved disease severity and nephritis in murine lupus models. These findings underscore the pathogenic role of CXCR4/SDF-1 in lymphoproliferative lupus and lupus nephritis, and highlight this axis as a promising therapeutic target for treating this disease, particularly lupus nephritis [90].

Acute Lung Injury

In patients with ALI increased local SDF-1 concentration and increased CXCR4 expression was associated with aggravated tissue damage which could be attenuated by SDF-1 or CXCR4 blockade suggesting a role of the CXCR4/SDF-1 axis in local inflammation in the lung [101]. A similar increase in SDF-1 levels was also seen in mice with LPS-induced pneumonitis. Additionally, upregulation of CXCR4 expression has been noted on the cell surface of the neutrophils that have migrated into the lung. Neutrophil migration is ameliorated by the use of a SDF-1 blocking antibody [101]. This effect may be in addition to the above therapeutic benefits from MSCs.

Asthma

The CXCR4/SDF-1 axis plays also a critical role in the recruitment of inflammatory leukocytes to the lung and the subsequent induction of pathophysiological manifestations which are characteristic for allergic, antigen-induced asthmatic responses [102]. There is a correlation between the influx of CXCR4$^+$ cells and the progression of the inflammatory phenotype: the neutralization of CXCR4-mediated signals with either anti-CXCR4 or anti-SDF-1a mAbs or CXCR4 antagonists leads to a reduced T_H2 type inflammatory and airway hyper-responsiveness in challenges with ovalbumin [103]. It is unclear whether this is a direct effect on inflammatory cells or mediated via the migration and influx of mobilized BM-derived stem cells.

Idiopathic Pulmonary Fibrosis

Treatment of mice with a CXCR4 antagonist (TN14003) in a bleomycin-induced lung injury model significantly attenuated lung fibrosis. Lung tissue from patients with IPF reveals higher numbers of cells expressing both SDF-1 and CXCR4 than did normal lungs. These results suggest that the CXCR4/SDF-1 axis is important in the complex sequence of events triggered by bleomycin exposure that results in lung repair [78].

Rheumatoid Arthritis

Accumulating evidence suggests the involvement of the CXCR4/SDF-1 system in the pathogenesis of RA. It was reported that RA is caused by the accumulation of CD4 memory T cell (increased CXCR4 expression) in the inflamed synovium with an increased SDF-1 expression. SDF-1 stimulates the migration of memory T cells and inhibits T-cell apoptosis. The incidence of CIA was significantly decreased in T-cell-specific CXCR4-deficient mice [104]. In addition, CXCR4 antagonists reduced the incidence [104] and progression [105] of arthritic signs and clinical symptoms and inhibited the migration and accumulation of rheumatoid T cells in experimental arthritis models in mice [106].

Skin Wound Healing

SDF-1 is similarly expressed in human, swine and rat skin by pericytes and endothelial cells, fibroblasts, and axons. Following burn wounds, the levels of SDF-1 rapidly and markedly increase in human burn blister fluids, hair follicles, and in blood vessel endothelium surrounding the burn wound. Three to eleven days following burns, an increased number of fibroblasts expressing SDF-1 were observed in the recovering dermis of rat, swine, and human skin. In contrast to SDF-1, CXCR4 expression was detected in proliferating epithelial cells as well as in eosinophil and mononuclear cells infiltrating the skin. Treatment of burn wounds in a rat model with antibodies to CXCR4 or the peptidic CXCR4 antagonist 4F-benzoyl-TN14003 resulted in improved epithelization and reduced eosinophilia. Thus, blocking CXCR4/SDF-1 interaction may significantly improve skin recovery after burns [107].

Neuroscience

SDF-1 and its receptor CXCR4 are also expressed in the hypothalamus in neurons expressing melanin-concentrating hormone (MCH) with possible neuroendocrine functions like feeding behavior. Patch clamp recordings of rat lateral hypothalamic area (LHA) slices demonstrated that SDF-1 has a direct effect on voltage-dependent membrane currents of MCH neurons suggesting that SDF-1 may directly regulate MCH neuronal activity [108].

Ophthalmology

CXCR4 plays a critical role in antigen-induced ocular inflammation (uveitis) by facilitating leukocyte infiltration providing the rationale to target CXCR4 as an anti-inflammatory strategy to treat uveitis [88].

Sjögren's Syndrome

Primary Sjögren's syndrome (pSS) is an autoimmune disorder characterized by B-cell hyperactivity as manifested by the production of auto-antibodies, hypergammaglobulinemia, formation of ectopic lymphoid structures within inflamed tissues, and enhanced risk of B-cell lymphoma. SDF-1 provides one mechanism for the prominent accumulation of $CXCR4^+$ memory B cells in the inflamed glands. These findings add to our understanding of the pathogenesis of this autoimmune inflammatory disorder and may result in new therapeutic approaches [109].

CXCR4 Receptor in Oncology

The chemokine receptor CXCR4 has been shown to be overexpressed in a large variety of human cancer types compared to the corresponding normal tissue, e.g., breast, prostate, and lung cancer [110, 111].

Several mechanisms are now known to explain why CXCR4 is expressed at high levels in tumors. The transcription factor HIF-1α is upregulated under hypoxic conditions in expanding tumors. HIF-1α induces VEGF promoted tumor vascularization which leads to enhanced expression of CXCR4 and subsequently to enhanced tumor cell survival and metastasis. In line with these findings, CXCR4 upregulation induced by HIF-1α was shown in glioblastoma to protect from apoptosis and to promote proliferation and invasion into the normal brain tissue [112]. In a xenograft prostate cancer model of CXCR4 overexpression, the density and function of tumor-associated blood vessels was significantly increased. SDF-1 was reported to trigger an angiogenic switch through the upregulation of VEGF and CXCL8 and down-regulation of the glycolytic enzyme phosphoglycerate kinase 1, a negative regulator of VEGF and CXCL8 expression [113]. Besides HIF-1α in hypoxia, an autocrine pathway for increased CXCR4 expression in prostate cancer with another transcription factor, NFκB, was described. In this model, SDF-1 activation led to IκBα phosphorylation and translocation of NFκB to the nucleus followed by transcription and expression of CXCR4 [114].

SDF-1 plays another important role in the motility of tumor cells. Breast cancer cell lines migrate towards gradients of SDF-1 [111]. High SDF-1 levels have been detected at preferred sites of breast cancer cell metastasis such as in the bone marrow and lung tissue. Additional experimental findings in breast cancer animal models support the hypothesis that the CXCR4/SDF-1 axis is relevant for the metastatic process. Upregulation or overexpression of CXCR4 alone leads to a significant increase in bone metastases [115], whereas repression or silencing of CXCR4 by siRNA or inhibition of the function of CXCR4 by antagonists decreased metastatic bone lesions [116].

Recent studies suggest that an efficient functional coupling of the CXCR4 signaling in mammary cancer cells is more relevant for the migration and metastasis than the level of CXCR4 receptor expression on the cell surface. In metastatic tumor cells, binding of SDF-1 to CXCR4 leads to activation of downstream kinases such as ERK1/2, JNK, Akt, and p38 MAPK as a consequence of Gαi dissociation from the Gβγ subunit in the Gαβγ heterotrimer. In nonmetastatic cells, however, CXCR4 forms complexes with both Gαi and Gβ subunits, but not with the Gαβγ heterotrimer leading to a less efficient activation of downstream kinase pathways [117]. Thus, high protein levels of CXCR4 are not necessarily leading to efficient CXCR4-mediated signaling and to tumor cell migration [118]. Nevertheless, high levels of CXCR4 are positively linked to poor prognosis in many cancer types.

Receptor tyrosine kinases (RTKs) are important factors of tumorigenesis and metastasis. There is increasing evidence of a crosstalk between CXCR4 and RTKs. For example, insulin growth factor 1 not only activates the RTK IGF-1R, but also transactivates CXCR4 signaling in CXCR4 positive metastatic cells, but not in CXCR4 positive nonmetastatic cells [119]. On the other hand, SDF-1 produced by stromal cells has been shown to activate the RTK Her2/neu which is an important oncogene in breast tumors [120]. The CXCR4 antagonist plerixafor decreased VEGF protein expression in colon cancer cell lines in a dose-dependent manner.

CXCR4 and SDF-1 have not only a function in migration, but also in adhesion and homing of tumor cells. The peptidomimetic antagonist of CXCR4 T140 blocks the CXCR4-mediated adhesion of tumor cells to components of the extracellular matrix through repression of the activation of integrins. Several studies now point toward an improved chemosensitivity of tumor cells which are hindered to adhere in presence of CXCR4 antagonist [121].

$CD133^+$ cancer stem cells are present at the invasive front of tumors. At this site, a subpopulation of $CD133^+CXCR4^+$ cancer stem cells has been identified in pancreatic tumors which showed a high metastatic potential. Interestingly, depletion of this subpopulation of migrating $CD133^+$ $CXCR4^+$ cancer stem cells from the cancer stem cell pool significantly reduces the metastatic phenotype without affecting their tumorigenic potential suggesting that CXCR4 may be a key factor in the switch to a more aggressive tumor phenotype [122].

Conclusions and Outlook

In the last years, CXCR4 antagonists have been important tools for preclinical and clinical research. A major focus is on the optimized use of different CXCR4 antagonists for autologous and allogeneic stem cell transplantation. Although drugs and cytokines are available for this indication, there is still considerable room for improvement. We tried to outline in this summary that CXCR4 antagonists may also bear considerable potential for additional indications and disease areas in the wide fields of tissue repair and regeneration and oncology. For tissue repair research on CXCR4, antagonists will certainly benefit from the activities in stem cell based research. In oncology current data and evidence suggests that CXCR4 antagonists may find a place in adjuvant (or eventually neoadjuvant) chemotherapy.

References

1. Zlotnik A, Yoshie O, Nomiyama H (2006) The chemokine and chemokine receptor superfamilies and their molecular evolution. Genome Biol 7(12):243
2. Moser B, Wolf M, Walz A, Loetscher P (2004) Chemokines: multiple levels of leukocyte migration control. Trends Immunol 25(2):75–84
3. Zaruba MM, Franz WM (2010) Role of the SDF-1-CXCR4 axis in stem cell-based therapies for ischemic cardiomyopathy1. Expert Opin Biol Ther 10(3):321–335
4. Liang Z, Brooks J, Willard M, Liang K, Yoon Y, Kang S, Shim H (2007) CXCR4/CXCL12 axis promotes VEGF-mediated tumor angiogenesis through Akt signaling pathway. Biochem Biophys Res Commun 359(3):716–722
5. Cheng ZJ, Zhao J, Sun Y, Hu W, Wu YL, Cen B, Wu GX, Pei G (2000) beta-arrestin differentially regulates the chemokine receptor CXCR4-mediated signaling and receptor internalization, and this implicates multiple interaction sites between beta-arrestin and CXCR4. J Biol Chem 275(4):2479–2485
6. Sun Y, Cheng Z, Ma L, Pei G (2002) Beta-arrestin2 is critically involved in CXCR4-mediated chemotaxis, and this is mediated by its enhancement of p38 MAPK activation. J Biol Chem 277(51):49212–49219
7. Naumann U, Cameroni E, Pruenster M, Mahabaleshwar H, Raz E, Zerwes HG, Rot A, Thelen M (2010) CXCR7 Functions as a Scavenger for CXCL12 and CXCL11. PLoS ONE 5(2):e9175
8. Grymula K, Tarnowski M, Wysoczynski M, Drukala J, Barr FG, Ratajczak J, Kucia M, Ratajczak MZ (2010) Overlapping and distinct role of CXCR7-SDF-1/ITAC and CXCR4-SDF-1 axes in regulating metastatic behavior of human rhabdomyosarcomas. Int J Cancer 127:2554–2568
9. Rajagopal S, Kim J, Ahn S, Craig S, Lam CM, Gerard NP, Gerard C, Lefkowitz RJ (2010) {beta}-arrestin-but not G protein-mediated signaling by the "decoy" receptor CXCR7 Proc. Natl Acad Sci U S A 107:628–632
10. Thelen M, Thelen S (2008) CXCR7, CXCR4 and CXCL12: an eccentric trio? J Neuroimmunol 198(1–2):9–13
11. Levoye A, Balabanian K, Baleux F, Bachelerie F, Lagane B (2009) CXCR7 heterodimerizes with CXCR4 and regulates CXCL12-mediated G protein signaling. Blood 113(24): 6085–6093
12. Zou YR, Kottmann AH, Kuroda M, Taniuchi I, Littman DR (1998) Function of the chemokine receptor CXCR4 in haematopoiesis and in cerebellar development. Nature 393(6685):595–599

13. Balabanian K, Lagane B, Pablos JL, Laurent L, Planchenault T, Verola O, Lebbe C, Kerob D, Dupuy A, Hermine O, Nicolas JF, Latger-Cannard V, Bensoussan D, Bordigoni P, Baleux F, Le DF, Virelizier JL, Renzana-Seisdedos F, Bachelerie F (2005) WHIM syndromes with different genetic anomalies are accounted for by impaired CXCR4 desensitization to CXCL12. Blood 105(6):2449–2457
14. Cho SY, Xu M, Roboz J, Lu M, Mascarenhas J, Hoffman R (2010) The effect of CXCL12 processing on CD34+ cell migration in myeloproliferative neoplasms. Cancer Res 70(8): 3402–3410
15. Khan A, Greenman J, Archibald SJ (2007) Small molecule CXCR4 chemokine receptor antagonists: developing drug candidates. Curr Med Chem 14(21):2257–2277
16. Lavrovsky Y, Ivanenkov YA, Balakin KV, Medvedeva DA, Ivachtchenko AV (2008) CXCR4 receptor as a promising target for oncolytic drugs 1. Mini Rev Med Chem 8(11):1075–1087
17. Muller A, Homey B, Soto H, Ge N, Catron D, Buchanan ME, McClanahan T, Murphy E, Yuan W, Wagner SN, Barrera JL, Mohar A, Verastegui E, Zlotnik A (2001) Involvement of chemokine receptors in breast cancer metastasis. Nature 410(6824):50–56
18. Rubin JB, Kung AL, Klein RS, Chan JA, Sun Y, Schmidt K, Kieran MW, Luster AD, Segal RA (2003) A small-molecule antagonist of CXCR4 inhibits intracranial growth of primary brain tumors. Proc Natl Acad Sci U S A 100(23):13513–13518
19. Chabot DJ, Broder CC (2000) Substitutions in a homologous region of extracellular loop 2 of CXCR4 and CCR5 alter coreceptor activities for HIV-1 membrane fusion and virus entry. J Biol Chem 275(31):23774–23782
20. Feng Y, Broder CC, Kennedy PE, Berger EA (1996) HIV-1 entry cofactor: functional cDNA cloning of a seven-transmembrane, G protein-coupled receptor. Science 272(5263):872–877
21. Wu B, Chien EY, Mol CD, Fenalti G, Liu W, Katritch V, Abagyan R, Brooun A, Wells P, Bi FC, Hamel DJ, Kuhn P, Handel TM, Cherezov V, Stevens RC (2010) Structures of the CXCR4 chemokine GPCR with small-molecule and cyclic peptide antagonists. Science 330(6007): 1066–1071
22. DeMarco SJ, Henze H, Lederer A, Moehle K, Mukherjee R, Romagnoli B, Robinson JA, Brianza F, Gombert FO, Lociuro S, Ludin C, Vrijbloed JW, Zumbrunn J, Obrecht JP, Obrecht D, Brondani V, Hamy F, Klimkait T (2006) Discovery of novel, highly potent and selective beta-hairpin mimetic CXCR4 inhibitors with excellent anti-HIV activity and pharmacokinetic profiles. Bioorg Med Chem 14:8396–8404
23. Doranz BJ, Grovit-Ferbas K, Sharron MP, Mao SH, Goetz MB, Daar ES, Doms RW, O'Brien WA (1997) A small-molecule inhibitor directed against the chemokine receptor CXCR4 prevents its use as an HIV-1 coreceptor. J Exp Med 186(8):1395–1400
24. Doranz BJ, Filion LG, Az-Mitoma F, Sitar DS, Sahai J, Baribaud F, Orsini MJ, Benovic JL, Cameron W, Doms RW (2001) Safe use of the CXCR4 inhibitor ALX40-4C in humans. AIDS Res Hum Retroviruses 17(6):475–486
25. Murakami T, Nakajima T, Koyanagi Y, Tachibana K, Fujii N, Tamamura H, Yoshida N, Waki M, Matsumoto A, Yoshie O, Kishimoto T, Yamamoto N, Nagasawa T (1997) A small molecule CXCR4 inhibitor that blocks T cell line-tropic HIV-1 infection. J Exp Med 186(8): 1389–1393
26. Nakashima H, Masuda M, Murakami T, Koyanagi Y, Matsumoto A, Fujii N, Yamamoto N (1992) Anti-human immunodeficiency virus activity of a novel synthetic peptide, T22 ([Tyr-5,12, Lys-7]polyphemusin II): a possible inhibitor of virus-cell fusion. Antimicrob Agents Chemother 36(6):1249–1255
27. Tamamura H, Kuroda M, Masuda M, Otaka A, Funakoshi S, Nakashima H, Yamamoto N, Waki M, Matsumoto A, Lancelin JM (1993) A comparative study of the solution structures of tachyplesin I and a novel anti-HIV synthetic peptide, T22 ([Tyr5,12, Lys7]-polyphemusin II), determined by nuclear magnetic resonance. Biochim Biophys Acta 1163(2):209–216
28. Tamamura H, Xu Y, Hattori T, Zhang X, Arakaki R, Kanbara K, Omagari A, Otaka A, Ibuka T, Yamamoto N, Nakashima H, Fujii N (1998) A low-molecular-weight inhibitor against the chemokine receptor CXCR4: a strong anti-HIV peptide T140. Biochem Biophys Res Commun 253(3):877–882

29. Tamamura H, Hiramatsu K, Mizumoto M, Ueda S, Kusano S, Terakubo S, Akamatsu M, Yamamoto N, Trent JO, Wang Z, Peiper SC, Nakashima H, Otaka A, Fujii N (2003) Enhancement of the T140-based pharmacophores leads to the development of more potent and bio-stable CXCR4 antagonists. Org Biomol Chem 1(21):3663–3669
30. Tamamura H, Hiramatsu K, Kusano S, Terakubo S, Yamamoto N, Trent JO, Wang Z, Peiper SC, Nakashima H, Otaka A, Fujii N (2003) Synthesis of potent CXCR4 inhibitors possessing low cytotoxicity and improved biostability based on T140 derivatives. Org Biomol Chem 1(21):3656–3662
31. Tamamura H, Hori A, Kanzaki N, Hiramatsu K, Mizumoto M, Nakashima H, Yamamoto N, Otaka A, Fujii N (2003) T140 analogs as CXCR4 antagonists identified as anti-metastatic agents in the treatment of breast cancer. FEBS Lett 550(1–3):79–83
32. Zhang WB, Navenot JM, Haribabu B, Tamamura H, Hiramatu K, Omagari A, Pei G, Manfredi JP, Fujii N, Broach JR, Peiper SC (2002) A point mutation that confers constitutive activity to CXCR4 reveals that T140 is an inverse agonist and that AMD3100 and ALX40-4C are weak partial agonists. J Biol Chem 277(27):24515–24521
33. Tamamura H, Araki T, Ueda S, Wang Z, Oishi S, Esaka A, Trent JO, Nakashima H, Yamamoto N, Peiper SC, Otaka A, Fujii N (2005) Identification of novel low molecular weight CXCR4 antagonists by structural tuning of cyclic tetrapeptide scaffolds. J Med Chem 48(9):3280–3289
34. DeMarco SJ, Henze H, Lederer A, Moehle K, Mukherjee R, Romagnoli B, Robinson JA, Brianza F, Gombert FO, Lociuro S, Ludin C, Vrijbloed JW, Zumbrunn J, Obrecht JP, Obrecht D, Brondani V, Hamy F, Klimkait T (2006) Discovery of novel, highly potent and selective beta-hairpin mimetic CXCR4 inhibitors with excellent anti-HIV activity and pharmacokinetic profiles. Bioorg Med Chem 14:8396–8404
35. Moncunill G, rmand-Ugon M, Clotet-Codina I, Pauls E, Ballana E, Llano A, Romagnoli B, Vrijbloed JW, Gombert FO, Clotet B, De MS, Este JA (2008) Anti-HIV activity and resistance profile of the CXC chemokine receptor 4 antagonist POL3026. Mol Pharmacol 73(4): 1264–1273
36. Wu B, Chien EYT, Mol CD, Fenalti G, Liu W, Katritch V, Abagyan R, Brooun A, Wells P, Bi FC, Hamel DJ, Kuhn P, Handel TM, Cherezov V, Stevens RC (2010) Structures of the CXCR4 chemokine GPCR with small-molecule and cyclic peptide antagonists. Science 330: 1066–1071
37. Wong D, Korz W (2008) Translating an antagonist of chemokine receptor CXCR4: from bench to bedside, 2. Clin Cancer Res 14(24):7975–7980
38. Singh B, Cook KR, Martin C, Huang EH, Mosalpuria K, Krishnamurthy S, Cristofanilli M, Lucci A (2010) Evaluation of a CXCR4 antagonist in a xenograft mouse model of inflammatory breast cancer. Clin Exp Metastasis 27(4):233–240
39. Tchernychev B, Ren Y, Sachdev P, Janz JM, Haggis L, O'Shea A, McBride E, Looby R, Deng Q, McMurry T, Kazmi MA, Sakmar TP, Hunt S III, Carlson KE (2010) Discovery of a CXCR4 agonist pepducin that mobilizes bone marrow hematopoietic cells. Proc Natl Acad Sci U S A 107(51):22255–22259
40. Donzella GA, Schols D, Lin SW, Este JA, Nagashima KA, Maddon PJ, Allaway GP, Sakmar TP, Henson G, De CE, Moore JP (1998) AMD3100, a small molecule inhibitor of HIV-1 entry via the CXCR4 co-receptor. Nat Med 4(1):72–77
41. Hendrix CW, Collier AM, Lederman MM, Flexner C, Macfarland RT, Giandomenico C, Fuchs EJ, Redpath E, Bridger G, Henson GW, Calandra G (2004) Safety, pharmacokinetics, and antiviral activity of AMD3100, a selective CXCR4 receptor inhibitor, in HIV-1 infection. J Acquir Immune Defic Syndr 37(2):1253–1262
42. Stone ND, Dunaway SB, Flexner CW, Tierney C, Calandra GB, Becker S, Cao YJ, Wiggins IP, Conley J, Macfarland RT, Park JG, Lalama C, Snyder S, Kallungal B, Klingman KL, Hendrix CW (2007) Multiple dose escalation study of the safety, pharmacokinetics, and biologic activity of oral AMD070, a selective CXCR4 receptor inhibitor, in human subjects (ACTG A5191). Antimicrob Agents Chemother 51(7):2351–2358
43. Bridger GJ, Skerlj RT, Hernandez-Abad PE, Bogucki DE, Wang Z, Zhou Y, Nan S, Boehringer EM, Wilson T, Crawford J, Metz M, Hatse S, Princen K, De Clercq E, Schols D (2010)

Synthesis and structure activity relationships of azamacrocyclic C-X-C chemokine receptor 4 antagonists: analogues containing a single azamacrocyclic ring are potent inhibitors of T-cell tropic (X4) HIV-1 replication. J Med Chem 53:1250–1260

44. Ichiyama K, Yokoyama-Kumakura S, Tanaka Y, Tanaka R, Hirose K, Bannai K, Edamatsu T, Yanaka M, Niitani Y, Miyano-Kurosaki N, Takaku H, Koyanagi Y, Yamamoto N (2003) A duodenally absorbable CXC chemokine receptor 4 antagonist, KRH-1636, exhibits a potent and selective anti-HIV-1 activity. Proc Natl Acad Sci U S A 100(7):4185–4190
45. Gudmundsson KS, Sebahar PR, Richardson LDA, Miller JF, Turner EM, Catalano JG, Spaltenstein A, Lawrence W, Thomson M, Jenkinson S (2009) Amine substituted N-(1H-benzimidazol-2yl-methyl)-5, 6, 7, 8-tetrahydro-8-quinolinamines as CXCR4 antagonists with potent activity against HIV-1. Bioorg Med Chem Lett 19(17):5048–5052
46. Juarez J, Bendall L, Bradstock K (2004) Chemokines and their receptors as therapeutic targets: the role of the SDF-1/CXCR4 axis. Curr Pharm Des 10(11):1245–1259
47. Albanese P, Caruelle D, Frescaline G, Delbe J, Petit-Cocault L, Huet E, Charnaux N, Uzan G, Papy-Garcia D, Courty J (2009) Glycosaminoglycan mimetics-induced mobilization of hematopoietic progenitors and stem cells into mouse peripheral blood: structure/function insights. Exp Hematol 37:1072–1083
48. Points to consider concerning endpoints in clinical studies with haematopoietic growth factors for mobilisation of autologous stem cells. Committee for Proprietary Medicinal Products (CPMP), The European Agency for the Evaluation of Medicinal Products (EMA), February 2000.
49. Rettig MP, Ramirez P, Nervi P, DiPersio JF (2009) CXCR4 and mobilization of hematopoietic precursors. Methods Enzymol 460:57–90
50. Rettig, MP, Ansstas G, DiPersio JF. Mobilization of hematopoietic stem and progenitor cells using inhibitors of CXCR4 and VLA-4. Leukemia 2011 Sep 2 [Epub ahead of print]
51. Bensinger W, DiPersio JF, McCarty JM (2009) Improving stem cell mobilization strategies: future directions. Bone Marrow Transplant 43:181–195
52. Giralt S, Stadtmauer EA, Harousseau JL, Palumbo A, Bensinger W, Comenzo RL, Kumar S, Munshi NC, Dispenzieri A, Kyle R, Merlini G, San Miguel J, Ludwig H, Hajek R, Jagannath S, Blade J, Lonial S, Dimopoulos MA, Einsele H, Barlogie B, Anderson KC, Gertz M, Attal M, Tosi P, Sonneveld P, Boccadoro M, Morgan G, Sezer O, Mateos MV, Cavo M, Joshua D, Turesson I, Chen W, Shimizu K, Powles R, Richardson PG, Niesvizky R, Raikumar SV, Durie BGM (2009) International myeloma working group (IMWG) consensus statement and guidelines regarding the current status of stem cell colelction and high dose therapy for multiple myeloma and the role of plerixafor (AMD3100). Leukemia 23:1904–1912
53. DiPersio JF, Micallef IN, Stiff PJ, Bolwell BJ, Maziarz RT, Jacobsen E et al (2009) Phase III prospective randomized double-blind placebo-controlled trial of plerixafor plus granulocyte colony-stimulating factor compared with placebo plus granulocyte colony-stimulating factor for autologous stem-cell mobilization and transplantation for patients with non-Hodgkin's lymphoma. J Clin Oncol 27:4767–4773
54. DiPersio JF, Stadtmauer EA, Nademanee A, Micallef IN, Stiff PJ, Kaufman JL et al (2009) Plerixafor and G-CSF versus placebo and G-CSF to mobilize hematopoietic stem cells for autologous stem cell transplantation in patients with multiple myeloma. Blood 113: 5720–5726
55. Bonig H, Wundes A, Chang KH, Lucas S, Papayannopoulou T (2008) Increased numbers of circulating hematopoietic stem/progenitor cells are chronically maintained in patients treated with the CD49d blocking antibody natalizumab. Blood 111:3439–3441
56. Bonig H, Watts KL, Chang KH, Kiem HP, Papayannopoulou T (2009) Concurrent blockade of alpha4-integrin and CXCR4 in hematopoietic stem/progenitor cell mobilization. Stem Cells 27:836–837
57. Liles WC, Broxmeyer HE, Rodger E, Wood B, Hübel K, Cooper S, Hangoc G, Bridger GJ, Henson GW, Calandra G, Dale DC (2003) Mobilization of hematopoietic progenitor cells in healthy volunteers by AMD3100, a CXCR4 antagonist. Blood 102:2728–2730
58. Devine SM, Flomenberg N, Vesole DH, Liesveld J, Weisdorf D, Badel K, Calandra G, DiPersio JF (2004) Rapid mobilization of CD34+ cells following administration of the CXCR4

antagonist AMD3100 to patients with multiple myeloma and non-Hodgkin's lymphoma. J Clin Oncol 22:1095–1102
59. Christopher MJ, Liu F, Hilton MJ, Long F, Link DC (2009) Suppression of CXCL12 production by bone marrow osteoblasts is a common and critical pathway for cytokine-induced mobilization. Blood 114:1331–1339
60. Flomenberg N, Comenzo RL, Badel K, Calandra G (2010) Plerixafor (Mozobil®) alone to mobilize hematopoietic stem cells from multiple myeloma patients for autologous transplantation. Biol Bone Marrow Transplant 16:695–700
61. Schmitt S, Weinhold N, Dembowsky K, Neben K, Witzens-Harig M, Braun M, Klemmer J, Wuchter P, Ludin C, Ho A, Goldschmidt H (2010) First results of a Phase-II study with the new CXCR4 antagonist POL6326 to mobilize hematopoietic stem cells (HSC) in multiple myeloma (MM). Blood 116:824 (ASH Annual Meeting Abstracts)
62. Taubert I, Saffrich R, Zepeda-Moreno A, Hellwig I, Eckstein V, Bruckner T, Ho AD, Wuchter P (2011) Characterization of hematopoietic stem cell subsets from patients with multiple myeloma after mobilization with plerixafor. Cytotherapy 13:459–466
63. Chung DT, Chang LW, Huang YH, Tsai CY, Hsu CH, King CHR, Yuan JH, Yen CF, Chen YM, Lu YC, Hsu MC (2009) TH-0054, a novel and potent stem cell mobilizer, displays excellent PK/PD and safety profile in Phase I trial. Blood 114:866 (ASH Annual Meeting Abstracts)
64. DiPersio JF, Ho AD, Hanrahan J, Hsu FJ, Fruehauf S (2011) Relevance and clinical implications of tumor cell mobilization in the autologous transplant setting. Biol Blood Marrow Transplant 17:943–955
65. Nervi B, Ramirez P, Rettig MP, Uy GL, Holt MS, Ritchey JK, Prior JL, Piwnica-Worms D, Bridger G, Ley TJ, DiPersio JF (2009) Chemosensitization of acute myeloid leukemia (AML) following mobilization by the CXCR4 antagonist AMD3100. Blood 113:6206–62014
66. Chen YC, Zeng Z, Shi Y, Jacamo R, Ludin C, Dembowsky K, Frenette PS, Konopleva M, Andreeff M (2010) Targeting CXCR4, SDF1 and beta-adrenergic receptors in the AML microenvironment by novel antagonist POL6326, G-CSF and isoproterenol. Blood 116:2179 (ASH Annual Meeting)
67. Uy GL, Rettig MP, McFarland K, Hladnik L, Kulkarni S, Abboud CN, Cashen AF, Stockerl-Goldstein K, Vij R, Westervelt P, DiPersio JF (2009) A Phase I/II study of chemosensitization with the CXCR4 antagonist plerixafor in relapsed or refractory AML. Blood 114:787 (ASH Annual Meeting Abstracts)
68. Summers C et al (2010) Neutrophil kinetics in health and disease. Trends Immunol 31(8):318–324
69. Tang YL et al (2009) Hypoxic preconditioning enhances the benefit of cardiac progenitor cell therapy for treatment of myocardial infarction by inducing CXCR4 expression. Circ Res 104:1209
70. Takahashi M (2010) Role of the SDF-1/CXCR4 system in myocardial infarction. Circ J 74:418–423
71. Zernecke A et al (2010) Chemokines in the vascular inflammatory response of atherosclerosis. Cardiovasc Res 86:192–201
72. Schober A (2008) Chemokines in vascular dysfunction and remodeling. Arterioscler Thromb Vasc Biol 28:1950–1959
73. Kitaori T et al (2009) Stromal cell–derived factor 1/CXCR4 signaling is critical for the recruitment of mesenchymal stem cells to the fracture site during skeletal repair in a mouse model. Arthritis Rheum 60(3):813–823
74. Granero-Moltó F et al (2009) Regenerative effects of transplanted mesenchymal stem cells in fracture healing. Stem Cells 27(8):1887–1898
75. Leng Q (2008) Elevated CXCL12 expression in the bone marrow of NOD mice is associated with altered T cell and stem cell trafficking and diabetes development. BMC Immunol 9:51
76. Fiorina P (2011) Targeting the CXCR4–CXCL12 Axis Mobilizes Autologous Hematopoietic Stem Cells and Prolongs Islet Allograft Survival via Programmed Death Ligand 1. J Immunol 186:121–131

77. Randell SH et al (2006) Airway epithelial stem cells and the pathophysiology of chronic obstructive pulmonary disease. Proc Am Thorac Soc 3(8):718–725
78. Xu J et al (2007) Role of the SDF-1/CXCR4 axis in the pathogenesis of lung injury and fibrosis. Am J Respir Cell Mol Biol 37:291–299
79. Song JS et al (2010) Inhibitory effect of CXC chemokine receptor 4 antagonist AMD3100 on bleomycin induced murine pulmonary fibrosis. Exp Mol Med 42(6):465–472
80. Cao J et al (2010) Effect of intratracheal transplantation of bone marrow-derived endothelial progenitor cell on cigarette smoking-induced emphysema in mice, Eur Respir J 36 Suppl. 54, 429s, P2436
81. Bonfield TL (2010) Adult mesenchymal stem cells: an innovative therapeutic for lung diseases. Discov Med 9(47):337–345
82. Young K et al (2009) Inhibition of the SDF-1/CXCR4 axis attenuates neonatal hypoxia-induced pulmonary hypertension. Circ Res 104(11):1293–1301
83. Lunyin Yu et al (2011) Effect of chemokine receptor CXCR4 on hypoxia-induced pulmonary hypertension and vascular remodeling in rats. Respir Res 12:21
84. Li B et al (2010) Mobilized human hematopoietic stem/progenitor cells promote kidney repair after ischemia/reperfusion injury. Circulation 121:2211–2220
85. Shin JW et al (2011) Combined effects of hematopoietic progenitor cell mobilization from bone marrow by G-CSF and AMD3100, and chemotaxis into the brain using SDF-1α in an Alzheimer's disease mouse model. Stem Cells 29(7):1075–1089
86. Siqueira RC et al (2010) Possible mechanisms of retinal function recovery with the use of cell therapy with bone marrow-derived stem cells. Arq Bras Oftalmol 73:474–479
87. Lee E et al (2010) Evaluation of CXCR4 Inhibition in the Prevention and Intervention Model of Laser-Induced Choroidal Neovascularization. Invest Ophthalmol Vis Sci 51:3666–3672
88. Zhang Z et al (2009) CXCR4 but not CXCR7 is mainly implicated in ocular leukocyte trafficking during ovalbumin-induced acute uveitis. Exp Eye Res 89(4):522–531
89. De Silva RL et al (2007) The SDF-1/CXCR4 ligand/receptor pair is an important contributor to several types of ocular neovascularization. FASEB J 21:3219–3230
90. Chong BF et al (2009) Targeting the CXCR4/CXCL12 axis in systemic lupus erythematosus. Expert Opin Ther Targets 13(10):1147–1153
91. Liang J et al (2010) Allogenic mesenchymal stem cells transplantation in refractory systemic lupus erythematosus: a pilot clinical study. Ann Rheum Dis 69(8):1423–1429
92. Singh UP (2010) Stem cells as potential therapeutic targets for inflammatory bowel disease. Front Biosci (Schol Ed) 2:993–1008
93. Tyndall A et al (2010) Stem cells in the treatment of inflammatory arthritis. Best Pract Res Clin Rheumatol 24(4):565–574
94. González MA et al (2009) Treatment of experimental arthritis by inducing immune tolerance with human adipose-derived mesenchymal stem cells. Arthritis Rheum 60(4):1006–1019
95. Lazennec G et al (2010) Chemokines and chemokine receptors: new insights into cancer-related inflammation. Trends Mol Med 16(3):133–144
96. Proudfoot AE et al (2010) Anti-chemokine small molecule drugs: a promising future? Expert Opin Investig Drugs 19(3):345–355
97. Ratajczak MZ et al (2006) The pleiotropic effects of the SDF-1–CXCR4 axis in organogenesis, regeneration and tumorigenesis. Leukemia 20:1915–1924
98. Devine SM et al (2008) Rapid mobilization of functional donor hematopoietic cells without G-CSF using AMD3100, an antagonist of the CXCR4-SDF-1 interaction. Blood 112:990–998
99. Xia XM et al (2010) CXCR4 antagonist AMD3100 attenuates colonic damage in mice with experimental colitis. World J Gastroenterol 16(23):2873–2880
100. Mikami S et al (2008) Blockade of CXCL12/CXCR4 axis ameliorates murine experimental colitis. J Pharmacol Exp Ther 327:383–392
101. Joseph MP et al (2007) Pulmonary stromal-derived factor-1 expression and effect on neutrophil recruitment during acute lung injury. J Immunol 178:8148–8157
102. Lukacs NW et al (2002) AMD3100, a CxCR4 antagonist, attenuates allergic lung inflammation and airway hyperreactivity. Am J Pathol 160:1353–1360

103. Gonzalo JA et al (2000) Critical Involvement of the chemotactic axis CXCR4/stromal cell-derived factor-1α in the inflammatory component of allergic airway disease. J Immunol 165:499–508
104. Chung SH et al (2010) CXC chemokine receptor 4 expressed in T cells plays an important role in the development of collagen-induced arthritis. Arthritis Res Ther 12(5):R188
105. Klerck BD et al (2005) Pro-inflammatory properties of stromal cell-derived factor-1 (CXCL12) in collagen-induced arthritis. Arthritis Res Ther 7:R1208–R1220
106. Tamamura H et al (2004) Identification of a CXCR4 antagonist, a T140 analog, as an anti-rheumatoid arthritis agent. FEBS Lett 569:99–104
107. Avniel S et al (2006) Involvement of the CXCL12/CXCR4 pathway in the recovery of skin following burns. J Invest Dermatol 126:468–476
108. Callewaere C et al (2007) Chemokines and chemokine receptors in the brain: implication in neuroendocrine regulation. J Mol Endocrinol 38:355–363
109. Hansen A et al (2007) B cells in Sjögren's syndrome: indications for disturbed selection and differentiation in ectopic lymphoid tissue. Arthritis Res Ther 9:218
110. Balkwill F (2004) Cancer and the chemokine network. Nat Rev Cancer 4(7):540–550
111. Muller A, Homey B, Soto H, Ge N, Catron D, Buchanan ME et al (2001) Involvement of chemokine receptors in breast cancer metastasis. Nature 410(6824):50–56
112. Zagzag D, Lukyanov Y, Lan L, Ali MA, Esencay M, Mendez O et al (2006) Hypoxia-inducible factor 1 and VEGF upregulate CXCR4 in glioblastoma: Implications for angiogenesis and glioma cell invasion. Lab Invest 86(12):1221–1232
113. Wang J, Dai J, Jung Y, Wei CL, Wang Y, Havens AM et al (2007) A glycolytic mechanism regulating an angiogenic switch in prostate cancer. Cancer Res 67(1):149–159
114. Fernandis AZ, Cherla RP, Chernock RD, Ganju RK (2002) CXCR4/CCR5 down-modulation and chemotaxis are regulated by the proteasome pathway. J Biol Chem 277(20):18111–18117
115. Kang Y, Siegel PM, Shu W, Drobnjak M, Kakonen SM, Cordon-Cardo C et al (2003) A multigenic program mediating breast cancer metastasis to bone. Cancer Cell 3(6):537–549
116. Liang Z, Yoon Y, Votaw J, Goodman MM, Williams L, Shim H (2005) Silencing of CXCR4 blocks breast cancer metastasis. Cancer Res 65(3):967–971
117. Holland JD, Kochetkova M, Akekawatchai C, Dottore M, Lopez A, McColl SR (2006) Differential functional activation of chemokine receptor CXCR4 is mediated by G proteins in breast cancer cells. Cancer Res 66(8):4117–4124
118. Fulton AM (2009) The chemokine receptors CXCR4 and CXCR3 in cancer. Curr Oncol Rep 11(2):125–131
119. Akekawatchai C, Holland JD, Kochetkova M, Wallace JC, McColl SR (2005) Transactivation of CXCR4 by the insulin-like growth factor-1 receptor (IGF-1R) in human mda-mb-231 breast cancer epithelial cells. J Biol Chem 280(48):39701–39708
120. Cabioglu N, Summy J, Miller C, Parikh NU, Sahin AA, Tuzlali S et al (2005) CXCL12/stromal cell-derived factor-1alpha transactivates her2-neu in breast cancer cells by a novel pathway involving src kinase activation. Cancer Res 65(15):6493–6497
121. Hartmann TN, Burger JA, Glodek A, Fujii N, Burger M (2005) CXCR4 chemokine receptor and integrin signaling co-operate in mediating adhesion and chemoresistance in small cell lung cancer (SCLC) cells. Oncogene 24(27):4462–4471
122. Hermann PC, Huber SL, Herrler T, Aicher A, Ellwart JW, Guba M et al (2007) Distinct populations of cancer stem cells determine tumor growth and metastatic activity in human pancreatic cancer. Cell Stem Cell 1(3):313–323

Part III
CXCR4 Antagonists for Treatment of Leukemias and Solid Tumors

Chapter 17
Application of CXCR4 Inhibitors in Leukemia

George Ansstas, Fazia Mir, Michael P. Rettig, Mark Schroeder, Linda Eissenberg, and John F. DiPersio

Abstract Hematopoietic and cancer cells express the CXCR4 receptor, which in conjunction with its SDF-1/CXCL12 ligand mediates leukemia cell trafficking and homing to the marrow microenvironment. This interaction brings CXCR4-bearing cells within close proximity to marrow stromal cells, thus providing a niche for leukemic cell growth and contributing to drug resistance. Historically, CXCR4 antagonists were developed for the treatment of human immunodeficiency virus (HIV), but were also found to induce leukocytosis upon administration. This led to their use in hematopoietic stem cell mobilization. However, since CXCR4 plays a key role in homing and retention of normal and leukemic stem cells as well as other cancer cells to their microenvironments, the use of CXCR4 antagonists may provide for a novel therapeutic approach to interrupt these protective interactions and thus sensitize AML blasts to chemotherapy in vivo. Preclinical and/or clinical studies have shown that these novel drugs mobilize both normal hematopoietic progenitors and AML blasts into the peripheral circulation and that they are synergistic with G-CSF. In this chapter we will discuss CXCR4 inhibitors and their effects on mobilizing normal and leukemic cells when given alone or with G-CSF in preclinical models and in the clinic.

Keywords Leukemia • CXCR4 antagonists • AMD 3100 • Hematopoietic stem cell mobilization • CXCR4 • Plerixafor • SDF-1 • CXCL12 • G-CSF • CD34⁺ cells

G. Ansstas, MD • F. Mir, MD • M.P. Rettig, PhD • M. Schroeder, MD • L. Eissenberg, PhD • J.F. DiPersio, MD, PhD (✉)
Division of Oncology, Siteman Cancer Center, Washington University School of Medicine, 660 South Euclid Avenue, Campus Box 8007, Saint Louis, MO 63110, USA
e-mail: jdipersi@dom.wustl.edu

S. Fruehauf et al. (eds.), *Novel Developments in Stem Cell Mobilization: Focus on CXCR4*, DOI 10.1007/978-1-4614-1960-0_17,

Introduction

Hematopoietic stem and progenitor cells (HSPCs) first arise in the yolk sac, then migrate to and come to reside in the bone marrow, a highly regulated microenvironment. The microenvironment is composed of marrow stromal cells, osteoblasts, osteoclasts and other extracellular matrix proteins (e.g., collagens, fibronectins, and proteoglycans) [1]. HSPCs express a number of cell surface molecules involved in signaling such as very late antigen 4 (VLA-4), CXCR4, CXCR2, CD44, CD62L, lymphocyte function-associated antigen-1 (LFA-1), and CD117 (c-kit) [2–4]. The presence of these molecules enables HSPCs to proliferate, migrate, adhere, and differentiate appropriately [5]. Regulated migration and homing of stem cells is not only critical during the embryonic period but also for the trafficking of normal stem cells during periods of stress. This process can also be corrupted by many cancers resulting in the promotion of both invasion and metastasis.

CXCR4 is a member of the large family of seven transmembrane domain receptors coupled to heterotrimeric G_i proteins and functions as a coreceptor for human immunodeficiency virus type 1 (HIV-1) cell entry [6, 7]. CXCR4 exists in different isoforms as the result of differential splicing that affects the length of its N-terminus [8]. The binding of CXCR4 to CXCL12 (also known as stromal derived factor-1, SDF-1) results in activation of multiple signal transduction pathways ultimately triggering chemotaxis. More recently, both trefoil factor family 2 (TFF2) [9] and macrophage migration inhibitory factor (MIF) were described as additional ligands of CXCR4 [10].

The expression of CXCR4 on human $CD34^+$ stem cells is dynamic: Flt3-ligand [9], SCF, IL-3, IL-8 [11, 12], hepatocyte growth factor, and granulocyte colony stimulating factor (G-CSF) [13] are all known to modulate the SDF-1/CXCR4 pathway. CXCL12 has direct growth promoting effects on many cancer cells and supports tumor progression by recruiting endothelial progenitor cells for tumor angiogenesis [14]. Because leukemic blasts localize to vascular and endosteal niches which provide a survival stimulus, CXCR4 antagonists potentially play a role in both mobilizing and/or detaching leukemic blasts from this protective microenvironment thus "sensitizing" them to the genotoxic effects of conventional anticancer drugs.

Standard Approaches to Hematopoietic Stem and Progenitor Cell Mobilization

The observation that the recovery phase after chemotherapy was associated with increased numbers of circulating progenitor cells, the surrogate marker of HSPCs in humans, which led to their use for stem cell collection in preparation for autologous transplantation, was first described in the 1980s [15, 16]. These early trials were followed by the use of colony-stimulating factors, such as granulocyte colony-stimulating factor (G-CSF) and granulocyte–macrophage colony-stimulating factor (GM-CSF), either alone or following chemotherapy (chemomobilization), providing potent stimuli to the bone marrow resulting in increased levels of circulating $CD34^+$ HSPCs within 7–14 days [17]. A minimum dose of $\geq 2\times 10^6$ $CD34^+$ cells/kg is generally considered necessary to ensure successful and sustained trilineage engraftment, whereas the optimal dose is $\geq 5\times 10^6$ $CD34^+$ cells/kg [18–20]. Unfortunately, up to 30% of patients with lymphoma do not reach the minimum dose either after mobilization with cytokine alone or after mobilization with chemotherapy and cytokines [20]. There are multiple potential factors that could limit the collection of an adequate amount of $CD34^+$ HSPC including age, sex, previous use of immunomodulatory drugs (lenalidomide), previous exposure to radiation, extent and type of chemotherapy, depressed peripheral blood $CD34^+$ HSPC counts before mobilization, previous attempts at mobilization, disease status, and involvement of bone marrow in the disease process [21–24].

Currently G-CSF alone or G-CSF plus chemotherapy are the most commonly used methods for autologous stem cell mobilization with approximately 5–10% of myeloma and 20–30% of lymphoma patients failing to reach the minimum target of 2×10^6 $CD34^+$ cells/kg after 4–5 apheresis procedures emphasizing the need for newer and more effective strategies to optimize stem cell mobilization in especially those patients who are at high risk of failure and for those patients who have failed an initial attempt at mobilization. One approach is to pharmacologically block the CXCR4-SDF-1 axis using both small molecules and antibodies resulting in rapid progenitor cell mobilization in mouse and man. CXCR4 antagonists can be broadly categorized as peptides, antibodies to CXCR4, agonists and antagonists to SDF-1, and bicyclams. Multiple CXCR4 antagonists are being tested in clinical trials while one, plerixafor, has been FDA-approved for stem cell mobilization in the United States.

Plerixafor

Plerixafor (AMD3100, Mozobil; Genzyme, MA, USA) is a small bicyclam molecule that reversibly and selectively competes with and inhibits CXCL12 binding to its receptor CXCR4. Plerixafor was originally developed as a potential agent for treatment of HIV infection by blocking virus entry into $CD4^+$ T cells [25, 26]. First studies in healthy volunteers showed good tolerability with minimal and reversible side effects [27, 28]. Administration of a single dose of plerixafor resulted in rapid mobilization of neutrophils, monocytes, as well as $CD34^+$ cells. Administration of a single subcutaneous dose of plerixafor at 160–240 μg/kg led to a six- to tenfold increase in peripheral blood $CD34^+$ cells starting 1 h, peaking at 9 h after injection, and declining to baseline by 24 h with similar pharmacokinetic studies between older and younger patients [29]. Plerixafor is not absorbed after oral administration. Bioavailability after 80 μg/kg subcutaneous (sc) injection is 87% with a dose-dependent increase in $CD34^+$ cells in the peripheral blood. The drug distributes in the extravascular space with 60% of it being bound to human plasma protein.

Plerixafor is renally excreted; thus, the dose needs to be adjusted for individuals with impaired kidney function. The use of plerixafor has not been studied in individuals aged <18 years. The most frequent reported side effects were transient pain and injection site erythema, headache, nausea, paresthesias, bloating, and diarrhea. Plerixafor combination with G-CSF augmented CD34$^+$ cells mobilization from normal human volunteers [30]. Based on these results, plerixafor is currently indicated for patients with multiple myeloma and non-Hodgkin's lymphoma; experimental and clinical studies are ongoing for targeting acute myeloid leukemia, chronic leukemias, and other hematologic malignancies [31].

Phase I Studies with Plerixafor

Devine et al. [32] performed a phase I study and assessed safety and clinical effects of plerixafor in patients with non-Hodgkin's lymphoma (NHL) and multiple myeloma (MM). A single dose of plerixafor let to a rapid and statistically significant increase in the total white blood cell (WBC) and peripheral blood CD34$^+$ cell counts at both 4 and 6 h. A dose-dependent increase in the absolute number of circulating CD34$^+$ cells at 4 and 6 h of plerixafor administration was noted with higher CD34$^+$ cells count in the 240 μg/kg group compared to the 160 μg/kg group with a maximum sixfold increase in circulating CD34$^+$ cells.

Phase II Studies with Plerixafor

Flomenberg et al. [33] led the first phase II clinical trial of plerixafor for human HSPC mobilization with the hypothesis that the combination of plerixafor plus G-CSF would be superior to G-CSF alone and that the plerixafor plus G-CSF-mobilized cells would engraft at least as well as their G-CSF-mobilized counterparts. The trial randomly assigned patients with MM or NHL in first or second complete or partial remission to receive plerixafor plus G-CSF or G-CSF alone as initial mobilizing regimen followed by a 2-week washout period and remobilization with the alternate regimen so patients can serve as their own controls. Subsequently, randomization was discontinued and all patients received G-CSF alone as the initial mobilizing regimen since all patients who were initially mobilized with G-CSF + plerixafor had extremely poor yields when remobilized with G-CSF alone. G-CSF mobilization regimen included daily subcutaneous administration at a dose of 10 μg/kg and apheresis was begun on day 5 of administration. In plerixafor plus G-CSF mobilization regimen, plerixafor was given subcutaneously at a dose of 160–240 μg/kg beginning on day 5 followed 6 h later by apheresis. Aphereses were limited to three blood volumes per day and a maximum of 4 days. The plerixafor plus G-CSF mobilized patients had more CD34$^+$ cells/kg per apheresis, required fewer aphereses to reach the target CD34$^+$ cell count (5×10^6 CD34$^+$ cells/kg), and mobilized higher total $CD34^+$ cell yield. Fifty-six percent of patients mobilized with plerixafor plus G-CSF yielded at least 2×10^6 $CD34^+$ cells/kg after one leukapheresis and 100% after two leukaphereses (compared to 64% with G-CSF alone). Nine out of 25 patients failed to yield the minimum $CD34^+$ cells/kg after four leukaphereses with G-CSF alone (2×10^6 $CD34^+$ cells/kg). Of the nine patients who mobilized less than 2×10^6 $CD34^+$ cells/kg with G-CSF alone, four mobilized at least 2×10^6 but less than 5×10^6 $CD34^+$ cells/kg, whereas five mobilized at least 5×10^6 $CD34^+$ cells/kg with plerixafor plus G-CSF.

The combination of plerixafor and G-CSF has also been used to salvage NHL, multiple myeloma, and Hodgkin's disease (HD) patients who were mobilization failures after treatment with G-CSF alone or G-CSF post chemotherapy. In one study, remobilization with G-CSF and plerixafor of 115 documented poor mobilizers (those that had failed an initial attempt of mobilization with either G-CSF or G-CSF + chemotherapy) resulted in successful mobilization in 60% of NHL patients, 71% of MM patients, and 77% of HD patients (>2×10^6 $CD34^+$ cells/kg in four or fewer aphereses). These cells, when transplanted resulted in neutrophil and platelet engraftment at a median of 11 and 18 days post-transplant, respectively [34].

Other studies in heavily pretreated patients with MM, NHL, and Hodgkin's lymphoma showed similar results, confirming that plerixafor is an effective and a well-tolerated mobilizing agent when administered alone or in combination with G-CSF [35–38]. The above studies also showed that plerixafor plus G-CSF can salvage patients who failed initial mobilization trials with G-CSF or chemotherapy plus G-CSF. The addition of plerixafor to chemotherapy plus G-CSF for HSPC mobilization in patients with multiple myeloma and NHL resulted in only modestly enhanced mobilization of $CD34^+$ cells when compared to mobilization with G-CSF and chemotherapy [39]. A retrospective study comparing plerixafor plus G-CSF to cyclophosphamide plus G-CSF for upfront mobilization showed similar $CD34^+$ cell yields, similar costs, but more predictable days of collection, no weekend apheresis procedures and less hospitalization in the plerixafor plus G-CSF group [40].

Phase III Studies with Plerixafor

Mobilization of stem cells in patients with NHL and MM with plerixafor plus G-CSF or G-CSF alone was performed in two phase III, multicenter, randomized, double-blind, and placebo-controlled studies [41, 42]. G-CSF at 10 μg/kg/day was administered subcutaneously daily in the morning for up to 8 days. Either plerixafor at 240 μg/kg or placebo was administered subcutaneously in the evening of the fourth day and continued daily for up to 4 days. On day 5, patients began daily apheresis until the total $CD34^+$ cell count was $\geq5\times10^6$/kg (NHL) or $\geq6\times10^6$/kg (MM) or until a total of four leukaphereses were performed. Patients who failed to collect $\geq2\times10^6$ $CD34^+$ cells/kg with G-CSF alone were eligible for rescue with plerixafor plus G-CSF. In the NHL trial 59% of patients in the plerixafor arm met the primary endpoint of $\geq5\times10^6$ $CD34^+$ cells/kg compared to 20% in the placebo arm ($N=298$, $P<0.001$). Another important finding was that 130/150 (87%) of patients in the plerixafor arm and only 70/148 (47%) in the placebo arm met the secondary endpoint of $\geq 2\times 10^6$ $CD34^+$ cells/kg ($P<0.001$). Patients who failed to collect at least $\geq 2\times 10^6$ $CD34^+$ cells/kg had the option of entering an open-label rescue mobilization with plerixafor plus G-CSF. Rescue mobilization was able to salvage 33/52 patients from the placebo arm and 4/10 patients from the plerixafor arm [43]. A total of 35% of patients in the placebo arm failed the mobilization process versus 7% of patients in the plerixafor arm. In the multiple myeloma trial the primary endpoint of $\geq 6\times 10^6$ $CD34^+$ cells/kg was reached in 72% of patients from the plerixafor group and in only 34% from the placebo group ($N=302$, $P<0.001$). Importantly, 95% of patients in the plerixafor arm and 88% in the placebo arm met the secondary endpoint of $\geq 2\times 10^6$ $CD34^+$ cells/kg in four or fewer apheresis days ($P=0.031$).

NHL and MM clinical trials have showed that plerixafor was well tolerated with few adverse effects. The $CD34^+$ cells mobilized by plerixafor plus G-CSF led to prompt hematopoietic recovery with durable grafts. Based on the results of the aforementioned clinical trials, the FDA approved plerixafor to be used in combination with G-CSF to mobilize HSPC in patients with NHL and multiple myeloma in December 2008.

Use of Plerixafor in Allogeneic Transplantation

Plerixafor was also studied as a stand-alone rapid HSPC mobilizing agent from healthy HLA-matched sibling donors in the allogeneic stem cell transplant setting [44]. Matched sibling donors ($N=25$) were treated with plerixafor at a dose of 240 μg/kg subcutaneously and underwent a 20 L apheresis 4 h later. A G-CSF mobilized backup product was also collected from the first eight patients after a 10-day washout period as required by FDA. Two-thirds (17/25) of the donors mobilized with plerixafor alone collected $\geq 2\times 10^6$ $CD34^+$ cells/kg after a single apheresis (100% after two collections). In comparison to G-CSF mobilized allografts, plerixafor mobilized allografts had fewer $CD34^+$ cells and higher numbers of T, B, and NK cells. Twenty patients with hematologic malignancies received only plerixafor mobilized allografts. All patients engrafted neutrophils and platelets rapidly with a median of 10 and 12 days, respectively. Fourteen patients had robust trilineage hematopoiesis and durable remission with a median follow-up of 277 days (range, 139–964 days). It was postulated that plerixafor mobilized allografts might have more $CD34^+$ cells if leukapheresis were to be initiated 6–10 h after plerixafor since this is the time of peak of mobilization in both patients and healthy allogeneic donors. Currently, there are multiple ongoing studies testing different doses, routes of administration (intravenous vs. subcutaneous) and schedules of plerixafor alone or in combination with G-CSF and GM-CSF for HSPC mobilization of allogeneic stem cell donors.

Investigators have looked at the kinetics of HSPC mobilization with intravenous plerixafor due to inconvenient schedule with subcutaneous injection of pleraxifor that requires its administration the night before leukapheresis to ensure a lapse of 6–10-h interval after injection to maximize HSPC mobilization harvest. In a phase I trial, 21 healthy donors were initially mobilized with increasing doses of IV plerixafor (80, 160, 240, 320, 400, or 480 μg/kg) [45]. The donors then had 4 days of drug washout before they were remobilized with a single subcutaneous dose of 240 μg/kg plerixafor followed by leukapheresis 4 h later. The number of $CD34^+$ cells/mm^3 peaked at 4–6 h after intravenous dosing compared to 6–9 h after subcutaneous dosing, and the magnitude of $CD34^+$ cells/mm^3 was modestly higher after intravenous dosing. Intravenous plerixafor administration showed a clear dose–response effect on mobilizing $CD34^+$ HSPCs. The 320 μg/kg intravenous dose yielded a maximum $CD34^+$ cells/mm^3 at 4 h after injection, representing a median eightfold increase from baseline. Interestingly, the intravenous dosing (especially doses >240 μg/kg) caused prolonged mobilization of $CD34^+$ cells such that levels approached 20 $CD34^+$ cells/mm^3 at 24 h after injection. Based on the above results, a total of 28 sibling donors were enrolled in the Phase II trial, with all donors mobilized using IV plerixafor at a dose of 320 μg/kg by intravenous injection, followed 4 h later by apheresis. Six of 23 evaluable donors (26%) did not achieve the minimum cell dose of 2×10^6 $CD34^+$ cells/kg in a single 20 L apheresis procedure. This mobilization failure rate of 26% (6/23) with 320 μg plerixafor/kg administered intravenously is similar to the observed failure rate of 33% (15/45) following subcutaneous administration of 240 μg plerixafor/kg. Four of the six patients who failed to yield $\geq 2.0 \times 10^6$ $CD34^+$ cells/kg after their first apheresis procedure reached the goal with their second mobilization and collection procedure. Plerixafor has shown to be a potent HSPC mobilizer after both subcutaneous and intravenous dosing with only 3/68 normal allogeneic donors failing to mobilize at least 2×10^6 $CD34^+$ cells/kg after two 20 L apheresis procedures.

Preclinical Models of Acute Myelogenous Leukemia

The association of acute myelogenous leukemia (AML) cells with the bone marrow microenvironment may be mediated by CXCR4, which is invariably expressed on AML blasts [46]. The survival of AML blasts in vitro is increased upon co-culture with primary bone marrow stromal cells or stromal cell lines that express CXCL12. This anti-apoptotic effect of stroma can be partially reversed by antibodies to CXCR4 or SDF-1 [47]. Burger et al. showed that CXCR4 and a4b1 integrins (also known as Very Late Antigen 4 or VLA-4) mediate spontaneous migration of AML cells through marrow stromal cells (pseudoemperipolesis). In comparison to AML cells that did not interact and bind to stroma, AML blasts that bound to stroma proliferated less and accumulated in G1 of the cell cycle. The property of stroma-induced cell cycle arrest suggests another mechanism by which the physical interaction of AML blasts with stroma might promote resistance to proliferation-based chemotherapy [48]. Tavor et al. [47] found that pretreating human AML cells with neutralizing CXCR4 antibodies inhibited their homing and retention in the marrow and spleen of transplanted NOD/SCID/β2m mice, thus implicating the CXCR4-SDF-1 axis as a target for anti-leukemic therapies.

To facilitate further investigation Westervelt et al. [49] created a mouse model in which the human PML-RARα fusion cDNA expressed in acute promyelocytic leukemia (APL) was knocked-in to the 5′ UTR of the mouse cathepsin G locus. Fatal myeloid leukemia occurs in 90–100% of these mice with a latency period of 150–400 days. Because CXCR4 is also expressed on the surface of mouse AML cells, administering plerixafor to the leukemic mice induced a 1.6-fold increase in total leukocytes and a ninefold increase of circulating APL blast counts, peaking at 3 h and returning to baseline by 12 h. When leukemic mice were pretreated with plerixafor, the efficacy of the Ara-C chemotherapy was significantly increased and their leukemic burden was decreased as measured by overall survival, leukemia free survival and bioluminescent imaging (BLI) (murine APL cells carried the click beetle red luciferase gene and could be tracked by non-invasive BLI) [50].

Patients with FLT3-ITD mutations, one of the most frequent mutations in AML, express higher levels of CXCR4 [51]. These patients respond poorly to chemotherapy and FLT3 inhibitors. Co-culture of FLT-3-ITD over-expressing AML cell lines with stromal cells provided protection from the antileukemia effects of FLT3 inhibitors. Furthermore by inhibiting CXCR4 interactions, the FLT3-ITD+AML cells became more sensitive to the lethal effects of the FLT3 inhibitor, sorafenib [52]. These data again support the importance of disrupting the CXCR4/CXCL12 interactions as a novel strategy for targeting leukemia.

Preclinical Models of Acute Lymphoblastic Leukemia

There is a tendency for acute lymphoblastic leukemia (ALL) blasts to infiltrate extramedullary sites, such as the central nervous system, liver, spleen, and lymph nodes. This process appears to be selectively mediated by specific chemokine receptor–ligand pairs, such as CXCR4-SDF-1 [53]. Both the 14-mer peptide, T140, and plerixafor inhibit CXCL12 binding to CXCR4 on pre-B ALL cells, and can modulate their localization and trafficking. Combining these CXCL12 inhibitors with cytotoxic agents had an additive effect, inhibiting the pre-B-ALL cell proliferation and decreasing their viability [54].

Spiegel et al. [55] showed major differences between precursor-B ALL cells and normal CD34+ HSPCs regarding their in vivo migration and homing to the bone marrow of NOD/SCID mice. Precursor-B ALL cells expressed higher levels of cell surface CXCR4 compared with CD34+ cells. In fact most of the CXCR4 expressed in CD34+ cells remains intracellular, while more of CXCR4 in pre-B cell ALL is expressed on the surface and immediately accessible to CXCR4 inhibitors. In addition, pertussis toxin (inhibits CXCR4-associated G-protein signaling) had a more potent inhibitory effect on homing of precursor-B ALL cells to the marrow microenvironment compared to normal CD34+ HSPC or normal CD10+/CD19+ precursor-B cells suggesting differences in CXCR4 signaling pathways in these cell types. Administration of plerixafore to NOD/SCID mice inhibited the engraftment of the human precursor-B ALL cell line, G2 cells and could effectively and rapidly mobilize G2 cells into the peripheral blood after a single subcutaneous injection [56]. Phenotypically, mice that lack CXR4 or CXCL12 have impaired B-cell lymphopoiesis and lack of bone marrow seeding by hematopoietic progenitors, whereas human mutations of CXCR4 lead to WHIM syndrome (warts, hypogammaglobulinemia, immunodeficiency, and myelokathexis), a rare hematological disorder in which mature neutrophils fail to exit the bone marrow and in which B and T cells are quantitatively and functionally deficient [57, 58].

Clinical Implication of CXCR4/CXCL12 Pathway in Leukemia Prognosis and Treatment

The proportion of CD34+ cells expressing CXCR4 is a prognostic indicator for adult AML patients. Rombouts et al. [59] found in a study of 90 AML patients that improved patient outcomes were associated with reduced expression of CXCR4 on AML blasts. Patients with a greater proportion of CD34+ AML blasts expressing CXCR4 had a median overall survival (OS) of 11 months and relapse free survival (RFS) of 8.3 months. In contrast the median OS and RFS for a subset of patients with reduced expression of CXCR4 on CD34+ AML blasts were >96 months ($P<0.01$). Patients with a high CXCR4 expression also tended to relapse by 18 months even following a complete remission (22 out of 33). Factors predicting a relapse and thus a reduced OS and RFS included the percentage of CD34+CXCR4+ AML blasts, age, unfavorable cytogenetics, and the presence of FLT3/ITDs (multivariate Cox regression analysis) [59].

Spoo et al. [60] found that the surface expression of CXCR4 in CD34+ and/or CD117+ AML cells strongly correlated with OS and RFS, confirming the correlation between CXCR4 expression on AML cells and poor outcome demonstrated by Rombout et al. [59]. However, Spoo's study used fresh marrow aspirates and a whole blood lysis method during preparation for flow cytometry in contrast to the frozen-thawed and T cell depleted samples that Rombout's study used.

In 122 AML patients with normal karyotype and wild type FLT3, Konoplev et al. [61] also found CXCR4 expression to be prognostic. All patients received intensive chemotherapy according to institutional protocols. High CXCR4 expression again correlated with shorter OS [hazard ratio (HR) = 2.04, $P=0.008$] as well as with shorter event-free survival (EFS; HR = 1.80, $P=0.01$). In addition to CXCR4 expression, a multivariate analysis demonstrated that the presence of multilineage dysplasia and an elevated serum creatinine predicted poorer OS and EFS [61]. Using G-CSF ± cytoxan, three patients with AML failed to mobilize a sufficient number of CD34+ cells for an autologous stem cell transplant. However, when Plerixafor was administered (240 μg/kg/day for 3–4 days) starting on day 4 of G-CSF treatment (G-CSF 10 μg/kg/day) significant numbers of leukemic cells were released into the circulation suggesting the role of the SDF-1-CXCR4 axis in leukemic cell retention in the bone marrow and trafficking to the peripheral blood [62].

Prompted by these observations, Uy et al. [63] conducted an open label, phase I/II study of 40 patients with relapsed or refractory AML to determine the extent to which plerixafor could mobilize leukemic cells when administered prior to salvage chemotherapy. Baseline characteristics of patients included a median age of 49 years, secondary AML (15%), prior transplant (10%), intermediate risk cytogenetics (60%) and poor risk cytogenetics (25%). To determine how well subcutaneous plerixafor could mobilize AML blasts in the absence of chemotherapy, a test dose of plerixafor was administrated followed by a 24 h observation period during which pharmacokinetic and pharmacodynamic studies were performed. AML blasts were released into the peripheral circulation (mean 2.5-fold increase, range 0.9- to 7.3-fold) peaking at 6–8 h after administration. AML blasts with higher baseline surface CXCR4 had an increased mobilization (Pearson's $r=0.53$, $P=0.023$). Subsequently in a phase I dose escalation trial (80, 160 and 240 μg/kg) plerixafor given 4 h prior to MEC chemotherapy (mitoxantrone 8 mg/m^2/day, etoposide 100 mg/m^2/day, and cytarabine 1,000 mg/m^2/day) daily for 5 days. Thirty-six patients (90%) received plerixafor + MEC as their first salvage regimen for relapsed disease and the remaining 4 pts (10%) received plerixafor + MEC as their second salvage regimen. A total of 34 patients were treated in the phase II study at the 240 μg/kg dose level. No evidence of hyperleukocytosis or significant delays in neutrophil or platelet recovery was noted. Of 32 patients who were evaluable for response at the 240 μg/kg dose level, 50% achieved a complete remission (CR + CRp). This is compared to historical complete remission rates of 25–35%. The overall survival at 1 year was estimated to be 56%. These encouraging data will need to be confirmed by others. Table 17.1 shows open clinical trials utilizing the inhibition of CXCR4/CXCL12 axis to sensitize AML to chemotherapy in vivo. If these confirmatory and exploratory studies are again consistent and encouraging definitive randomized phase III prospective clinical trials will need to be performed in patients with relapsed AMLto determine the role of CXCR4 blockade in improving CR rates in these high risk patients.

Similar to AML, blockade of the CXCR4/CXCL12 pathway by plerixafor is being investigated in multiple myeloma and chronic lymphocytic leukemia (CLL). Ghobrial et al. [64] conducted a phase I study in 13 patients with relapsed or refractory MM to assess the ability of plerixafor to both mobilize malignant plasma cells and sensitize them to bortezomib in vivo and to determine the maximum tolerated dose (MTD) of plerixafor in combination with bortezomib. Patients included those with previous therapy if they had measurable disease. Patients of median age of 60 years, median lines of prior therapy of 2, median number of cycles on therapy of 5, and previous bortezomib exposure (100%). To determine the safety and efficacy of plerixafor in combination with bortezomib, five dose levels of 160, 240, 320, 400, and 480 μg/kg of plerixafor were tested. Plerixafor was given subcutaneously 60–90 min prior to bortezomib on days 1–6 of every cycle for a total of eight cycles as long as patients responded or had stable disease. Bortezomib was given at the recommended dose twice weekly for 2 weeks every 3 weeks. The combination therapy was well tolerated

Table 17.1 Ongoing clinical trials using CXCR4/CXCL12 antagonists in leukemia treatment

Study title	Clinical trial. gov identifier	Institution
A Phase I, Open-Label, Multicenter Study of MDX-1338 (BMS-936564) in Subjects with Relapsed/Refractory Acute Myelogenous Leukemia	NCT01120457	Multicenter
Chemosensitization with Plerixafor Plus G-CSF in Relapsed or Refractory Acute Myeloid Leukemia	NCT00906945	Washington University School of Medicine
A Phase I Study of Intravenous Plerixafor in Combination with Mitoxantrone Etoposide and Cytarabine for Relapsed or Refractory Acute Myeloid Leukemia	NCT01027923	Washington University School of Medicine
A Phase I/II Study of AMD3100 With Mitoxantrone, Etoposide and Cytarabine (AMD3100+MEC) in Relapsed or Refractory AML	NCT00512252	Washington University School of Medicine
Mobilization of Leukemic Cells Using Plerixafor as Part of a Myeloablative Preparative Regimen for Patients with AML Undergoing Allografting: Assessment of Feasibility and Efficacy	NCT01141543	Princess Margaret Hospital
G-CSF and Plerixafor with Sorafenib for Acute Myelogenous Leukemia with FLT3 Mutations	NCT00943943	MD Anderson Cancer Center
G-CSF and Plerixafor with Busulfan and Fludarabine for Allogeneic Stem Cell Transplantation for Myeloid Leukemias	NCT00822770	MD Anderson Cancer Center
Phase I/II Study of Plerixafor and Clofarabine in Previously Untreated Older (≥60 Years) Adult Patients with Acute Myelogenous Leukemia (AML) with Two Or More Unfavorable Prognostic Factors for Whom Standard Induction Chemotherapy Is Unlikely to Be of Benefit	NCT01160354	MD Anderson Cancer Center

G-CSF granulocyte colony stimulating factor, *AMD3100* plerixafor

with no dose-limiting toxicities associated with plerixafor. Twelve patients were evaluable for response with response rate of 16% (one complete remission and one minimal response). Eight patients had stable disease.

In addition, Andritsos et al. [65] reported a phase I study in 17 patients with intermediate or high risk CLL not refractory to rituximab to determine MTD and safety of plerixafor when combined with rituximab. Patients were enrolled if they had white blood cell count $\leq 50 \times 10^9$/L with active disease by NCI criteria. Basic characteristics of patients were median age of 64 years, males 88%, and Rai Stage IV of 53%. To determine the safety and efficacy of plerixafor in combination with rituximab, four dose levels of 80, 160, 240, and 320 μg/kg of plerixafor were tested. Plerixafor was administered subcutaneously prior to rituximab starting at the fourth rituximab dose for nine total doses, whereas rituximab was given three times weekly with 100 mg fixed dose on day 1, and subsequently 375 mg/m^2 IV for 12 total doses. The combination therapy had minimal side effects with no dose-limiting toxicities noted. Of 14 evaluable patients, five had partial response, three had stable disease for ≥2 months, and six had progressive disease.

In this review we have described the preclinical and early clinical data suggesting that the CXCR4/CXCL12 axis plays a key role in leukemic cell homing and retention in tissue microenvironments. Blocking of this axis using CXCR4/CXCL12 antagonist may abrogate stroma-mediated drug resistance, and enhance sensitivity of leukemic cells to chemotherapy.

References

1. Wilson A, Trumpp A (2006) Bone-marrow haematopoietic-stem-cell niches. Nat Rev Immunol 6(2):93–106
2. Lapidot T, Dar A, Kollet O (2005) How do stem cells find their way home? Blood 106(6): 1901–1910
3. Kollet O, Dar A, Lapidot T (2007) The multiple roles of osteoclasts in host defense: bone remodeling and hematopoietic stem cell mobilization. Annu Rev Immunol 25:51–69
4. Kollet O, Shivtiel S, Chen YQ et al (2003) HGF, SDF-1, and MMP-9 are involved in stress-induced human CD34+ stem cell recruitment to the liver. J Clin Invest 112(2):160–169
5. Kiel MJ, Morrison SJ (2008) Uncertainty in the niches that maintain haematopoietic stem cells. Nat Rev Immunol 8(4):290–301
6. Hartmann O, Le Corroller AG, Blaise D, et al (1997) Peripheral blood stem cell and bone marrow transplantation for solid tumors and lymphomas: hematologic recovery and costs. A randomized, controlled trial. Ann Intern Med 126(8):600–607
7. Beyer J, Schwella N, Zingsem J et al (1995) Hematopoietic rescue after high-dose chemotherapy using autologous peripheral-blood progenitor cells or bone marrow: a randomized comparison. J Clin Oncol 13(6):1328–1335
8. Bensinger WI, Martin PJ, Storer B et al (2001) Transplantation of bone marrow as compared with peripheral-blood cells from HLA-identical relatives in patients with hematologic cancers. N Engl J Med 344(3):175–181
9. Schmitz N, Linch DC, Dreger P et al (1996) Randomised trial of filgrastim-mobilised peripheral blood progenitor cell transplantation versus autologous bone-marrow transplantation in lymphoma patients. Lancet 347(8998):353–357
10. Bernhagen J, Krohn R, Lue H et al (2007) MIF is a noncognate ligand of CXC chemokine receptors in inflammatory and atherogenic cell recruitment. Nat Med 13:587–596
11. Pruijt JF, Fibbe WE, Laterveer L et al (1999) Prevention of interleukin-8-induced mobilization of hematopoietic progenitor cells in rhesus monkeys by inhibitory antibodies against the metalloproteinase gelatinase B (MMP-9). Proc Natl Acad Sci USA 96(19):10863–10868
12. Bensinger W, DiPersio JF, McCarty JM (2009) Improving stem cell mobilization strategies: future directions. Bone Marrow Transplant 43(3):181–195
13. Levesque JP, Hendy J, Takamatsu Y, Simmons PJ, Bendall LJ (2003) Disruption of the CXCR4/CXCL12 chemotactic interaction during hematopoietic stem cell mobilization induced by GCSF or cyclophosphamide. J Clin Invest 111(2):187–196
14. Burger JA, Tsukada N, Burger M, Zvaifler NJ, Dell'Aquila M, Kipps TJ (2000) Blood-derived nurse-like cells protect chronic lymphocytic leukemia B cells from spontaneous apoptosis through stromal cell-derived factor-1. Blood 96(8):2655–2663
15. Kessinger A, Armitage JO, Landmark JD, Weisenburger DD (1986) Reconstitution of human hematopoietic function with autologous cryopreserved circulating stem cells. Exp Hematol 14(3):192–196
16. Korbling M, Dorken B, Ho AD, Pezzutto A, Hunstein W, Fliedner TM (1986) Autologous transplantation of blood-derived hemopoietic stem cells after myeloablative therapy in a patient with Burkitt's lymphoma. Blood 67(2):529–532

17. Bensinger W, Dipersio JF, McCarty JM (2009) Improving stem cell mobilization strategies: future directions. Bone Marrow Transplant 43(3):181–195
18. Bensinger W, Appelbaum F, Rowley S et al (1995) Factors that influence collection and engraftment of autologous peripheral-blood stem cells. J Clin Oncol 13(10):2547–2555
19. Reiffers J, Faberes C, Boiron JM et al (1994) Peripheral blood progenitor cell transplantation in 118 patients with hematological malignancies: analysis of factors affecting the rate of engraftment. J Hematother Fall 3(3):185–191
20. Weaver CH, Hazelton B, Birch R et al (1995) An analysis of engraftment kinetics as a function of the CD34 content of peripheral blood progenitor cell collections in 692 patients after the administration of myeloablative chemotherapy. Blood 86(10):3961–3969
21. Haas R, Mohle R, Fruhauf S et al (1994) Patient characteristics associated with successful mobilizing and autografting of peripheral blood progenitor cells in malignant lymphoma. Blood 83(12):3787–3794
22. Sugrue MW, Williams K, Pollock BH et al (2000) Characterization and outcome of "hard to mobilize" lymphoma patients undergoing autologous stem cell transplantation. Leuk Lymphoma 39(5–6):509–519
23. Ozkurt ZN, Yegin ZA, Suyani E et al (2010) Factors affecting stem cell mobilization for autologous hematopoietic stem cell transplantation. J Clin Apher 25(5):280–286
24. de la Rubia J, Arbona C, de Arriba F et al (2002) Analysis of factors associated with low peripheral blood progenitor cell collection in normal donors. Transfusion 42(1):4–9
25. De Clercq E (2003) The bicyclam AMD3100 story. Nat Rev Drug Discov 2(7):581–587
26. Donzella GA, Schols D, Lin SW et al (1998) AMD3100, a small molecule inhibitor of HIV-1 entry via the CXCR4 co-receptor. Nat Med 4(1):72–77
27. Hendrix CW, Flexner C, MacFarland RT et al (2000) Pharmacokinetics and safety of AMD-3100, a novel antagonist of the CXCR-4 chemokine receptor, in human volunteers. Antimicrob Agents Chemother 44(6):1667–1673
28. Lack NA, Green B, Dale DC et al (2005) A pharmacokinetic-pharmacodynamic model for the mobilization of CD34+ hematopoietic progenitor cells by AMD3100. Clin Pharmacol Ther 77(5):427–436
29. Liles WC, Broxmeyer HE, Rodger E et al (2003) Mobilization of hematopoietic progenitor cells in healthy volunteers by AMD3100, a CXCR4 antagonist. Blood 102(8):2728–2730
30. Liles WC, Rodger E, Broxmeyer HE et al (2005) Augmented mobilization and collection of CD34+ hematopoietic cells from normal human volunteers stimulated with granulocyte-colony-stimulating factor by single-dose administration of AMD3100, a CXCR4 antagonist. Transfusion 45(3):295–300
31. Choi HY, Yong CS, Yoo BK (2010) Plerixafor for stem cell mobilization in patients with non-Hodgkin's lymphoma and multiple myeloma. Ann Pharmacother 44(1):117–126
32. Devine SM, Flomenberg N, Vesole DH et al (2004) Rapid mobilization of CD34+ cells following administration of the CXCR4 antagonist AMD3100 to patients with multiple myeloma and non-Hodgkin's lymphoma. J Clin Oncol 22(6):1095–1102
33. Flomenberg N, Devine SM, Dipersio JF et al (2005) The use of AMD3100 plus G-CSF for autologous hematopoietic progenitor cell mobilization is superior to G-CSF alone. Blood 106(5):1867–1874
34. Calandra G, McCarty J, McGuirk J et al (2008) AMD3100 plus G-CSF can successfully mobilize CD34+ cells from non-Hodgkin's lymphoma, Hodgkin's disease and multiple myeloma patients previously failing mobilization with chemotherapy and/or cytokine treatment: compassionate use data. Bone Marrow Transplant 41(4):331–338
35. Cashen A, Lopez S, Gao F et al (2008) A phase II study of plerixafor (AMD3100) plus G-CSF for autologous hematopoietic progenitor cell mobilization in patients with Hodgkin lymphoma. Biol Blood Marrow Transplant 14(11):1253–1261
36. Fowler CJ, Dunn A, Hayes-Lattin B et al (2009) Rescue from failed growth factor and/or chemotherapy HSC mobilization with G-CSF and plerixafor (AMD3100): an institutional experience. Bone Marrow Transplant 43(12):909–917

37. Stiff P, Micallef I, McCarthy P et al (2009) Treatment with plerixafor in non-Hodgkin's lymphoma and multiple myeloma patients to increase the number of peripheral blood stem cells when given a mobilizing regimen of G-CSF: implications for the heavily pretreated patient. Biol Blood Marrow Transplant 15(2):249–256
38. Stewart DA, Smith C, MacFarland R, Calandra G (2009) Pharmacokinetics and pharmacodynamics of plerixafor in patients with non-Hodgkin lymphoma and multiple myeloma. Biol Blood Marrow Transplant 15(1):39–46
39. Dugan MJ, Maziarz RT, Bensinger WI et al (2010) Safety and preliminary efficacy of plerixafor (Mozobil) in combination with chemotherapy and G-CSF: an open-label, multicenter, exploratory trial in patients with multiple myeloma and non-Hodgkin's lymphoma undergoing stem cell mobilization. Bone Marrow Transplant 45(1):39–47
40. Shaughnessy P, Islas-Ohlmayer M, Murphy J, et al (2009) Plerixafor plus G-CSF compared to chemotherapy plus G-CSF for mobilization of autologous CD34+ cells resulted in similar cost but more predictable days of apheresis and less hospitalization. Blood (ASH Annual Meeting Abstracts) 114(22): http://abstracts.hematologylibrary.org/cgi/content/abstract/114/22/2277?maxtoshow=&hits=10&RESULTFORMAT=&fulltext=2277&searchid=1&FIRSTINDEX=0&volume=114&issue=22&resourcetype=HWCIT abstract [2277]
41. DiPersio JF, Micallef IN, Stiff PJ et al (2009) Phase III prospective randomized double-blind placebo-controlled trial of plerixafor plus granulocyte colony-stimulating factor compared with placebo plus granulocyte colony-stimulating factor for autologous stem-cell mobilization and transplantation for patients with non-Hodgkin's lymphoma. J Clin Oncol 27(28):4767–4773
42. DiPersio JF, Stadtmauer EA, Nademanee A et al (2009) Plerixafor and G-CSF versus placebo and G-CSF to mobilize hematopoietic stem cells for autologous stem cell transplantation in patients with multiple myeloma. Blood 113(23):5720–5726
43. Micallef IN, Stiff PJ, DiPersio JF et al (2009) Successful stem cell remobilization using plerixafor (mozobil) plus granulocyte colony-stimulating factor in patients with non-hodgkin lymphoma: results from the plerixafor NHL phase 3 study rescue protocol. Biol Blood Marrow Transplant 15(12):1578–1586
44. Devine SM, Vij R, Rettig M et al (2008) Rapid mobilization of functional donor hematopoietic cells without G-CSF using AMD3100, an antagonist of the CXCR4/SDF-1 interaction. Blood 112(4):990–998
45. Rettig MP, Lopez S, McFarland K, et al (2010) Rapid and prolonged mobilization of human CD34+ hematopoietic stem cells following intravenous (IV) administration of plerixafor. Blood (ASH Annual Meeting Abstracts) 116:abstract [2261]
46. Peled A, Petit I, Kollet O et al (1999) Dependence of human stem cell engraftment and repopulation of NOD/SCID mice on CXCR4. Science 283:845–848
47. Tavor S, Petit I, Proozov S et al (2004) CXCR4 regulates migration and development of human acute myelogenous leukemia stem cells in transplanted NOD/SCID mice. Cancer Res 64:12817–12824
48. Burger JA, Spoo A, Dwenger A et al (2003) CXCR4 chemokine receptors (CD184) and alpha-4beta1 integrins mediate spontaneous migration of human CD34+ progenitors and acute myeloid leukaemia cells beneath marrow stromal cells (pseudoemperipolesis). Br J Haematol 122:579–589
49. Westervelt P, Lane AA, Pollock JL et al (2003) High-penetrance mouse model of acute promyelocytic leukemia with very low levels of PML-RARalpha expression. Blood 102:1857–1865
50. Nervi B, Ramirez P, Rettig MP et al (2009) Chemosensitization of AML following mobilization by the CXCR4 antagonist AMD3100. Blood 113(24):6206–6214
51. Fukudas S, Broxmeyer HE, Pelus LM (2005) Flt3 ligand and the Flt3 receptor regulate hematopoietic cell migration by modulating the SDF-1α(CXCL12)/CXCR4 axis. Blood 105:3117–3126
52. Zeng Z, Shi YX, Samudio IJ et al (2009) Targeting the leukemia microenvironment by CXCR4 inhibition overcomes resistance to kinase inhibitors and chemotherapy in AML. Blood 113(24):6215–6224

53. Bradostock KF, Makrynikola V, Bianchi A et al (2000) Effects of the chemokine stromal cell-derived factor-1 on the migration and localization of precursor-B acute lymphoblastic leukemia cells within bone marrow stromal layers. Leukemia 14(5):882–888
54. Juarez J, Bradotock KF, Gottlieb DJ, Bendall LJ (2003) Effects of inhibitors of the chemokine receptor CXCR4 on acute lymphoblastic leukemia cells in vitro. Leukemia 17(7):1294–300
55. Spiegel A, Kollet O, Peled A et al (2004) Unique SDF-1-induced activation of human precursor-B ALL cells as a result of altered CXCR4 expression and signaling. Blood 103(8): 2900–2907
56. Juarez J, Dela Pena A, Baraz R, et al (2007) CXCR4 antagonists mobilize childhood acute lymphoblastic leukemia cells into the peripheral blood and inhibit engraftment. Leukemia 21(6):1249–1257
57. Nagasawa T, Hirota S, Tachibana K et al (1996) Defects of B-cell lymphopoiesis and bone-marrow myelopoiesis in mice lacking the CXC chemokine PBSF/SDF-1. Nature 382: 635–638
58. Hernandez PA, Gorlin RJ, Lukens JN et al (2003) Mutations in the chemokine receptor gene CXCR4 are associated with WHIM syndrome, a combined immunodeficiency disease. Nat Genet 34:70–74
59. Rombouts EJ, Pavic B, Lowenberg B et al (2004) Relation between CXCR-4 expression, Flt3 mutations, and unfavorable prognosis of adult acute myeloid leukemia. Blood 104(2): 550–557
60. Spoo AC, Lubbert M, Wierda WG et al (2007) CXCR4 is a prognostic marker in acute myelogenous leukemia. Blood 109:786–791
61. Konoplev S, Rassidakis GZ, Estey E et al (2007) Overexpression of CXCR4 predicts adverse overall and event-free survival in patients with unmutated FLT3 acute myeloid leukemia with normal karyotype. Cancer 109(6):1152–1156
62. Andreeff M, Konoplev S, Wang R, et al (2006) Massive mobilization of AML cells into circulation by disruption of leukemia/stroma cell interactions using CXCR4 antagonist AMD3100: first evidence in patients and potential for abolishing bone marrow microenvironment-mediated resistance. Blood (ASH Annual Meeting Abstracts) 108–171A: abstract [568]
63. Uy GL, Rettig MP, Mc Farland K, et al (2009) A phase I/II study of chemosensitization with the CXCR4 antagonist plerixafor in relapsed or refractory AML. Blood (ASH Annual Meeting Abstracts) 114(22): http://abstracts.hematologylibrary.org/cgi/content/abstract/114/22/787?maxtoshow=&hits=10&RESULTFORMAT=&fulltext=787&searchid=1&FIRSTINDEX=0&sortspec=relevance&resourcetype=HWCIT abstract [787]
64. Ghobrial I, Azab AA, Laubch JP, et al (2010) Phase I trial of plerixafor and bortezomib as a chemosensitization strategy in relapsed or relapsed/refractory multiple myeloma. Blood (ASH Annual Meeting Abstracts) 116(21): http://abstracts.hematologylibrary.org/cgi/content/abstract/116/21/1943?maxtoshow=&hits=10&RESULTFORMAT=&fulltext=1943&searchid=1&FIRSTINDEX=0&volume=116&issue=21&resourcetype=HWCIT abstract [1943]
65. Andritsos L, Byrd JC, Jones JA, et al (2010) Preliminary results from a phase I dose escalation study to determine the maximum tolerated dose of plerixafor in combination with rituximab in patients with relapsed chronic lymphocytic leukemia. Blood (ASH Annual Meeting Abstracts) 116(21): http://abstracts.hematologylibrary.org/cgi/content/abstract/116/21/2450?maxtoshow=&hits=10&RESULTFORMAT=&fulltext=2450&searchid=1&FIRSTINDEX=0&sortspec=relevance&resourcetype=HWCIT abstract [2450]

Chapter 18
CXCR4 Antagonists for the Treatment of CML

Anupriya Agarwal*, Thomas O'Hare*, and Michael Deininger

Abstract Tyrosine kinase inhibitor (TKI)-based targeted therapy has improved clinical outcomes in chronic myeloid leukemia (CML) to an extent unrivaled in other hematologic malignancies. Targeted therapy elicits durable remissions but does not eradicate leukemic stem cells (LSCs), the reservoir of CML. Recurrence of active leukemia is the predictable result upon cessation of therapy, even in the best responders. Interactions between LSCs and the bone marrow microenvironment are thought to mediate disease persistence in vivo, despite effective inhibition of BCR-ABL tyrosine kinase, the molecular driver of CML. Homing and engraftment of CML LSCs in the absence of therapy is characterized by an exaggerated dependence on the CD44 homing receptor and reduced dependence on C-X-C chemokine receptor 4 (CXCR4) compared to normal hematopoietic stem cells (HSCs). In fact, high-level BCR-ABL expression leads to downregulation of CXCR4. Recent evidence suggests that successful TKI-based targeting of BCR-ABL restores reliance on CXCR4 and its ligand, stromal cell-derived factor 1 (SDF-1), for trafficking and homing of CML LSCs to the bone marrow. Perturbation of the CXCR4/SDF-1 interaction with CXCR4 antagonists can promote egress of CML LSCs and progenitor cells from the bone marrow niche, potentially increasing their susceptibility to targeted and conventional purging strategies. Targeting of CXCR4/SDF-1 interactions represents a promising therapeutic avenue and is currently being evaluated in clinical trials. Here, we explore the role of CXCR4/SDF-1 signaling in the navigation of CML LSCs

* A.A and T.O. contributed equally to this study

A. Agarwal
Division of Hematology and Medical Oncology, Oregon Health & Science University, Knight Cancer Institute, Portland, OR 97239, USA
e-mail: agarwala@ohsu.edu

T. O'Hare • M. Deininger (✉)
Division of Hematology and Hematologic Malignancies, Huntsman Cancer Institute, University of Utah, Salt Lake City, UT 84112, USA
e-mail: Thomas.ohare@hci.utah.edu; Michael.Deininger@hci.utah.edu

S. Fruehauf et al. (eds.), *Novel Developments in Stem Cell Mobilization: Focus on CXCR4*, DOI 10.1007/978-1-4614-1960-0_18,

within the bone marrow microenvironment and summarize pre-clinical and clinical development of CXCR4 antagonists for use in extending the practical limit of targeted therapy to disease eradication, the ultimate goal in the treatment of CML.

Keywords CML • CXCR4 • SDF-1 • Plerixafor (AMD3100) • Disease persistence

Chronic Myeloid Leukemia

Chronic myeloid leukemia (CML) is a hematopoietic neoplasm characterized by the t(9;22)(q34;q11) translocation, karyotypically visible as the Philadelphia chromosome (Ph) [1, 2]. This translocation gives rise to the BCR-ABL fusion protein, which has constitutive tyrosine kinase activity that drives survival and proliferation of CML cells through multiple downstream signaling pathways and is causative for CML [3–6].

CML is typically diagnosed in the chronic phase, characterized by expansion of functionally normal myeloid cells. If untreated, the disease progresses to blastic phase, a rapidly fatal acute leukemia of myeloid or lymphoid phenotype in which the capacity for terminal differentiation is lost [7]. Imatinib (Gleevec), an ABL tyrosine kinase inhibitor (TKI), is highly effective in newly diagnosed CML patients in chronic phase, with complete cytogenetic responses (CCyR) in more than 80% of patients [8]. However, imatinib is not a curative therapy and the fact that active disease recurs upon discontinuation of drug represents a significant challenge for clinical management.

In CML, the mechanisms that govern homing and engraftment of LSCs to the bone marrow are not yet fully elucidated. Unlike normal hematopoietic stem cells (HSCs), in which prominent roles for C-X-C receptor 4 (CXCR4) and its ligand stromal cell-derived factor-1 (SDF-1) have been established in these processes, leukemic stem cells (LSCs) in CML exhibit functional defects in β1 integrin [9] and CXCR4 signaling [10]. In a landmark set of papers in 2006, Krause et al. [11] demonstrated that the lymphocyte homing receptor CD44 is a critical alternative adhesive pathway for homing and engraftment of CML LSCs; Jin et al. [12] reported similar data for acute myeloid leukemia (AML).

Given the reduced importance of the CXCR4/SDF-1 system in CML as compared to normal HSCs, one could reasonably ask why CXCR4 antagonists are of potential utility for treatment of CML. The particular application that captures most of our interest is transforming deep, sustained remission (a level of response known as minimal residual disease (MRD) in which the *BCR-ABL* transcript, assessed by real-time polymerase chain reaction (RT-PCR), is at very low levels or undetectable) and cure, defined as sustained remission despite continuation of therapy. The impediments to this goal are several, but can be summarized by stating that the protective environment of the bone marrow provides CML LSCs with a safe place to persist. One strategy for eradicating this reservoir of disease is to force or trick the LSCs out into the open where they can be more effectively targeted. A clear lesson learned so far is that these cells and their surrounding environment cooperate in sophisticated ways to achieve self-preservation. In many respects, HSCs and LSCs are indistinguishable [13], making therapeutic elimination of LSCs a difficult endeavor.

Recurrence upon therapy discontinuation is usually observed even in the small subset of patients with consistently undetectable *BCR-ABL* transcripts, and while some patients have maintained responses, it is undisputed that the vast majority of patients must continue therapy indefinitely to avoid recurrence, suggesting that fully leukemogenic cells survive imatinib therapy, a phenomenon commonly referred to a disease persistence [14–16]. Several approaches are being evaluated to overcome diseases persistence, including higher doses of imatinib, more potent second-line ABL TKIs disease such as dasatinib [17], nilotinib [18], and ponatinib (reviewed in ref. [19]), and combining of ABL TKIs with other agents such as interferon-alpha (IFN) or histone deacetylase inhibitors [20–22]. It is not yet known whether any of these strategies will eliminate disease persistence in a larger proportion of patients than imatinib.

Various mechanisms have been proposed for the persistence of CML LSCs, including quiescence [23, 24], high expression of BCR-ABL, mutations in the kinase domain of BCR-ABL [25], drug transport [26, 27], and protection by the bone marrow microenvironment [28, 29]. The last of these mechanism has considerable precedent in other hematologic malignancies, including myeloma [30] and AML [29]. The niche is a well-accepted concept in stem cell biology and implies an arrangement in which the marrow microenvironment provides critical protective factors to stem cells, including HSCs. Chemokines play key roles in regulating the homing and niche retention of normal and leukemic progenitors. It has been suggested that chemokine-dependent interactions between CML LSCs and the microenvironment mediate disease persistence despite effective inhibition of BCR-ABL kinase activity [29]. Here we review the role of the chemokine receptor CXCR4 and its ligand SDF-1 in CML.

Physiological Roles and Downstream Signaling Mediated by CXCR4 and Its Ligand SDF-1

Migration and homing of stem cells to their niches are tightly controlled processes during embryonic development and tissue repair but also in cancer stem cell dissemination. In this context, chemokine networks orchestrate directional migration of cells along a concentration gradient (chemotaxis) through binding to chemokine receptors [31, 32]. The CXCR4/SDF-1 chemokine signaling axis has attracted considerable attention as a mechanism of stem cell homing to the bone marrow niche, both for normal HSCs and LSCs [33–39].

CXCR4 is a G-protein-coupled receptor [40] constitutively expressed on the plasma membrane of hematopoietic cells including lymphocytes, monocytes, stem cells, and progenitors (reviewed in ref. [41]). The major physiological CXCR4 ligand is SDF-1, also known as CXCL12, an evolutionarily conserved chemokine that plays an important role in hematopoiesis, development, and organization of the immune system [42, 43] initially identified as a growth factor for pre-B-cell progenitors and as a chemotactic factor for T cells and monocytes [44]. Subsequently, it was noted that *Cxcr4* and *Cxcl12* gene-deleted mice displayed an identical, lethal phenotype characterized by deficient B-lymphopoiesis and myelopoiesis with abnormal neuronal and cardiovascular development [45].

The bone marrow (BM) niche is anatomically and functionally organized into endosteal (osteoblastic) and perivascular compartments (Fig. 18.1). The endosteal niche is in immediate proximity to trabecular or cortical bone and, with its abundant bone-forming osteoblasts, provides a long-term refuge for quiescent HSCs [46, 47]. Perivascular structures are defined by proximity to the sinusoidal vascular endothelium and surrounding supportive structures such as mesenchymal stem or stromal cells (MSCs). MSCs constitutively secrete high levels of SDF-1 that are essential for chemotaxis-mediated trafficking and homing of circulating stem and progenitor cells to distinct perivascular and endosteal niches [48]. In addition, SDF-1-abundant reticular cells may function in the shuttling of HSCs between the osteoblastic and perivascular niches [49, 50]. There is in vivo evidence that pre-treatment of $CD34^+$ cells with SDF-1 or a CXCR4 antibody increases their migration and repopulation potential in NOD-SCID mice, consistent with a role for CXCR4/SDF-1 signaling in modulation of homing and migration [51].

The CXCR4/SDF-1 axis activates several signaling pathways (reviewed in ref. [52]) by specifying the transcription of various genes and by increasing intracellular calcium. Cellular processes influenced by CXCR4/SDF-1 signaling include chemotaxis, trafficking, cell survival, and interaction of cells with the intercellular environment [53]. It has been suggested that SDF-1 binding triggers CXCR4 dimerization. Additionally, SDF-1 can stimulate tyrosine phosphorylation of each of the JAK family kinases, leading to association with and tyrosine phosphorylation of CXCR4. Consequently, several members of the STAT family of transcription factors including STAT2 and STAT4 are recruited and phosphorylated depending on cell type [54]. Besides its function in activating STATs, JAK2 is required for activation of PI3K and the MEK–MAPK p42/44 kinase cascade [55]. PI3K activation can result in the phosphorylation of several focal adhesion components such as proline-rich kinase-2 (PYK-2), Crk-associated substrate (p130Cas), focal adhesion kinase (FAK), paxillin, Nck, Crk, and Crk-L [56]. CXCR4 signaling also involves the RAS-activated signaling pathway, several SRC family kinases (SRC, LYN, FYN, LCK), the T-cell activating kinase ZAP-70, the adaptor VAV, and small GTPases [52].

SDF-1 can also promote cell survival by post-translational inactivation of cell death-related proteins and by increased transcription of cell survival-related genes, for example, through JAK2-mediated PI3K activation of the serine-threonine kinase AKT, which plays a key role in cell survival and proliferation [57]. Additionally, SDF-1 can promote inactivation of the proapoptotic protein BAD through the MAPK/MEK, S6K or PI3K pathways. CXCR4 signaling is complex and involves several complementary signaling cascades in a cell type-dependent fashion.

CXCR4 intracellular signaling through the PI3K pathway also regulates integrin-mediated cell adhesion. A recent study has shown that in SDF-1 stimulated

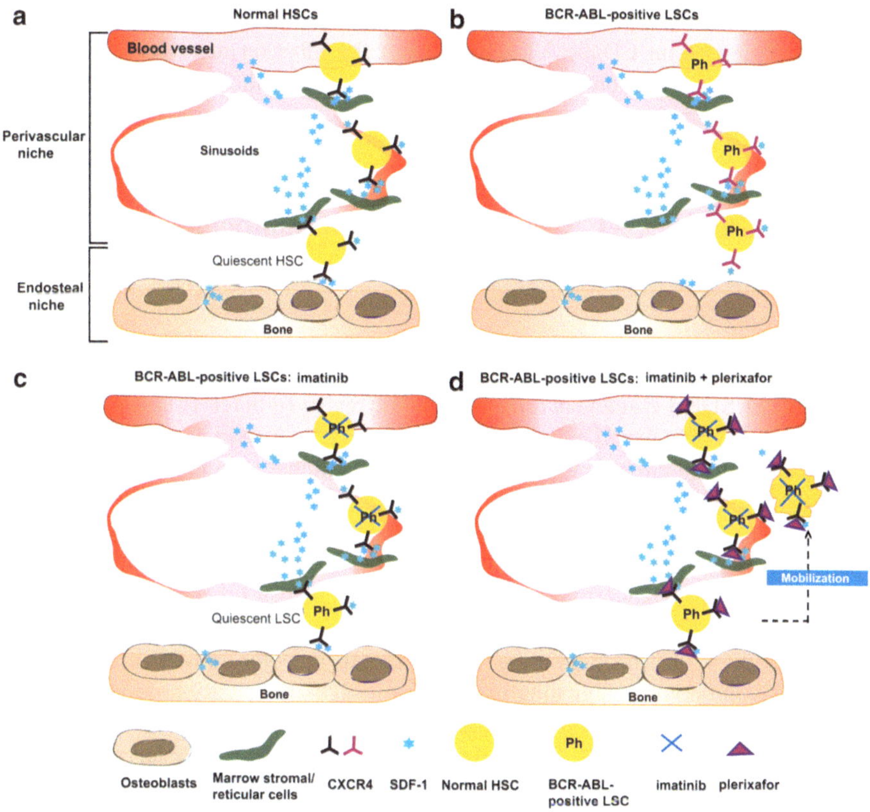

Fig. 18.1 CXCR4/SDF-1 signaling in homing of hematopoietic stem cells (HSCs) and CML leukemic stem cells (LSCs) to the bone marrow microenvironment. The perivascular niche is composed of a network of sinusoids (*white*) and adjacent reticular stromal cells (*green*) that constitutively secrete SDF-1. Osteoblasts are specialized, SDF-1-secreting fibroblasts critical for bone marrow formation that also provide niches for stem cell homing. (**a**) CXCR4 (*black*) expressing HSCs (*yellow*) migrate along the chemotactic gradient of SDF-1 towards the perivascular and endosteal niches. (**b**) In CML, BCR-ABL-positive LSCs (*yellow*) may exploit the same mechanism as HSCs to access niches. However, BCR-ABL downregulates CXCR4 expression (*purple*), leading to migration and adhesion defects. (**c**) BCR-ABL kinase inhibition after treatment with ABL tyrosine kinase inhibitors (TKIs; e.g., imatinib) restores CXCR4 expression (*black*), allowing the SDF-1 gradient to serve as a guide for these LSCs as they migrate across the perivascular wall to the stromal niche. CXCR4/SDF-1-mediated interactions between CML LSCs and the stromal niche activate pro-survival pathways, induce quiescence, and shelter LSCs from the cytotoxic effects of TKIs. (**d**) Interruption of CXCR4/SDF-1 interactions by small-molecule CXCR4 antagonists (e.g., plerixafor) may promote expulsion of quiescent LSCs from their niche and render them more accessible to targeted therapeutic agents

HSCs, LYN kinase is a positive regulator of cell movement while negatively regulating adhesion to stromal cells by inhibiting the binding of β_2 integrin to its ligand, intracellular adhesion molecule-1 (ICAM-1), there by providing a molecular mechanism for crosstalk between CXCR4 and β_2 integrins [58]. For stem cell homing, additional important roles were demonstrated for CD49d [very late antigen (VLA-4)], fibronectin, CD49e (VLA-5), and vascular adhesion molecule-1 (VCAM-1), which mediates initial contact of leukocytes with the endothelium through CXCR4/SDF-1-based signaling [59, 60].

The Role of the CXCR4/SDF-1 Axis in Hematopoietic Malignancies Including CML

CXCR4 is constitutively expressed on the surface of LSCs and progenitors from patients with acute and chronic leukemias, and several observations have implicated the CXCR1/SDF-1 cascade in leukemogenesis (reviewed in ref. [41]). For example, a polymorphism in the SDF-1 gene (*CXCL12* G801A) is associated with extremly elevated counts of circulating blasts in AML and a higher frequency of extramedullary disease [61]. In CML, a pathogenesis-associated polymorphism within the 3′-untranslated region of SDF-1 (SDF1-3′A) has been reported. 44% of CML patients had the heterozygous genotype, and 16% were homozygous for the variant allele, which was shown to have an important regulatory function in homing and maintenance of blasts through the increased production of SDF-1 [62]. More recently, CXCR7 has been described as an alternate receptor for SDF-1. Rather than displaying autonomous signaling in response to SDF-1, CXCR7 appears to modulate or fine-tune CXCR4/SDF-1 signaling output by sequestering SDF-1 [63]. CXCR7 is expressed at very low levels on normal human HSCs and has a minor role in normal cell migration. In contrast, it is directly involved in trafficking and adhesion of human leukemic cells including pre B-ALL cells [64].

Leukemic cells lodged in the sanctuary of BM niches are largely dependent on the CXCR4/SDF-1 cascade to provide growth and survival factors (reviewed in ref. [65, 66]). For example, leukemic hematopoietic progenitors from CML [67] and AML [68, 69] patients and leukemic B cells from chronic lymphocytic leukemia (CLL) [70] and acute lymphoblastic leukemia (ALL) [71, 72] patients utilize CXCR4 for homing and migration to locations beneath the SDF-1 secreting marrow stromal cells both in vitro and in vivo. During drug treatment, LSCs may hijack homeostatic mechanisms used by HSCs to take refuge within the niche, sparing them for a subsequent role in disease relapse [73]. Increased survival of LSCs in contact with BM stroma involves reduced proliferation, cell cycle arrest and decreased apoptosis. A primary cell xenograft study using AML and ALL samples demonstrated that leukemic cell proliferation in the BM microenvironment disrupts the HSC niche and creates malignant niches that outcompete the native niche with respect to $CD34^{+}$ cell engraftment by downregulating SDF-1 levels in areas of leukemic infiltration [74]. Interestingly, CXCR4 and SDF-1 levels are subject to circadian oscillations, which may have implications for the timing of anti-leukemic therapy to maximize disruption of niche interactions during therapy [75, 76].

In CML, several studies have shown that BCR-ABL impairs highly coordinated CXCR4 signaling, leading to altered adhesive interactions of CML progenitor cells with the marrow stroma (Fig. 18.1) [77]. As a result, the migratory response to SDF-1 is blunted compared to normal CD34⁺ cells, in blast crisis as well as chronic phase CML [10, 36, 78]. In vivo studies in NOD/SCID mice confirmed lower migratory responses as well as defective adhesion and engraftment of the Ph⁺ CD34⁺ cells as compared with Ph⁻ CD34⁺ progenitor cells from the same patients [67]. BCR-ABL appears to interfere with CXCR4/SDF-1 signaling in several different ways. In terms of mechanism, high-level BCR-ABL expression is correlated with decreased CXCR4 transcription in a BCR-ABL kinase-independent manner [36]. Additionally, consistent with the possibility that impaired SDF-1 mediated chemotaxis of CML CD34⁺ cells is due to signaling defects downstream of the CXCR4 receptor [78], LYN-mediated crosstalk between BCR-ABL and CXCR4 has been implicated in deregulated CXCR4 signaling [79]. Thus BCR-ABL directly activates LYN kinase, which is localized in both the lipid raft and non-raft fractions of the plasma membrane. Specifically, the active, phosphorylated PLYN(Tyr396) form is present within lipid rafts, while the inactive PLYN(Tyr507) form is localized in non-raft fractions. In CML cells, CXCR4 is primarily localized to non-raft cell surface regions. Under co-culture conditions, imatinib treatment inhibited LYN phosphorylation at Tyr507 but failed to reduce PLYN(Tyr396) levels. Further, BCR-ABL inhibition induces CXCR4 clustering in lipid rafts where it co-localizes with activated LYN and facilitates migration of CML cells to the BM niche [80].

The BM microenvironment in leukemia, including CML [81], is relatively hypoxic and the CXCR4/SDF-1 axis also controls trafficking and homing of progenitor cells to hypoxic tumor niches. In CML, high level BCR-ABL expression is correlated with induction of the transcription factor hypoxia-inducible factor-1 (HIF-1), which contributes to maintenance of cell viability by enhancing glycolysis with reduced glucose flux [81]. Hypoxic conditions in the BM niche induce stabilization of HIF-1, which in turn induces the local expression of SDF-1 in direct proportion to reduced oxygen tension. HIF-1-induced SDF-1 expression in endothelial cells attracts circulating stem and progenitor cells to areas of tissue damage [82]. Thus, hypoxia-induced HIF-1 accumulation leads to the activation of the CXCR4/SDF-1 axis, providing a survival benefit for tumor cells expressing high levels of CXCR4 [83].

Ph⁺ CML progenitors also exhibit reduced VLA-4 and VLA-5 dependent adhesion to stromal cells and to fibronectin (FN) [84], which leads to impaired chemotaxis of CML cells [67]. Several studies reported increased spontaneous motility of CML progenitors on FN-coated plates [10] and in extracellular matrix (ECM)-like gels, together with a reduction in their migration to SDF-1 through the ECM, possibly resulting from inappropriate activation of integrins. Subsequently, it was reported that Ph⁺ CD34⁺ cells are impaired in β1-integrin capping [85] and other CXCR4-mediated functions. Consequently, this may impede the binding of VLA-4 and VLA-5 to their endothelial/stromal and ECM ligands, VCAM-1 and FN, respectively, and may contribute to impaired retention of Ph⁺ CD34⁺ within the BM microenvironment. Overall this suggests that Ph⁺ CD34⁺ cells have a reduced ability to interact with BM endothelial/stromal cells and ECM in response to SDF-1. These deficiencies could affect their homing to the BM and retention within the stromal microenvironment (Fig. 18.1b) [67].

Despite their impaired interaction with BM stroma, there is evidence that pluripotent CML progenitors are protected by the BM environment, which allows them to persist despite imatinib therapy. Inhibition of BCR-ABL with TKIs including imatinib and dasatinib in primary $CD34^+$ cells markedly increases CXCR4 mRNA and membrane expression, thereby restoring the CXCR4/SDF-1 interaction. As a consequence, the CML cells lodge within the supportive BM microenvironment, where they enter quiescence, further enhancing their survival (Fig. 18.1c) [79, 86]. Thus, a paradoxical effect of BCR-ABL kinase inhibition by TKIs may be to increase survival of CML LSCs by driving them into a CXCR4-mediated quiescent state. Since these quiescent CML progenitor cells are likely the source of relapse and recurrence, targeting them by combining CXCR4 antagonists with TKIs may lead to improvements in CML therapy. Although normal HSCs will also be subject to the mobilizing properties of CXCR4 antagonists, they should not be adversely affected by exposure to ABL TKIs. The key question is whether CML LSCs, once deprived of the extrinsic protective effects provided by the BM microenvironment, will be sensitive to TKI therapy. Recent studies with a stroma co-culture assay have shown that blockade of CXCR4/SDF-1 interaction by the small-molecule CXCR4 antagonist plerixafor (AMD3100) resulted in dissociation of CML cells from BM feeder cells and sensitization of the CML cells to TKIs (Fig. 18.1d). In co-culture studies of CML cell lines and primary CML cells with MSC stroma, the presence of stroma correlates with decreased apoptosis, possibly by reducing caspase-3 activation in a CXCR4-dependent manner and by modulating the expression of anti-apoptotic proteins [87]. When CML cells are exposed to TKIs while in contact with MSCs, their ability to engraft NOD/SCID mice is preserved, indicating that MSCs protect SCID leukemia-repopulating cells and CML progenitors from the effects of targeted therapy. Another study has shown that SDF-1 produced by stromal cells protects BCR-ABL^+ lymphoblasts from imatinib-induced cell death [88]. Altogether, these data show that extrinsic signals provided by the microenvironment are instrumental for CML persistence despite inhibition of BCR-ABL kinase, and that the CXCR4/SDF-1 system plays an important role in this process [73].

CXCR4 Receptor Antagonists for the Treatment of CML

The discovery that CXCR4 has critical roles in normal and leukemic cell adhesion, migration, and homing to the BM microenvironment has prompted interest in using CXCR4 antagonists to promote HSC mobilization for the treatment of cancer and autoimmune disease. The approach for targeting the CXCR4/SDF-1 axis using CXCR4 antagonists in CML entails three coordinated objectives: (1) disruption of stroma-mediated adhesion and blocking of stroma-mediated survival signals; (2) expulsion of leukemic cells from their niche, resulting in increased susceptibility to conventional chemotherapy and to targeted agents such as ABL TKIs; and (3) blockade of paracrine growth and survival signals transmitted through the CXCR4/SDF-1 axis.

Currently, several CXCR4 antagonists and agonists are being evaluated as therapeutic agents in preclinical and clinical studies for various cancers and as a means for mobilization of normal HSCs (reviewed in ref. [89]). These agents can be divided into four major classes: (a) small-molecule CXCR4 antagonists such as plerixafor (formerly AMD3100; Mozobil); (b) peptide natural product antagonists of CXCR4 such as self-defense peptides tachyplesin and polyphemusin (e.g., T140, TN14003, TC14012, ALX40-4C and RCP168); (c) blocking antibodies to CXCR4; and (d) modified agonists and antagonists for SDF-1, including CTCE-9908 and CTCE-0214.

Comparative studies of two peptide antagonists of CXCR4, T140 and ALX40-4C, and the small-molecule CXCR4 antagonist plerixafor revealed that plerixafor and ALX40-4C have weak, SDF-1-like partial agonist activity and induce G-protein activation in CXCR4-expressing cells. In contrast, T140 functions as an inert or inverse agonist, binding to CXCR4 but not inducing signaling. Further experimentation revealed that T140 binds within the extracellular domain and the hydrophobic core of CXCR4, regions that are distinct from the SDF-1 binding site. At present, the data in CML are limited to small-molecule antagonists of CXCR4, and we will therefore highlight this class of molecules.

Small-Molecule Antagonists of CXCR4

Plerixafor is a bicyclam that specifically blocks SDF-1 binding to CXCR4, inhibits SDF-1-mediated calcium mobilization, chemotaxis and GTP binding, and does not cross-react with other chemokine receptors. Among small-molecule CXCR4 antagonists, plerixafor is at the most advanced stage of pre-clinical and clinical development. Plerixafor was initially investigated for a potential role in interfering with HIV-1 fusion or uncoating. However, an unexpected rapid, transient leukocytosis was noticed during phase I/II clinical trials in healthy subjects and HIV-infected patients, and further investigation revealed that this was caused by the mobilization to the blood of various hematopoietic cells, including $CD34^+$ HSCs. Overall, the anti-HIV activity of plerixafor was low and this application was not pursued further [90, 91]. Instead, the agent is now under intense scrutiny as an agent for controlled, convenient HSC mobilization, alone and in combination with granulocyte-colony stimulating factor (G-CSF). Liles et al. reported on 26 healthy volunteers in whom a single subcutaneous injection of plerixafor at doses up to 240 μg/kg/day induced a rapid, generalized leukocytosis associated with a transient increase (up to tenfold) in peripheral blood $CD34^+$ cells [92]. In a phase III study of patients with non-Hodgkin's lymphoma, plerixafor and G-CSF were well tolerated and resulted in a significantly higher rate of successful mobilizations with fewer apheresis sessions required as compared with G-CSF alone [93]. Recently, the FDA approved plerixafor for stem cell mobilization in combination with G-CSF in patients with non-Hodgkin's lymphoma and multiple myeloma [94, 95].

Several preclinical studies have explored the role of CXCR4 antagonists for inhibition of SDF-1-induced tumor cell migration and downstream signaling using various in vitro and in vivo tumor models [34, 35, 39, 41], specially in multiple myeloma [34] and AML [33, 38, 39]. For example, studies in a murine model of acute promyelocytic leukemia (APL) convincingly showed that dislodgement of APL cells from their niche and/or the interruption of CXCR4 signaling by plerixafor increased cytarabine or anthracycline-induced cell death [38]. Similarly, another in vivo study using a mutant FLT3-based murine AML model demonstrated that treatment with a derivative of plerixafor, AMD3465, induced mobilization of progenitors into the circulation, enhanced the anti-leukemic effects of the multi-kinase inhibitor sorafenib whose target profile includes FLT3, reduced leukemia burden, and prolonged survival [39]. Recently, a newly developed polypeptide RCP168 was shown to exhibit a very strong antagonistic effect on SDF-1-induced extracellular signaling and significantly enhanced chemotherapy-induced apoptosis in AML cells harboring a FLT3 mutation. In a comparative study, equivalent results were obtained with RCP168 or AMD3465, suggesting that disruption of CXCR4/SDF-1 interaction may represent a novel strategy for targeting leukemic cells within the BM microenvironment. These results provided the rationale for an ongoing proof-of-concept clinical trial (NCT00906945) in which relapsed/refractory AML patients are treated with MEC chemotherapy (mitoxantrone, etoposide, and cytarabine) plus escalating doses of plerixafor [96]. The complete response rate stands at 50%, which compares favorably with historical controls [97].

In CML, in vitro studies suggest that plerixafor binding to CXCR4 significantly inhibits SDF-1-mediated chemotaxis and cell migration toward the stroma and increases the detachment rate of cells reliant on SDF-1-mediated/VCAM-1-associated cell adherence. Thus Giuntoli et al. [86] showed that culturing of primitive CML cells in hypoxic conditions confers imatinib resistance. An in vitro co-culture study showed that cell migration was partially inhibited by AMD3465, implying that blocking of the CXCR4/SDF-1 axis might sensitize CML cells to TKI therapy by depriving them of the protective effect of the BM environment [98]. In vivo data are sparse and limited to a study using the Ph^+ pre-B cell line BV173 in a NOD-SCID xenograft model. In this study, BV173 cells co-cultured with stromal cells were pretreated with imatinib in the presence or absence of plerixafor, followed by injection into mice. Combined treatment with plerixafor and imatinib led to a significant reduction of engraftment compared to imatinib only, suggesting plerixafor-mobilized SCID leukemia repopulating cells are sensitive to ABL TKIs [87].

To more closely mimic CML, we recently tested plerixafor in combination with imatinib or dasatinib in a retroviral bone marrow transplantation/transduction model of CML [99]. In this aggressive disease model, We observed no difference in leukemia burden upon inclusion of plerixafor in addition to TKIs despite clear evidence for the mobilization of CXCR4-positive cells into the blood. Our study and the BV173 xenograft study described differed with respect to disease model and experimental design. For example, we used continuous plerixafor dosing, while in the BV173 xenograft study, cells were treated in vitro before transplantation. In our study using an extremely aggressive CML mouse model, TKI therapy induced hematologic responses only, and not the profound suppression of disease seen in many CML patients treated with ABL TKIs. Thus, it remains entirely possible that plerixafor may be effective in targeting residual leukemia in patients with well-controlled CML. This possibility could be investigated in recently developed mouse models of residual disease in which oncogene expression is limited to the stem cell compartment [100].

Although no clinical data is available so far in patients with CML, a number of clinical trials are underway to evaluate the ability of plerixafor to sensitize leukemic cells to chemotherapy and improve clinical outcomes in patients with various other hematologic malignancies. As mentioned above, plerixafor is under investigation in combination with MEC chemotherapy in patients with relapsed or refractory AML (NCT00512252); another study combines plerixafor with rituximab in patients with CLL or small lymphocytic lymphoma (NCT00694590). Further, orally bioavailable small-molecule CXCR4 antagonists such as AMD070 [101] and KRH-1636 [102], which could be clinically more effective than plerixafor, are currently under development. Overall, these different CXCR4 antagonists have shown activity in animal models for solid tumors [103, 104], hematopoietic malignancies [36, 38, 39, 70], and autoimmune diseases [105], providing a basis for future clinical development. However, the different mechanisms through which CXCR4 antagonists may display activity in treatment of neoplastic diseases raise questions about when during the course of the disease and for how long they should be administered, and whether CXCR4 antagonists should be given alone or in combination with conventional or targeted anticancer drugs. These questions will need to be addressed in further clinical trials.

Side Effects of CXCR4 Receptor Antagonists in the Context of Cancer Therapy

There are several concerns regarding potential side effects from antagonizing CXCR4 in patients with malignant disorders. During the treatment of cancer patients with CXCR4 antagonists, normal HSCs that would otherwise be protected in marrow niches could be mobilized, which could increase the toxicity of simultaneously administered cytotoxic drugs, with prolonged cytopenias as a possible result. Preliminary results from the study in relapsed AML have thus far not demonstrated increased hematopoietic toxicity. It is also possible that increased mobilization of leukemic cells may promote the homing of leukemic cells to extramedullary sites. For instance, in our studies described above we observed increased extramedullary hematopoiesis in liver, lungs, and spleen in mice receiving imatinib or dasatinib plus plerixafor as compared to mice treated with either TKI alone. Of note, mice treated with plerixafor in combination with dasatinib were more likely to develop neurological deficits in association with central nervous system infiltration by hematopoietic cells [99]. While these observations may be related to the specifics of the model, particularly the continuous plerixafor treatment in the context of active leukemia, they also call for careful patient selection and study design.

Summary

A large body of data has implicated the CXCR4/SDF-1 axis as a bona fide target for cancer therapy. CXCR4 antagonists designed to dislodge leukemia cells from their sanctuary in the bone marrow microenvironment may promote the elimination of residual disease in CML and other hematologic malignancies. Early data from clinical trials in AML are promising, but need more follow up. In CML, where most patients achieve profound responses, the key potential application will be the elimination of persistent disease, thereby moving patients from MRD status closer to cure. Studies in CML are in planning and will clarify whether the rationale for combining CXCR4 antagonists with TKIs can be translated into a clinical benefit. One appeal of CML as a model system is that for patients reaching and maintaining MRD, the remaining reservoir of disease is small. Lessons learned in this well-controlled situation may be applicable to AML and other hematologic malignancies. The co-release of HSCs is a potential concern when utilizing CXCR4 antagonists to mobilize LSCs from the niche. In the case of CML, interrupting niche-based, extrinsically mediated resistance to ABL TKIs provides a means of selectively eliminating CML LSCs, providing that the mobilized leukemic cells are sufficiently BCR-ABL addicted upon mobilization.

Acknowledgments We thank Sarah Bowden and Suzanne Wickens for administrative support. This study was supported by NIH grants HL082978-01 (M.W.D.) and CA04963920A2 (M.W.D.), Leukemia and Lymphoma Society grant 7036–01 (M.W.D.), and a grant from Genzyme Pharmaceuticals (M.W.D.). M.W.D. is a Leukemia and Lymphoma Society Scholar in Clinical Research. A.A. is a recipient of Lady Tata Memorial Trust and OHSU Knight Cancer Institute Cancer Research Development Awards.

References

1. Rowley JD (1973) Letter: A new consistent chromosomal abnormality in chronic myelogenous leukaemia identified by quinacrine fluorescence and Giemsa staining. Nature 243(5405): 290–293
2. Nowell PC, Hungerford DA (1960) Chromosome studies on normal and leukemic human leukocytes. J Natl Cancer Inst 25:85–109
3. Daley GQ, Van Etten RA, Baltimore D (1990) Induction of chronic myelogenous leukemia in mice by the P210bcr/abl gene of the Philadelphia chromosome. Science 247(4944): 824–830
4. Groffen J, Stephenson JR, Heisterkamp N, de Klein A, Bartram CR, Grosveld G (1984) Philadelphia chromosomal breakpoints are clustered within a limited region, bcr, on chromosome 22. Cell 36(1):93–99
5. Cowan-Jacob SW, Guez V, Fendrich G et al (2004) Imatinib (STI571) resistance in chronic myelogenous leukemia: molecular basis of the underlying mechanisms and potential strategies for treatment. Mini Rev Med Chem 4(3):285–299
6. Quintas-Cardama A, Cortes J (2009) Molecular biology of bcr-abl1-positive chronic myeloid leukemia. Blood 113(8):1619–1630
7. Calabretta B, Perrotti D (2004) The biology of CML blast crisis. Blood 103(11):4010–4022

8. Druker BJ, Guilhot F, O'Brien SG et al (2006) Five-year follow-up of patients receiving imatinib for chronic myeloid leukemia. N Engl J Med 355(23):2408–2417
9. Bhatia R, Verfaillie CM (1998) Inhibition of BCR-ABL expression with antisense oligodeoxynucleotides restores beta1 integrin-mediated adhesion and proliferation inhibition in chronic myelogenous leukemia hematopoietic progenitors. Blood 91(9):3414–3422
10. Salgia R, Quackenbush E, Lin J et al (1999) The BCR/ABL oncogene alters the chemotactic response to stromal-derived factor-1alpha. Blood 94(12):4233–4246
11. Krause DS, Lazarides K, von Andrian UH, Van Etten RA (2006) Requirement for CD44 in homing and engraftment of BCR-ABL-expressing leukemic stem cells. Nat Med 12(10):1175–1180
12. Jin L, Hope KJ, Zhai Q, Smadja-Joffe F, Dick JE (2006) Targeting of CD44 eradicates human acute myeloid leukemic stem cells. Nat Med 12(10):1167–1174
13. Goardon N, Marchi E, Atzberger A et al (2011) Coexistence of LMPP-like and GMP-like leukemia stem cells in acute myeloid leukemia. Cancer Cell 19(1):138–152
14. Hughes TP, Kaeda J, Branford S et al (2003) Frequency of major molecular responses to imatinib or interferon alfa plus cytarabine in newly diagnosed chronic myeloid leukemia. N Engl J Med 349(15):1423–1432
15. Rousselot P, Huguet F, Rea D et al (2007) Imatinib mesylate discontinuation in patients with chronic myelogenous leukemia in complete molecular remission for more than 2 years. Blood 109(1):58–60
16. Mahon FX, Rea D, Guilhot J, et al. (2010) Discontinuation of imatinib in patients with chronic myeloid leukaemia who have maintained complete molecular remission for at least 2 years: the prospective, multicentre Stop Imatinib (STIM) trial. Lancet Oncol 11(11):1029–1035.
17. Copland M, Hamilton A, Elrick LJ et al (2006) Dasatinib (BMS-354825) targets an earlier progenitor population than imatinib in primary CML but does not eliminate the quiescent fraction. Blood 107(11):4532–4539
18. Jorgensen HG, Allan EK, Jordanides NE, Mountford JC, Holyoake TL (2007) Nilotinib exerts equipotent anti-proliferative effects to imatinib and does not induce apoptosis in CD34+ CML cells. Blood 109:4016–4019
19. O'Hare T, Deininger MW, Eide CA, Clackson T, Druker BJ. (2011) Targeting the BCR-ABL signaling pathway in therapy-resistant Philadelphia chromosome-positive leukemia. Clin Cancer Res 17(2):212–221
20. Preudhomme C, Guilhot J, Nicolini FE, et al. (2010) Imatinib plus peginterferon alfa-2a in chronic myeloid leukemia. N Engl J Med 363(26):2511–2521.
21. Zhang B, Strauss AC, Chu S et al (2010) Effective targeting of quiescent chronic myelogenous leukemia stem cells by histone deacetylase inhibitors in combination with imatinib mesylate. Cancer Cell 17(5):427–442
22. Helgason GV, Young GA, Holyoake TL (2010) Targeting chronic myeloid leukemia stem cells. Curr Hematol Malig Rep 5(2):81–87
23. Corbin AS, Agarwal A, Loriaux M, Cortes J, Deininger MW, Druker BJ. (2011) Human chronic myeloid leukemia stem cells are insensitive to imatinib despite inhibition of BCR-ABL activity. J Clin Invest 121(1):396–409
24. Graham SM, Jorgensen HG, Allan E et al (2002) Primitive, quiescent, Philadelphia-positive stem cells from patients with chronic myeloid leukemia are insensitive to STI571 in vitro. Blood 99(1):319–325
25. Chu S, Xu H, Shah NP et al (2005) Detection of BCR-ABL kinase mutations in CD34+ cells from chronic myelogenous leukemia patients in complete cytogenetic remission on imatinib mesylate treatment. Blood 105(5):2093–2098
26. White DL, Saunders VA, Dang P et al (2007) Most CML patients who have a suboptimal response to imatinib have low OCT-1 activity: higher doses of imatinib may overcome the negative impact of low OCT-1 activity. Blood 110(12):4064–4072
27. Mahon FX, Belloc F, Lagarde V et al (2003) MDR1 gene overexpression confers resistance to imatinib mesylate in leukemia cell line models. Blood 101(6):2368–2373

28. Damiano JS, Hazlehurst LA, Dalton WS (2001) Cell adhesion-mediated drug resistance (CAM-DR) protects the K562 chronic myelogenous leukemia cell line from apoptosis induced by BCR/ABL inhibition, cytotoxic drugs, and gamma-irradiation. Leukemia 15(8):1232–1239
29. Lane SW, Scadden DT, Gilliland DG (2009) The leukemic stem cell niche: current concepts and therapeutic opportunities. Blood 114(6):1150–1157
30. Damiano JS, Cress AE, Hazlehurst LA, Shtil AA, Dalton WS (1999) Cell adhesion mediated drug resistance (CAM-DR): role of integrins and resistance to apoptosis in human myeloma cell lines. Blood 93(5):1658–1667
31. Luster AD (1998) Chemokines–chemotactic cytokines that mediate inflammation. N Engl J Med 338(7):436–445
32. Baggiolini M (1998) Chemokines and leukocyte traffic. Nature 392(6676):565–568
33. Tavor S, Eisenbach M, Jacob-Hirsch J et al (2008) The CXCR4 antagonist AMD3100 impairs survival of human AML cells and induces their differentiation. Leukemia 22(12): 2151–5158
34. Azab AK, Runnels JM, Pitsillides C et al (2009) CXCR4 inhibitor AMD3100 disrupts the interaction of multiple myeloma cells with the bone marrow microenvironment and enhances their sensitivity to therapy. Blood 113(18):4341–4351
35. Burger JA, Burkle A (2007) The CXCR4 chemokine receptor in acute and chronic leukaemia: a marrow homing receptor and potential therapeutic target. Br J Haematol 137(4):288–296
36. Geay JF, Buet D, Zhang Y et al (2005) p210BCR-ABL inhibits SDF-1 chemotactic response via alteration of CXCR4 signaling and down-regulation of CXCR4 expression. Cancer Res 65(7):2676–2683
37. Jin L, Tabe Y, Konoplev S et al (2008) CXCR4 up-regulation by imatinib induces chronic myelogenous leukemia (CML) cell migration to bone marrow stroma and promotes survival of quiescent CML cells. Mol Cancer Ther 7(1):48–58
38. Nervi B, Ramirez P, Rettig MP et al (2009) Chemosensitization of acute myeloid leukemia (AML) following mobilization by the CXCR4 antagonist AMD3100. Blood 113(24): 6206–6214
39. Zeng Z, Shi YX, Samudio IJ et al (2009) Targeting the leukemia microenvironment by CXCR4 inhibition overcomes resistance to kinase inhibitors and chemotherapy in AML. Blood 113(24):6215–6224
40. Oberlin E, Amara A, Bachelerie F et al (1996) The CXC chemokine SDF-1 is the ligand for LESTR/fusin and prevents infection by T-cell-line-adapted HIV-1. Nature 382(6594):833–835
41. Burger JA, Kipps TJ (2006) CXCR4: a key receptor in the crosstalk between tumor cells and their microenvironment. Blood 107(5):1761–1767
42. Bleul CC, Fuhlbrigge RC, Casasnovas JM, Aiuti A, Springer TA (1996) A highly efficacious lymphocyte chemoattractant, stromal cell-derived factor 1 (SDF-1). J Exp Med 184(3): 1101–1109
43. Shirozu M, Nakano T, Inazawa J et al (1995) Structure and chromosomal localization of the human stromal cell-derived factor 1 (SDF1) gene. Genomics 28(3):495–500
44. Nagasawa T, Hirota S, Tachibana K et al (1996) Defects of B-cell lymphopoiesis and bone-marrow myelopoiesis in mice lacking the CXC chemokine PBSF/SDF-1. Nature 382(6592): 635–638
45. Ma Q, Jones D, Borghesani PR et al (1998) Impaired B-lymphopoiesis, myelopoiesis, and derailed cerebellar neuron migration in CXCR4$^-$ and SDF-1-deficient mice. Proc Natl Acad Sci USA 95(16):9448–9453
46. Mayack SR, Wagers AJ (2008) Osteolineage niche cells initiate hematopoietic stem cell mobilization. Blood 112(3):519–531
47. Nilsson SK, Johnston HM, Coverdale JA (2001) Spatial localization of transplanted hemopoietic stem cells: inferences for the localization of stem cell niches. Blood 97(8):2293–2299
48. Netelenbos T, van den Born J, Kessler FL et al (2003) Proteoglycans on bone marrow endothelial cells bind and present SDF-1 towards hematopoietic progenitor cells. Leukemia 17(1): 175–184

49. Kiel MJ, Yilmaz OH, Iwashita T, Yilmaz OH, Terhorst C, Morrison SJ (2005) SLAM family receptors distinguish hematopoietic stem and progenitor cells and reveal endothelial niches for stem cells. Cell 121(7):1109–1121
50. Lo Celso C, Fleming HE, Wu JW, et al (2009) Live-animal tracking of individual haematopoietic stem/progenitor cells in their niche. Nature 457(7225):92–96
51. Plett PA, Frankovitz SM, Wolber FM, Abonour R, Orschell-Traycoff CM (2002) Treatment of circulating CD34(+) cells with SDF-1alpha or anti-CXCR4 antibody enhances migration and NOD/SCID repopulating potential. Exp Hematol 30(9):1061–1069
52. Teicher BA, Fricker SP. (2010) CXCL12 (SDF-1)/CXCR4 pathway in cancer. Clin Cancer Res 16(11):2927–2931
53. Durig J, Testa NG, Heyworth CM (1999) Distinct biological effects of macrophage inflammatory protein-1alpha and stroma-derived factor-1alpha on CD34+ hemopoietic cells. Stem Cells 17(2):62–71
54. Kijowski J, Baj-Krzyworzeka M, Majka M et al (2001) The SDF-1-CXCR4 axis stimulates VEGF secretion and activates integrins but does not affect proliferation and survival in lymphohematopoietic cells. Stem Cells 19(5):453–466
55. Mellado M, Rodriguez-Frade JM, Manes S, Martinez AC (2001) Chemokine signaling and functional responses: the role of receptor dimerization and TK pathway activation. Annu Rev Immunol 19:397–421
56. Zhang XF, Wang JF, Matczak E, Proper JA, Groopman JE (2001) Janus kinase 2 is involved in stromal cell-derived factor-1alpha-induced tyrosine phosphorylation of focal adhesion proteins and migration of hematopoietic progenitor cells. Blood 97(11):3342–3348
57. Barbero S, Bonavia R, Bajetto A et al (2003) Stromal cell-derived factor 1alpha stimulates human glioblastoma cell growth through the activation of both extracellular signal-regulated kinases 1/2 and Akt. Cancer Res 63(8):1969–1974
58. Nakata Y, Tomkowicz B, Gewirtz AM, Ptasznik A (2006) Integrin inhibition through Lyn-dependent cross talk from CXCR4 chemokine receptors in normal human CD34+ marrow cells. Blood 107(11):4234–4239
59. Peled A, Kollet O, Ponomaryov T et al (2000) The chemokine SDF-1 activates the integrins LFA-1, VLA-4, and VLA-5 on immature human CD34(+) cells: role in transendothelial/stromal migration and engraftment of NOD/SCID mice. Blood 95(11):3289–3296
60. Avecilla ST, Hattori K, Heissig B et al (2004) Chemokine-mediated interaction of hematopoietic progenitors with the bone marrow vascular niche is required for thrombopoiesis. Nat Med 10(1):64–71
61. Dommange F, Cartron G, Espanel C et al (2006) CXCL12 polymorphism and malignant cell dissemination/tissue infiltration in acute myeloid leukemia. FASEB J 20(11):1913–1915
62. de Oliveira CE, Cavassin GG, Perim Ade L, et al (2007) Stromal cell-derived factor-1 chemokine gene variant in blood donors and chronic myelogenous leukemia patients. J Clin Lab Anal 21(1):49–54
63. Odemis V, Boosmann K, Heinen A, Kury P, Engele J. (2010) CXCR7 is an active component of SDF-1 signalling in astrocytes and Schwann cells. J Cell Sci 123(Pt 7):1081–1088
64. Tarnowski M, Liu R, Wysoczynski M, Ratajczak J, Kucia M, Ratajczak MZ. (2010) CXCR7: a new SDF-1-binding receptor in contrast to normal CD34(+) progenitors is functional and is expressed at higher level in human malignant hematopoietic cells. Eur J Haematol 85(6): 472–483
65. Kucia M, Reca R, Miekus K, et al (2005) Trafficking of normal stem cells and metastasis of cancer stem cells involve similar mechanisms: pivotal role of the SDF-1-CXCR4 axis. Stem cells (Dayton, Ohio) 23(7):879–894
66. Kucia M, Jankowski K, Reca R et al (2004) CXCR4-SDF-1 signalling, locomotion, chemotaxis and adhesion. J Mol Histol 35(3):233–245
67. Peled A, Hardan I, Trakhtenbrot L et al (2002) Immature leukemic CD34+CXCR4+ cells from CML patients have lower integrin-dependent migration and adhesion in response to the chemokine SDF-1. Stem Cells 20(3):259–266

68. Wen Q, Chen RL, Cai KR, Lin YW. (2011) [Level of SDF-1/CXCR4 in children with acute leukemia and its significance]. Zhongguo Shi Yan Xue Ye Xue Za Zhi 19(2):324–326
69. Kalinkovich A, Tavor S, Avigdor A et al (2006) Functional CXCR4-expressing microparticles and SDF-1 correlate with circulating acute myelogenous leukemia cells. Cancer Res 66(22): 11013–11020
70. Burger JA. (2010) Chemokines and chemokine receptors in chronic lymphocytic leukemia (CLL): from understanding the basics towards therapeutic targeting. Semin Cancer Biol 20(6): 424–430
71. Sipkins DA, Wei X, Wu JW et al (2005) In vivo imaging of specialized bone marrow endothelial microdomains for tumour engraftment. Nature 435(7044):969–973
72. Spiegel A, Kollet O, Peled A et al (2004) Unique SDF-1-induced activation of human precursor-B ALL cells as a result of altered CXCR4 expression and signaling. Blood 103(8): 2900–2907
73. Cashman J, Clark-Lewis I, Eaves A, Eaves C (2002) Stromal-derived factor 1 inhibits the cycling of very primitive human hematopoietic cells in vitro and in NOD/SCID mice. Blood 99(3):792–799
74. Colmone A, Amorim M, Pontier AL, Wang S, Jablonski E, Sipkins DA (2008) Leukemic cells create bone marrow niches that disrupt the behavior of normal hematopoietic progenitor cells. Science 322(5909):1861–1865
75. Mendez-Ferrer S, Lucas D, Battista M, Frenette PS (2008) Haematopoietic stem cell release is regulated by circadian oscillations. Nature 452(7186):442–447
76. Williams SA, Harata-Lee Y, Comerford I, Anderson RL, Smyth MJ, McColl SR. (2010) Multiple functions of CXCL12 in a syngeneic model of breast cancer. Mol Cancer 9:250
77. Gordon MY, Dowding CR, Riley GP, Goldman JM, Greaves MF (1987) Altered adhesive interactions with marrow stroma of haematopoietic progenitor cells in chronic myeloid leukaemia. Nature 328(6128):342–344
78. Durig J, Rosenthal C, Elmaagacli A et al (2000) Biological effects of stroma-derived factor-1 alpha on normal and CML CD34+ haemopoietic cells. Leukemia 14(9):1652–1660
79. Ptasznik A, Urbanowska E, Chinta S et al (2002) Crosstalk between BCR/ABL oncoprotein and CXCR4 signaling through a Src family kinase in human leukemia cells. J Exp Med 196(5):667–678
80. Tabe Y, Jin L, Yixin Z, et al. Role of stromal microenvironment in non-pharmacological resistance of CML to tyrosine kinase inhibitors through Lyn/CXCR4 interactions in lipid rafts. Annuual Meeting of American Society of Hematology Vol. 2010
81. Zhao F, Mancuso A, Bui TV, et al. (2010) Imatinib resistance associated with BCR-ABL upregulation is dependent on HIF-1alpha-induced metabolic reprograming. Oncogene 29(20): 2962–2972
82. Ceradini DJ, Kulkarni AR, Callaghan MJ et al (2004) Progenitor cell trafficking is regulated by hypoxic gradients through HIF-1 induction of SDF-1. Nat Med 10(8):858–864
83. Staller P, Sulitkova J, Lisztwan J, Moch H, Oakeley EJ, Krek W (2003) Chemokine receptor CXCR4 downregulated by von Hippel-Lindau tumour suppressor pVHL. Nature 425(6955): 307–311
84. Bhatia R, McGlave PB, Verfaillie CM (1995) Treatment of marrow stroma with interferon-alpha restores normal beta 1 integrin-dependent adhesion of chronic myelogenous leukemia hematopoietic progenitors. Role of MIP-1 alpha. J Clin Invest 96(2):931–939
85. Bhatia R, Munthe HA, Verfaillie CM (1999) Role of abnormal integrin-cytoskeletal interactions in impaired beta1 integrin function in chronic myelogenous leukemia hematopoietic progenitors. Exp Hematol 27(9):1384–1396
86. Giuntoli S, Rovida E, Barbetti V (2006) Cipolleschi MG, Olivotto M. Dello Sbarba P Hypoxia suppresses BCR/Abl and selects imatinib-insensitive progenitors within clonal CML populations Leukemia 20(7):1291–1293
87. Vianello F, Villanova F, Tisato V, et al. (2010) Bone marrow mesenchymal stromal cells non-selectively protect chronic myeloid leukemia cells from imatinib-induced apoptosis via the CXCR4/CXCL12 axis. Haematologica 95(7):1081–1089

88. Mishra S, Zhang B, Cunnick JM, Heisterkamp N, Groffen J (2006) Resistance to imatinib of bcr/abl p190 lymphoblastic leukemia cells. Cancer Res 66(10):5387–5393
89. Juarez J, Bendall L, Bradstock K (2004) Chemokines and their receptors as therapeutic targets: the role of the SDF-1/CXCR4 axis. Curr Pharm Des 10(11):1245–1259
90. De Clercq E (2003) The bicyclam AMD3100 story. Nature reviews 2(7):581–587
91. De Clercq E. (2010) Recent advances on the use of the CXCR4 antagonist plerixafor (AMD3100, Mozobil) and potential of other CXCR4 antagonists as stem cell mobilizers. Pharmacol Ther 128(3):509–518
92. Liles WC, Broxmeyer HE, Rodger E et al (2003) Mobilization of hematopoietic progenitor cells in healthy volunteers by AMD3100, a CXCR4 antagonist. Blood 102(8):2728–2730
93. DiPersio JF, Micallef IN, Stiff PJ et al (2009) Phase III prospective randomized double-blind placebo-controlled trial of plerixafor plus granulocyte colony-stimulating factor compared with placebo plus granulocyte colony-stimulating factor for autologous stem-cell mobilization and transplantation for patients with non-Hodgkin's lymphoma. J Clin Oncol 27(28): 4767–4773
94. Brave M, Farrell A, Ching Lin S, et al. (2010) FDA review summary: Mozobil in combination with granulocyte colony-stimulating factor to mobilize hematopoietic stem cells to the peripheral blood for collection and subsequent autologous transplantation. Oncology 78(3–4):282–288
95. Pusic I, DiPersio JF. (2010) Update on clinical experience with AMD3100, an SDF-1/CXCL12-CXCR4 inhibitor, in mobilization of hematopoietic stem and progenitor cells. Curr Opin Hematol 17(4):319–326
96. Uy GL, Rettig MP, McFarland KM (2008) Mobilization and chemosensitization of AMLwith the CXCR4 antagonist plerixafor (AMD3100): a phase I/II study of AMD3100+MEC in patients with relapsed or refractory disease. Blood 112:(11):678–679
97. Uy GL, Rettig MP, McFarland K, et al (2009) A phase I/II study of chemosensitization with the CXCR4 antagonist plerixafor in relapsed or refractory AML. Blood 114:abstract 787(22):325
98. Dillmann F, Veldwijk MR, Laufs S et al (2009) Plerixafor inhibits chemotaxis toward SDF-1 and CXCR4-mediated stroma contact in a dose-dependent manner resulting in increased susceptibility of BCR-ABL+ cell to Imatinib and Nilotinib. Leuk Lymphoma 50(10): 1676–1686
99. Agarwal A, Fleischman AG, Petersen CL, et al (2010) Effects of plerixafor (AMD3100) in combination with tyrosine kinase inhibition In a murine model of CML. Blood 116:(21):1387–1388
100. Perez-Caro M, Cobaleda C, Gonzalez-Herrero I et al (2009) Cancer induction by restriction of oncogene expression to the stem cell compartment. EMBO J 28(1):8–20
101. Stone ND, Dunaway SB, Flexner C et al (2007) Multiple-dose escalation study of the safety, pharmacokinetics, and biologic activity of oral AMD070, a selective CXCR4 receptor inhibitor, in human subjects. Antimicrob Agents Chemother 51(7):2351–2358
102. Murakami T, Kumakura S, Yamazaki T et al (2009) The novel CXCR4 antagonist KRH-3955 is an orally bioavailable and extremely potent inhibitor of human immunodeficiency virus type 1 infection: comparative studies with AMD3100. Antimicrob Agents Chemother 53(7): 2940–2948
103. Tamamura H, Hori A, Kanzaki N et al (2003) T140 analogs as CXCR4 antagonists identified as anti-metastatic agents in the treatment of breast cancer. FEBS Lett 550(1–3):79–83
104. Takenaga M, Tamamura H, Hiramatsu K et al (2004) A single treatment with microcapsules containing a CXCR4 antagonist suppresses pulmonary metastasis of murine melanoma. Biochem Biophys Res Commun 320(1):226–232
105. Tamamura H, Fujisawa M, Hiramatsu K et al (2004) Identification of a CXCR4 antagonist, a T140 analog, as an anti-rheumatoid arthritis agent. FEBS Lett 569(1–3):99–104

Chapter 19
Targeting CXCR4 in Chronic Lymphocytic Leukemia: Preclinical Rationale and Early Clinical Experience

Jan A. Burger

Abstract Chronic lymphocytic leukemia (CLL) cells express high levels of CXCR4, a seven transmembrane G-protein coupled chemokine receptor. Bone marrow stromal cells (BMSCs) and other mesenchymal stromal cells (MSCs) at extramedullary sites constitutively secrete stromal cell-derived factor-1 (SDF-1, now called CXCL12), the ligand for CXCR4. Activation of CXCR4 induces CLL cell migration and homing to the marrow microenvironment, where CXCL12 retains leukemia cells in close contact with BMSC which provide growth and drug-resistance signals. CXCR4 antagonists, such as plerixafor (Mozobil®, AMD3100) and T140 analogs, can disrupt adhesive tumor–stroma interactions and mobilize CLL cells from their protective niches into the blood, making them more accessible to conventional drugs. This approach, to mobilize and then target tumor cells outside of their microenvironment, is also called "chemo-sensitization." The CXCR4–CXCL12 axis is now targeted in a first, ongoing clinical trial in CLL patients who are treated with plerixafor in combination with the anti-CD20 antibody rituximab. The fact that CLL cells express high levels of CXCR4 and readily respond to CXCL12, along with easy access to circulating leukemia cells for monitoring of leukemia cell mobilization, makes CLL a particularly well-suited disease model for studying the effects of CXCR4 antagonists in leukemia. This chapter summarizes preclinical and preliminary clinical experience with CXCR4 antagonists in CLL.

Keywords CXCR4 • CXCR4 antagonists • Leukemia microenvironment • Leukemia stem cells • CXCL12

J.A. Burger (✉)
Department of Leukemia, Unit 428, The University of Texas M.D. Anderson Cancer Center, PO Box 301402, Houston, TX 77230-1402, USA
e-mail: jaburger@mdanderson.org

S. Fruehauf et al. (eds.), *Novel Developments in Stem Cell Mobilization: Focus on CXCR4*, DOI 10.1007/978-1-4614-1960-0_19,

Chemokines and Their Receptors: Introduction

The chemokine receptor CXCR4 is part of the family of heterotrimeric guanine nucleotide-binding protein (G-protein)-coupled receptors (GPCRs). Its ligand CXCL12 belongs to the family of *chemo*-attractant cyto*kines* (chemokines), which are small (~5–20 kDa) proteins that are either constitutively secreted or inducible, for example, during inflammation [1, 2]. The term chemokines was coined in 1992 as a short form of "chemotactic cytokines," only a few years after discovery and characterization of the first chemokine, interleukine-8 (IL-8) [3, 4]. Subsequently, chemokines were characterized as a family of cytokines that regulate cell trafficking and homing of various immune cells. Besides their role in cell migration and tissue homing, chemokines are also implicated in a broad range of other biological functions, including angiogenesis, angiostasis, embryogenesis, hematopoiesis, lymphopoiesis, wound healing, cancer, inflammatory disease, and human immunodeficiency virus (HIV)-1 pathogenesis [5–8]. The human chemokine system currently includes more than 40 chemokines and 18 chemokine receptors [9]. Chemokines released either constitutively or in response to stimulation cause migration of cells toward a gradient of the chemokine (chemotaxis). Based upon whether or not two conserved cysteine residues present in all chemokines are separated by an intervening amino acid, chemokines can be segregated into two main subfamilies, accounting for CXC or CC chemokines [9].

Chemokines bind to chemokine receptors, which belong to the large family of seven transmembrane domain GPCRs. Chemokine receptors are designated CXCR1 through 5, CCR1 through 11, XCR1, and CX3CR1, based on their specific preference for certain chemokines. Chemokines bind to the extracellular domain of chemokine receptors, comprising the N-terminus and three extracellular loops. Following activation, the intracellular domains (three loops and the C-terminus) cause dissociation of G-proteins, which are composed of three distinct subunits (α, β, γ heterotrimers). This leads to formation of the second messengers inositol triphosphate (IP3) and diacylglycerol (DAG), resulting in cytoplasmatic calcium mobilization, and activation of multiple downstream signaling cascades, such as the phosphatidylinositol 3-kinase (PI3K)/Akt and the Ras/mitogen-activated protein kinase (MAPK, also called ERK 1/2) signaling pathways.

The CXCR4–CXCL12 Axis for Hematopoietic Cell Migration and Bone Marrow Homing

Stromal cell-derived factor 1 (SDF-1), now designated CXCL12 [9], signals through the CXCR4 chemokine receptor [10, 11], and initially was described as a pre-B-cell growth factor in 1994 [12]. In 1996, the co-receptor function of CXCR4 for entry of T-tropic (X4) HIV-1 strains into CD4 positive T cells was discovered [11, 13, 14]. Subsequently, CXCL12 and CXCR4 gene-deleted mice were described with an identical, lethal phenotype, suggesting a monogamous relationship between this chemokine and its receptor. The phenotype of these mice is characterized by deficient hematopoiesis with defects in B-cell development and myelopoiesis, and abnormal neuronal and cardiovascular development [15–18]. More recently, CXCR7 has been described as an alternate receptor for CXCL12, which appears to function by sequestering CXCL12 [19, 20] and modifying CXCR4 signaling rather than inducing the typical functional and signaling responses after ligand binding [21].

Mesenchymal stromal cells (MSCs), in particularly bone marrow stromal cell (BMSC), are considered a major source for CXCL12 in the adult organism. CXCL12-secreting MSC can be found in various tissues, such as the liver, lungs, lymphatic tissues, and the marrow (BMSC) [6]. Constitutive high-level CXCL12 secretion by BMSC is essential for homing [22] and maintenance of hematopoietic stem cells (HSCs) in distinct vascular and endosteal niches for their development and growth [23]. Via CXCL12, these stromal cells also attract circulating hematopoietic progenitor cells [24] or leukemia cells [25] for homing to the marrow. Actually, CXCR4 is the only functional chemokine receptor on hematopoietic progenitor cells [26], emphasizing the predominant role of this chemokine receptor for homing and maintenance of HSC in the marrow niches. More recently, the architecture of niches for hematopoietic and other tissue stem cells (i.e., germline stem cells, follicle cell stem cell, intestinal stem cell, central nervous system stem cell, and others), and the mechanism that govern stem cell homeostasis within these niches are emerging [27, 28].

In the bone marrow, at least two HSC niches have been described, one endosteal and one perivascular. Specialized osteoblasts lining the bone surface form endosteal niches. These osteoblasts are spindle-shaped N-cadherin^{+}CD45^{-} osteoblastic (SNO) cells, and express high amounts of N-cadherin. The relevance of SNO cells as HSC niches has been debated, based on the fact that hematopoiesis can be sustained at extramedullary sites, and by observations that selective osteoblast depletion or expansion do not acutely affect HSC numbers [29]. On the other hand, sinusoidal endothelial cells and a small population of perivascular reticular cells with long processes, expressing high amounts of CXCL12 (called CXCL12-abundant reticular or CAR cells) create vascular niches, which are scattered throughout the marrow cavity. Because most HSC, B-cell precursors, and plasma cells also are scattered throughout the marrow cavity and are in contact with CAR cells, it was proposed that CAR cells are a key component of HSC and B-cell niches [30]. This hypothesis is strengthened by recent in vivo studies that demonstrated that CAR ablation resulted in depletion of hematopoietic, and particularly of lymphoid progenitors [31]. Another group recently defined MSC critical for hematopoietic niches based on the expression of nestin, a type VI intermediate filament protein [29]. There appears to be a substantial overlap between CAR cells and nestin^{+} MSC. CXCL12 transcripts were high in nestin^{+} MSC [29], and depletion of both CAR cells and nestin^{+} MSC reduced numbers of HSCs by approximately 50% [29, 31]. Also, both types of BMSC have mesenchymal stem cell characteristics, as they can undergo osteogenic and adipogenic differentiation. Functionally, the proximity to CAR/nestin^{+} BMSCs likely influences lineage choice decisions as well as HSC cycling. Another layer of complexity in the marrow microenvironment is introduced by neural (e.g., from the sympathetic nervous system) [32] and hormonal (e.g., parathormone) input into the regulation of HSC and MSC maintenance, proliferation, and

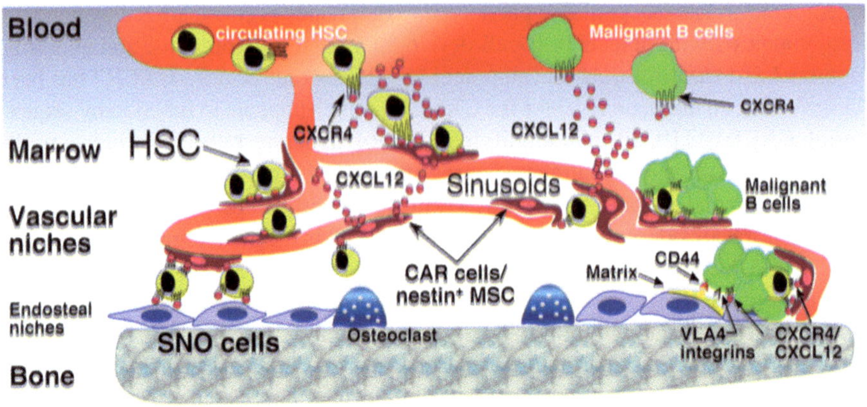

Fig. 19.1 Cellular and molecular interactions between malignant B cells (i.e., CLL cells) and the marrow microenvironment. Both hematopoietic stem cells (HSC, *left-hand side*) and CLL cells (*right-hand side*) express CXCR4, which directs chemotaxis of hematopoietic progenitor cells (HPC) and CLL from the circulation to the marrow. During this process, both cell types follow gradients of CXCL12 (SDF-1), the ligand for CXCR4, which is constitutively secreted by marrow stromal cells. Reticular stromal cells with high CXCL12 expression are called CXCL12-abundant reticular (CAR) cells. CAR cells are often located adjacent to a vascular network termed "sinusoids" and are scattered throughout the marrow cavity. Via CXCR4, HSC migrate to these reticular stromal cells, and this marrow compartment composed of sinusoids and reticular stromal cells is also referred to as "vascular niches." On the one hand, osteoblasts, lining the bone surface, form endosteal niches. These osteoblasts are spindle-shaped N-cadherin$^+$CD45$^-$ osteoblastic (SNO) cells, and express high amounts of N-cadherin. Malignant B cells utilize the CXCR4–CXCL12 axis to access niches that normally are restricted to HSC. Thus, CXCR4 allows malignant B cells to compete with HPC for niches that provide conditions that favor their survival. However, other mechanisms are also important in cross-talk between HSC or CLL cells and the marrow microenvironment. CLL cells interact with extracellular matrix molecules, such as fibronectin and hyaluronan, through corresponding receptors expressed on the CLL cells (CD49d/VLA-4 and CD44, respectively). These interactions not only confer adhesion, but also provide survival and drug-resistance signals to the CLL cells (adapted after [74])

differentiation [29]. The relative importance of these distinct niches and mechanism for B-cell malignancies have not been defined at this time, but a number of in vitro and in vivo studies suggest that malignant B cells utilize the marrow microenvironment to gain growth support and protection from chemotherapeutic agents (Fig. 19.1) (reviewed in ref. [33]).

CXCR4: Ligand Binding Sites and Signaling

Being a GPCR, CXCR4 signals through heterotrimeric GTP-binding G-proteins, involving α and βγ subunits, which in case of CXCR4 includes members of the Gi (pertussis toxin-sensitive), Gq, and $G\alpha_{12/13}$ subfamilies [34–36]. Activation of the $G\alpha_{13}$-Rho signaling axis downstream of CXCR4 seems to play a dominant role in

CXCL12-induced migration [35]. Multiple other signaling molecules modulate CXCR4 signaling, depending on cell type and maturation stage and the cellular environment. For example, B-cell antigen receptor (BCR) signaling modulates CXCR4 responsiveness in normal [37, 38] and malignant B cell [39].

The crystal structure of CXCR4 has recently been described, using surrogate ligands for precise definition of ligand binding sites. These studies revealed that ligands (natural and pharmacological) bind to CXCR4 via helices V and VI [40]. Compared to other GPCRs, such as rhodopsin, the β_2-adrenergic receptor, and the A_{2A} adenosine receptor, these CXCR4 ligand binding sites are larger, more open and located closer to the extracellular surface, providing new insight into the interactions between CXCR4 and its natural ligand CXCL12, and with the HIV-1 glycoprotein gp120 [41]. Upon CXCL12 stimulation, CXCR4 receptors become internalized from the cell surface via endocytosis and localize to $Rab11^+$ vesicles, a recycling compartment near the microtubule organizing center and Golgi apparatus. This CXCR4 trafficking requires Gα13 and Rho activation and presence of the CXCR4 C-terminal tail domain [42].

The responsiveness to CXCL12 significantly changes during differentiation of hematopoietic cells, as demonstrated for lymphoid [43, 44] and myeloid [45] cells. These maturation-dependent changes in CXCL12 responsiveness, which are not necessary accompanied by changes in CXCR4 expression levels [43], are thought to regulate trafficking and homing to distinct tissue microenvironments. For example, high CXCL12 responsiveness allows for the retention and homing of immature and mature B cells (pre- and pro-B cells, and plasma cells) to the marrow [46–48]. This maturation-dependent CXCL12 responsiveness appears to be retained in malignancies that correspond to respective maturation stages of their normal counterparts; i.e., pre- and pro-B-cell acute lymphoblastic leukemia (ALL) cells and multiple myeloma cells utilize the CXCR4/CXCL12 axis for bone marrow homing [25, 49].

The clinical features related to increased CXCR4 sensitivity in patients with WHIM syndrome also illustrates the critical role of CXCR4 signaling for homing and retention of hematopoietic cells in the marrow microenvironment. The WHIM syndrome is characterized by human papilloma virus-induced *W*arts, *H*ypogammaglobulinemia, recurrent bacterial *I*nfections, and *M*yelokathexis due to retention of neutrophils in the bone marrow. This syndrome is caused by dominant mutations in the C-terminal region of CXCR4 [50], leading to increased sensitivity to CXCL12 by preventing the internalization, and subsequent downregulation of CXCR4 [50, 51].

CXCR4 in Chronic Lymphocytic Leukemia

The CXCR4 chemokine receptor was among the first chemokine receptors characterized in chronic lymphocytic leukemia (CLL) [52, 53]. CXCR4 is expressed at high levels on the surface of peripheral blood CLL cells [52–55], and surface expression correlated with the clinical stage of the disease in one study [56], but not in another one [55]. CXCR4 expression is downregulated by its ligand CXCL12 (previously called stromal cell-derived factor 1 (SDF-1)) via receptor endocytosis [52]. This characteristic can be used to distinguish tissue (lymphatic tissue- and marrow-derived) from blood CLL cells, which express low or high CXCR4 levels, respectively [52, 57, 58]. Proliferating, Ki-67$^+$ CLL cells isolated from marrow and lymphatic tissue displayed significantly lower levels of CXCR4 and CXCR5 than nonproliferating CLL cells [59]. Moreover, in vivo deuterium (^{2}H) labeling of CLL cells revealed that patients with higher CXCR4 expression on their CLL cells had delayed appearance of newly produced CD38$^+$ cells in the blood, and increased risk for lymphoid organ infiltration and poor outcome [57]. These ^{2}H studies also revealed intraclonal heterogeneity of CXCR4 expression, with an enrichment of CLL cells expressing lower CXCR4 surface levels in the CD38$^+$/CD5^{bright} fraction, along with increased ^{2}H incorporation [57]. These in vivo data indicate that lower blood CXCR4 surface levels label a fraction of CLL cells that has recently exited the tissues into the blood.

Functionally, CXCR4 mediates CLL cell chemotaxis, migration across vascular endothelium, actin polymerization, and migration beneath and underneath BMSCs that secrete CXCL12, an in vitro phenomenon termed "pseudoemperipolesis" [52, 60, 61]. Besides its effects on CLL cell migration, CXCL12 also has a pro-survival effect on CLL cells, as demonstrated by using recombinant CXCL12 and the nurse-like cell (NLC) model in which NLC constitutively secrete CXCL12 [62–64]. This is not too surprising, given that CXCL12 initially was characterized as a pre-B-cell growth factor [12]. CLL cell responsiveness to CXCL12 can be modulated by accessory signals from the CLL microenvironment. BCR signaling results in down modulation of CXCR4 [39, 65], along with enhanced chemotaxis toward CXCL12 and CXCL13, at least in our hands [39]. This may explain why ZAP-70$^+$ CLL cells display increased chemotaxis and survival in response to CXCL12 when compared to ZAP-70-negative CLL cells [64], given that ZAP-70 expression is associated with a higher responsiveness to BCR stimulation [66]. CD38$^+$ CLL cell also displays higher levels of chemotaxis [67], and CD38 activation with an agonistic monoclonal antibody (mAb) enhanced chemotaxis toward CXCL12, whereas a blocking anti-CD38 mAbs inhibited chemotaxis [68]. CXCR4 signaling in CLL cells is pertussis toxin-sensitive and induces calcium mobilization, activation of PI3 kinases [52], p44/42 MAP kinases [62], and serine phosphorylation of signal transducer and activator of transcription 3 (STAT3) [69]. Inhibition of CXCR4 signaling with isoform-selective PI3 kinase inhibitors [70] or a Syk inhibitor [39] resulted in a reduction of chemotaxis and actin polymerization and reduced CLL cell migration beneath MSC.

Collectively, these data indicate that CXCR4 is involved in CLL cell migration and homing to tissue niches, where stromal cell-derived CXCL12 functions as a retention signal. Clinically, this mechanism may be involved in drug-resistance and minimal residual disease (MRD), given that CLL cells become highly resistant to conventional cytotoxic drugs (fludarabine, cyclophosphamide, and dexamethasone) when cultured in the presence of BMSC [69, 71]. Conceivably, stromal cell niches in the marrow and lymphatic tissues may provide a sanctuary in which CLL cells are protected them from (immuno-) chemotherapy, accounting for MRD and relapses invariably seen after current CLL therapies [72]. CXCR4 can specifically be blocked by CXCR4 antagonists (reviewed in ref. [33]), and we reported that CXCR4 antagonists inhibit CLL cell activation by CXCL12, and reverse, at least in parts, BMSC-mediated drug resistance [69].

Blocking CXCR4 in the Treatment of Leukemia and Other Cancers

CXCR4 chemokine receptors are expressed by leukemia cells from patients with acute and chronic leukemias and also various solid tumors, such as breast cancer, lung cancer, prostate cancer, and others [73, 74]. In general, CXCR4 expression by the tumor cells allows for tumor cell migration, and homing of the neoplastic cells to sites where nonmalignant stromal cells express CXCL12, the ligand for CXCR4 [75]. This concept implies that tumor cell metastasis is not random, but guided by the expression of chemokine receptors and adhesion molecules on the neoplastic cells, and respective ligands in the target organs [6, 76]. Tumor cells apparently utilize this mechanism to access microenvironments, such as the marrow, that provide factors that favor their growth. For example, the importance of CXCR4 for breast cancer metastasis to different target organs was demonstrated in vitro and in vivo [6]. Leukemia cells from patients with CLL and ALL utilize CXCR4 for homing to marrow stromal cells in vitro [52] and in vivo [25]. Moreover, CXCL12 has a direct growth- and survival-promoting effect for various cancer cells, such as breast cancer cells [77] or CLL cells [62]. CXCL12 also promotes tumor progression by recruiting endothelial progenitor cells to tumors for tumor angiogenesis [77]. Stromal fibroblasts, also called carcinoma-associated fibroblasts (CAFs) or MSCs, are part of the tumor microenvironment. These stromal fibroblasts constitutively secrete CXCL12, and contact between tumor cells and stromal cells is largely dependent upon the CXCR4–CXCL12 axis. For example, co-culture between CLL cells [52] or lung cancer cells [78] and CXCL12-secreting stromal cells induce strong adhesion and spontaneous migration of the neoplastic cells beneath the stromal cells (pseudoemperipolesis) in a CXCR4-dependent fashion. Nonspecific and specific CXCR4 antagonists, such as pertussis toxin and CXCR4 antagonists, (T140, AMD3100) can block this adhesion and migration [69]. Adhesion to stromal cells confers resistance to spontaneous and drug-induced cell death of tumor cells, and therefore also is termed cell adhesion-mediated drug-resistance (CAM-DR) [79, 80]. Tumor cells that adhere to stromal cells via CXCR4 therefore are, at least partially, protected from the effects of cytotoxic chemotherapy and represent a reservoir for MRD and relapses commonly seen in the treatment of patients with various cancers. However, the overall role of MSC in the tumor microenvironment remains controversial. While on the one hand MSC can provide survival, growth, and drug-resistance signals [69, 77], MSC can also induce cell cycle- and growth-arrest in epithelial cancer [81–83] and leukemia cells [78]. Based upon these findings, the therapeutic use of MSC to decelerate tumor growth has been proposed [84, 85]. These controversial findings regarding the capacity of MSC to induce tumor progression (in vivo) but also to induce tumor cell growth arrest (in vitro) could, at least in parts, be due to the ability of MSC to provide niches for CSCs in vivo. In these tissue niches, MSC are thought to maintain and support a subpopulation of growth-arrested tumor cells/CSCs that are resistant to cytotoxic treatments and function as a reservoir of the disease with the potential to proliferate and sustain the malignant process [86].

CXCR4 Antagonists

CXCR4 antagonists initially were developed as new drugs for the treatment of HIV-1 infection. At the time of their discovery in the early 1990s, the mechanism of anti-HIV activity of the most prominent CXCR4 antagonists, T140 and its analogs [87, 88], AMD3100 [89, 90], and ALX-4C [91], was unknown. After the discovery of the co-receptor function of CXCR4 for T-tropic HIV-1, the specific CXCR4 blocking function of the different CXCR4 antagonists was rapidly demonstrated [92–94]. With the rapid increase in our knowledge of other, non-HIV related functions of CXCR4 over the past 11 years, other potential applications such as HSC mobilization and treatment of cancer and autoimmune disease are emerging and gradually have replaced the original intent to use CXCR4 antagonists as anti-HIV drugs.

In general, four major classes of CXCR4 antagonists and agonists can be distinguished: (a) small peptide CXCR4 antagonists, such as T140 and its analogs (TN14003 and others), (b) nonpeptide CXCR4 antagonists, such as the bicyclam AMD3100, (c) antibodies to CXCR4, and (d) modified agonists and antagonists for SDF-1. Below, we summarize the current status of preclinical and clinical development for CXCR4 antagonists (Table 19.1).

Small Peptide Antagonist of CXCR4

Initially, this group of small peptide CXCR4 antagonists was discovered screening naturally occurring peptides for anti-HIV activity. In that process, self-defense peptides from horseshoe crabs, called tachyplesin (from the Japanese horseshoe crab *Tachypleus tridentatus*) and polyphemusin (from the American horseshoe crab *Limulus polyphemus*), were identified and chemically modified, leading to the synthesis of anti-HIV peptides T22 [88], T134, and T140 [95]. Initially, these compounds were thought to function by inhibiting HIV-1–T cell fusion or the viral uncoating [87]. However, the precise mechanism of anti-HIV activity remained unclear until the discovery that T-tropic HIV-1 (X4-HIV-1) utilizes CXCR4 as a co-receptor for cellular entry into CD4-positive T cells. Soon after this, it was demonstrated the T22 specifically binds to CXCR4 and blocks CXCR4 receptor regions that are critical for HIV-1 viral entry and for activation by its natural ligand,

Table 19.1 CXCR4 antagonists that currently are in preclinical and clinical development

Product name	Company	Structure	Administration	Indication	Study phase
Plerixafor (AMD3100)	Genzyme (now: Sanofi-Aventis)	Bicyclam	s.c.	Stem cell mobilization	ad 1: FDA approved
				Chemo-sensitization in leukemia (CLL, AML)	ad 2: Phase I/II
AMD070	Genzyme (now: Sanofi-Aventis)	Bicyclam derived	Oral	HIV	Phase I/II
MDX-1338 (BMS-936564)	Bristol-Myers Squibb	CXCR4 antibody	i.v.	Leukemia (AML)	Phase I/II
CTCE-9908 Antagonist	Chemokine Therapeutics Corp.	Modified SDF-1	s.c./i.v.	Solid tumors	Phase I/II
CTCE-0214-Agonist	Chemokine Therapeutics Corp.	Modified SDF-1	s.c./i.v.	Mobilization BM recovery	Phase I
BKT140	Biokine Therapeutics	Modified Peptide	s.c./oral	MM and leukemia	Phase I
POL6326	Polyphor Ltd.	Protein epitope mimetic (PEM)	i.v.	Stem cell mobilization in multiple myeloma	Phase II

CXCL12 [94]. T140 is considered the most active CXCR4 peptide antagonist among the initially synthesized peptides, but lacks serum stability due to cleavage of the C-terminal Arg. Therefore, C-terminally amidated T140 analogs were developed to overcome serum instability [96], leading to the synthesis of TN14003 and TC14012. Further work revealed the binding regions for T140 within the extracellular domains and regions of the hydrophobic core of CXCR4, which are distinct from the binding region for AMD3100 [97]. Also, in a series of experiments to elucidate the mechanism of CXCR4 signaling, it was noticed that T140 decreased autonomous CXCR4 signaling in CXCR4 wild-type or constitutively active CXCR4 mutants, characterizing T140 as an inverse CXCR4 agonist, whereas AMD3100 and ALX40-4C displayed partial agonist activity in this study [98]. Clinical trials will help to determine whether this characteristic of CXCR4 peptide antagonists correlates with a profile of activities and/or side effects that is distinct from AMD3100.

The efficacy of T140 and its analogs for blocking CXCR4 in vitro and in vivo has been documented in numerous preclinical studies, including in vivo models for breast cancer and melanoma [99, 100], rheumatoid arthritis [101], and stem cell mobilization [102]. Other studies explored the activity of these agents in acute [103, 104] and chronic leukemias [69], multiple myeloma [105], small cell lung cancer [78], malignant melanoma [100], and pancreatic cancer [106]. Besides these disease-oriented studies, T140 and its analogs have been used in basic studies exploring the function of CXCR4 in dendritic cell development [107] and migration [108], B-cell homing and germinal center positioning within lymphatic tissues [109], and HSC homing [110]. Currently, the T140 analog TN14003 is under clinical development by Biokine Therapeutics Ltd., Rehovot, Israel.

ALX40-4C is a polypeptide of nine Arg residues that is stabilized by terminal protection and inclusion of D-amino acids. ALX40-4C is a specific CXCR4 antagonist [92], and was the first CXCR4 antagonist clinically used in Phase I and Phase I/II trials in HIV patients conducted by the Canadian company Allelix Biopharmaceuticals [91]. This peptide is no longer under development, particularly because of formulation difficulties, lack of efficacy, and because it is unlikely that an oral formulation of this complex peptide can be produced.

Nonpeptide CXCR4 Antagonists

AMD3100 is a bicyclam, in which two cyclam rings are connected through an aromatic bridge. AMD3100 possesses the highest anti-HIV activity among a series of bicyclams that were synthesized in the early 1990s [90, 111]. AMD3100 is a specific antagonist of CXCL12 binding to CXCR4, inhibiting CXCL12-mediated calcium mobilization, chemotaxis, and GTP binding, and does not cross-react with other chemokine receptors [112]. AMD3100 initially was considered to interfere with HIV-1 fusion or uncoating [89]. Initially developed at Johnson Matthey in collaboration with the Rega Institute for Medical Research (Leuven University, Belgium), this compound was first called JM3100, which changed to AMD3100 after a new company (AnorMED) took over the development. The anti-HIV-1 activity of AMD3100 restricted to X4-HIV-1 strains, and the blocking function of AMD3100 on gp120 interaction with CXCR4 during viral entry [113] was the initial focus during the early development of this drug. However, an unexpected rapid, transient leukocytosis was noticed during phase I/II clinical trials of AMD3100 in volunteers and HIV-infected patients, caused by the mobilization of various hematopoietic cells, including CD34-positive HSC, to the blood [114, 115]. In the second trial in HIV patients, one patient receiving the highest dose of AMD3100 (160 μg/kg/h) had a significant drop in his viral load, but overall the efficacy of AMD3100 affecting disease activity in HIV-1 patients was considered low and therefore this application was not further pursued for AMD3100. Instead, AnorMED explored AMD3100 as a mobilizing agent for HSC [115], and a subsequent series of preclinical and clinical trials demonstrated that AMD3100 alone and in combination with G-CSF mobilizes HSC [116–118]. AMD3100 (recently re-named as Plerixafor or Mozobil™) is now owned by Genzyme after a recent takeover of AnorMED by Genzyme in late 2006. Plerixafor currently is used in phase III trials in lymphoma and multiple myeloma patients undergoing autologous stem cell mobilization, and current plans are to file for USA and European approval of the drug in 2008. The activity of Plerixafor to inhibit CXCR4 activation in various in vitro and in vivo tumor models, such as inhibition of CXCL12-induced tumor cell migration and downstream signaling and activity in murine tumor models has been reported.

Preliminary Clinical Experience with the CXCR4 Antagonist Plerixafor in CLL

Because of the central role of the CXCR4/CXCL12 axis in CLL cell homing and retention in tissue microenvironments, it was hypothesized that plerixafor may abrogate stroma-mediated drug resistance and enhance sensitivity of CLL cells to rituximab. Therefore, a phase 1 trial of plerixafor in combination with rituximab in previously treated patients with CLL was initiated; this study is still ongoing, and preliminary results were reported at the 2010 meetings of the European and American Societies of Hematology (EHA, ASH) [119, 120]. The clinical endpoints in this trial are to determine the maximum tolerated dose (MTD), the principal toxicities, and dose limiting toxicities (DLTs) of the combination of plerixafor and rituximab, along with exploratory analyses to determine mobilization of $CD34^+$ cells, WBCs, and CLL cells by plerixafor. Patients were treated with rituximab three times weekly, administered as a 100 mg flat dose on day 1, and thereafter at 375 mg/m^2 i.v. for 12 total doses. Plerixafor was administered, beginning with the fourth rituximab dose. Four cohorts of patients were treated subcutaneously (s.c.) at doses of 0.08, 0.16, 0.24, or 0.32 mg/kg. A fifth cohort was treated intravenously (i.v.) at 0.42 mg/kg. At the time of the last update (ASH 2010), the investigators reported preliminarily that the combination of plerixafor plus rituximab in CLL patients appears to be well tolerated and safe at doses up to 0.32 mg/kg s.c. Adverse events apparently were mild to moderate in the majority of cases; one DLT (grade 3 nausea) was observed. The majority of responses were observed at higher (≥0.32 mg/kg) plerixafor doses; while preliminary, these data suggest a possible dose-dependent relationship. Also, plerixafor treatment mobilized CLL cells to the peripheral blood, justifying further investigation into its use as a potential sensitizing agent to enhance the activity of other agents utilized in the treatment of CLL.

Collectively, CXCR4 antagonists provide a new, targeted tool to mobilize leukemia cells from their protective marrow microenvironment. Mobilized leukemia cells then become better accessible to conventional drugs, and therefore this strategy may help to overcome MRD and relapses commonly seen in the treatment of CLL patients. Currently, CXCR4 antagonists are explored in proof-of-principle studies in leukemia patients in which leukemia cell mobilization can easily be assessed and monitored. However, given the expression of functional CXCR4 receptors by a variety of other hematopoietic and epithelial cancers [73], a broader use of CXCR4 antagonists in other cancers will be a logical next step.

Acknowledgments This study was supported by an ASCO Career Development Award, a CLL Global Research Foundation grant, and a Cancer Prevention and Research Institute of Texas (CPRIT) research award (to J.A.B.).

References

1. Murphy PM (2001) Chemokines and the molecular basis of cancer metastasis. N Engl J Med 345(11):833–835
2. Moser B, Wolf M, Walz A, Loetscher P (2004) Chemokines: multiple levels of leukocyte migration control. Trends Immunol 25(2):75–84
3. Thelen M, Peveri P, Kernen P, von Tscharner V, Walz A, Baggiolini M (1988) Mechanism of neutrophil activation by NAF, a novel monocyte-derived peptide agonist. FASEB J 2(11):2702–2706
4. Kunkel SL, Strieter RM, Lindley IJ, Westwick J (1995) Chemokines: new ligands, receptors and activities. Immunol Today 16(12):559–561
5. Rossi D, Zlotnik A (2000) The biology of chemokines and their receptors. Annu Rev Immunol 18:217–242
6. Muller A, Homey B, Soto H et al (2001) Involvement of chemokine receptors in breast cancer metastasis. Nature 410(6824):50–56
7. Zlotnik A (2006) Chemokines and cancer. Int J Cancer 119(9):2026–2029
8. Balkwill F (2004) Cancer and the chemokine network. Nat Rev Cancer 4(7):540–550
9. Zlotnik A, Yoshie O (2000) Chemokines: a new classification system and their role in immunity. Immunity 12(2):121–127
10. Bleul CC, Farzan M, Choe H et al (1996) The lymphocyte chemoattractant SDF-1 is a ligand for LESTR/fusin and blocks HIV-1 entry. Nature 382(6594):829–833
11. Oberlin E, Amara A, Bachelerie F et al (1996) The CXC chemokine SDF-1 is the ligand for LESTR/fusin and prevents infection by T-cell-line-adapted HIV-1 [published erratum appears in Nature 1996 Nov 21;384(6606):288]. Nature 382(6594):833–835
12. Nagasawa T, Kikutani H, Kishimoto T (1994) Molecular cloning and structure of a pre-B-cell growth-stimulating factor. Proc Natl Acad Sci USA 91(6):2305–2309
13. Bleul CC, Fuhlbrigge RC, Casasnovas JM, Aiuti A, Springer TA (1996) A highly efficacious lymphocyte chemoattractant, stromal cell-derived factor 1 (SDF-1) [see comments]. J Exp Med 184(3):1101–1109

14. Feng Y, Broder CC, Kennedy PE, Berger EA (1996) HIV-1 entry cofactor: functional cDNA cloning of a seven-transmembrane, G protein-coupled receptor [see comments]. Science 272(5263):872–877
15. Nagasawa T, Hirota S, Tachibana K et al (1996) Defects of B-cell lymphopoiesis and bone-marrow myelopoiesis in mice lacking the CXC chemokine PBSF/SDF-1. Nature 382(6592):635–638
16. Nagasawa T, Tachibana K, Kishimoto T (1998) A novel CXC chemokine PBSF/SDF-1 and its receptor CXCR4: their functions in development, hematopoiesis and HIV infection. Semin Immunol 10(3):179–185
17. Zou YR, Kottmann AH, Kuroda M, Taniuchi I, Littman DR (1998) Function of the chemokine receptor CXCR4 in haematopoiesis and in cerebellar development [see comments]. Nature 393(6685):595–599
18. Ma Q, Jones D, Borghesani PR et al (1998) Impaired B-lymphopoiesis, myelopoiesis, and derailed cerebellar neuron migration in CXCR4- and SDF-1-deficient mice. Proc Natl Acad Sci USA 95(16):9448–9453
19. Boldajipour B, Mahabaleshwar H, Kardash E et al (2008) Control of chemokine-guided cell migration by ligand sequestration. Cell 132(3):463–473
20. Naumann U, Cameroni E, Pruenster M et al (2010) CXCR7 functions as a scavenger for CXCL12 and CXCL11. PLoS One 5(2):e9175
21. Rajagopal S, Kim J, Ahn S et al (2010) Beta-arrestin- but not G protein-mediated signaling by the "decoy" receptor CXCR7. Proc Natl Acad Sci USA 107(2):628–632
22. Peled A, Grabovsky V, Habler L et al (1999) The chemokine SDF-1 stimulates integrin-mediated arrest of $CD34^+$ cells on vascular endothelium under shear flow. J Clin Invest 104(9):1199–1211
23. Sugiyama T, Kohara H, Noda M, Nagasawa T (2006) Maintenance of the hematopoietic stem cell pool by CXCL12-CXCR4 chemokine signaling in bone marrow stromal cell niches. Immunity 25(6):977–988
24. Peled A, Petit I, Kollet O et al (1999) Dependence of human stem cell engraftment and repopulation of NOD/SCID mice on CXCR4. Science 283(5403):845–848
25. Sipkins DA, Wei X, Wu JW et al (2005) In vivo imaging of specialized bone marrow endothelial microdomains for tumour engraftment. Nature 435(7044):969–973
26. Wright DE, Bowman EP, Wagers AJ, Butcher EC, Weissman IL (2002) Hematopoietic stem cells are uniquely selective in their migratory response to chemokines. J Exp Med 195(9):1145–1154
27. Moore KA, Lemischka IR (2006) Stem cells and their niches. Science 311(5769):1880–1885
28. Morrison SJ, Spradling AC (2008) Stem cells and niches: mechanisms that promote stem cell maintenance throughout life. Cell 132(4):598–611
29. Mendez-Ferrer S, Michurina TV, Ferraro F et al (2010) Mesenchymal and haematopoietic stem cells form a unique bone marrow niche. Nature 466(7308):829–834
30. Nagasawa T (2008) New niches for B cells. Nat Immunol 9(4):345–346
31. Omatsu Y, Sugiyama T, Kohara H et al (2010) The essential functions of adipo-osteogenic progenitors as the hematopoietic stem and progenitor cell niche. Immunity 33(3):387–399
32. Katayama Y, Battista M, Kao WM et al (2006) Signals from the sympathetic nervous system regulate hematopoietic stem cell egress from bone marrow. Cell 124(2):407–421
33. Burger JA, Peled A (2009) CXCR4 antagonists: targeting the microenvironment in leukemia and other cancers. Leukemia 23(1):43–52
34. Thelen M (2001) Dancing to the tune of chemokines. Nat Immunol 2(2):129–134
35. Tan W, Martin D, Gutkind JS (2006) The Galpha13-Rho signaling axis is required for SDF-1-induced migration through CXCR4. J Biol Chem 281(51):39542–39549
36. Soede RD, Zeelenberg IS, Wijnands YM, Kamp M, Roos E (2001) Stromal cell-derived factor-1-induced LFA-1 activation during in vivo migration of T cell hybridoma cells requires Gq/11, RhoA, and myosin, as well as Gi and Cdc42. J Immunol 166(7):4293–4301
37. Bleul CC, Schultze JL, Springer TA (1998) B lymphocyte chemotaxis regulated in association with microanatomic localization, differentiation state, and B cell receptor engagement. J Exp Med 187(5):753–762

38. Guinamard R, Signoret N, Masamichi I, Marsh M, Kurosaki T, Ravetch JV (1999) B cell antigen receptor engagement inhibits stromal cell-derived factor (SDF)-1alpha chemotaxis and promotes protein kinase C (PKC)-induced internalization of CXCR4. J Exp Med 189(9):1461–1466
39. Quiroga MP, Balakrishnan K, Kurtova AV et al (2009) B-cell antigen receptor signaling enhances chronic lymphocytic leukemia cell migration and survival: specific targeting with a novel spleen tyrosine kinase inhibitor, R406. Blood 114(5):1029–1037
40. Wu B, Chien EY, Mol CD et al (2010) Structures of the CXCR4 chemokine GPCR with small-molecule and cyclic peptide antagonists. Science 330(6007):1066–1071
41. Harrison C (2010) G protein-coupled receptors: insights into chemokine receptors. Nat Rev Drug Discov 9(12):920
42. Kumar A, Kremer KN, Dominguez D, Tadi M, Hedin KE (2011) Galpha13 and Rho mediate endosomal trafficking of CXCR4 into Rab11+ vesicles upon stromal cell-derived factor-1 stimulation. J Immunol 186(2):951–958
43. Honczarenko M, Douglas RS, Mathias C, Lee B, Ratajczak MZ, Silberstein LE (1999) SDF-1 responsiveness does not correlate with CXCR4 expression levels of developing human bone marrow B cells. Blood 94(9):2990–2998
44. Le Y, Zhu BM, Harley B et al (2007) SOCS3 protein developmentally regulates the chemokine receptor CXCR4-FAK signaling pathway during B lymphopoiesis. Immunity 27(5):811–823
45. Martin C, Burdon PC, Bridger G, Gutierrez-Ramos JC, Williams TJ, Rankin SM (2003) Chemokines acting via CXCR2 and CXCR4 control the release of neutrophils from the bone marrow and their return following senescence. Immunity 19(4):583–593
46. Ma Q, Jones D, Springer TA (1999) The chemokine receptor CXCR4 is required for the retention of B lineage and granulocytic precursors within the bone marrow microenvironment. Immunity 10(4):463–471
47. Hargreaves DC, Hyman PL, Lu TT et al (2001) A coordinated change in chemokine responsiveness guides plasma cell movements. J Exp Med 194(1):45–56
48. Cyster JG (2003) Homing of antibody secreting cells. Immunol Rev 194:48–60
49. Alsayed Y, Ngo H, Runnels J et al (2007) Mechanisms of regulation of CXCR4/SDF-1 (CXCL12)-dependent migration and homing in multiple myeloma. Blood 109(7):2708–2717
50. Hernandez PA, Gorlin RJ, Lukens JN et al (2003) Mutations in the chemokine receptor gene CXCR4 are associated with WHIM syndrome, a combined immunodeficiency disease. Nat Genet 34(1):70–74
51. Kawai T, Choi U, Cardwell L et al (2007) WHIM syndrome myelokathexis reproduced in the NOD/SCID mouse xenotransplant model engrafted with healthy human stem cells transduced with C-terminus-truncated CXCR4. Blood 109(1):78–84
52. Burger JA, Burger M, Kipps TJ (1999) Chronic lymphocytic leukemia B cells express functional CXCR4 chemokine receptors that mediate spontaneous migration beneath bone marrow stromal cells. Blood 94(11):3658–3667
53. Mohle R, Failenschmid C, Bautz F, Kanz L (1999) Overexpression of the chemokine receptor CXCR4 in B cell chronic lymphocytic leukemia is associated with increased functional response to stromal cell-derived factor-1 (SDF-1). Leukemia 13(12):1954–1959
54. Durig J, Schmucker U, Duhrsen U (2001) Differential expression of chemokine receptors in B cell malignancies. Leukemia 15(5):752–756
55. Barretina J, Junca J, Llano A et al (2003) CXCR4 and SDF-1 expression in B-cell chronic lymphocytic leukemia and stage of the disease. Ann Hematol 82(8):500–505
56. Ghobrial IM, Bone ND, Stenson MJ et al (2004) Expression of the chemokine receptors CXCR4 and CCR7 and disease progression in B-cell chronic lymphocytic leukemia/ small lymphocytic lymphoma. Mayo Clin Proc 79(3):318–325
57. Calissano C, Damle RN, Hayes G et al (2009) In vivo intraclonal and interclonal kinetic heterogeneity in B-cell chronic lymphocytic leukemia. Blood 114(23):4832–4842
58. Herishanu Y, Perez-Galan P, Liu D et al (2011) The lymph node microenvironment promotes B-cell receptor signaling, NF-{kappa}B activation, and tumor proliferation in chronic lymphocytic leukemia. Blood 117(2):563–574

59. Bennett F, Rawstron A, Plummer M et al (2007) B-cell chronic lymphocytic leukaemia cells show specific changes in membrane protein expression during different stages of cell cycle. Br J Haematol 139(4):600–604
60. Till KJ, Lin K, Zuzel M, Cawley JC (2002) The chemokine receptor CCR7 and alpha4 integrin are important for migration of chronic lymphocytic leukemia cells into lymph nodes. Blood 99(8):2977–2984
61. Trentin L, Cabrelle A, Facco M et al (2004) Homeostatic chemokines drive migration of malignant B cells in patients with non-Hodgkin lymphomas. Blood 104(2):502–508
62. Burger JA, Tsukada N, Burger M, Zvaifler NJ, Dell'Aquila M, Kipps TJ (2000) Blood-derived nurse-like cells protect chronic lymphocytic leukemia B cells from spontaneous apoptosis through stromal cell-derived factor-1. Blood 96(8):2655–2663
63. Nishio M, Endo T, Tsukada N et al (2005) Nurselike cells express BAFF and APRIL, which can promote survival of chronic lymphocytic leukemia cells via a paracrine pathway distinct from that of SDF-1alpha. Blood 106(3):1012–1020
64. Richardson SJ, Matthews C, Catherwood MA et al (2006) ZAP-70 expression is associated with enhanced ability to respond to migratory and survival signals in B-cell chronic lymphocytic leukemia (B-CLL). Blood 107(9):3584–3592
65. Vlad A, Deglesne PA, Letestu R et al (2009) Down-regulation of CXCR4 and CD62L in chronic lymphocytic leukemia cells is triggered by B-cell receptor ligation and associated with progressive disease. Cancer Res 69(16):6387–6395
66. Chen L, Widhopf G, Huynh L et al (2002) Expression of ZAP-70 is associated with increased B-cell receptor signaling in chronic lymphocytic leukemia. Blood 100(13):4609–4614
67. Deaglio S, Vaisitti T, Aydin S et al (2007) CD38 and ZAP-70 are functionally linked and mark CLL cells with high migratory potential. Blood 110(12):4012–4021
68. Vaisitti T, Aydin S, Rossi D, et al (2010) CD38 increases CXCL12-mediated signals and homing of chronic lymphocytic leukemia cells. Leukemia 24(5):958–969
69. Burger M, Hartmann T, Krome M et al (2005) Small peptide inhibitors of the CXCR4 chemokine receptor (CD184) antagonize the activation, migration, and antiapoptotic responses of CXCL12 in chronic lymphocytic leukemia B cells. Blood 106(5):1824–1830
70. Niedermeier M, Hennessy BT, Knight ZA et al (2009) Isoform-selective phosphoinositide 3′-kinase inhibitors inhibit CXCR4 signaling and overcome stromal cell-mediated drug resistance in chronic lymphocytic leukemia: a novel therapeutic approach. Blood 113(22):5549–5557
71. Kurtova AV, Balakrishnan K, Chen R et al (2009) Diverse marrow stromal cells protect CLL cells from spontaneous and drug-induced apoptosis: development of a reliable and reproducible system to assess stromal cell adhesion-mediated drug resistance. Blood 114(20):4441–4450
72. Rawstron AC, Kennedy B, Evans PA et al (2001) Quantitation of minimal disease levels in chronic lymphocytic leukemia using a sensitive flow cytometric assay improves the prediction of outcome and can be used to optimize therapy. Blood 98(1):29–35
73. Burger JA, Kipps TJ (2006) CXCR4: a key receptor in the crosstalk between tumor cells and their microenvironment. Blood 107(5):1761–1767
74. Burger JA, Burkle A (2007) The CXCR4 chemokine receptor in acute and chronic leukaemia: a marrow homing receptor and potential therapeutic target. Br J Haematol 137(4):288–296
75. Orimo A, Weinberg RA (2006) Stromal fibroblasts in cancer: a novel tumor-promoting cell type. Cell Cycle 5(15):1597–1601
76. Liotta LA (2001) An attractive force in metastasis. Nature 410(6824):24–25
77. Orimo A, Gupta PB, Sgroi DC et al (2005) Stromal fibroblasts present in invasive human breast carcinomas promote tumor growth and angiogenesis through elevated SDF-1/CXCL12 secretion. Cell 121(3):335–348
78. Burger M, Glodek A, Hartmann T et al (2003) Functional expression of CXCR4 (CD184) on small-cell lung cancer cells mediates migration, integrin activation, and adhesion to stromal cells. Oncogene 22(50):8093–8101
79. Damiano JS, Cress AE, Hazlehurst LA, Shtil AA, Dalton WS (1999) Cell adhesion mediated drug resistance (CAM-DR): role of integrins and resistance to apoptosis in human myeloma cell lines. Blood 93(5):1658–1667

80. Li ZW, Dalton WS (2006) Tumor microenvironment and drug resistance in hematologic malignancies. Blood Rev 20(6):333–342
81. Ramasamy R, Lam EW, Soeiro I, Tisato V, Bonnet D, Dazzi F (2007) Mesenchymal stem cells inhibit proliferation and apoptosis of tumor cells: impact on in vivo tumor growth. Leukemia 21(2):304–310
82. Maestroni GJ, Hertens E, Galli P (1999) Factor(s) from nonmacrophage bone marrow stromal cells inhibit Lewis lung carcinoma and B16 melanoma growth in mice. Cell Mol Life Sci 55(4):663–667
83. Ohlsson LB, Varas L, Kjellman C, Edvardsen K, Lindvall M (2003) Mesenchymal progenitor cell-mediated inhibition of tumor growth in vivo and in vitro in gelatin matrix. Exp Mol Pathol 75(3):248–255
84. Pisati F, Belicchi M, Acerbi F et al (2007) Effect of human skin-derived stem cells on vessel architecture, tumor growth, and tumor invasion in brain tumor animal models. Cancer Res 67(7):3054–3063
85. Khakoo AY, Pati S, Anderson SA et al (2006) Human mesenchymal stem cells exert potent antitumorigenic effects in a model of Kaposi's sarcoma. J Exp Med 203(5):1235–1247
86. Laird DJ, von Andrian UH, Wagers AJ (2008) Stem cell trafficking in tissue development, growth, and disease. Cell 132(4):612–630
87. Nakashima H, Masuda M, Murakami T et al (1992) Anti-human immunodeficiency virus activity of a novel synthetic peptide, T22 ([Tyr-5,12, Lys-7]polyphemusin II): a possible inhibitor of virus-cell fusion. Antimicrob Agent Chemother 36(6):1249–1255
88. Masuda M, Nakashima H, Ueda T et al (1992) A novel anti-HIV synthetic peptide, T-22 ([Tyr5,12, Lys7]-polyphemusin II). Biochem Biophys Res Commun 189(2):845–850
89. De Clercq E, Yamamoto N, Pauwels R et al (1992) Potent and selective inhibition of human immunodeficiency virus (HIV)-1 and HIV-2 replication by a class of bicyclams interacting with a viral uncoating event. Proc Natl Acad Sci USA 89(12):5286–5290
90. De Clercq E, Yamamoto N, Pauwels R et al (1994) Highly potent and selective inhibition of human immunodeficiency virus by the bicyclam derivative JM3100. Antimicrob Agent Chemother 38(4):668–674
91. Doranz BJ, Filion LG, Diaz-Mitoma F et al (2001) Safe use of the CXCR4 inhibitor ALX40-4C in humans. AIDS Res Hum Retroviruses 17(6):475–486
92. Doranz BJ, Grovit-Ferbas K, Sharron MP et al (1997) A small-molecule inhibitor directed against the chemokine receptor CXCR4 prevents its use as an HIV-1 coreceptor. J Exp Med 186(8):1395–1400
93. Schols D, Struyf S, Van Damme J, Este JA, Henson G, De Clercq E (1997) Inhibition of T-tropic HIV strains by selective antagonization of the chemokine receptor CXCR4. J Exp Med 186(8):1383–1388
94. Murakami T, Nakajima T, Koyanagi Y et al (1997) A small molecule CXCR4 inhibitor that blocks T cell line-tropic HIV-1 infection. J Exp Med 186(8):1389–1393
95. Tamamura H, Xu Y, Hattori T et al (1998) A low-molecular-weight inhibitor against the chemokine receptor CXCR4: a strong anti-HIV peptide T140. Biochem Biophys Res Commun 253(3):877–882
96. Tamamura H, Omagari A, Hiramatsu K et al (2001) Development of specific CXCR4 inhibitors possessing high selectivity indexes as well as complete stability in serum based on an anti-HIV peptide T140. Bioorg Med Chem Lett 11(14):1897–1902
97. Trent JO, Wang ZX, Murray JL et al (2003) Lipid bilayer simulations of CXCR4 with inverse agonists and weak partial agonists. J Biol Chem 278(47):47136–47144
98. Zhang WB, Navenot JM, Haribabu B et al (2002) A point mutation that confers constitutive activity to CXCR4 reveals that T140 is an inverse agonist and that AMD3100 and ALX40-4C are weak partial agonists. J Biol Chem 277(27):24515–24521
99. Tamamura H, Hori A, Kanzaki N et al (2003) T140 analogs as CXCR4 antagonists identified as anti-metastatic agents in the treatment of breast cancer. FEBS Lett 550(1–3):79–83

100. Takenaga M, Tamamura H, Hiramatsu K et al (2004) A single treatment with microcapsules containing a CXCR4 antagonist suppresses pulmonary metastasis of murine melanoma. Biochem Biophys Res Commun 320(1):226–232
101. Tamamura H, Fujisawa M, Hiramatsu K et al (2004) Identification of a CXCR4 antagonist, a T140 analog, as an anti-rheumatoid arthritis agent. FEBS Lett 569(1–3):99–104
102. Abraham M, Biyder K, Begin M et al (2007) Enhanced unique pattern of hematopoietic cell mobilization induced by the CXCR4 antagonist 4F-benzoyl-TN14003. Stem Cell 25(9):2158–2166
103. Juarez J, Bradstock KF, Gottlieb DJ, Bendall LJ (2003) Effects of inhibitors of the chemokine receptor CXCR4 on acute lymphoblastic leukemia cells in vitro. Leukemia 17(7): 1294–1300
104. Juarez J, Dela Pena A, Baraz R et al (2007) CXCR4 antagonists mobilize childhood acute lymphoblastic leukemia cells into the peripheral blood and inhibit engraftment. Leukemia 21(6):1249–1257
105. Zannettino AC, Farrugia AN, Kortesidis A et al (2005) Elevated serum levels of stromal-derived factor-1alpha are associated with increased osteoclast activity and osteolytic bone disease in multiple myeloma patients. Cancer Res 65(5):1700–1709
106. Mori Y, Shimizu N, Dallas M et al (2004) Anti-alpha4 integrin antibody suppresses the development of multiple myeloma and associated osteoclastic osteolysis. Blood 104(7): 2149–2154
107. Kohara H, Omatsu Y, Sugiyama T, Noda M, Fujii N, Nagasawa T (2007) Development of plasmacytoid dendritic cells in bone marrow stromal cell niches requires CXCL12-CXCR4 chemokine signaling. Blood 110(13):4153–4160.
108. Kabashima K, Shiraishi N, Sugita K et al (2007) CXCL12–CXCR4 engagement is required for migration of cutaneous dendritic cells. Am J Pathol 171(4):1249–1257
109. Allen CD, Ansel KM, Low C et al (2004) Germinal center dark and light zone organization is mediated by CXCR4 and CXCR5. Nat Immunol 5(9):943–952
110. Petit I, Szyper-Kravitz M, Nagler A et al (2002) G-CSF induces stem cell mobilization by decreasing bone marrow SDF-1 and up-regulating CXCR4. Nat Immunol 3(7):687–694
111. De Clercq E (2003) The bicyclam AMD3100 story. Nat Rev Drug Discov 2(7):581–587
112. Fricker SP, Anastassov V, Cox J et al (2006) Characterization of the molecular pharmacology of AMD3100: a specific antagonist of the G-protein coupled chemokine receptor, CXCR4. Biochem Pharmacol 72(5):588–596
113. Donzella GA, Schols D, Lin SW et al (1998) AMD3100, a small molecule inhibitor of HIV-1 entry via the CXCR4 co-receptor. Nat Med 4(1):72–77
114. Hendrix CW, Flexner C, MacFarland RT et al (2000) Pharmacokinetics and safety of AMD-3100, a novel antagonist of the CXCR-4 chemokine receptor, in human volunteers. Antimicrob Agent Chemother 44(6):1667–1673
115. Hendrix CW, Collier AC, Lederman MM et al (2004) Safety, pharmacokinetics, and antiviral activity of AMD3100, a selective CXCR4 receptor inhibitor, in HIV-1 infection. J Acquir Immune Defic Syndr 37(2):1253–1262
116. Broxmeyer HE, Orschell CM, Clapp DW et al (2005) Rapid mobilization of murine and human hematopoietic stem and progenitor cells with AMD3100, a CXCR4 antagonist. J Exp Med 201(8):1307–1318
117. Liles WC, Broxmeyer HE, Rodger E et al (2003) Mobilization of hematopoietic progenitor cells in healthy volunteers by AMD3100, a CXCR4 antagonist. Blood 102(8):2728–2730
118. Devine SM, Flomenberg N, Vesole DH et al (2004) Rapid mobilization of CD34+ cells following administration of the CXCR4 antagonist AMD3100 to patients with multiple myeloma and non-Hodgkin's lymphoma. J Clin Oncol 22(6):1095–1102
119. Andritsos LA, Byrd JC, Hewes B, Kipps TJ, Johns D, Burger JA (2010) Preliminary results from a phase I/II dose escalation study to determine the maximum tolerated dose of plerixafor in combination with rituximab in patients with relapsed chronic lymphocytic leukemia. Haematologica 95(suppl. 2):Abstract 0772; p. 321
120. Andritsos L, Byrd JC, Jones JA et al (2010) Preliminary results from a phase I dose escalation study to determine the maximum tolerated dose of plerixafor in combination with rituximab in patients with relapsed chronic lymphocytic leukemia. Blood 116(21):1017a

Chapter 20
CXCR4-Blockade for Treatment of Breast Cancer

Patricia A. Cronin and H. Paul Redmond

Abstract Breast cancer is the most commonly diagnosed malignancy in women worldwide. The chemokine receptor CXCR4 has been implicated in the pathogenesis of many cancers including breast cancer. It has been shown to be involved in primary tumour growth and particularly in the metastatic potential of breast cancer. In treatment models of breast cancer, CXCR4 attenuation has shown promise as a monotherapy and potentially as a dual agent with other therapies. It may be particularly relevant in the management of bone metastases of breast cancer. Crosstalk between the oestrogen receptor (ER) and stromal derived factor-1 (SDF1), the unique ligand of CXCR4, has been implicated in the development of ER independence in ER-positive breast cancers. This highlights CXCR4 as a potential therapeutic target for this population of breast cancers that progress. CXCR4 blockade may be used as a possible adjuvant or palliative therapy. It could be exploited as a preventative strategy in the perioperative period.

Introduction

Breast cancer is by far the most frequent cancer among women with an estimated 1.38 million new cancer cases diagnosed in 2008 (23% of all cancers), and ranks second overall (10.9% of all cancers) [16]. It ranks fifth as a cause of death with mortality rates ranging from 6 to 19 per 100,000. It is still however is the leading cause of cancer-related mortality in women in the developing and developed world. There have been increases in incidence worldwide in most countries particularly since 1990 with an approximate 0.5% per year increase in incidence [50]. Although there have been increase in incidence, there has been significant improvements in mortality.

P.A. Cronin (✉) • H.P. Redmond
Department of Academic Surgery, Cork University Hospital, Cork, Ireland
e-mail: PatCronin@rcsi.ie

S. Fruehauf et al. (eds.), *Novel Developments in Stem Cell Mobilization: Focus on CXCR4*, DOI 10.1007/978-1-4614-1960-0_20,

The reasons for this are multifactorial and include breast screening programmes, improved surgical technique, radiotherapy and adjuvant treatment protocols.

The success of its adjuvant treatment protocols has benefited from specific targeted therapies. Breast cancer treatment pioneered patient tailored management and therapeutic plans. Endocrine manipulation for oestrogen receptor (ER) and/or progesterone receptor (PR) positive breast cancer has proved invaluable in the treatment of hormone sensitive breast cancers [1, 14]. More recently, targeted therapies directed at epidermal growth factor receptor 2 (EGFR2, also known as Her2/neu) have created gains in survival for breast cancers overexpressing that receptor [20, 29]. Breast cancer research continues to investigate and seek out new biomarkers that may prove to be useful as a target for future therapies.

CXCR4 in Breast Cancer Metastases

Although early stage breast cancers are not life threatening, development of metastatic breast cancer is responsible for the majority of cancer-related death. Metastasis is the result of several sequential steps and represents a highly organized, non-random and organ-selective process. It has been proposed that molecules regulating the metastatic dissemination of tumour cells in an organ-specific manner would need to fulfil certain criteria [48, 71]. They would have to be constitutively expressed in the target organs of metastasis. Adhesion of the circulating tumour cells to the endothelium and their transendothelial migration would need to be promoted. These molecules would need to be capable of mediating the invasion of tumour cells into tissues that would provide supportive microenvironments. Lastly, this process would require the expression of a distinct receptor repertoire by the target cells, depending on their metastatic profile. Given their well-established roles in leukocyte trafficking and homeostasis, chemokines are perfectly positioned to fulfil these criteria [51, 73].

Because of these similarities between the preferential localization of tumour metastases in specific sites and the trafficking of immune cells, Muller et al. [47] investigated the functions of chemokines and chemokine receptors in breast cancer. These investigators found that high levels of stromal derived factor-1 (SDF1) are produced in many organs and tissues commonly affected by metastatic breast cancer, e.g. bone, lung, liver, etc., while CXCR4 appears to be expressed in human breast cancer cells and metastatic lesions. CXCR4 signalling in response to SDF1 induces chemotaxis and migration of breast cancer cells. These data were the first to identify a key function for SDF1-CXCR4 in metastatic breast cancer. Subsequent studies have validated these initial observations and expanded upon functions of CXCR4 in metastatic breast cancer. Kang et al. [34] used left ventricular injection of MD-MBA-231 human breast cancer cells to produce experimental metastases in mice and recovered cells that preferentially formed bone metastases. Microarray analysis identified CXCR4 as one of a limited number of genes that were enriched in this subpopulation of breast cancer cells, and overexpression of CXCR4 alone significantly increased numbers of bone metastases in vivo. CXCR4 also has essential functions in metastasis of breast cancer cells to lung. In a mouse model of breast cancer, amounts of CXCR4 in tumour cells recovered from lung metastases were greater than levels of the receptor in primary tumours or cells maintained in culture [25].

The hypothesis now proposed in relation to chemokines, specifically SDF1 and its receptor CXCR4, is that organ-specific attractant molecules such as SDF1 stimulate the migrating tumour cells that express CXCR4 to invade the walls in blood vessels and enter the target organs. This theory is widely known as "chemoattraction" theory [45]. This echoes Paget's original paper looking at the site-specific pattern of breast cancer metastases proposing "seed and soil theory" [49].

CXCR4 Signalling and Function in Breast Cancer

As shown by Muller et al. [47], CXCR4 is expressed in breast cancer cells but not in normal mammary epithelial cells. This most likely a result of factors in the tumour microenvironment such as hypoxia, loss of PTEN, increased vascular endothelial growth factor (VEGF) and Her2/neu expression. Hypoxia induces the activation of hypoxia-inducible factor-1 (HIF-1) which has been shown to promote the expression of CXCR4 [13, 61]. Increased levels of VEGF in the tumour and activation of nuclear factor kappa B (NF-κB) have both been found to increase CXCR4 expression particularly during cancer progression [4, 25]. Interestingly in Her2/neu expressing breast cancer, it has been found that Her2 enhances CXCR4 expression which could account for the aggressive nature of these tumours [41].

CXCR4 activates several different intracellular events such as cell survival, proliferation, chemotaxis, invasion and adhesion, all of which are properties that correlate with metastatic behaviour of cancer cells in vivo. The large number of downstream effector molecules regulated by CXCR4 likely account for the multiple effects of this receptor in the pathobiology of breast cancer.

SDF1 binding to CXCR4 leads to the activation of pro-metastatic and tumorigenic pathways within tumours. SDF1 and CXCR4 stimulate the phosphatidylinositol-3-kinase pathway that subsequently activates the protein kinase Akt. The principal role of Akt is to facilitate growth factor-mediated cell survival and to suppress apoptosis induced by various stimuli [18]. Beyond functions in promoting cell survival, Akt also has been implicated in effects of CXCR4 on proliferation of cells [5] and migration toward a chemotactic gradient of SDF1 [52, 72]. Based on the diverse functions of Akt in breast cancer cells in culture, it is very likely that Akt is a key effector of CXCR4 in breast cancer in vivo.

The mitogen-activated protein kinase pathway (MAP kinase pathway) is another signal transduction pathway regulated by CXCR4. In response to SDF1, CXCR4 activates the kinase MEK, the upstream activator of the p42/44 MAP kinases (also known as ERK 1/2) [57]. Activated p42/44 MAP kinases phosphorylate transcription factors including Elk-1 to increase expression of genes that promote proliferation and survival of cancer cells [69].

The JAK/STAT (Janus kinase/signal transducer and activator of transcription) pathway is a third potential effector of CXCR4 in breast cancer. Following activation by SDF1, JAK kinases, including JAK 2 and JAK 3, associate with CXCR4 [2, 68]. JAK kinases then recruit and activate members of the STAT family of transcription factors, which translocate to the nucleus and drive expression of a variety of genes. The JAK/STAT pathway is implicated in enhancing motility of normally stationary epithelial cells, thereby promoting migration and invasion of cancer cells [65]. This signalling pathway has also been shown to promote proliferation and survival of breast cancer cells in vitro [40]. However, the significance of the JAK/STAT pathway for biological effects of CXCR4 in breast cancer currently is uncertain because one study suggested that CXCR4 signalling is independent of the JAK/STAT pathway in cultured cells [46].

CXCR4 also activates members of the src family of protein tyrosine kinases, thereby producing phosphorylation and activation of components of focal adhesion complexes such as RAFTK/Pyk2, focal adhesion kinase, Crk and paxillin [17]. CXCR4 also promotes adhesion to components of the extracellular matrix, including collagen and fibronectin, through integrins α2, α4, α5 and β1 [22]. Focal adhesion complexes and integrins have been shown to promote migration of cells and interactions with extracellular matrix molecules. Activated CXCR4 also increases secretion of matrix metalloproteinases (MMP) 2 and 9 in MD-MBA-231 breast cancer cells. MMPs are involved in degradation of extracellular matrix molecules, thereby providing a mechanism for invasion and metastases of breast cancer cells. These various processes are dependent upon SDF1 activation of CXCR4, as shown by significantly greater invasion of cultured breast cancer cells engineered to overexpress SDF1 to allow autocrine signalling through CXCR4 [32].

CXCR4 also appears to directly regulate angiogenesis, which is essential for normal physiology as well as formation and growth of primary and metastatic tumours [53]. Genetically engineered mice lacking CXCR4 or SDF1 have defective formation of blood vessels in the gastrointestinal tract, indicating that this signalling pathway is essential for embryonic vascularization. Studies have demonstrated that CXCR4 is a key mediator of normal microvascular angiogenesis in epithelial cells in the colon, and SDF1–CXCR4 also stimulates mature endothelial cells to migrate and form capillary-like structures [59]. Pro-angiogenic effects of CXCR4 signalling may be mediated through upregulation of VEGF, an established pro-angiogenic molecule [36]. VEGF itself has been shown to increase expression of CXCR4 in breast cancer cells, thereby forming a potential positive feedback loop for promoting angiogenesis [4].

There is now growing evidence that interactions between the SDF1–CXCR4 signalling pathway and other genes and pathways play a significant role not only in primary breast cancer development and growth but also in the promotion of metastasis. These studies identify CXCR4 as a valuable potential therapeutic marker in the management of breast cancer.

CXCR4 as Therapeutic Target in Breast Cancer

In human breast cancer, CXCR4 is the most abundantly expressed chemokine receptor [47] and is observed in over half of primary breast carcinomas [7]. Several papers looking at CXCR4 expression in primary human breast cancers have shown an association with tumour grade [58], the degree of lymph node metastases [8, 33, 35], bone metastases [6, 34] and poor patient overall survival [10, 28, 44]. These data also support the role of the SDF1–CXCR4 ligand receptor pathway in the pathogenesis of breast cancer metastases and encourage investigation into the usefulness of disrupting this pathway for the treatment of breast cancer.

Breast cancer cell proliferation has been shown to be promoted by the effect of SDF1 on CXCR4 in vitro and in vivo [21, 39, 64]. Similarly, Muller et al. [47] reported that SDF1–CXCR4 signalling induced chemotaxis and migration of cancer cells. The importance of these specific chemokine interactions in breast cancer growth and metastases is supported by the success of targeted therapies in murine models of breast cancer. In Muller et al.'s original paper, they showed that an anti-CXCR4 antibody produced a 61–68% reduction in the number of lung metastases. As well as CXCR4 inhibition with an antibody, silencing CXCR4 expression using small interfering RNA has also had successful results with a decrease in both breast cancer growth and metastases in multiple studies [39, 43, 64]. CXCR4 antagonists, e.g. AMD3100, TN14003 and CTCE-9908 have also been used in similar experiment models with similar results [13, 42, 64].

These results are promising for developing a role for CXCR4 blockade in the management of breast cancer. A recent phase I/II study of CTCE-9908, a novel anticancer agent and CXCR4 antagonist, in patients with advanced solid cancers including breast cancer indicated that CTCE-9908 has been tolerated well as a single agent and shown some preliminary signs of efficacy. Thirty percent of patients had stable disease after one cycle of treatment [30, 31].

As with all new therapies, the next challenge will be to establish how CXCR4 could enhance current breast cancer management strategies and to identify those patients who would benefit most from CXCR4 blockade.

CXCR4 Blockade in Bone Metastases

There are several studies and data now available that indicate a close link between SDF1–CXCR4 signalling and development of bone metastases. In vivo studies have shown that overexpression of CXR4 is associated with increased bone metastases [34], and it has been observed that overexpression of CXCR4 in human primary breast cancer is associated with increased isolated tumour cells in the bone marrow [6]. In a further recent paper, Cabioglu et al. [7] observed that the majority of bone metastases in breast cancer patients expressed a high level of CXCR4. Several other papers have also suggested this relationship between CXCR4 expression and bone metastases [37, 63, 70]. Bone stromal cells and bone tissue-conditioned media induced migration of prostate cells through a SDF1–CXCR4 signalling pathway that could be abrogated by a CXCR4 antibody [9]. In an in vivo model of prostate cancer bone metastases, the intraosseous growth of tumour cells following intratibial injection was attenuated by antibody neutralization of CXCR4 [66].

CXCR4 expression and SDF1 signalling appears to preferentially promote bone metastases, with bone metastases three times more likely to express CXCR4 than visceral metastases [7]. This evidence from a population of clinical samples of human metastases supports the findings of earlier in vivo studies that demonstrated that selected bone-metastatic sub-populations of MDA-MB-231 breast cancer cells express high levels of CXCR4 relative to other poorly metastatic sub-populations [34].

The relationship between CXCR4 expression and the development of bone metastases could be exploited in patients for targeted treatment with CXCR4 blockade [56]. The only concern that has been raised with CXCR4 inhibition is a possible negative effect on the turnover of normal bone [26, 27].

CXCR4 Crosstalk in ER-Positive Breast Cancer

Up to 70% of all breast cancers are oestrogen receptor (ER) positive, meaning they are reliant on oestrogen for their growth. They are generally associated with a favourable prognosis and are amenable to endocrine therapies. Although hormonal manipulation can be a successful treatment in these patients, as many as half can get tumour progression with de novo resistance to these treatments [11]. SDF1 is a known ER-regulated gene suggesting an association between ER-mediated signalling and the SDF1–CXCR4 receptor ligand axis [21, 60]. Tamoxifen-treated MCF-7 cells have downregulation of CXCR4 expression [38].

CXCR4 overexpression in primary tumours has been reported to be predictive of recurrence and poorer outcome [10]. It has been postulated that this could be due to CXCR4 expression driving oestrogen independence in ER-positive breast cancers [54, 55]. Authors found that CXCR4 activation in MCF-7 breast cancer cells led to enhanced tumorigenesis and metastases, and promoted oestrogen independence and that the inhibitory effect of anti-oestrogen therapy could be negated by exogenous treatment with SDF1. This suggests that CXCR4 signalling alone may be sufficient to drive ER-positive breast cancer.

Given that CXCR4 activation may be implicated when ER-positive tumours progress and develop resistance to endocrine therapies, this population could benefit from strategies that target the SDF1–CXCR4 axis.

CXCR4 in Her2-Mediated Breast Cancer

Overexpression of Her2, a receptor tyrosine kinase of the epidermal growth factor receptor family, is associated with enhanced growth and the metastatic phenotype of breast cancers. Amplification of Her2 is found in approximately 30% of breast cancers and is frequently associated with poor prognosis. Her2 is a known inducer of the CXCR4 receptor, and CXCR4 is essential for Her2-mediated metastasis [41]. A small study demonstrated that CXCR4 may be implicated in Her2-amplified breast cancer metastases to brain [15]. Interestingly, Trastuzumab, an anti-Her2 monoclonal antibody, involves downregulation of the CXCR4 receptor [3]. CXCR4 blockade may be a beneficial strategy for Her2 amplified breast cancers.

Despite the links between ER/Her2 and CXCR4 that identify both ER-positive and Her2-amplified breast cancers as suitable target populations, CXCR4 has also been shown to be an independent predictor of outcome in triple negative breast cancers. Further research and data are required to delineate whether there are target populations that would benefit from CXCR4-targeted therapies or whether it is a more universal target.

Clinical Application of CXCR4-Targeted Therapies

As previously described, CXCR4 attenuation as a monotherapy in murine models and in early phase I/II trials has shown a therapeutic benefit in the prevention or treatment of breast cancer and breast cancer metastases. In combination treatment regimes with known chemotherapeutic agents, there have been mixed results. One study with Paclitaxel [62] did not show any improvement in the primary tumour or lung metastases with the addition of CTCE-9908, a CXCR4 antagonist. However, CTCE-9908 in addition to Docetaxel, or DC101 (an anti-VEGFR2 monoclonal antibody) did show enhanced results as dual therapies as opposed to those agents as monotherapies in another paper [24].

As well as the potential for adjuvant or palliative treatment of breast cancer, interference with the SDF1–CXCR4 axis, could be of potential therapeutic benefit in the prevention of breast cancer metastases. The perioperative period may afford a window of opportunity for treatment using interference of the CXCR4–SDF1α axis. There are many factors during the perioperative period that are thought to affect tumour development [12]. One of these is the possibility of increased circulating tumour cells postoperatively [19, 67]. A preclinical trial looked at heparinoids in the prevention of breast cancer lung metastases [23]. Heparinoids antagonize the effects of SDF1 on cancer cells. The authors found that 28 days of treatment commenced 4 h before tail injection of breast cancer cells led to a significant reduction in the number and area of lung metastases. These data are encouraging from a preventative strategy view.

Conclusion

The chemokine receptor, CXCR4, and its unique ligand SDF1 play an important role in the tumorigenesis and metastatic ability of breast cancer. It is therefore the subject of ongoing research to exploit its therapeutic potential. Certainly from in vivo studies there have been significant results from CXCR4 attenuation, prompting hope for future clinical trials. It has possibilities both as a monotherapy or dual therapy with existing chemotherapeutic agents for the adjuvant and palliative treatment of breast cancer. It could also have a role in perioperative regimes for the prevention of breast cancer metastases.

References

1. Davies, C., et al (2011) Relevance of breast cancer hormone receptors and other factors to the efficacy of adjuvant tamoxifen: patient-level meta-analysis of randomised trials. Lancet 378(9793): 771–784
2. Ahr B, Denizot M et al (2005) Identification of the cytoplasmic domains of CXCR4 involved in Jak2 and STAT3 phosphorylation. J Biol Chem 280(8):6692–6700
3. Arya M, Ahmed H et al (2007) Clinical importance and therapeutic implications of the pivotal CXCL12-CXCR4 (chemokine ligand-receptor) interaction in cancer cell migration. Tumour Biol 28(3):123–131
4. Bachelder RE, Wendt MA et al (2002) Vascular endothelial growth factor promotes breast carcinoma invasion in an autocrine manner by regulating the chemokine receptor CXCR4. Cancer Res 62(24):7203–7206
5. Barbero S, Bonavia R et al (2003) Stromal cell-derived factor 1alpha stimulates human glioblastoma cell growth through the activation of both extracellular signal-regulated kinases 1/2 and Akt. Cancer Res 63(8):1969–1974
6. Cabioglu N, Sahin A et al (2005) Chemokine receptor CXCR4 expression in breast cancer as a potential predictive marker of isolated tumor cells in bone marrow. Clin Exp Metastasis 22(1):39–46
7. Cabioglu N, Sahin AA et al (2009) Chemokine receptors in advanced breast cancer: differential expression in metastatic disease sites with diagnostic and therapeutic implications. Ann Oncol 20(6):1013–1019
8. Cabioglu N, Yazici MS et al (2005) CCR7 and CXCR4 as novel biomarkers predicting axillary lymph node metastasis in T1 breast cancer. Clin Cancer Res 11(16):5686–5693
9. Chinni SR, Sivalogan S et al (2006) CXCL12/CXCR4 signaling activates Akt-1 and MMP-9 expression in prostate cancer cells: the role of bone microenvironment-associated CXCL12. Prostate 66(1):32–48
10. Chu QD, Holm NT et al (2011) Chemokine receptor CXCR4 overexpression predicts recurrence for hormone receptor-positive, node-negative breast cancer patients. Surgery 149(2): 193–199
11. Clarke R, Liu MC et al (2003) Antiestrogen resistance in breast cancer and the role of estrogen receptor signaling. Oncogene 22(47):7316–7339
12. Coffey JC, Wang JH et al (2003) Excisional surgery for cancer cure: therapy at a cost. Lancet Oncol 4(12):760–768
13. Cronin PA, Wang JH et al (2010) Hypoxia increases the metastatic ability of breast cancer cells via upregulation of CXCR4. BMC Cancer 10:225
14. Cuzick J, Sestak I et al (2010) Effect of anastrozole and tamoxifen as adjuvant treatment for early-stage breast cancer: 10-year analysis of the ATAC trial. Lancet Oncol 11(12):1135–1141
15. Dawood S, Gong Y et al (2010) Trastuzumab in primary inflammatory breast cancer (IBC): high pathological response rates and improved outcome. Breast J 16(5):529–532
16. Ferlay J, Shin HR et al (2010) Estimates of worldwide burden of cancer in 2008: GLOBOCAN 2008. Int J Cancer 127(12):2893–2917
17. Fernandis AZ, Prasad A et al (2004) Regulation of CXCR4-mediated chemotaxis and chemoinvasion of breast cancer cells. Oncogene 23(1):157–167

18. Fresno Vara JA, Casado E et al (2004) PI3K/Akt signalling pathway and cancer. Cancer Treat Rev 30(2):193–204
19. Galan M, Vinolas N et al (2002) Detection of occult breast cancer cells by amplification of CK19 mRNA by reverse transcriptase-polymerase chain reaction: role of surgical manipulation. Anticancer Res 22(5):2877–2884
20. Geyer CE, Forster J et al (2006) Lapatinib plus capecitabine for HER2-positive advanced breast cancer. N Engl J Med 355(26):2733–2743
21. Hall JM, Korach KS (2003) Stromal cell-derived factor 1, a novel target of estrogen receptor action, mediates the mitogenic effects of estradiol in ovarian and breast cancer cells. Mol Endocrinol 17(5):792–803
22. Hartmann TN, Burger JA et al (2005) CXCR4 chemokine receptor and integrin signaling co-operate in mediating adhesion and chemoresistance in small cell lung cancer (SCLC) cells. Oncogene 24(27):4462–4471
23. Harvey JR, Mellor P et al (2007) Inhibition of CXCR4-mediated breast cancer metastasis: a potential role for heparinoids? Clin Cancer Res 13(5):1562–1570
24. Hassan S, Buchanan M et al (2011) CXCR4 peptide antagonist inhibits primary breast tumor growth, metastasis and enhances the efficacy of anti-VEGF treatment or docetaxel in a transgenic mouse model. Int J Cancer 129(1):225–232
25. Helbig G, Christopherson KW II et al (2003) NF-kappaB promotes breast cancer cell migration and metastasis by inducing the expression of the chemokine receptor CXCR4. J Biol Chem 278(24):21631–21638
26. Hirbe AC, Morgan EA et al (2010) The CXCR4/SDF-1 chemokine axis: a potential therapeutic target for bone metastases? Curr Pharm Des 16(11):1284–1290
27. Hirbe AC, Rubin J et al (2007) Disruption of CXCR4 enhances osteoclastogenesis and tumor growth in bone. Proc Natl Acad Sci U S A 104(35):14062–14067
28. Holm NT, Abreo F et al (2009) Elevated chemokine receptor CXCR4 expression in primary tumors following neoadjuvant chemotherapy predicts poor outcomes for patients with locally advanced breast cancer (LABC). Breast Cancer Res Treat 113(2):293–299
29. Hortobagyi GN (2005) Trastuzumab in the treatment of breast cancer. N Engl J Med 353(16):1734–1736
30. Hotte SJ, Hirte HW et al (2007) Phase I/II study of CTCE-9908, a novel anticancer agent that inhibits CXCR4, in patients with advanced solid cancers. Mol Cancer Ther 6(12):3385s–3386s
31. Hotte SJ, Hirte HW et al (2008) Final results of a phase I/II study of CTCE-9908, a novel anticancer agent that inhibits CXCR4, in patients with advanced solid cancers. Ejc Supplements 6(12):127–127
32. Kang H, Mansel RE et al (2005) Genetic manipulation of stromal cell-derived factor-1 attests the pivotal role of the autocrine SDF-1-CXCR4 pathway in the aggressiveness of breast cancer cells. Int J Oncol 26(5):1429–1434
33. Kang H, Watkins G et al (2005) Stromal cell derived factor-1: its influence on invasiveness and migration of breast cancer cells in vitro, and its association with prognosis and survival in human breast cancer. Breast Cancer Res 7(4):R402–R410
34. Kang Y, Siegel PM et al (2003) A multigenic program mediating breast cancer metastasis to bone. Cancer Cell 3(6):537–549
35. Kato M, Kitayama J et al (2003) Expression pattern of CXC chemokine receptor-4 is correlated with lymph node metastasis in human invasive ductal carcinoma. Breast Cancer Res 5(5):R144–R150
36. Kijowski J, Baj-Krzyworzeka M et al (2001) The SDF-1-CXCR4 axis stimulates VEGF secretion and activates integrins but does not affect proliferation and survival in lymphohematopoietic cells. Stem Cells 19(5):453–466
37. Kozlow W, Guise TA (2005) Breast cancer metastasis to bone: mechanisms of osteolysis and implications for therapy. J Mammary Gland Biol Neoplasia 10(2):169–180
38. Kubarek L, Kozlowska A et al (2009) Down-regulation of CXCR4 expression by tamoxifen is associated with DNA methyltransferase 3B up-regulation in MCF-7 breast cancer cells. Biomed Pharmacother 63(8):586–591

39. Lapteva N, Yang AG et al (2005) CXCR4 knockdown by small interfering RNA abrogates breast tumor growth in vivo. Cancer Gene Ther 12(1):84–89
40. Li L, Hooi D et al (2004) Bacterial *N*-acylhomoserine lactone-induced apoptosis in breast carcinoma cells correlated with down-modulation of STAT3. Oncogene 23(28):4894–4902
41. Li YM, Pan Y et al (2004) Upregulation of CXCR4 is essential for HER2-mediated tumor metastasis. Cancer Cell 6(5):459–469
42. Liang Z, Wu T et al (2004) Inhibition of breast cancer metastasis by selective synthetic polypeptide against CXCR4. Cancer Res 64(12):4302–4308
43. Liang Z, Yoon Y et al (2005) Silencing of CXCR4 blocks breast cancer metastasis. Cancer Res 65(3):967–971
44. Mirisola V, Zuccarino A et al (2009) CXCL12/SDF1 expression by breast cancers is an independent prognostic marker of disease-free and overall survival. Eur J Cancer 45(14):2579–2587
45. Moore MA (2001) The role of chemoattraction in cancer metastases. Bioessays 23(8): 674–676
46. Moriguchi M, Hissong BD et al (2005) CXCL12 signaling is independent of Jak2 and Jak3. J Biol Chem 280(17):17408–17414
47. Muller A, Homey B et al (2001) Involvement of chemokine receptors in breast cancer metastasis. Nature 410(6824):50–56
48. Nicolson GL (1993) Paracrine and autocrine growth mechanisms in tumor metastasis to specific sites with particular emphasis on brain and lung metastasis. Cancer Metastasis Rev 12(3–4):325–343
49. Paget S (1989) The distribution of secondary growths in cancer of the breast. 1889. Cancer Metastasis Rev 8(2):98–101
50. Parkin DM, Bray FI et al (2001) Cancer burden in the year 2000. The global picture. Eur J Cancer 37(Suppl 8):S4–S66
51. Peled A, Petit I et al (1999) Dependence of human stem cell engraftment and repopulation of NOD/SCID mice on CXCR4. Science 283(5403):845–848
52. Peng SB, Peek V et al (2005) Akt activation, but not extracellular signal-regulated kinase activation, is required for SDF-1alpha/CXCR4-mediated migration of epitheloid carcinoma cells. Mol Cancer Res 3(4):227–236
53. Pinto MP, Badtke MM et al (2010) Vascular endothelial growth factor secreted by activated stroma enhances angiogenesis and hormone-independent growth of estrogen receptor-positive breast cancer. Cancer Res 70(7):2655–2664
54. Rhodes LV, Antoon JW et al (2010) Effects of human mesenchymal stem cells on ER-positive human breast carcinoma cells mediated through ER-SDF-1/CXCR4 crosstalk. Mol Cancer 9:295
55. Rhodes LV, Short SP et al (2011) Cytokine receptor CXCR4 mediates estrogen-independent tumorigenesis, metastasis, and resistance to endocrine therapy in human breast cancer. Cancer Res 71(2):603–613
56. Rose AA, Siegel PM (2010) Emerging therapeutic targets in breast cancer bone metastasis. Future Oncol 6(1):55–74
57. Rubin JB, Kung AL et al (2003) A small-molecule antagonist of CXCR4 inhibits intracranial growth of primary brain tumors. Proc Natl Acad Sci U S A 100(23):13513–13518
58. Salvucci O, Bouchard A et al (2006) The role of CXCR4 receptor expression in breast cancer: a large tissue microarray study. Breast Cancer Res Treat 97(3):275–283
59. Salvucci O, Yao L et al (2002) Regulation of endothelial cell branching morphogenesis by endogenous chemokine stromal-derived factor-1. Blood 99(8):2703–2711
60. Sauve K, Lepage J et al (2009) Positive feedback activation of estrogen receptors by the CXCL12-CXCR4 pathway. Cancer Res 69(14):5793–5800
61. Schioppa T, Uranchimeg B et al (2003) Regulation of the chemokine receptor CXCR4 by hypoxia. J Exp Med 198(9):1391–1402
62. Singh B, Cook KR et al (2010) Evaluation of a CXCR4 antagonist in a xenograft mouse model of inflammatory breast cancer. Clin Exp Metastasis 27(4):233–240

63. Sloan EK, Anderson RL (2002) Genes involved in breast cancer metastasis to bone. Cell Mol Life Sci 59(9):1491–1502
64. Smith MC, Luker KE et al (2004) CXCR4 regulates growth of both primary and metastatic breast cancer. Cancer Res 64(23):8604–8612
65. Soriano SF, Serrano A et al (2003) Chemokines integrate JAK/STAT and G-protein pathways during chemotaxis and calcium flux responses. Eur J Immunol 33(5):1328–1333
66. Sun YX, Schneider A et al (2005) Skeletal localization and neutralization of the SDF-1(CXCL12)/CXCR4 axis blocks prostate cancer metastasis and growth in osseous sites in vivo. J Bone Miner Res 20(2):318–329
67. Topal B, Aerts JL et al (2005) Cancer cell dissemination during curative surgery for colorectal liver metastases. Eur J Surg Oncol 31(5):506–511
68. Vila-Coro AJ, Rodriguez-Frade JM et al (1999) The chemokine SDF-1alpha triggers CXCR4 receptor dimerization and activates the JAK/STAT pathway. FASEB J 13(13):1699–1710
69. Vlahakis SR, Villasis-Keever A et al (2002) G protein-coupled chemokine receptors induce both survival and apoptotic signaling pathways. J Immunol 169(10):5546–5554
70. Wang J, Loberg R et al (2006) The pivotal role of CXCL12 (SDF-1)/CXCR4 axis in bone metastasis. Cancer Metastasis Rev 25(4):573–587
71. Wang JM, Deng X et al (1998) Chemokines and their role in tumor growth and metastasis. J Immunol Methods 220(1–2):1–17
72. Zhao M, Mueller BM et al (2008) Akt plays an important role in breast cancer cell chemotaxis to CXCL12. Breast Cancer Res Treat 110(2):211–222
73. Zlotnik A, Yoshie O (2000) Chemokines: a new classification system and their role in immunity. Immunity 12(2):121–127

Chapter 21
Molecular Imaging of CXCR4 Receptor Expression in Tumors

Lauren E. Woodard and Sridhar Nimmagadda

Abstract Metastasis is responsible for most cancer-related deaths. Chemokine receptors have been shown to aid tumor propagation at the key steps of metastasis, including the adherence of tumor cells to the endothelium, extravasation from blood vessels, colonization, angiogenesis, proliferation, and protection from the host immune response. The CXCR4/CXCL12 axis plays a major role in the homing of CXCR4 positive tumor cells to distant metastatic sites. Over the last few years, several agents have been evaluated for monitoring CXCR4 expression using PET, SPECT, and optical imaging modalities in preclinical models. This chapter discusses the current status of CXCR4-targeted probe development. As these agents become clinically available, CXCR4-based imaging could play an important role in detecting tumors with high risk for metastasis, in the early detection of metastases and in therapeutic monitoring.

Abbreviations

TME	Tumor microenvironment
CXCR4	Chemokine receptor 4
CXCL12	Chemokine ligand 12
PET	Positron emission tomography
SPECT	Single photon emission computed tomography
CT	Computed tomography
SCID	Severe combined immunodeficiency

L.E. Woodard • S. Nimmagadda (✉)
Russell H. Morgan Department of Radiology and Radiological Science,
Johns Hopkins University, Baltimore, MD, USA
e-mail: snimmag1@ihmi.edu

S. Fruehauf et al. (eds.), *Novel Developments in Stem Cell Mobilization: Focus on CXCR4*, DOI 10.1007/978-1-4614-1960-0_21,

FOLFOX	Folinic acid, fluorouracil, and oxaliplatin
CHO	Chinese hamster ovarian
Dde	1-(4,4′-Dimethyl-2,6-dioxocyclohexylidene) ethyl
mAbs	Monoclonal antibodies
FII	Fluorescence intensity imaging
BBN	*N*-Butyl-*N*-(4-hydroxybutyl) nitrosamine

Introduction

Metastasis, not the primary tumor, is the major cause of morbidity and mortality. Identifying the metastatic potential of the primary tumor and detecting micrometastases early on, therefore, is of paramount importance for the therapeutic outcome and overall survival. Biopsies represent only a snapshot of the highly heterogeneous tumor, are invasive and are impractical for monitoring therapy. Appropriately chosen molecular imaging technologies on the other hand provide functional information on the whole tumor, on all the tumors in the body and at multiple time points. The microenvironment of the tumor, consisting of cancer cells and the stroma, plays a critical role in the cancer cell survival, growth, adaptation to lethal conditions, and migration to newer fertile grounds. In recent years, chemokines and chemokine receptors have been established as key players of the tumor microenvironment (TME) [1]. In particular, the interaction between chemokine CXCL12 and chemokine receptor 4 (CXCR4) is extensively studied within the context of TME [2]. CXCR4 is overexpressed in nearly 23 different cancers and its expression is elevated at the sites of metastases [3, 4]. Binding of CXCL12 to CXCR4 activates several major signaling pathways related to cell survival, proliferation, and migration of cancer cells to the distant sites (i.e., the main sites of cancer metastasis). CXCR4 inhibitors are shown to reduce the metastasis and are considered a therapeutic option [5–7]. As blocking the CXCR4-CXCL12 pathway becomes a viable strategy to target various solid tumors, development and evaluation of imaging agents for tracking this pathway in vivo is critical, which will be the focus of this chapter.

Molecular Imaging

Molecular imaging is the visualization, characterization, and measurement of biological processes at the molecular and cellular levels in humans and other living systems [8]. Nuclear (PET and SPECT), optical, ultrasound, computed tomography, and magnetic resonance imaging comprise the most commonly used molecular imaging modalities. Each modality has strengths and weaknesses and provides complementary diagnostic information [9]. The detection limits and spatial resolution of these modalities are given in Table 21.1.

CXCR4-based imaging probe development so far has been focused on nuclear and optical imaging modalities.

Table 21.1 Detection limits and spatial resolutions of PET, SPECT, MRI, and FII (from [9–11])

Modality	Detection limit	Small animal scanner resolution	Clinical scanner resolution
PET	10^{-12} to 10^{-10} M	1–2 mm	4–7 mm
SPECT	10^{-11} to 10^{-10} M	1–2 mm	8–12 mm
MRI	10^{-5} to 10^{-3} M	25–100 μm	10–100 μm
FII	10^{-12} to 10^{-9} M	2–3 mm	1–2 mm

Nuclear Imaging

Positron Emission Tomography

Positron emission tomography (PET) is a noninvasive functional imaging technique that uses tracer levels of radiolabeled molecules to interrogate the biochemical information in living systems. PET tracers, injected in nano to picomolar concentrations, decay in the body by positron emission. The collision of an emitted positron with a nearby electron produces two 511 eV photons at an angle of 180° with each other, which will be detected by scintillation detectors [12]. The signals from these temporal photon pairs are then reconstructed into a three-dimensional image corresponding to the spatial distribution of the radiotracer in the body. The spatial resolution of PET scanners is low, about 4–5 mm for clinical scanners. For this reason, PET images are usually co-registered with computed tomography (CT) images, which provide intricate anatomical detail with high spatial resolution.

Commonly used PET radionuclides include ^{11}C ($t_{1/2}$=20.4 min), ^{13}N ($t_{1/2}$=9.9 min), ^{15}O ($t_{1/2}$=2 min), ^{68}Ga ($t_{1/2}$=68 min), ^{18}F ($t_{1/2}$=109.8 min), ^{64}Cu ($t_{1/2}$=12.7 h) and ^{124}I ($t_{1/2}$=4.12 d). In order to obtain images with good target to background ratios, when choosing an appropriate radionuclide, it is important to match the timescale of the biological process being studied or the biological half-life of the tracer to the half-life of the radionuclide [12]. For example, when using peptides, which are rapidly cleared from the body, short-lived radionuclides, such as ^{18}F, ^{68}Ga, and ^{64}Cu, should be used. Another parameter to consider is the length of the radiolabeling procedure. If the procedure is lengthy, the use of short-lived radionuclides may not be an option.

PET Imaging Agents

Cyclams

AMD3100 (Fig. 21.1), a bicyclam discovered by Bridger et al. in 1995, was the first nonpeptide CXCR4 inhibitor [13]. AMD3100 has been shown to be a specific inhibitor of CXCR4 with an IC_{50} of 651±37 nM for CXCL12 displacement [14]. It has been postulated that the four protonated nitrogens of AMD3100 at physiological pH closely interact with negatively charged amino acid residues, such as Asp187,

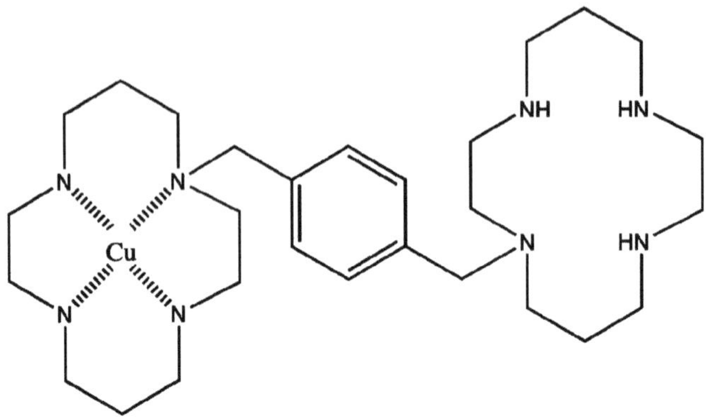

Fig. 21.1 Structure of Cu-AMD3100

Table 21.2 In vitro analysis of CXCR4 receptor expression and [^{64}Cu]AMD3100 binding

Cell line	Receptors/cell	Percentage of incubated dose
U87-stb-CXCR4	134,999 ± 20,341	13.1 ± 1.6
U87	3,664 ± 802	0.1 ± 0.0
DU4475	16,640 ± 5,128	0.3 ± 0.0
MDA-MB-231	6,833 ± 1,570	0.1 ± 1.0

Asp97, and Glu288 [15]. Cyclam moieties have the ability to form strong complexes with transition metals, such as copper and zinc. Interestingly, previous studies have shown that when bound to copper, the affinity of AMD3100 for CXCR4 increases by sevenfold [16], opening the door for radiolabeling and CXCR4 expression imaging in cancers.

The first radiochemical synthesis and evaluation of [^{64}Cu]AMD3100 as a possible PET imaging agent was performed by Jacobson and colleagues [17]. These authors verified that [^{64}Cu]AMD3100 was as potent as AMD3100 as a CXCR4 inhibitor. Biodistribution studies of [^{64}Cu]AMD3100 in immune competent C57BL/6 mice showed highest uptake of radioactivity in the liver (41 %ID/g) and in immune-related organs, such as the spleen (13 %ID/g), bone marrow (14 %ID/g), and lymph nodes (10 %ID/g). Coinjection of nonradioactive AMD3100 with the radiotracer resulted in a 60–80% reduction in uptake in all immune-related organs and in the liver, suggesting CXCR4-specific binding and accumulation in these organs. This was an expected result given that multiple immune cells express CXCR4 [18].

Further evaluation and applicability of this agent for imaging graded levels of tumor CXCR4 expression was demonstrated by Nimmagadda et al. using subcutaneous brain tumor models stably expressing CXCR4 [19]. Preclinical and clinical studies have detected high concentrations of CXCR4 receptors in the primary brain tumors compared to normal brain parenchyma [20, 21]. The invading regions of glioblastomas and satellite tumors, which are the primary reason for recurrence, have also been observed to express high levels of CXCR4 [22]. Using mice harboring U87

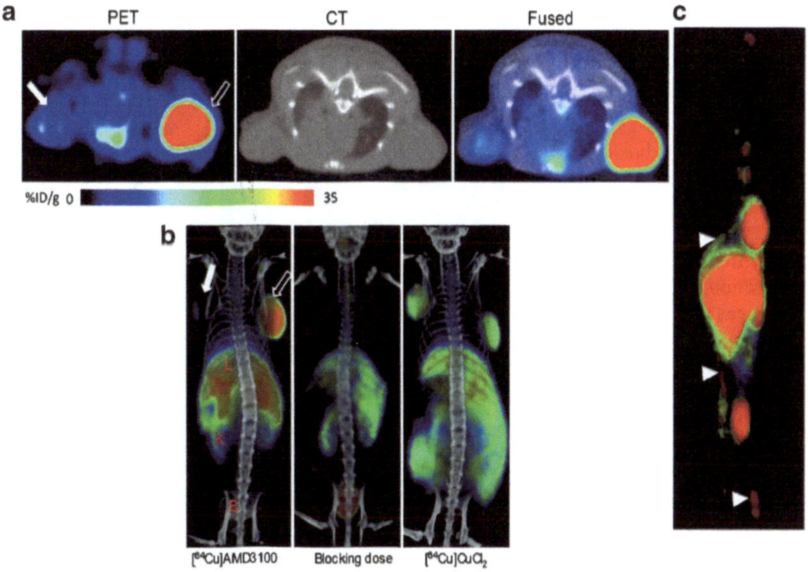

Fig. 21.2 PET/CT imaging of CXCR4 expression in subcutaneous brain tumor xenografts with [^{64}Cu]AMD3100. NOD/SCID mice bearing U87 and U87-stb-CXCR4 glioblastoma xenografts on the left and right flanks, respectively, were given <11.1 MBq (300 μCi) of ^{64}Cu-labeled radiotracers via tail vein injection, and PET/CT images were acquired. (**a**) Representative transaxial PET, CT, and fused sections of both the tumors from a [^{64}Cu]AMD3100-injected mouse at 90 min postinjection. (**b**) Volume-rendered whole body images of [^{64}Cu]AMD3100 (*left*), 50 mg/kg of AMD3100 blocking dose followed by [^{64}Cu]AMD3100 (*middle*), and [^{64}Cu]$CuCl_2$ alone (*right*). All images were scaled to the same maximum threshold value. (**c**) PET image of bone marrow uptake of [^{64}Cu]AMD3100 at 90 min postinjection. Scale was adjusted for clear visualization of bone marrow. *Solid arrow*, U87 tumor; *unfilled arrow*, U87-stb-CXCR4 tumor; *arrow head*, bone marrow; *L* liver, *K* kidney, *B* bladder (from [19])

and U87 cells stably expressing CXCR4 (U87-stb-CXCR4) (Table 21.2) glioblastoma brain tumors, the authors showed that at 90 min postinjection of [^{64}Cu]AMD3100, PET images displayed distinct accumulation of radioactivity in the U87-stb-CXCR4 tumors (Fig. 21.2a). Considerable uptake was also observed in the kidneys, liver, bladder, and bone marrow (Fig. 21.2b, c). Injection of a pharmacological dose (50 mg/kg) of nonradioactive AMD3100 prior to [^{64}Cu]AMD3100 resulted in greater than 90% reduction in activity accumulation in both tumors and also significantly reduced the accumulation of radioactivity in the liver and kidneys (Fig. 21.2b). Transchelation of copper is a known phenomenon with certain chelators [23]. Even though ^{64}Cu-cyclam complexes are thermodynamically stable in vitro, several studies suggest that ^{64}Cu may dissociate and subsequently transchelate to superoxide dismutase, resulting in increased accumulation in the blood and liver [23–25]. However, unlike the specific uptake observed with [^{64}Cu]AMD3100, in [^{64}Cu]$CuCl_2$ injected mice radiotracer distribution was rather uniform (Fig. 21.2b).

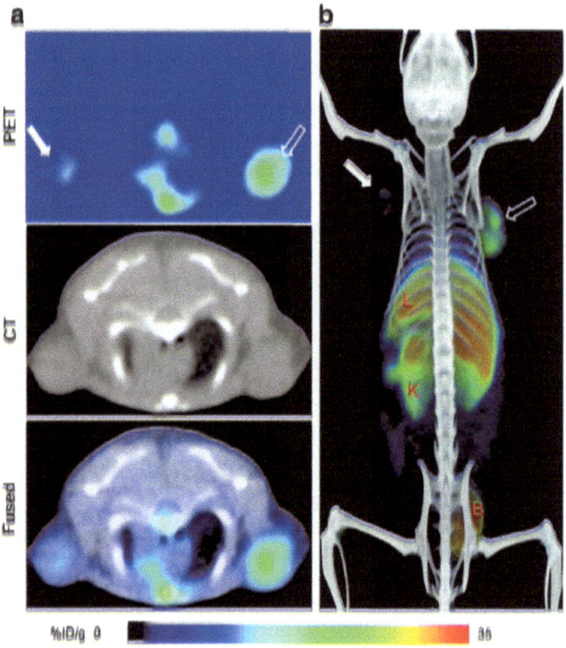

Fig. 21.3 CXCR4 imaging in orthotopic breast tumor xenografts with [^{64}Cu]AMD3100. NOD/SCID mice harboring MDA-MB-231 and DU4475 orthotopic breast tumor xenografts in the upper thoracic mammary fat pad received 11 MBq (300 μCi) of [^{64}Cu]AMD3100 via tail vein injection, and whole body images were acquired at 90 min postinjection. (**a**) Transaxial PET, CT, and fused sections of both the tumors. (**b**) Volume-rendered whole body image showing clear accumulation of radioactivity in DU4475 tumor from ([19]) Solid arrow, MDA-MB-231 tumor; open arrow, DU4475 tumor; L, liver; K, kidney; B, bladder

To further validate the use of [^{64}Cu]AMD3100 in tumor models with variable CXCR4 expression, well-characterized breast tumor models were pursued [19]. CXCR4 expression in breast cancers has been well characterized. Overexpression of CXCR4 in primary tumors is directly correlated to the degree of lymph node metastasis and poor survival rates in breast cancer patients [26–28]. A study by Holm et al., demonstrated that CXCR4 overexpression occurs in most breast cancer patients and HER2-negative breast tumors with CXCR4 overexpression demonstrate more aggressive behavior and are more likely to recur than tumors that do not express elevated levels of CXCR4 [29]. Similarly, estrogen and progesterone receptor negative breast cancers and triple negative breast cancers with elevated CXCR4 expression are associated with high possibility of lymph node metastasis [30]. To evaluate the applicability of AMD3100 imaging for breast cancers, MDA-MB-231 (CXCR4^{low}) and DU4475 (CXCR4^{high}) (Table 21.2) tumor bearing mice were injected with [^{64}Cu]AMD3100 and imaged at 90 min postinjection. These whole-body images showed selective accumulation of radioactivity in the DU4475 tumors (Fig. 21.3a, b) demonstrating that detection of graded levels of CXCR4 expression is feasible in tumors.

Metastases have elevated levels of CXCR4 expression compared to the primary tumor [31–33], which could therefore be used as a novel strategy for the detection of metastatic disease. Lung, bone, brain, and liver xenograft metastatic models of breast cancer can be developed by intravenous, intracardiac, and intraspenic injection of MDA-MB-231 cells [34, 35]. In an experimental model of lung metastasis

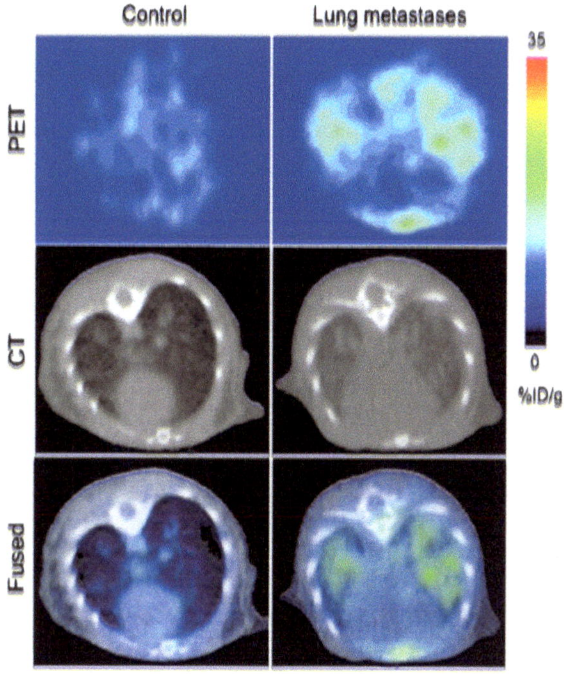

Fig. 21.4 CXCR4 imaging of MDA-MB-231–derived lung metastases with [^{64}Cu]AMD3100. NOD/SCID mice that received either 2×10^6 MDA-MB-231 cells or HBSS received 11 MBq (300 micro Ci) of [^{64}Cu]AMD3100 at 35 day after inoculation. Images were acquired at 90 min after injection. Transaxial PET, CT, and fused sections of lung metastasis and control mice (adapted from [19])

generated by tail vein injection of MDA-MB-231 cells into SCID mice, a clear accumulation of radioactivity was observed in the lung metastases (Fig. 21.4, [19]). Ex vivo biodistribution studies showed a statistically significant increase in uptake of radioactivity in the metastases bearing lungs. Further analysis of the single cell suspension of the metastases-derived cells showed an increase in the CXCR4 expression levels compared to the parental MDA-MB-231 cells. Wide variation in CXCR4 expression was observed suggesting that evaluation of CXCR4 receptor density contribution to the establishment of metastasis and the ability to detect these metastases by PET imaging needs further investigation. Given these promising results, it is reasonable to predict that stable copper-based imaging agents would be potentially useful in a clinical setting.

While AMD3100 showed promise as a PET imaging agent, its use also has disadvantages. Namely, it has relatively low affinity for CXCR4 and its structural scaffold is not amenable to modification. AMD3465 (Fig. 21.5), a second generation cyclam-based CXCR4 inhibitor, has been demonstrated to have high affinity (41.7 ± 1.2 nM), reduced charge and is smaller in size compared to AMD3100 [36]. Recently, De Silva et al. evaluated AMD3465, which was chelated to Copper-64, as a PET imaging agent for imaging CXCR4 expression in brain and colon cancer xenograft models [37].

Utilizing the abovementioned U87 and U87-stb-CXCR4 model, the authors demonstrated that at 65 min postinjection, radioactivity uptake in U87-stb-CXCR4 tumors reached 110 %ID/g, which was nearly threefold greater than those of the

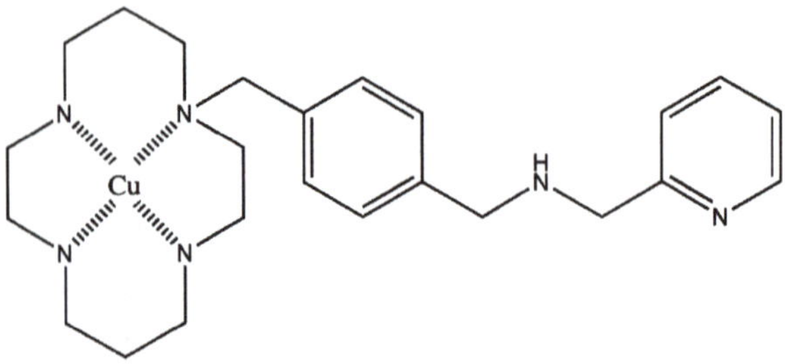

Fig. 21.5 Structure of Cu-AMD3465

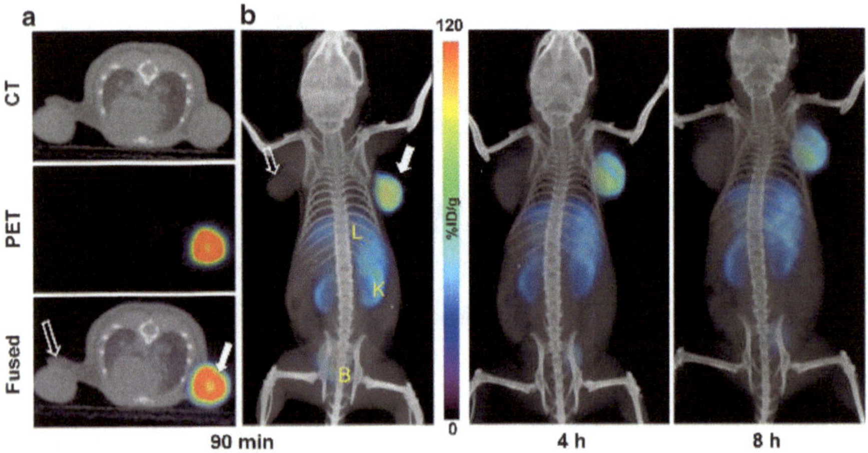

Fig. 21.6 PET/CT imaging of CXCR4 expression in subcutaneous brain tumor xenografts with [^{64}Cu]AMD3465. NOD/SCID mice bearing U87 and U87-stb-CXCR4 glioblastoma xenografts on the left and right flanks, respectively, were given approximately 9.25 MBq (250 μCi) of ^{64}Cu-labeled radiotracers *via* tail vein injection and PET/CT images were acquired. (**a**) representative transaxial PET, CT, and fused sections of both the tumors from a [^{64}Cu]AMD3465 injected mouse at 90 min postinjection; (**b**) Representative volume rendered whole body images of [^{64}Cu]AMD3465 at 90 min (*right panel*), 4 h (*middle panel*) and 8 h (*left panel*) postinjection. All images were decay corrected and scaled to the same maximum threshold value. *Unfilled arrow*, U87 tumor; *solid arrow*, U87-stb-CXCR4 tumor; *L* liver, *K* kidney, *B* bladder (from [37])

kidneys and liver and almost 18-fold greater than the U87 tumors. The highest uptake was consistently observed in the U87-stb-CXCR4 tumors and the best image contrast was reached at 90 min postinjection (Fig. 21.6). The liver and kidneys were the only other organs with any appreciable uptake. A blocking dose of 25 mg/kg AMD3465 resulted in a greater than 95% reduction in radiotracer uptake in both U87 and U87-stb-CXCR4 tumors (Fig. 21.7), confirming the specificity of the agent. Mice given a blocking dose also showed an approximately 50% decrease in %ID/g values for the kidneys, liver, spleen, and bone marrow, suggesting that a significant portion of that uptake is CXCR4 mediated. Ex vivo biodistribution studies performed at 30, 60, 90, 240, and 600 min postinjection of [^{64}Cu]AMD3465 (Table 21.3) showed the highest uptake in the U87-stb-CXCR4 tumors at all time

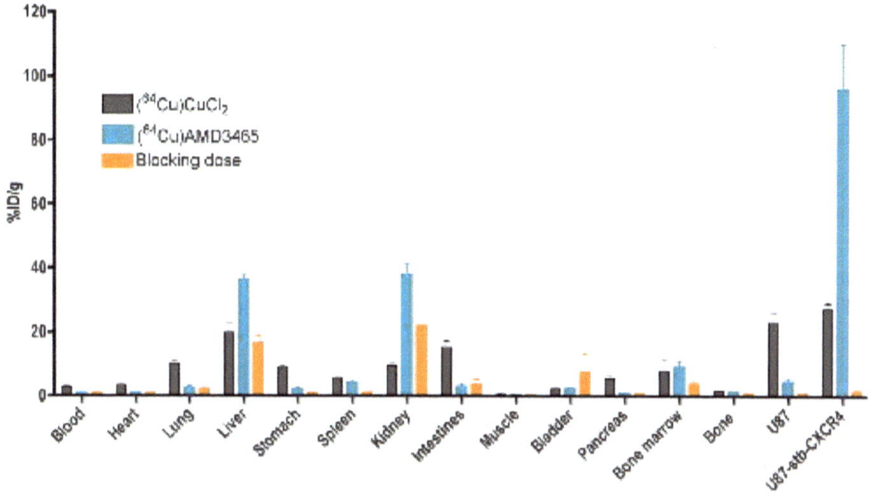

Fig. 21.7 In vivo specificity of [^{64}Cu]AMD3465 in subcutaneous brain tumor xenografts. NOD/SCID mice bearing U87 and U87-stb-CXCR4 glioblastoma xenografts on the left and right flanks, respectively, were used for biodistribution. Biodistribution analysis of selected tissues from mice injected with 740 kBq (20 μCi) of radiotracers and sacrificed at 90 min postinjection. All radioactivity values were converted into percentage of injected dose per gram of tissue (%ID/g). Biodistribution data are means ± SD of four to five animals (from [37])

Table 21.3 [^{64}Cu]AMD3465 ex vivo biodistribution studies for s.c. brain tumor xenografts

	30 min	60 min	90 min	240 min	600 min
Blood	1.93 ± 0.30	0.90 ± 0.08	0.73 ± 0.23	0.61 ± 0.09	1.20 ± 0.36
Heart	1.19 ± 0.16	1.00 ± 0.20	0.90 ± 0.25	0.93 ± 0.06	0.72 ± 0.07
Lung	4.48 ± 0.56	3.70 ± 0.99	2.78 ± 0.47	3.39 ± 0.85	2.10 ± 0.13
Liver	32.08 ± 2.03	35.06 ± 7.77	36.15 ± 1.79	33.65 ± 3.13	27.27 ± 2.57
Stomach	1.91 ± 0.31	2.02 ± 0.76	2.17 ± 0.65	1.98 ± 0.102	1.21 ± 0.03
Spleen	6.23 ± 1.17	5.68 ± 1.75	4.28 ± ± 1.00	4.88 ± 0.42	2.64 ± 0.12
Kidney	32.45 ± 2.33	32.05 ± 4.03	37.93 ± 3.57	33.57 ± 6.39	25.15 ± 3.29
Small intestines	3.12 ± 0.53	3.33 ± 0.87	2.99 ± 1.01	2.77 ± 0.69	1.79 ± 0.19
Muscle	0.75 ± 0.52	0.37 ± 0.12	0.30 ± 0.13	0.23 ± 0.03	0.19 ± 0.02
Bladder	2.65 ± 0.32	4.75 ± 3.43	2.41 ± 0.51	2.17 ± 0.71	0.96 ± 0.21
Pancreas	1.19 ± 0.18	1.53 ± 0.32	1.13 ± 0.22	1.47 ± 0.62	0.68 ± 0.05
Bone	2.79 ± 0.74	1.53 ± 0.44	1.38 ± 0.19	1.12 ± 0.19	0.80 ± 0.36
Bone marrow	6.39 ± 0.00	10.22 ± 4.97	9.18 ± 2.04	8.10 ± 3.38	9.42 ± 3.88
U87	3.34 ± 0.59	2.56 ± 0.20	4.15 ± 0.94	4.23 ± 1.30	4.03 ± 0.94
U87-stb-CXCR4	106.58 ± 5.99[a]	102.70 ± 20.80[a]	96.29 ± 13.98[a]	50.95 ± 6.38[a]	28.92 ± 2.65[a]

[a]Signifies a $P < 0.0001$ and the comparative reference is U87 tumor uptake

points, which is similar to the results seen with imaging. The liver, kidneys, and bone marrow were the only other tissues with notable uptake of the radiotracer. The tumor-to-muscle ratios, which are an indicator of image contrast, reached a maximum of 362.56 ± 153.51 at 90 min after injection of the [^{64}Cu]AMD3465.

Validation of CXCR4-based imaging agents in various tumor models is advantageous for further clinical translation. Colon carcinoma is one of the nearly 23 different cancers in which CXCR4 expression is well characterized. CXCR4 is differentially expressed in CRC and is required for the outgrowth of colon cancer metastasis [38, 39]. CXCR4 expression in primary CRC is often associated with recurrence, poor survival, and liver metastases [38]. In patients treated with the folinic acid, fluorouracil and oxaliplatin (FOLFOX) regimen, enhanced CXCR4 expression in resected liver metastases was observed suggesting that CXCR4 may be contributing to drug resistance and indicating an expanding role of CXCR4 in cancer biology [40]. Using an HT-29 colon cancer model that has 30% of cells positive for CXCR4 expression as determined by flow cytometry, De Silva et al. showed that detection of graded levels of CXCR4 expression is feasible in tumors. The %ID/g for the HT-29 tumors at 90 min postinjection was 5.62 ± 0.90 and the tumor-to-muscle and tumor-to-blood ratios were 24.78 ± 2.38 and 8.05 ± 0.60, respectively.

The same research group also investigated AMD3100 as a PET imaging agent [19] in the glioblastoma model (U87), as mentioned previously in this chapter, allowing for further comparison between these two imaging agents. The tissue-to-muscle and tissue-to-blood ratios for [^{64}Cu]AMD3465 at 90 min postinjection are seven to eight times higher than those of [^{64}Cu]AMD3100. These studies combined with specificity observed in the HT-29 tumor model indicate that [^{64}Cu]AMD3465 has good target selectivity, produces better image contrast and is suitable for the detection of graded levels of CXCR4 expression in tumors.

Peptide-Based CXCR4 Imaging Agents

Peptides have frequently been radiolabeled and used as imaging agents by targeting cell surface receptors that are overexpressed in human cancers [41, 42]. These peptides are usually shorter than 40 amino acids, are easy to synthesize and are stable to radiolabeling conditions. In addition, peptides are typically highly specific for their targets and have high binding affinities [43, 44].

T140, a 14-residue peptide with a disulfide bridge, was found to be a potent CXCR4 antagonist [45, 46]. However, it is unstable in serum due to cleavage of the C-terminal Arg, which is required for its anti-HIV activity. Derivatives in which the C-terminus was amidated were synthesized in order to overcome this serum instability, which led to the discovery of TN14003 [46]. TN14003 was found to be highly stable in serum and retained high selectivity for CXCR4. Several TN14003 analogs conjugated with PET, SPECT, and optical probes have been used for imaging.

An ^{18}F-labeled derivative of TN14003 was synthesized by Jacobson et al. for the PET imaging of CXCR4 expression in Chinese hamster ovarian (CHO)-CXCR4 tumors (Fig. 21.8, [47]). The synthesis of *N*-succinimidyl 4-^{18}F-fluorobenzoate (^{18}F-SFB) was automated in three steps using a 2-reaction-vial module (Fig. 21.9). ^{18}F-SFB was then conjugated to 1-(4,4′-dimethyl-2,6-dioxocyclohexylidene) ethyl (Dde) protected T140 and the protecting groups were hydrolyzed to yield 4-F-benzoyl-TN14003 (4-F-T140). 4-F-T140 was then evaluated for its ability to image CXCR4 expression

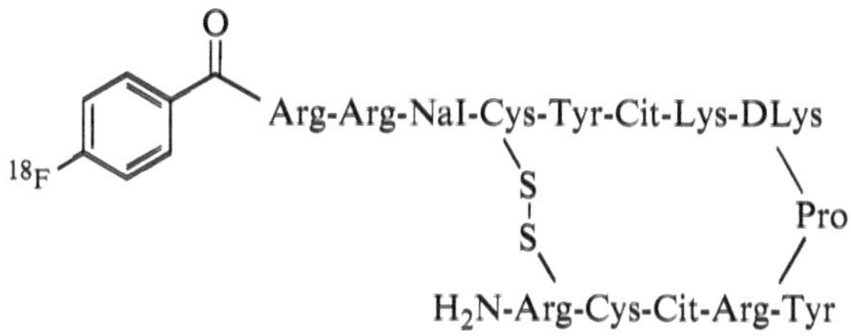

Fig. 21.8 Schematic structure of 4-F-T140 (adapted from [47])

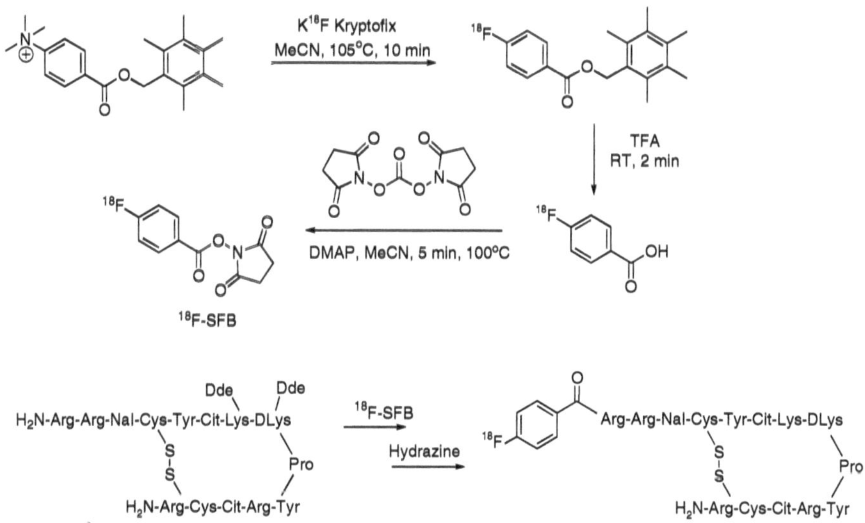

Fig. 21.9 Radiosynthesis of 4-^{18}F-T140. *MeCN* acetonitrile, *DMAP* 4-(dimethylamino)pyridine, *RT* room temperature (adapted from [47])

levels in mice subcutaneously harboring CXCR4-positive and CXCR4-negative CHO tumor cells. Initially, extremely high blood uptake was observed, and the slightly higher uptake seen in the CHO-CXCR4 tumors compared to the CXCR4-negative tumors was not statistically significant. Coinjection of 10 μg of cold 4-F-T140 with 4-^{18}F-T140 resulted in a decrease in activity seen in the blood and the CXCR4-negative tumors, while activity increased in the CXCR4-positive tumors, thereby improving the tumor-to-background ratios. Even though these results imply that 4-^{18}F-T140 binding is CXCR4 specific, the translational potential of this peptide is limited.

Single Photon Emission Computed Tomography

Single photon emission computed tomography (SPECT) imaging, like PET, involves the use of radiolabeled probes to gather functional information from a biological system. SPECT radionuclides, however, decay by emitting gamma radiation, which is measured directly by a rotating gamma camera with an attached collimator.

The gamma emissions from these radionuclides are lower in energy than those for PET imaging, and the use of a collimator results in sensitivity that is two to three orders of magnitude lower than PET, yielding lower resolution images (spatial resolution = 8–15 mm). SPECT isotopes are often longer-lived and the most commonly used radionuclides are ^{123}I ($t_{1/2}$ = 13.1 h), ^{111}In ($t_{1/2}$ = 2.8 day), ^{99m}Tc ($t_{1/2}$ = 6 h), and ^{67}Ga ($t_{1/2}$ = 78.3 h) [48]. The long half-lives of these radionuclides allow for the observation of biological processes several hours or even days after tracer administration. Co-registration of SPECT and CT images yields a combination of functional and anatomic information.

SPECT Imaging Agents

Peptides

Development of the first SPECT-based radiolabeled probe for in vivo imaging of CXCR4 expression was reported by Koglin et al. [49]. A cyclic pentapeptide, CPCR4 (*cyclo*(D-Tyr-Arg-Arg-Nal-Gly)), was radiolabeled with Iodine-125 and used for SPECT and biodistribution studies in mice. In mice bearing CMS5/CXCR4$^+$ and CMS5/CXCR4$^-$ fibrosarcoma tumors, at 1 h postinjection of ^{125}I-CPCR4, CXCR4$^+$ tumors showed 5.5 ± 1.5 %ID/g compared to 0.6 ± 0.2 %ID/g in the control tumor. However, ^{125}I-CPCR4 also accumulated at high concentration in the liver (19.5 ± 2.8 %ID/g), intestine (17.2 ± 2.9 %ID/g), and kidneys (12.2 ± 2.3 %ID/g) limiting further applicability of the agent.

Soon after, Hanaoka et al. developed an Indium-111 labeled radiotracer for the in vivo imaging of tumors using SPECT [50]. The group had previously discovered that T22, a peptide with anti-HIV activity, inhibited CXCR4. Based on T22, a truncated analog (Ac-TZ14011) was synthesized in which the four amino acid residues necessary for the inhibitory activity against CXCR4 were conserved (Fig. 21.10). In order to promote site-selective radiolabeling, a single amino acid (D-Lys) was installed at a reasonable distance from the pharmacophore. Diethylenetriaminepentaacetic

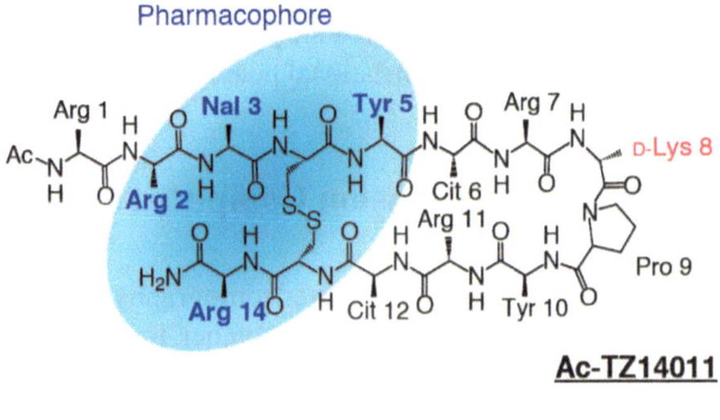

Fig. 21.10 Structure of Ac-TZ14011 and its pharmacophore (from [50])

Table 21.4 Biodistribution of radioactivity after intravenous injection of ^{111}In-DTPA-Ac-TZ14011 in nude mice bearing pancreatic carcinoma, AsPC-1 (from [50])

	1 h	6 h	24 h	1 h+ Ac-TZ14011[a]
Blood[b]	0.39 (0.06)	0.05 (0.01)	0.03 (0.01)	2.06** (0.61)
Liver[b]	27.0 (2.9)	25.2 (2.0)	19.3 (2.5)	1.95** (0.25)
Kidney[b]	50.9 (4.3)	43.4 (6.3)	29.5 (5.7)	45.4 (6.8)
Spleen[b]	8.22 (0.70)	7.57 (0.54)	5.83 (0.99)	2.66** (1.21)
Pancreas[b]	0.15 (0.03)	0.05 (0.01)	0.05 (0.02)	1.07** (0.46)
Muscle[b]	0.17 (0.05)	0.07 (0.02)	0.07 (0.01)	1.35** (0.26)
Tumor[b]	0.51 (0.08)	0.20 (0.03)	0.14 (0.03)	1.70** (0.27)
T/B ratio[c]	1.31 (0.14)	4.05 (0.79)	5.65 (2.89)	0.88* (0.31)
T/M ratio[d]	3.17 (0.99)	4.43 (1.89)	3.23 (1.08)	1.31** (0.41)

Each value represents the mean (S.D.) for five animals

*$P<0.05$, comparison between ^{111}In-DTPA-Ac-TZ14011 with or without unlabeled Ac-TZ14011 at 1 h

**$P<0.005$, comparison between ^{111}In-DTPA-Ac-TZ14011 with or without unlabeled Ac-TZ14011 at 1 h

[a]Coinjection with unlabeled Ac-TZ14011 (10 mg/kg)

[b]Expressed as % injected dose per gram

[c]Tumor-to-blood ratio

[d]Tumor-to-muscle ratio

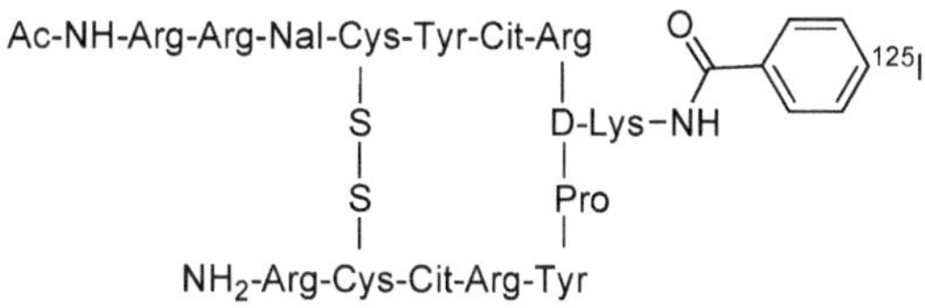

Fig. 21.11 Structure of ^{125}I-labeled Ac-TZ14011 (adapted from [51])

acid (DTPA) was then conjugated to Ac-TZ14011, which was subsequently reacted with $^{111}InCl_3$ to yield the radiolabeled product.

Biodistribution of ^{111}In-DTPA-Ac-TZ14011 in athymic nude BALB/c mice with s.c. AsPC-1 pancreatic carcinoma xenografts was determined at 1, 6, and 24 h postinjection (Table 21.4). While ^{111}In-DTPA-Ac-TZ14011 uptake was higher in the tumor than in the muscle or blood, 15- to 200-fold increase in uptake was observed in the liver, kidneys, and spleen. Coinjection of unlabeled Ac-TZ14011 with ^{111}In-DTPA-Ac-TZ14011 resulted in decreased uptake in the liver and spleen and increased activity in the tumors. However, coinjection also produced higher uptake in the blood, which markedly lowered the tumor-to-blood ratio. The high kidney uptake, which appears to be nonspecific, was attributed to the highly positive charge created by five arginine residues. The low tumor-to-muscle ratios and the high nonspecific uptake observed would most likely limit the use of ^{111}In-DTPA-Ac-TZ14011 as a CXCR4 imaging agent.

The same research group also took advantage of the specific binding of Ac-TZ14011 to CXCR4 and completed the preliminary evaluation of an ^{125}I-labeled radiopharmaceutical for the in vivo imaging of CXCR4-expressing tumors [51]. *N*-succinimidyl-3-[^{125}I]iodobenzoate (^{125}I-SIB) was synthesized and conjugated with Ac-TZ14011 (Fig. 21.11). MCF-7 breast cancer cells incubated for scheduled

Table 21.5 Biodistribution of ^{125}I-IB-Ac-TZ14011 in normal mice (from [51])

Tissue	Injected dose/organ percent at different intervals of time postinjection (%ID/g)		
	10 min	120 min	240 min
Heart	1.482±0.282	0.133±0.034	0.038±0.008
Liver	1.749±0.468	0.197±0.066	0.04±0.009
Lung	1.747±0.566	0.168±0.058	0.043±0.007
Spleen	0.755±0.329	0.073±0.014	0.023±0.002
Stomach	1.071±0.249	0.432±0.15	0.086±0.027
Kidney	16.152±4.121	0.866±0.352	0.116±0.042
Intestine	1.911±0.657	0.182±0.371	0.03±0.005
Muscle	2.02±0.292	0.232±0.046	0.043±0.006
Bone	2.558±0.508	0.23±0.054	0.07±0.006
Blood	6.737±1.179	0.51±0.118	0.115±0.017
Brain	0.159±0.053	0.022±0.009	0.008±0.001
Thyroid	1.91±0.542	0.185±0.031	0.059±0.014

intervals of time with ^{125}I-IB-Ac-TZ14011 showed a 7% incubated radioactivity binding by 30 min that reached a plateau by 120 min.

Similar to the distribution profile observed with the aforementioned In-111 labeled analog, biodistribution studies performed in female Chinese Kunming mice showed the highest radiotracer uptake in the kidneys at 10 min (16.152±4.121 %ID/g), which cleared slowly over 2 h (Table 21.5). The spleen, liver, intestines, and thyroid all displayed relatively low uptake of ^{125}I-IB-Ac-TZ14011.

Low activity seen in the thyroid in these biodistribution studies indicates low deiodination of ^{125}I-IB-Ac-TZ14011 in vivo. Relatively low liver and intestine radioactivity uptake observed suggest that the introduction of the 3-[^{125}I]iodobenzoyl group does not increase the ligand lipophilicity. These preliminary results reported by Han et al. are promising and further evaluation of ^{125}I-IB-Ac-TZ14011 in in vivo tumor models would be desirable.

Monoclonal Antibodies

Monoclonal antibodies (mAbs), because of their target-binding specificity, provide an attractive choice as a molecular scaffold for therapy as well as radiopharmaceutical-based imaging. Unlike peptides, which often require the presence of an active site for a high-affinity interaction, antibodies are unrivaled in their ability to recognize almost any target of interest [52]. This potential has largely gone unrealized due to the large size of these agents, which results in relatively poor pharmacokinetics with long circulation times and mitigating solid tumor penetration. However, mAbs are gaining attention as viable clinical imaging agents [52]. Even though intracellular targets are inaccessible with the use of monoclonal antibodies, they can be used to detect cell surface receptor expression on tumor cells, such as CXCR4 expression.

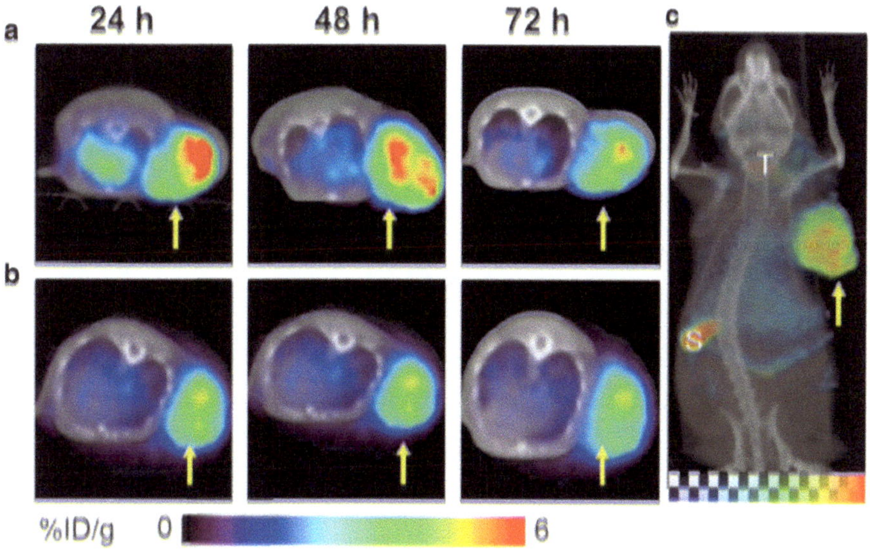

Fig. 21.12 SPECT/CT of CXCR4 expression in subcutaneous U87 xenografts with mAbs. Severe combined immunodeficient mice bearing U87 glioblastoma xenografts were injected with 37 MBq (1 mCi) of either ^{125}I-12 G5 (**a**) or ^{125}I-IgG_{2A} (**b**) via tail vein. SPECT/CT images were acquired at 24, 48, and 72 h after injection of mAbs. All images were adjusted to same maximum value to show relative active concentrations of tracers. *Arrow* depicts tumor in coronal sections. (**c**) Maximum-intensity-projection image of ^{125}I-12 G5-injected mouse at 48 h after injection; *arrow* shows tumor. *%ID/g* percentage of injected dose per gram of tissue, *S* spleen; *T* thyroid (from [54])

The radiolabeled monoclonal CXCR4 antibody clone 12G5, which binds the same extracellular loop as CXCL12, is routinely used for screening CXCR4 inhibitors [53]. In 2009, Nimmagadda et al. reported the use of ^{125}I-12G5 for the imaging of CXCR4 expression in subcutaneous U87 brain tumors using SPECT/CT [54]. Images acquired at 24, 48, and 72 h postinjection in male BALB/c SCID mice implanted subcutaneously with U87 glioblastoma tumor cells showed that ^{125}I-12 G5 (Fig. 21.12a) clearly exhibited increased radioactivity compared to isotype matched 125I-IgG2A control antibody (Fig. 21.12b). The whole body maximum intensity projection also showed the highest radioactivity accumulation in the spleen (Fig. 21.12c).

Ex vivo biodistribution studies indicated that mice injected with ^{125}I-12G5 demonstrated consistently higher uptake of radioactivity compared to animals given ^{125}I-IgG_{2A} (Fig. 21.13). The nonspecific activity accumulation observed with ^{125}I-IgG_{2A} control antibody implies that at least part of the activity seen with ^{125}I-12G5 was nonspecific, which could account for the enhanced permeability and retention [55]. Similarly, high uptake in the spleen could be due to cross-reactivity of the antibody with the antigen-positive circulating cells and normal B cells in the blood or spleen [56]. Further analysis of the tumor-derived cells by flow cytometry

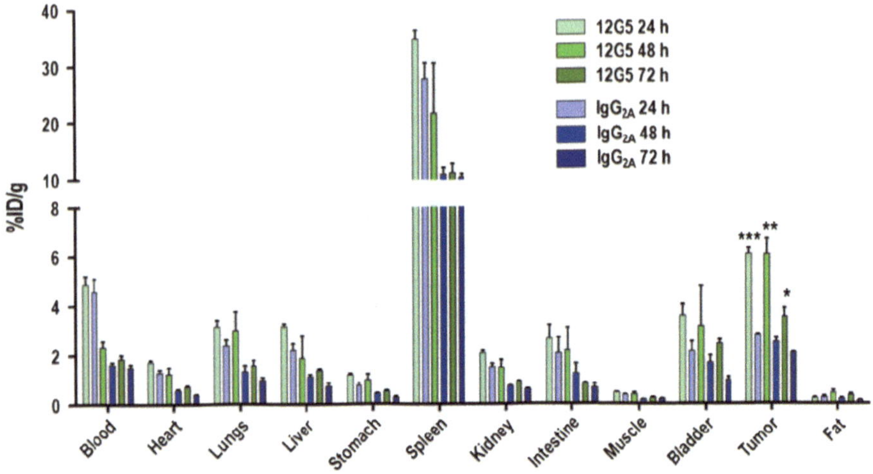

Fig. 21.13 Ex vivo biodistribution data for mAbs in tumor-bearing severe combined immunodeficient (SCID) mice. SCID mice harboring U87 glioblastoma xenografts were injected with 74 kBq (2 μCi) of either ^{125}I-12G5 or ^{125}I-IgG$_{2A}$ via tail vein. At 24, 48, and 72 h after injection, selected tissues and tumors were harvested and weighed, and radioactivity was counted in a spectrometer. All values were converted into percentage of injected dose per gram of tissue (%ID/g). Data are means ± SEM of 3 animals. Comparative reference is ^{125}I-IgG$_{2A}$ uptake. *$P<0.05$. **$P<0.01$. ***$P<0.001$ (from [54])

showed a two- to sevenfold increase in CXCR4 expression. Because U87 cells grown in hypoxic conditions display a five- to tenfold increase in CXCR4 expression, the authors hypothesized that the aforementioned increase in CXCR4 expression was due to either tumor hypoxia or to clonal selection of high CXCR4-expressing cells. As a whole, these results are promising and establish the viability of using radiolabeled mAbs for the imaging of CXCR4 expression in tumors.

Optical Imaging Agents

Optical imaging, consisting of bioluminescence and fluorescence intensity imaging (FII) modalities, allows the imaging of internally generated light linked to specific biological function [48]. Optical imaging techniques are based on the detection of photons both within and outside the visible spectrum with charge-coupled device cameras. Bioluminescence imaging detects enzymatically mediated light produced by chemical reactions in cells and tissues. The imaging of light produced by an injected or applied fluorophore when excited by an external light source is called fluorescence intensity imaging [9].

While very few optical imaging probes have been translated to the clinic, they offer multiple advantages over radionuclides. These probes do not subject the patient to harmful ionizing radiation and they are activatable, unlike radiotracers which are "always on" and therefore produce images with higher background noise [9]. However, optical probes suffer from poor penetration of light in tissue. Given this fact, optical probes have thus far been developed mainly for fluorescence-guided surgical techniques and endoscopic imaging [9].

Fluorescence Intensity Imaging

A pressing issue in oncologic surgery is the need for identification and complete resection of the primary tumor. This is much more challenging for a locally invasive disease. To assist in this endeavor, considerable effort is devoted to developing fluorescent probes, particularly near infrared emitting, that could be used intraoperatively for tumor boundary detection. Early detection and treatment of small or flat malignant urothelium is vital in those with high-grade bladder cancer, however, diagnosis using conventional methods is sometimes difficult. Several new methods for detecting bladder cancer using fluorescence cytoscopy have been developed, but these seem to suffer from high false-positive rates or low specificity [57–59]. CXCR4 was found to be the only chemokine receptor whose mRNA expression level was upregulated in bladder cancer cell lines [60], therefore, the development of a fluorescent antagonist of CXCR4 would be highly useful as an imaging agent for bladder cancer.

In 2010, Nishizawa et al. identified a carboxyfluorescein-labeled analog of T140, a CXCR4 antagonist, as an imaging agent for high-grade bladder cancer [61]. The T140 analog, TY14003, is 14 amino acid residues long (Ac-Arg-Arg-Nal-Cys-Tyr-Cit-Arg-D-Lys*-Pro-Tyr-Arg-Cit-Cys-Arg-NH_2; with carboxyfluorescein conjugated to D-Lys (D-Lys* indicates the carboxyfluorescein-labeled D-Lys). Because T140 is specific for CXCR4, the authors suspected that TY14003 might be used to label the bladder cancer cell line TCCSUP. Fluorescent TY14003 successfully stained the bladder cancer cell line TCCSUP (Fig. 21.14a) while two negative control peptides, TR14009 and TR14010, failed to stain the cells. In order to test the utility of TY14003 as a biomarker in a clinical setting, urine specimens taken from bladder cancer patients were analyzed. Urine sediments also stained positive with TY14003 (Fig. 21.14d) unlike specimens taken from patients without bladder cancer. While white blood cells in urine sediments did stain, this was an expected result and these cells were easily distinguished from urothelial cells (Fig. 21.14e).

For in vivo imaging of bladder cancer in mice, fluorescent TY14003 was instilled at 12 weeks of tumor growth in a mouse bladder cancer model induced by 0.025% *N*-butyl-*N*-(4-hydroxybutyl) nitrosamine (BBN). For microscopic analysis, mice were euthanized 5–10 min later and their bladders were harvested and sectioned (Fig. 21.15a, b). Cancer could not be detected by either direct vision or by phase-contrast microscopy because of flat tumors (Fig. 21.15c). Using endoscopy with fluorescent light, in vivo observation of the mouse bladder showed focal fluorescent staining with TY14003 (Fig. 21.15d, e).

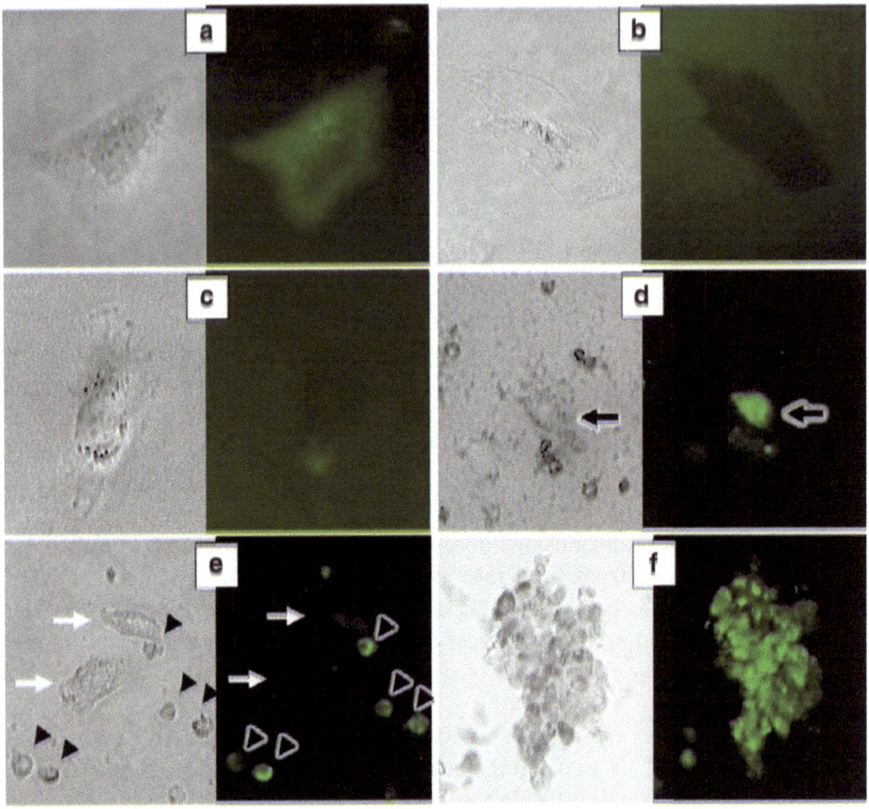

Fig. 21.14 Confocal laser microscopy with phase-contrast images and fluorescent images of the same fields of cells are shown in the left and right panels, respectively. (**a**) Fluorescent imaging of TCCSUP cells using TY14003 (×400). (**b**) Mouse fibroblast cells cultured from peritoneal connective tissue is not labeled by TY14003 (×400). (**c**) TY14003 cannot bind to internalized CXCR4, 5 min after administration of SDF-1 (×400) (**d**) Microscopic images of human urine sedimentation using TY14003 with a representative view of urothelial cells from patients with invasive bladder cancer. The urine cytology was class 4 (×200). (**e**) Urine sedimentation after sixth weekly intravesical BCG therapy. Urothelial cells are not labeled by TY14003 (*white arrow*), although white blood cells are labeled (*dark arrow head*). The urine sedimentation turned out to be class 2 (×200) (**f**) Ex vivo imaging of human bladder cancer using TY14003 (×50). Bladder cancer specimen was obtained by cold-cup biopsy (from [61])

The results obtained from these studies are easier to interpret than those obtained through conventional cytology, a method whose success largely depends on the skill of the pathologist. In the future, TY14003 may be useful as a diagnostic tool in the clinic for the detection of bladder cancer.

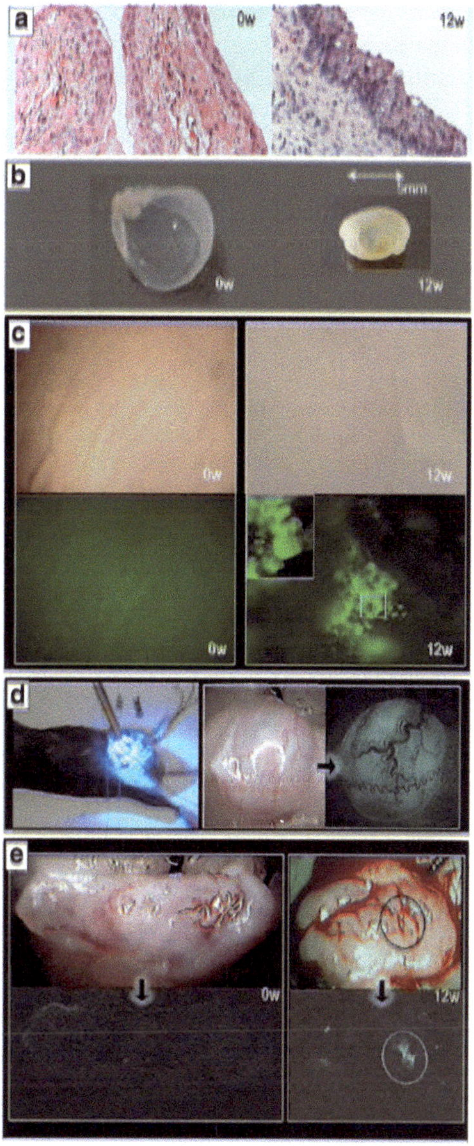

Fig. 21.15 Representative microscopic view (**a**) and macroscopic view (**b**) of cut surfaces of mouse bladders. 0w: normal bladder, 12w: carcinoma in situ (CIS) caused by BBN. (**c**) After 12-week BBN drinking, multiple CIS lesions were observed by confocal laser microscopy with fluorescent images. Confocal laser microscopy of mouse bladder mucosa with phase-contrast image (upper column, ×100) and fluorescent image using TY14003 (lower column, ×100 and ×400). (**d**) Mouse bladders were directly observed under anesthesia by endoscope with *white light* images and fluorescent images. TY14003 instilled into bladder was illuminated through the bladder wall (*right panel*). (**e**) After the anterior bladder walls were cut and opened, bladder mucosa was washed twice and observed by white light (*upper panels*) and fluorescent light (*lower panels*). Fluorescent stain for TY14003 was observed in mice after 12-weeks BBN drinking (*circle*) (from [61])

Conclusion

There is considerable enthusiasm in the research community for CXCR4-based imaging agents. However, success of CXCR4-based imaging agents will depend on detailed characterization of the changes in CXCR4 and CXCL12 expression profiles in tumors and metastases and also on our mechanistic understanding of the underlying biology in response to treatments. Another important consideration is desensitization of the receptor, which could be misleading if patients are simply stratified based on CXCR4 expression on tumor cells. As targeted molecular therapies become the "standard therapy," identification and validation of imaging biomarkers will lead to early detection, improved staging and monitoring of the disease. We are cautiously optimistic that CXCR4-based imaging has the potential to fulfill these criteria.

References

1. Sun X, Cheng G et al (2010) CXCL12/CXCR4/CXCR7 chemokine axis and cancer progression. Cancer Metastasis Rev 29:709
2. Hu M, Polyak K (2008) Molecular characterization of the tumor microenvironment in breast cancer. Eur J Cancer 44:2760
3. Balkwill F (2004) The significance of cancer cell expression of the receptor CXCR4. Semin Cancer Biol 14:171
4. Tanaka T, Bai Z et al (2005) Chemokines in tumor progression and metastasis. Cancer Sci 96:317
5. Wong D, Korz W (2008) Translating an antagonist of chemokine receptor CXCR4: from bench to bedside. Clin Cancer Res 14:7975
6. Teicher BA, Fricker SP (2010) CXCL12 (SDF-1)/CXCR4 pathway in cancer. Clin Cancer Res 16:2927
7. Duda DG, Kozin SV et al (2011) CXCL12 (SDF-1)-CXCR4/CXCR7 pathway inhibition: an emerging sensitizer for anticancer therapies? Clin Cancer Res 17:2074
8. Mankoff D (2007) A definition of molecular imaging. J Nucl Med 48:18N
9. Alford R, Ogawa M et al (2009) Molecular probes for the in vivo imaging of cancer. Mol Biosyst 5:1279
10. Mawlawi O, Townsend DW (2009) Multimodality imaging: an update on PET/CT technology. Eur J Nucl Med Mol Imaging 36:S15
11. Miller JC, Thrall JH (2004) Clinical molecular imaging. J Am Coll Radiol 1:S4
12. Li Z, Conti PS (2010) Radiopharmaceutical chemistry for positron emission tomography. Adv Drug Deliv Rev 62:1031
13. Bridger GJ, Skerlj RT et al (1995) Synthesis and structure-activity relationships of phenylenebis(methylene)-linked bis-tetraazamacrocycles that inhibit HIV replication. Effects of macrocyclic ring size and substituents on the aromatic linker. J Med Chem 38:366
14. Fricker SP, Anastassov V et al (2006) Characterization of the molecular pharmacology of AMD3100: a specific antagonist of the G-protein coupled chemokine receptor, CXCR4. Biochem Pharmacol 72:588
15. Brelot A, Heveler N, Montes M, Alizon M (2000) J Biol Chem 275:23736
16. Gerlach LO, Jakobsen JS et al (2003) Metal ion enhanced binding of AMD3100 to Asp262 in the CXCR4 receptor. Biochemistry 42:710
17. Jacobson O, Weiss ID et al (2009) 64Cu-AMD3100-A novel imaging agent for targeting chemokine receptor CXCR4. Bioorg Med Chem 17:1486
18. Wald O, Weiss I et al (2007) Chemokines in hepatitis C virus infections: pathogenesis, prognosis and therapeutics. Cytokine 39:50
19. Nimmagadda S, Pullambhatla M et al (2010) Molecular imaging of CXCR4 receptor expression in human cancer xenografts with [^{64}Cu]AMD3100 positron emission tomography. Cancer Res 70:3935
20. Rempel SA, Dudas S et al (2000) Indentification and localization of the cytokine SDF1 and its receptor, CXC chemokine receptor 4, to regions of necrosis and angiogenesis in human glioblastoma. Clin Cancer Res 6:102

21. Sehgal A, Keener C et al (1998) CXCR4, a chemokine receptor, is overexpressed in and required for proliferation of glioblastoma tumor cells. J Surg Oncol 69:99
22. Zagzag D, Esencay M, Mendez O et al (2008) Hypoxia- and vascular endothelial growth factor-induced stromal cell-derived factor-1α/CXCR4 expression in glioblastomas: one plausible explanation of Scherer's structures. Am J Pathol 173:545
23. Wadas TJ, Wong EH et al (2007) Copper chelation chemistry and its role in copper radiopharmaceuticals. Curr Pharm Des 13:3
24. Smith-Jones PM, Fridrich R et al (1991) Antibody labeling with copper-67 using the bifunctional macrocycle 4-[(1,4,8,11-tetraazacyclotetradec-1-yl)methyl]benzoic acid. Bioconjug Chem 2:415
25. Boswell CA, Sun X, Niu W et al (2004) Comparative in vivo stability of copper-64-labeled cross-bridged and conventional tetraazamacrocyclic complexes. J Med Chem 47:1465
26. Kato M, Kitayama J, Kazama S, Nagawa H (2003) Expression pattern of CXC chemokine receptor-4 is correlated with lymph node metastasis in human invasive ductal carcinoma. Breast Cancer Res 5:R144–R150
27. Kang H, Watkins G, Douglas-Jones A, Mansel RE, Jiang WG (2005) The elevated level of CXCR4 is correlated with nodal metastasis of human breast cancer. Breast 14:360–367
28. Holm NT, Abreo F, Johnson LW, Li BD, Chu QD (2009) Elevated chemokine receptor CXCR4 expression in primary tumors following neoadjuvant chemotherapy predicts poor outcomes for patients with locally advanced breast cancer (LABC). Breast Cancer Res Treat 113:293–299
29. Holm NT, Byrnes K, Li BD et al (2007) Elevated Levels of chemokine receptor CXCR4 in HER-2 negative breast cancer specimens predict recurrence. J Surg Res 141:53–59
30. Chu QD, Panu L, Holm NT, Li BD, Johnson LW, Zhang S (2010) High Chemokine receptor CXCR4 level in triple negative breast cancer specimens predicts poor clinical outcome. J Surg Res 159:689
31. Oda Y, Yamamoto H et al (2006) CXCR4 and VEGF expression in the primary site and the metastatic site of human osteosarcoma: analysis within a group of patients, all of whom developed lung metastasis. Mod Pathol 19:738
32. Salvucci O, Bouchard A et al (2006) The role of CXCR4 receptor expression in breast cancer: a large tissue microarray study. Breast Cancer Res Treat 97:275
33. Sun YX, Wang J et al (2003) Expression of CXCR4 and CXCL12 in human prostate cancers in vivo. J Cell Biochem 89:462
34. Minn AJ, Kang Y et al (2005) Distinct organ-specific metastatic potential of individual breast cancer cells and primary tumors. J Clin Invest 115:44
35. Robey IF, Baggett BK et al (2009) Bicarbonate increases tumor pH and inhibits spontaneous metastases. Cancer Res 69:2260
36. Wong RSY, Bodart V et al (2008) Comparison of the potential multiple binding modes of bicyclam, monocyclam, and noncyclam small-molecule CXC chemokine receptor 4 inhibitors. Mol Pharmacol 74:1485
37. De Silva RA, Peyre K et al (2011) Imaging CXCR4 expression in human cancer xenografts: evaluation of monocyclam [64Cu]AMD3465. J Nucl Med 52:986
38. Kim J, Takeuchi H et al (2005) Chemokine receptor CXCR4 expression in colorectal cancer patients increases the risk for recurrence and for poor survival. J Clin Oncol 23:2744
39. Zeelenberg IS, Ruuls-Van Stalle L et al (2003) The chemokine receptor CXCR4 is required for outgrowth of colon carcinoma micrometastases. Cancer Res 63:3833
40. Dessein AF, Stechly L et al (2010) Autocrine induction of invasive and metastatic phenotypes by the MIF-CXCR4 axis in drug-resistant human colon cancer cells. Cancer Res 70:4644
41. Smith-Jones PM, Stolz B et al (1994) Gallium-67/gallium-68-[DFO]-octreotide–a potential radiopharmaceutical for PET imaging of somatostatin receptor-positive tumors: synthesis and radiolabeling in vitro and preliminary in vivo studies. J Nucl Med 35:317
42. Chen K, Conti PS (2010) Target specific delivery of peptide-based probes for PET imaging. Adv Drug Deliv Rev 62:1005
43. Maina T, Nock BA et al (2005) Species differences of bombesin analog interactions with GRP-R define the choice of animal models in the development of GRP-R-targeting drugs. J Nucl Med 46:823

44. Cescato R, Maina T et al (2008) Bombesin receptor antagonists may be preferable to agonists for tumor targeting. J Nucl Med 49:318
45. Tamamura H, Xu Y et al (1998) A low-molecular-weight inhibitor against the chemokine receptor CXCR4: a strong anti-HIV peptide T140. Biochem Biophys Res Commun 253:877
46. Tamamura H, Omagari A et al (2001) Development of specific CXCR4 inhibitors possessing high selectivity indexes as well as complete stability in serum based on an anti-HIV peptide T140. Bioorg Med Chem Lett 11:1897
47. Jacobson O, Weiss ID et al (2010) PET of tumor CXCR4 expression with 4-^{18}F-T140. J Nucl Med 51:1796
48. Signore A, Mather SJ et al (2010) Molecular imaging of inflammation/infection: nuclear medicine and optical imaging agents and methods. Chem Rev 110:3112
49. Koglin N, Anton M et al (2006) CXCR4 chemokine receptor SPECT/PET imaging with radiolabeled CPCR4: a promising approach for imaging metastatic processes. J Nucl Med 47(Suppl 1): 505P
50. Hanaoka H, Mukai T et al (2006) Development of an ^{111}In-labeled peptide derivative targeting a chemokine receptor, CXCR4, for imaging tumors. Nucl Med Biol 33:489
51. Han Y, Yin D et al (2010) Synthesis and preliminary evaluation of a novel ^{125}I-labeled T140 analog for quantification of CXCR4 expression. J Radioanal Nucl Chem 284:279
52. Wu A (2009) Antibodies and antimatter: The resurgence of immuno-PET. J Nucl Med 50:2
53. McKnight A, Wilkinson D et al (1997) Inhibition of human immunodeficiency virus fusion by a monoclonal antibody to a coreceptor (CXCR4) is both cell type and virus strain dependent. J Virol 71:1692
54. Nimmagadda S, Pullambhatla M, Pomper MG (2009) Immunoimaging of CXCR4 expression in brain tumor xenografts using SPECT/CT. J Nucl Med 50:1124
55. Maeda H, Wu J et al (2000) Tumor vascular permeability and the EPR effect in macromolecular therapeutics: a review. J Control Release 65:271
56. Beatty JD, Beatty BG et al (1990) Mechanisms of tissue uptake and metabolism of radiolabeled antibody-role of antigen: antibody complex formation. Cancer Res 50(3, suppl):840s
57. Jichlinski P, Leisinger HJ (2005) Fluorescence cystoscopy in the management of bladder cancer: a help for the urologist. Urol Int 74:97
58. Witjes JA, Douglass J (2007) The role of hexaminolevulinate fluorescence cystoscopy in bladder cancer. Nat Clin Pract Urol 4:542
59. Herr HW, Donat SM (2008) A comparison of white-light cystoscopy and narrow-band imaging cystoscopy to detect bladder tumour recurrences. BJU Int 102:1111
60. Retz MM, Sidhu SS et al (2005) CXCR4 expression reflects tumor progression and regulates motility of bladder cancer cells. Int J Cancer 114:182
61. Nishizawa K, Nishiyama H et al (2010) Fluorescent imaging of high-grade bladder cancer using a specific antagonist for chemokine receptor CXCR4. Int J Cancer 127:1180

Part IV
Novel Applications

Chapter 22
Potential Use of CXCR4 Antagonists to Mobilize Endothelial and Mesenchymal Stem Cells

Sara M. Rankin*

Abstract In addition to hematopoietic stem and progenitors cells (HSPCs), the adult bone marrow contains a number of other distinct populations of stem cells, including mesenchymal stem cells (MSCs) and endothelial progenitor cells. HSPCs generate a lifelong supply of the cellular components of blood and have been used clinically for over 40 years to regenerate the bone marrow of patients with genetic blood disorders and leukemias. A critical function of MSCs in vivo is in the bone marrow where they support hematopoiesis, regulating the development of HSPCs. MSCs also have the capacity to differentiate into adipocytes, chondrocytes, and osteoblasts and secrete an array of growth factors, prosurvival factors, and anti-inflammatory factors. MSCs have been shown to drive tissue regeneration in the context of orthopedic injuries and heart disease, through their ability to directly incorporate into tissue and through their paracrine effects. EPCs play a role in post-natal vasculogenesis promoting the formation of new blood vessels in ischemic tissues. Therapies that mobilize MSCs and EPCs could, therefore, represent novel regenerative medicines and are the focus of this chapter.

Keywords Chemokines • Stem cells • Bone marrow • Mobilization

---

*Prof. Sara M Rankin has no conflicts of interest to disclose.

S.M. Rankin, PhD (✉)
Leukocyte Biology Section, NHLI Division, Faculty of Medicine,
Imperial College, Room 351, SAF Building, London SW7 2AZ, UK
e-mail: s.rankin@imperial.ac.uk

S. Fruehauf et al. (eds.), *Novel Developments in Stem Cell Mobilization: Focus on CXCR4*, DOI 10.1007/978-1-4614-1960-0_22,

Abbreviations

EOG EPC	Early outgrowth endothelial progenitor cell
HSPCs	Hematopoietic stem and progenitor cells
HPCs	Hematopoietic progenitor cells
HSCs	Hematopoietic stem cells
LOG EPC	Late outgrowth endothelial progenitor cell
MSC	Mesenchymal stem cell
MM	Multiple myeloma
NHL	Non-Hodgkin's lymphoma
VEGF	Vascular endothelial growth factor

Introduction

The adult bone marrow is a reservoir for a number of distinct populations of stem cells, including hematopoietic stem cells, mesenchymal stem cells, and endothelial progenitor cells. Hematopoietic stem and progenitor cells (HSPCs) provide a lifelong supply of blood cells and have been used clinically for many years to perform bone marrow transplants. Endothelial progenitor cells, also present in the bone marrow, are mobilized from the bone marrow into the blood in response to ischemia and recruited into ischemic tissues, where they play an important role in vasculogenesis. Mesenchymal stem cells have been shown to promote tissue regeneration, both through their capacity to differentiate into tissues such as bone and cartilage, but also through their secretion of growth factors, survival factors, and anti-inflammatory mediators.

Cytokines such as G-CSF are used clinically to mobilize HSPCs into the blood for bone marrow transplants. While they have proven to be safe and efficacious, in a proportion of patients and normal donors, classified as "poor mobilizers," G-CSF does not mobilize sufficient numbers of HSPCs to perform a bone marrow transplant. In recent years, the discovery that G-CSF acts by disrupting the CXCR4/CXCL12 retention mechanism has led to the development of CXCR4 antagonists as HSPC mobilizing therapies.

Therapies that mobilize endothelial and mesenchymal stem cells have potential as regenerative medicines. It is thought that by boosting numbers of these stem cells in the blood their recruitment to sites of tissue injury will be increased, thereby accelerating the regenerative process. In this chapter, the focus is on the role of CXCR4/CXCL12 chemokine axis in the mobilization of these distinct populations of stem cells.

CXCL12, CXCR4, and CXCR7

The chemokine CXCL12, originally isolated from supernatants of bone marrow stromal cells, binds exclusively to the chemokine receptors, CXCR4 and CXCR7 [1–3]. CXCR4 is a classical G protein coupled chemokine receptor that activates signaling molecules and pathways to stimulate chemotaxis of both leukocytes and stem cells. By contrast, CXCR7, while exhibiting a very high affinity for CXCL12, does not couple to the signaling pathways driving migration [4]. Indeed, CXCR7 appears to act as a sink for CXCL12, as on binding to CXCR7, CXCL12 is internalized and subsequently degraded [5]. CXCR7 is expressed on endothelial cells and genetic deletion of CXCR7 is embryonic lethal. The CXCR7–/– embryos exhibit aortic and pulmonary valve stenosis, with occasional ventricular septal defects [5–7]. Expression of CXCR7 on endothelial cells has been shown to regulate transendothelial migration of renal progenitor cells and tumor cells and entry of leukocytes into the CNS parenchyma during autoimmune diseases [7–10]. Evidence from elegant studies in the developing zebrafish suggests that expression of CXCR7 is critical to generate CXCL12 gradients thereby allowing migration of germinal stem cells using the CXCL12/CXCR4 chemokine axis [8].

CXCL12 and CXCR4 in HSPC Migration

Long-term maintenance of stem cell populations is dependent on their physical localization in stem cell niches. Within the bone marrow HSPCs are primarily localized within a stem cell niche, which has a specific cellular composition, designed to maintain these stem cells in a quiescent state. When this function is impaired the HSC pool is exhausted prematurely leading to hematological failure. Classically, the HSPC niche was thought to be physically located near the endosteal lining of the bone and osteoblasts were considered key cellular components of the niche. It is now recognized that there is also a vascular niche located in close proximity to bone marrow sinusoids and it is likely that the "mobilizable" pool of stem cells resides in this vascular niche. The chemokine CXCL12 is produced constitutively by ostoeblasts, endothelial cells, and reticular cells, and thus, stem cells in the niche are likely to be exposed to a high concentration of CXCL12 [11–13]. CXCL12 has been shown to inhibit the proliferation of HSCs in vitro, and when the CXCR4 gene was deleted in mice during adult hematopoiesis, the HSCs in the bone marrow became hyperproliferative [13, 14]. Similarly, it was found that in adult mice the loss of CXCL12 in the bone marrow led to proliferation of HPCs at the expense of quiescent HSCs and their relocalization from the endosteal niche to the vascular niches [15]. These studies indicate that under homeostatic conditions CXCL12 plays a critical role in maintaining HSCs in a quiescent state in the endosteal niche.

HSPCs express CXCR4, and it has been shown that CXCL12 is both a potent chemoattractant and prosurvival factor for HSPCs [16–18]. The CXCR4/CXCL12 chemokine axis is critical for migration of HSCs from the fetal liver to the bone marrow during development as this process is defective in CXCR4 and CXCL12 knockout mice [19, 20]. In adult mice, it has been reported that following their injection i.v. the trafficking of HSPCs from the blood back to the bone marrow is inhibited when CXCR4 is blocked with a mAb [21].

HSPCs are known to exit the bone marrow into the blood and then home back to the bone marrow, following a circadian rhythm, and it has recently been shown that this phenomenon can be explained by the change in CXCL12 levels in the bone marrow, with mobilization correlating with low levels of CXCL12 expression [22]. Thus, it appears that CXCL12 is an important retention factor for HSPCs in the bone marrow. Interestingly it has recently been shown that production of CXCL12 is regulated centrally by the sympathetic nervous system and follows a circadian rhythm [22, 23]. Noradrenaline released from sympathetic nerve fibers acts via β2 and β3 adrenoreceptors present on osteoblasts and nestin$^+$ MSCs respectively, to downregulate their production of CXCL12 [23, 24].

Bone Marrow Transplants

A reservoir of hematopoietic stem cells, present in the bone marrow, provides a lifelong supply of blood cells. In bone marrow transplants (BMTs) HSPCs harvested from the bone marrow of a donor can be used to reconstitute the bone marrow of a patient whose bone marrow has been destroyed by irradiation. BMTs have been used successfully for over 40 years to treat patients with genetic blood disorders or leukemias [25–27]. While the original BMTs were performed by directly harvesting bone marrow from donors for transplantation, more recently CD34$^+$ hematopoietic stem/progenitor cell (HSPCs) have been mobilized from the bone marrow into the blood using pharmacological agents, making the process of bone marrow donation far less invasive for the donor. Moreover, there is now scientific evidence that mobilized HSPCs reconstitute the bone marrow more rapidly and result in a lower long-term relapse rate compared to directly harvested stem cells [28]. Further on a practical note, these patients require a shorter period of hospitalization and more reduced costs.

Mobilization of HSPCs with G-CSF

The cytokine granulocyte colony-stimulating factor (G-CSF) is commonly used clinically to mobilize HSPCs for BMTs. Of note, G-CSF does not induce the acute release of HSPCs from the bone marrow into the blood, but requires treatment with G-CSF over 4–7 days. Surprisingly, studies with genetically manipulated mice showed that expression of G-CSFR on HSPCs was not required for their mobilization by G-CSF, implying that G-CSF acts indirectly to mobilize HSPCs (Fig. 22.1) [27, 29]. As neutrophils express G-CSFR it was first thought that G-CSF stimulated neutrophils in the bone marrow reserve to release proteases that would then degrade molecules such as CXCL12 and VCAM that are known to be critical for HSPC retention in the bone marrow [30]. However, subsequent studies utilizing protease-deficient mice did not support this hypothesis [31]. G-CSF treatment of mice results in a marked decrease in both mRNA and protein levels of the chemokine CXCL12 in the bone marrow and thus it was proposed that the CXCL12/CXCR4 chemokine

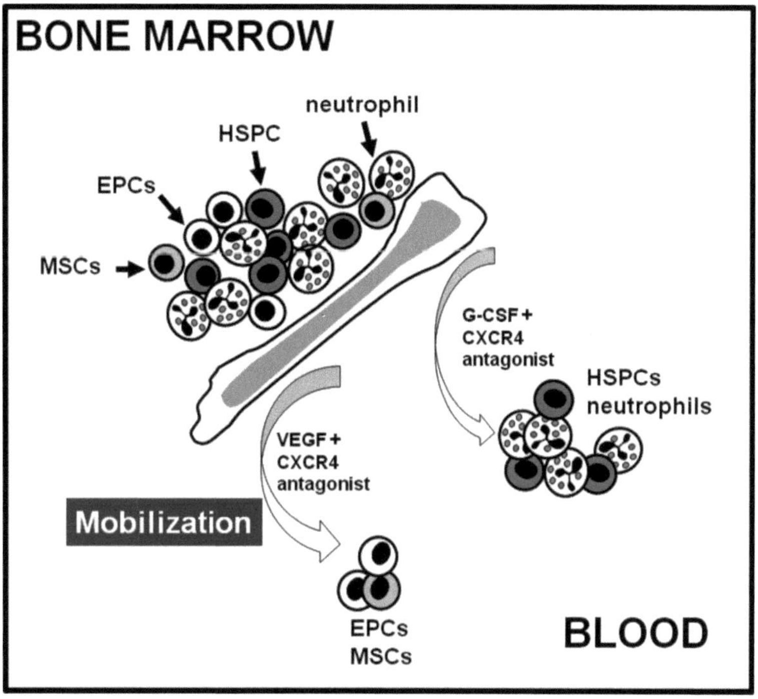

Fig. 22.1 Schematic of differential stem cell mobilization from the bone marrow. Mobilization of hematopoietic stem and progenitor cells (HSPCs), endothelial progenitor cells (EPCs), and mesenchymal stem cells (MSCs) by the CXCR4 antagonist AMD3100 in mice pretreated with either G-CSF or VEGF. G-CSF in combination with the CXCR4 antagonist mobilizes high numbers of HSPCs, and neutrophils and modest numbers of EPCs, but no MSCs. VEGF in combination with the CXCR4 antagonist stimulates the selective mobilization of EPCs and MSCs

axis may be important in the retention of HSPCs in the bone marrow [21, 32–34]. Further studies using the CXCR4–/– chimeric mice supported this hypothesis as in these mice HSPCs were constitutively mobilized into the blood and G-CSF treatment did not further enhance HSPC mobilization [35]. Other distinct studies investigating the role of CD26 in G-CSF-induced mobilization of HSPCs corroborate this view. CD26 is a protease expressed on the cell surface of HSPCs that degrades and thereby inactivates CXCL12. Pharmacologic inhibition or genetic deletion of CD26 has been shown to impair mobilization of HSPCs by G-CSF [36–38]. Following the discovery that CXCL12 production is regulated centrally via the sympathetic nervous system, it was also shown that G-CSF directly activates sympathetic neurons innervating the bone marrow, thereby releasing noradrenaline that acts via β2 and β3 receptors to downregulate CXCL12 production by osteoblasts and nestin^{+} MSCs, respectively [23, 24]. More recently, three independent studies have shown that mobilization of HSPCs by G-CSF is dependent on the monocytic lineage [39–41]. More specifically, evidence is provided that CD68^{+} bone marrow macrophages activated by G-CSF release a soluble factor that downregulates

CXCL12 production by bone marrow stromal cells [39, 40]. In summary, thus far at least three distinct mechanisms have been shown to reduce CXCL12 production and thereby mobilize HSPCs in response to G-CSF: (a) activation of CD26, (b) activation of bone marrow macrophages, and (c) activation of sympathetic neurons innervating the bone marrow. At present, the relative contribution of each of these mechanisms to HSPC mobilization by G-CSF is unclear. However, all studies to date are consistent with the idea that the CXCR4/CXCL12 chemokine axis is critical in the retention of HSPCs within the bone marrow. Identifying this retention pathway has been critically important in the development of novel therapies to efficiently mobilize HSPCs from the bone marrow, for bone marrow transplants, as discussed below.

Despite its extensive use in the clinic for HSPC mobilization in ~20% of patients and normal donors, treatment with G-CSF fails to mobilize sufficient numbers of HSPCs to perform a bone marrow transplant [27]. There is thus a clinical need to develop strategies to further enhance HSPC mobilization.

AMD3100: A CXCR4 Antagonist for HSPC Mobilization

Understanding the critical role of the CXCR4/CXCL12 chemokine axis in the retention of HSPCs within the bone marrow and the mechanism of action of G-CSF in disrupting this pathway to mobilize HSPCs led to the development of CXCR4 antagonists for HSPC mobilization.

One such CXCR4 antagonist is the bicyclam, AMD3100 (Mozobil, Plerixafor). AMD3100 is a short acting competitive antagonist with a half life in normal healthy volunteers of 3.6 h after i.v. injection. In contrast to G-CSF it induces a rapid tenfold increase in circulating numbers of $CD34^+$ cells, beginning after 1 h and peaking at 9 h [42]. In murine models, it was shown that the ability of structural analogs of AMD3100 to mobilize HSPCs correlated directly with their affinity for CXCR4, indicating that AMD3100 is indeed mobilizing HSPCs due to its activity as a CXCR4 antagonist [43].

In murine models and normal volunteers, it was shown that G-CSF acted synergistically with AMD3100, with respect to $CD34^+$ cell mobilization [43–46]. AMD3100 has now been assessed in a number of phase II and III trials for HSPC mobilization in combination with G-CSF in patients with NHL and MM. All trials have shown that AMD3100 plus G-CSF was more effective in mobilizing $CD34^+$ cells than G-CSF alone. Of particular note the clinical trials revealed a high success rate for the AMD3100/G-CSF combination therapy in patients that were poor mobilizers when treated with G-CSF alone. In all of these patients, engraftment of AMD3100/G-CSF-mobilized HSPCs was rapid and durable. As such AMD3100 was approved by the FDA in December 2008, for use in combination with G-CSF for the mobilization of HSPCs in patients with NHL and MM. AMD3100 is currently being evaluated for the mobilization of HSPCs from normal donors for allogenic transplants.

In addition to HSPCs, the adult bone marrow is a reservoir for other distinct populations of stem and progenitor cells including endothelial progenitor cells (EPCs), mesenchymal stem cells (MSCs). These subsets of stem cells are thought to play a role in tissue regeneration.

Endothelial Progenitor Cells

Endothelial progenitor cells (EPC) were first described by Asahara et al [47] as a population of VEGFR2$^+$ mononuclear cells detected in blood following treatment of mice with VEGF, that had the capacity to differentiate into mature endothelial cells in vitro. It was proposed that EPCs mobilized from the bone marrow in response to ischemia may contribute to the formation of new blood vessels (vasculogenesis) in ischemic tissues. Two distinct subsets of EPCs have been described the early outgrowth EPCs (EOG-EPCs) and the late outgrowth EPCs (LOG-EPCs). EOG-EPCs are monocytic cells expressing CD45 and CD115 that form colonies with characteristic spindle shaped cells after only 5 days in culture. EOG-EPCs do not form tubules in matrigel in vitro and are not thought to contribute directly to the formation of new blood vessels in vivo. However, they secrete proangiogenic factors including VEGF-A, CXCL12, and IGF-1, and there is evidence that they contribute to vasculogenesis through a paracrine mechanism [48]. In contrast LOG-EPCs express the endothelial markers vWF, CD31, VEGFR2, and CD34 and importantly do not express monocytic markers. LOG-EPCs form colonies with a characteristic cobblestone morphology after 21 days in culture [48]. Moreover, there is evidence that LOG-EPCs contribute directly to new vessel formation both in vitro and in vivo [48]. The absolute contribution of LOG-EPCs to the angiogenic response seen in either models of ischemia/reperfusion injury or tumor models is variable and appears to be both tissue and disease dependent [49, 50].

Mobilization of EPCs

LOG-EPCs like other HSPCs express CXCR4, and thus, it is likely that they are actively retained in the bone marrow via the CXCL12/CXCR4 retention axis. Indeed, the CXCR4 antagonist, AMD3100, has been reported to rapidly mobilize EPCs from the bone marrow into the blood [51–53]. G-CSF can also mobilize LOG-EPCs into the blood which may be an indirect effect of G-CSF due to its ability to reduce levels of CXCL12 in the bone marrow as EPCs do not express G-CSFR [52]. Further studies with mice under nitrous oxide-deficient conditions have shown that mobilization of EPCs by G-CSF is NO-dependent, while mobilization of HPCs by G-CSF does not require NO. This suggests that discrete molecular mechanisms may regulate the mobilization of EPCs and HPCs [54]. There is also evidence that induction of endothelial-NO synthase (eNOS) plays a critical role in

EPC mobilization by HMG-CoA reductase inhibitors (statins) [55–57]. Mobilization of EPCs by the cytokine erythropoietin (EPO) has been well-documented and has been shown to require activation of endothelial nitric oxide synthase [58, 59]. Numerous groups have reported that VEGF mobilizes EPCs from the bone marrow into the blood and it has been shown that VEGF-A does not affect levels of CXCL12 in the bone marrow or expression of CXCR4, thus mobilization of EPCs by VEGF is not mediated by disruption of the CXCL12 /CXCR4 retention axis. VEGF acting via VEGFR2 directly stimulates EPC migration and therefore may promote EPC mobilization in this way; however, interestingly it has also been shown that VEGF-stimulated mobilization of EPCs is dependent on eNOS [47, 53, 61]. It is clear, therefore, that a wide range of growth factors and pharmacological tools stimulate EPC mobilization through their ability to activate eNOS. What is not clear is how eNOS effects this mobilization. Importantly, in addition to studies in mice, it has also been shown that VEGF-A gene transfer also increases circulating numbers of EPCs in man [60].

Treatment of mice with AMD3100, further enhanced the rate of EPC mobilization in mice pretreated with VEGF, suggesting that such a combination therapy might maximize EPC mobilization [53]. Interestingly this VEGF/AMD3100 combination therapy did not mobilize HPCs into the blood. Indeed it was found that HPCs and EPCs express distinct VEGF receptors, HPCs expressing VEGFR1 and EPCs expressing VEGFR2. Activation of VEGRR1 on HPCs was shown to drive these cells into the G2/S phase of the cell cycle and reduce their migratory capacity, such that they could not be mobilized by the CXCR4 antagonist (Fig. 22.1) [53]. By contrast, mobilization of EPCs is VEGFR2-dependent [53]. We and others have shown that CXCL12 can stimulate EPCs to migrate, and in one study it has been shown that a prolonged increase in plasma levels of CXCL12, produced by administration of CXCL12-expressing adenovirus also mobilizes EPCs into the blood [61].

EPCs express receptors for GM-CSF and it has been shown that GM-CSF can mobilize EPCs in mice and rabbits [62]. The molecular pathways regulating this process have not been defined, but it is postulated the GM-CSF stimulates enhanced EPC motility.

The HSPC niche within the bone marrow has been well characterized and it has previously been shown that modulation of this stem cell niche can impact on HSPC mobilization [63]. While less is known about the nature of the EPC niche, it was recently shown that Wnt signaling antagonist Dickkopf (Dkk)-1 stimulates the mobilization of both HSPCs and EPCs by disrupting the niche. Specifically, it was shown that Dkk-1 induced the osteoclast differentiation factor RANKL, which subsequently stimulated the release of the major bone-resorbing protease cathepsin K [64].

Mobilized EPCs may facilitate postnatal neovascularization in adults and they might therefore be of therapeutic value in diseases where ischemic tissue requires reperfusion around existing occluded vessels in order to regain organ function [47, 48, 65, 66]. Recent elegant experiments using multiple model systems to evaluate angiogenesis in mice confirm that bone marrow stem cells make a significant contribution to neovascularization and that this is dependent on the nature of the extent of the disease. Thus, there is evidence that the more the severe the ischemia the greater the contribution of bone marrow stem cells to the vasculogenesis [67].

Mesenchymal Stem Cells

In adults, mesenchymal stem cells (MSCs) are concentrated primarily in the bone marrow (BM) and adipose tissue [68]. Their principal function in vivo is in the bone marrow where they support hematopoiesis, regulating the development of hematopoietic stem cells and progenitors. MSCs extracted from bone marrow or adipose tissue are plastic adherent cells that have the ability to self-renew and have a high proliferative capacity. MSCs can thus be expanded ex vivo with relative ease. Populations of MSCs are further characterized by their expression of markers including CD73, CD90, and CD105 and importantly are negative for markers of the hematopoietic lineage that include CD45, CD34, CD14, CD11b, CD79a, and HLA-DR. MSCs exhibit robust trilineage differentiation potential into tissues of mesodermal origin (osteoblasts, adipocytes, and chondrocytes), while there are some reports that they can also differentiate into skeletal muscle, smooth muscle, cardiac myocytes, and neurons, although this is somewhat controversial [68]. MSCs secrete an array of growth factors, survival factors, and anti-inflammatory mediators. The evidence to date suggests that MSCs contribute to tissue regeneration both through their ability to differentiate into a range of tissues and through their paracrine effects.

In addition to their regenerative capacity, there is an extensive literature documenting the immunomodulatory effects of MSCs [68, 69]. Ex vivo expanded MSCs have been shown to suppress immune cells both in vitro and in vivo. Specifically, they have been shown to inhibit the activation and proliferation of T cells, block the differentiation of monocytes into dendritic cells, to skew the cytokine profile of macrophages towards an anti-inflammatory M2 phenotype and inhibit antibody secretion by B cells. The immunosuppressive effects of MSCs are thought to be mediated primarily by a paracrine mechanism, for example in the mouse, the expression of nitric oxide (NO) is critical for the immunosuppression of murine T cells while in humans indoleamine 2,3-dioxygenase (IDO) is required for this activity [69].

MSCs are currently being evaluated in animal models and clinical trials for their capacity to promote tissue regeneration, for example following myocardial infarction or in the context of orthopedic injuries and for the treatment of autoimmune diseases, such as acute graft versus host disease [69–72]. Many studies have shown that MSCs delivered intravenously home to areas of tissue injury or inflammation and are effective in promoting tissue regeneration or immunosuppression [70–72]. Current therapeutic use of MSCs relies on their ex vivo expansion and is, therefore, associated with cost, regulatory and technical hurdles. Therapies that stimulate the mobilization of endogenous MSCs from the bone marrow into the blood would provide a cost effective an innovative approach to regenerative medicine, circumventing problems classically associated with stem cell therapy.

Mobilization of MSCs from the Bone Marrow

MSCs have been detection in the circulation in response to tissue injury [73, 74]. This suggests that MSCs in the bone marrow represent a reserve that can be mobilized into the blood in response to specific signals and recruited into damaged tissue to promote tissue repair. Identifying the signals and molecular mechanisms regulating MSC mobilization could lead to the development of novel regenerative therapies. A number of groups have investigated whether MSCs are mobilized from the bone marrow by G-CSF treatment, in both mouse models and man; however, the results have been negative [53, 75, 76]. Further studies in mice confirmed that G-CSF does not stimulate MSC mobilization, but showed that G-CSF stimulated the proliferation of MSCs in the bone marrow through its ability to promote osteoclast resorption [53, 77].

While MSCs have been reported to express high levels of the chemokine receptor CXCR4, administration of the CXCR4 antagonist, AMD3100, did not mobilize MSCs in mice, suggesting that MSC retention in the bone marrow is a tightly regulated process involving a number of distinct mechanisms [53]. Further, AMD3100 did not mobilize MSCs in mice pretreated with G-CSF.

MSCs have been reported to express VEGFR1 and R2 receptors; however, MSCs were not mobilized in mice treated with VEGF alone. By contrast, when mice pretreated with VEGF were administered the CXCR4 antagonist, AMD3100, MSCs were mobilized into the blood (Fig. 22.1) [53]. Thus, mobilization of MSCs requires a combination therapy, suggesting that this process involves a number of discrete molecular steps. Other studies have reported that hypoxia is sufficient to increase circulating MSC levels in rats [78]. The effect of hypoxia is dependent on the activation of HIF-1α probably due to increased levels of VEGF in the bone marrow and CXCL12 in the blood [78].

Together, the data support a model where mobilization of discrete subsets of progenitor cells by the CXCR4 antagonist can be achieved by preconditioning of the bone marrow with different cytokines. Thus HSPCs are maximally mobilized by AMD3100 in mice pretreated with G-CSF, while EPCs and MSCs are optimally mobilized in mice pretreated with VEGF. In terms of G-CSF this preconditioning disrupts the CXCR4/CXCL12 retention pathway, while it is currently not known how VEGF pretreatment augments the mobilization of EPCs and MSCs in response to AMD3100. The coordinated mobilization of MSCs and EPCs may reflect the role both these stem cells have in tissue regeneration. Understanding the molecular pathways regulating the mobilization of MSCs and EPCs is critical when considering progenitor cell trafficking in the context of tissue damage or disease and for the development of novel regenerative therapies.

References

1. Loetscher M, Geiser T, O'Reilly T, Zwahlen R, Baggiolini M, Moser B (1994) Cloning of a human seven-transmembrane domain receptor, LESTR, that is highly expressed in leukocytes. J Biol Chem 269:232–237
2. Balabanian K, Lagane B, Infantino S, Chow KY, Harriague J, Moepps B et al (2005) The chemokine SDF-1/CXCL12 binds to and signals through the orphan receptor RDC1 in T lymphocytes. J Biol Chem 280:35760–35766
3. Burns JM, Summers BC, Wang Y, Melikian A, Berahovich R, Miao Z et al (2006) A novel chemokine receptor for SDF-1 and I-TAC involved in cell survival, cell adhesion, and tumor development. J Exp Med 203:2201–2213
4. Rajagopal S, Kim J, Ahn S, Craig S, Lam CM, Gerard NP et al (2010) Beta-arrestin- but not G protein-mediated signaling by the "decoy" receptor CXCR7. Proc Natl Acad Sci USA 107: 628–632
5. Naumann U, Cameroni E, Pruenster M, Mahabaleshwar H, Raz E, Zerwes HG et al (2010) CXCR7 functions as a scavenger for CXCL12 and CXCL11. PLoS One 5:e9175
6. Sierro F, Biben C, Martinez-Munoz L, Mellado M, Ransohoff RM, Li M et al (2007) Disrupted cardiac development but normal hematopoiesis in mice deficient in the second CXCL12/ SDF-1 receptor, CXCR7. Proc Natl Acad Sci USA 104:14759–14764
7. Zabel BA, Wang Y, Lewen S, Berahovich RD, Penfold ME, Zhang P et al (2009) Elucidation of CXCR7-mediated signaling events and inhibition of CXCR4-mediated tumor cell transendothelial migration by CXCR7 ligands. J Immunol 183:3204–3211
8. Boldajipour B, Mahabaleshwar H, Kardash E, Reichman-Fried M, Blaser H, Minina S et al (2008) Control of chemokine-guided cell migration by ligand sequestration. Cell 132: 463–473
9. Mazzinghi B, Ronconi E, Lazzeri E, Sagrinati C, Ballerini L, Angelotti ML et al (2008) Essential but differential role for CXCR4 and CXCR7 in the therapeutic homing of human renal progenitor cells. J Exp Med 205:479–490
10. Cruz-Orengo L, Holman DW, Dorsey D, Zhou L, Zhang P, Wright M et al (2011) CXCR7 influences leukocyte entry into the CNS parenchyma by controlling abluminal CXCL12 abundance during autoimmunity. J Exp Med 208:327–339
11. Tashiro K, Tada H, Heilker R, Shirozu M, Nakano T, Honjo T (1993) Signal sequence trap: a cloning strategy for secreted proteins and type I membrane proteins. Science 261:600–603
12. Nagasawa T, Kikutani H, Kishimoto T (1994) Molecular cloning and structure of a pre-B-cell growth-stimulating factor. Proc Natl Acad Sci USA 91:2305–2309
13. Sugiyama T, Kohara H, Noda M, Nagasawa T (2006) Maintenance of the hematopoietic stem cell pool by CXCL12-CXCR4 chemokine signaling in bone marrow stromal cell niches. Immunity 25:977–988
14. Cashman J, Clark-Lewis I, Eaves A, Eaves C (2002) Stromal-derived factor 1 inhibits the cycling of very primitive human hematopoietic cells in vitro and in NOD/SCID mice. Blood 99:792–799
15. Tzeng YS, Li H, Kang YL, Chen WC, Cheng WC, Lai DM (2011) Loss of Cxcl12/Sdf-1 in adult mice decreases the quiescent state of hematopoietic stem/progenitor cells and alters the pattern of hematopoietic regeneration after myelosuppression. Blood 117:429–439
16. Broxmeyer HE, Kohli L, Kim CH, Lee Y, Mantel C, Cooper S et al (2003) Stromal cell-derived factor-1/CXCL12 directly enhances survival/antiapoptosis of myeloid progenitor cells through CXCR4 and G(alpha)i proteins and enhances engraftment of competitive, repopulating stem cells. J Leukoc Biol 73:630–638
17. Lee Y, Gotoh A, Kwon HJ, You M, Kohli L, Mantel C et al (2002) Enhancement of intracellular signaling associated with hematopoietic progenitor cell survival in response to SDF-1/ CXCL12 in synergy with other cytokines. Blood 99:4307–4317

18. Aiuti A, Webb IJ, Bleul C, Springer T, Gutierrez-Ramos JC (1997) The chemokine SDF-1 is a chemoattractant for human CD34+ hematopoietic progenitor cells and provides a new mechanism to explain the mobilization of CD34+ progenitors to peripheral blood. J Exp Med 185:111–120
19. Nagasawa T, Hirota S, Tachibana K, Takakura N, Nishikawa S, Kitamura Y et al (1996) Defects of B-cell lymphopoiesis and bone-marrow myelopoiesis in mice lacking the CXC chemokine PBSF/SDF-1. Nature 382:635–638
20. Ma Q, Jones D, Springer TA (1999) The chemokine receptor CXCR4 is required for the retention of B lineage and granulocytic precursors within the bone marrow microenvironment. Immunity 10:463–471
21. Peled A, Petit I, Kollet O, Magid M, Ponomaryov T, Byk T et al (1999) Dependence of human stem cell engraftment and repopulation of NOD/SCID mice on CXCR4. Science 283:845–848
22. Mendez-Ferrer S, Lucas D, Battista M, Frenette PS (2008) Haematopoietic stem cell release is regulated by circadian oscillations. Nature 452:442–447
23. Mendez-Ferrer S, Battista M, Frenette PS (2010) Cooperation of beta(2)- and beta(3)-adrenergic receptors in hematopoietic progenitor cell mobilization. Ann N Y Acad Sci 1192:139–144
24. Mendez-Ferrer S, Michurina TV, Ferraro F, Mazloom AR, Macarthur BD, Lira SA et al (2010) Mesenchymal and haematopoietic stem cells form a unique bone marrow niche. Nature 466:829–834
25. Thomas ED, Lochte HL Jr, Lu WC, Ferrebee JW (1957) Intravenous infusion of bone marrow in patients receiving radiation and chemotherapy. N Engl J Med 257:491–496
26. To LB, Haylock DN, Simmons PJ, Juttner CA (1997) The biology and clinical uses of blood stem cells. Blood 89:2233–2258
27. Cashen AF, Link D, Devine S, DiPersio J (2004) Cytokines and stem cell mobilization for autologous and allogeneic transplantation. Curr Hematol Rep 3:406–412
28. Ringden O, Remberger M, Runde V, Bornhauser M, Blau IW, Basara N et al (2000) Faster engraftment of neutrophils and platelets with peripheral blood stem cells from unrelated donors: a comparison with marrow transplantation. Bone Marrow Transplant 25(Suppl 2):S6–S8
29. Liu F, Poursine-Laurent J, Link DC (2000) Expression of the G-CSF receptor on hematopoietic progenitor cells is not required for their mobilization by G-CSF. Blood 95:3025–3031
30. Levesque JP, Takamatsu Y, Nilsson SK, Haylock DN, Simmons PJ (2001) Vascular cell adhesion molecule-1 (CD106) is cleaved by neutrophil proteases in the bone marrow following hematopoietic progenitor cell mobilization by granulocyte colony-stimulating factor. Blood 98:1289–1297
31. Levesque JP, Liu F, Simmons PJ, Betsuyaku T, Senior RM, Pham C et al (2004) Characterization of hematopoietic progenitor mobilization in protease-deficient mice. Blood 104:65–72
32. Levesque JP, Hendy J, Takamatsu Y, Simmons PJ, Bendall LJ (2003) Disruption of the CXCR4/CXCL12 chemotactic interaction during hematopoietic stem cell mobilization induced by GCSF or cyclophosphamide. J Clin Invest 111:187–196
33. Semerad CL, Christopher MJ, Liu F, Short B, Simmons PJ, Winkler I et al (2005) G-CSF potently inhibits osteoblast activity and CXCL12 mRNA expression in the bone marrow. Blood 106:3020–3027
34. Petit I, Szyper-Kravitz M, Nagler A, Lahav M, Peled A, Habler L et al (2002) G-CSF induces stem cell mobilization by decreasing bone marrow SDF-1 and up-regulating CXCR4. Nat Immunol 3:687–694
35. Christopher MJ, Liu F, Hilton MJ, Long F, Link DC (2009) Suppression of CXCL12 production by bone marrow osteoblasts is a common and critical pathway for cytokine-induced mobilization. Blood 114:1331–1339
36. Christopherson KW 2nd, Cooper S, Broxmeyer HE (2003) Cell surface peptidase CD26/DPPIV mediates G-CSF mobilization of mouse progenitor cells. Blood 101:4680–4686
37. Christopherson KW, Cooper S, Hangoc G, Broxmeyer HE (2003) CD26 is essential for normal G-CSF-induced progenitor cell mobilization as determined by CD26–/– mice. Exp Hematol 31:1126–1134

38. Marquez-Curtis L, Jalili A, Deiteren K, Shirvaikar N, Lambeir AM, Janowska-Wieczorek A (2008) Carboxypeptidase M expressed by human bone marrow cells cleaves the C-terminal lysine of stromal cell-derived factor-1alpha: another player in hematopoietic stem/progenitor cell mobilization? Stem Cells 26:1211–1220
39. Chow A, Lucas D, Hidalgo A, Mendez-Ferrer S, Hashimoto D, Scheiermann C et al (2011) Bone marrow CD169+ macrophages promote the retention of hematopoietic stem and progenitor cells in the mesenchymal stem cell niche. J Exp Med 208:261–271
40. Christopher MJ, Rao M, Liu F, Woloszynek JR, Link DC (2011) Expression of the G-CSF receptor in monocytic cells is sufficient to mediate hematopoietic progenitor mobilization by G-CSF in mice. J Exp Med 208:251–260
41. Winkler IG, Sims NA, Pettit AR, Barbier V, Nowlan B, Helwani F et al (2010) Bone marrow macrophages maintain hematopoietic stem cell (HSC) niches and their depletion mobilizes HSCs. Blood 116:4815–4828
42. Liles WC, Broxmeyer HE, Rodger E, Wood B, Hubel K, Cooper S et al (2003) Mobilization of hematopoietic progenitor cells in healthy volunteers by AMD3100, a CXCR4 antagonist. Blood 102:2728–2730
43. Martin C, Bridger GJ, Rankin SM (2006) Structural analogues of AMD3100 mobilise haematopoietic progenitor cells from bone marrow in vivo according to their ability to inhibit CXCL12 binding to CXCR4 in vitro. Br J Haematol 134:326–329
44. Broxmeyer HE, Orschell CM, Clapp DW, Hangoc G, Cooper S, Plett PA et al (2005) Rapid mobilization of murine and human hematopoietic stem and progenitor cells with AMD3100, a CXCR4 antagonist. J Exp Med 201:1307–1318
45. DiPersio JF, Micallef IN, Stiff PJ, Bolwell BJ, Maziarz RT, Jacobsen E et al (2009) Phase III prospective randomized double-blind placebo-controlled trial of plerixafor plus granulocyte colony-stimulating factor compared with placebo plus granulocyte colony-stimulating factor for autologous stem-cell mobilization and transplantation for patients with non-Hodgkin's lymphoma. J Clin Oncol 27:4767–4773
46. DiPersio JF, Stadtmauer EA, Nademanee A, Micallef IN, Stiff PJ, Kaufman JL et al (2009) Plerixafor and G-CSF versus placebo and G-CSF to mobilize hematopoietic stem cells for autologous stem cell transplantation in patients with multiple myeloma. Blood 113: 5720–5726
47. Asahara T, Murohara T, Sullivan A, Silver M, van der Zee R, Li T et al (1997) Isolation of putative progenitor endothelial cells for angiogenesis. Science 275:964–967
48. Yoder MC, Ingram DA (2009) Endothelial progenitor cell: ongoing controversy for defining these cells and their role in neoangiogenesis in the murine system. Curr Opin Hematol 16: 269–273
49. Critser PJ, Yoder MC (2010) Endothelial colony-forming cell role in neoangiogenesis and tissue repair. Curr Opin Organ Transplant 15:68–72
50. Li Calzi S, Neu MB, Shaw LC, Kielczewski JL, Moldovan NI, Grant MB (2010) EPCs and pathological angiogenesis: when good cells go bad. Microvasc Res 79:207–216
51. Capoccia BJ, Shepherd RM, Link DC (2006) G-CSF and AMD3100 mobilize monocytes into the blood that stimulate angiogenesis in vivo through a paracrine mechanism. Blood 108: 2438–2445
52. Shepherd RM, Capoccia BJ, Devine SM, Dipersio J, Trinkaus KM, Ingram D et al (2006) Angiogenic cells can be rapidly mobilized and efficiently harvested from the blood following treatment with AMD3100. Blood 108:3662–3667
53. Pitchford SC, Furze RC, Jones CP, Wengner AM, Rankin SM (2009) Differential mobilization of subsets of progenitor cells from the bone marrow. Cell Stem Cell 4:62–72
54. Ozuyaman B, Ebner P, Niesler U, Ziemann J, Kleinbongard P, Jax T et al (2005) Nitric oxide differentially regulates proliferation and mobilization of endothelial progenitor cells but not of hematopoietic stem cells. Thromb Haemost 94:770–772
55. Llevadot J, Murasawa S, Kureishi Y, Uchida S, Masuda H, Kawamoto A et al (2001) HMG-CoA reductase inhibitor mobilizes bone marrow-derived endothelial progenitor cells. J Clin Invest 108:399–405

56. Dimmeler S, Aicher A, Vasa M, Mildner-Rihm C, Adler K, Tiemann M et al (2001) HMG-CoA reductase inhibitors (statins) increase endothelial progenitor cells via the PI 3-kinase/Akt pathway. J Clin Invest 108:391–397
57. Aicher A, Heeschen C, Mildner-Rihm C, Urbich C, Ihling C, Technau-Ihling K et al (2003) Essential role of endothelial nitric oxide synthase for mobilization of stem and progenitor cells. Nat Med 9:1370–1376
58. Heeschen C, Aicher A, Lehmann R, Fichtlscherer S, Vasa M, Urbich C et al (2003) Erythropoietin is a potent physiologic stimulus for endothelial progenitor cell mobilization. Blood 102:1340–1346
59. Santhanam AV, d'Uscio LV, Peterson TE, Katusic ZS (2008) Activation of endothelial nitric oxide synthase is critical for erythropoietin-induced mobilization of progenitor cells. Peptides 29:1451–1455
60. Kalka C, Masuda H, Takahashi T, Gordon R, Tepper O, Gravereaux E et al (2000) Vascular endothelial growth factor(165) gene transfer augments circulating endothelial progenitor cells in human subjects. Circ Res 86:1198–1202
61. Moore MA, Hattori K, Heissig B, Shieh JH, Dias S, Crystal RG et al (2001) Mobilization of endothelial and hematopoietic stem and progenitor cells by adenovector-mediated elevation of serum levels of SDF-1, VEGF, and angiopoietin-1. Ann N Y Acad Sci 938:36–45, discussion 45–37
62. Takahashi T, Kalka C, Masuda H, Chen D, Silver M, Kearney M et al (1999) Ischemia- and cytokine-induced mobilization of bone marrow-derived endothelial progenitor cells for neovascularization. Nat Med 5:434–438
63. Kollet O, Dar A, Shivtiel S, Kalinkovich A, Lapid K, Sztainberg Y et al (2006) Osteoclasts degrade endosteal components and promote mobilization of hematopoietic progenitor cells. Nat Med 12:657–664
64. Aicher A, Kollet O, Heeschen C, Liebner S, Urbich C, Ihling C et al (2008) The Wnt antagonist Dickkopf-1 mobilizes vasculogenic progenitor cells via activation of the bone marrow endosteal stem cell niche. Circ Res 103:796–803
65. Nolan DJ, Ciarrocchi A, Mellick AS, Jaggi JS, Bambino K, Gupta S et al (2007) Bone marrow-derived endothelial progenitor cells are a major determinant of nascent tumor neovascularization. Genes Dev 21:1546–1558
66. Yoder MC, Mead LE, Prater D, Krier TR, Mroueh KN, Li F et al (2007) Redefining endothelial progenitor cells via clonal analysis and hematopoietic stem/progenitor cell principals. Blood 109:1801–1809
67. Madlambayan GJ, Butler JM, Hosaka K, Jorgensen M, Fu D, Guthrie SM et al (2009) Bone marrow stem and progenitor cell contribution to neovasculogenesis is dependent on model system with SDF-1 as a permissive trigger. Blood 114:4310–4319
68. Bernardo ME, Locatelli F, Fibbe WE (2009) Mesenchymal stromal cells. Ann N Y Acad Sci 1176:101–117
69. Tolar J, Le Blanc K, Keating A, Blazar BR (2010) Concise review: hitting the right spot with mesenchymal stromal cells. Stem Cells 28:1446–1455
70. Balabanian K, Lagane B, Pablos JL, Laurent L, Planchenault T, Verola O et al (2005) WHIM syndromes with different genetic anomalies are accounted for by impaired CXCR4 desensitization to CXCL12. Blood 105:2449–2457
71. Sung L, Dror Y (2007) Clinical applications of granulocyte-colony stimulating factor. Front Biosci 12:1988–2002
72. King AG, Wierda D, Landreth KS (1988) Bone marrow stromal cell regulation of B-lymphopoiesis. I. The role of macrophages, IL-1, and IL-4 in pre-B cell maturation. J Immunol 141:2016–2026
73. Mansilla E, Marin GH, Drago H, Sturla F, Salas E, Gardiner C et al (2006) Bloodstream cells phenotypically identical to human mesenchymal bone marrow stem cells circulate in large amounts under the influence of acute large skin damage: new evidence for their use in regenerative medicine. Transplant Proc 38:967–969

74. Wang Y, Johnsen HE, Mortensen S, Bindslev L, Ripa RS, Haack-Sorensen M et al (2006) Changes in circulating mesenchymal stem cells, stem cell homing factor, and vascular growth factors in patients with acute ST elevation myocardial infarction treated with primary percutaneous coronary intervention. Heart 92:768–774
75. Lazarus HM, Haynesworth SE, Gerson SL, Caplan AI (1997) Human bone marrow-derived mesenchymal (stromal) progenitor cells (MPCs) cannot be recovered from peripheral blood progenitor cell collections. J Hematother 6:447–455
76. Wexler SA, Donaldson C, Denning-Kendall P, Rice C, Bradley B, Hows JM (2003) Adult bone marrow is a rich source of human mesenchymal 'stem' cells but umbilical cord and mobilized adult blood are not. Br J Haematol 121:368–374
77. Brouard N, Driessen R, Short B, Simmons PJ (2010) G-CSF increases mesenchymal precursor cell numbers in the bone marrow via an indirect mechanism involving osteoclast-mediated bone resorption. Stem Cell Res 5:65–75
78. Liu L, Yu Q, Lin J, Lai X, Cao W, Du K, et al (2011) Hypoxia-inducible factor-1alpha is essential for hypoxia-induced mesenchymal stem cell mobilization into the peripheral blood. Stem Cells Dev 20:1961–1971

Chapter 23
Strategies to Enhance Hematopoietic Stem Cell Engraftment Following Transplantation

Yubin Kang and Nelson J. Chao

Abstract Following intravenous infusion of hematopoietic stem/progenitor cells (HSPCs) during hematopoietic cell transplantation (HCT), HSPCs home to and engraft in marrow niche microenvironment, which ultimately leads to reconstitution of whole immunological and hematological repertoire of the recipient. The homing and engraftment of HSPCs occur relatively early (during the initial stage of HCT), but have major impacts on the success and outcomes of transplantation. HSPC homing and engraftment require well-coordinated interplay involving various cells (endothelial cells, osteoblasts, osteoclasts, and other mesenchymal stem cells), cytokines and chemokines, soluble and membrane-bound factors, as well as extracellular matrix. Many aspects and the detailed mechanisms regulating HSPC homing and engraftment still remain to be elucidated. In this chapter, we first provide a brief overview of HSPC homing and engraftment processes and the interactions between HSPCs and various cell types and different molecules in the niche microenvironment. We then summarize several strategies to enhance HSPC homing and engraftment during HCT. In particular, we present ongoing studies in our laboratories using CXCR4 antagonists to enhance donor cell engraftment following HCT.

Y. Kang
Division of Hematology-Oncology, Medical University of South Carolina, Charleston, SC 29425, USA

N.J. Chao (✉)
Division of Cellular Therapy/BMT, Duke University, 2400 Pratt Street, Suite 1100, Box 3961, Durham, NC 27710, USA
e-mail: chao0002@mc.duke.edu

S. Fruehauf et al. (eds.), *Novel Developments in Stem Cell Mobilization: Focus on CXCR4*, DOI 10.1007/978-1-4614-1960-0_23,

Hematopoietic Stem Cell Homing and Engraftment: A Brief Overview

The homing and engraftment of hematopoietic stem/progenitor cells (HSPCs) are two separate, but intimately connected processes that ultimately determine the success of hematopoietic cell transplantation (HCT). Strategies to enhance hematopoietic stem cell engraftment include those enhancing HSPC homing efficiency. A brief overview of HSPC homing and engraftment and the role of CXCR4/SDF-1 interaction in HSPC homing and engraftment is provided first as a prelude to fully appreciate the development of novel strategies for enhanced HSPC engraftment.

Homing of Hematopoietic Stem Cells

HCT is currently performed by intravenous infusion of HSPCs into a preconditioned-host via a central line. Intraosseus infusion of HSPCs was tested in animal models and in a few medical centers, but has not been widely used in general clinical practice. Following intravenous infusion, HSPCs are initially widely distributed in blood circulation and in multiple organs including lung, kidney, liver, spleen, and bone marrow, but engraftment and hematopoiesis almost exclusively occur in bone marrow (and in spleen in mouse), suggesting that bone marrow provides a unique microenvironment for HSPCs to home to, to reside, and to expand [1]. The process of transplanted HSPC moving out of blood circulation and migrating into bone marrow space is termed as homing, and is a relatively inefficient process. At 24 h after HCT, only approximately 2% of transplanted HSPCs were detected in the bone marrow space [2]. The majority of the infused HSPCs are either sequestrated or extravasated in nonhematopoietic sites such as the lung tissue. These cells will eventually lose the capacity of hematopoietic reconstitution, and are eliminated by apoptosis.

The homing of HSPCs is a multistep process, involving rolling and adhesion of HSPCs on endothelial cells, transendothelial migration and subendothelial migration, interaction of HSPCs with marrow microenvironment, and eventually lodgment of HSPCs in appropriate niches [3]. For individual stem cell, the homing process usually takes a few hours to complete. Homing is not a random event, and transplanted HSPCs are not evenly distributed in the bone marrow space. Bone marrow space is compartmentalized as individual specialized microenvironment, termed as "niche," that provides cellular and molecular support for HSPCs to reside, proliferate, and differentiate [4]. There are two main types of niches: vascular niche in close proximity to the sinusoidal endothelium and osteoblastic niche in endosteal regions [5]. The difference between these two niches is currently not fully understood. It is unclear if these two niches represent two functionally distinct regulatory structures or simply two redundant, functionally overlapping compartments. It also remains to be elucidated whether HSPCs have preferences of homing to one type of niche over the other, and what signals guide this preference. However, studies using intravital animal imaging techniques have demonstrated that transplanted HSCs tended to home to the endosteum and were more frequently detected in the trabecular bone area compared with compact bone area [6]. More recently, it was found that HSCs tend to home to niches containing nestin$^+$ mesenchymal stem cells (MSCs) [7].

HSPC homing is orchestrated by coordinated interplay between HSPCs and endothelial cells as well as between HSPCs and marrow niche microenvironment. Several molecular interactions play critical roles in this process, in particular stromal-derived factor-1 (SDF-1)/CXCR4 [8]; selectins (L, P, and E) [9]; very late antigen-4 [VLA-4 ($\alpha_4\beta_1$)]/endothelial vascular cell adhesion molecule-1 (VCAM-1) [10]; lymphocyte function-associated antigen-1 [LFA-1 ($\alpha_L\beta_2$)]/intracellular adhesion molecule-1 (ICAM-1), etc. The binding of HSPCs to bone marrow endothelial selectins (P and E) and VCAM-1 results in rolling and adhesion of circulating HSPCs to endothelial cells. This adhesion is further enhanced by the interactions between VLA-4 ($\alpha_4\beta_1$)/VCAM-1 and LFA-1 ($\alpha_L\beta_2$)/ICAM-1, which then lead to transendothelial migration of HSPCs toward bone marrow niches. Matrix metalloproteinases (MMP)-2 and MMP-9 degrade basement membrane and facilitate the transendothelial and subendothelial migration of HSPCs. Finally, the ligands of stromal cells and the niche extracellular matrix (VCAM-1, ICAM-1, and fibronectin) interact with HSPC integrins (VLA-4, VLA-5, and LFA-1) and hold HSPCs in the niche. Serum response factor was recently found to be an essential factor in anchoring HSPCs in niche microenvironment [11]. SDF-1/CXCR4 interaction plays an indispensable role in HSPC homing (see below for details).

Engraftment of Hematopoietic Stem Cells

Once HSPCs home to the marrow niches, they seed in the space, interact with the niche microenvironment, and undergo expansion, self-renewal, and differentiation, which ultimately lead to reconstitution of hematopoiesis. This process is termed as HSC engraftment. Successful engraftment requires HSPCs to establish extensive, well-coordinated interactions with niche microenvironment and these HSC–niche interactions influence the self-renewal, quiescence, or survival of HSPCs. Hematopoietic niche microenvironment is comprised of various supporting cells, namely mesenchymal stromal cells, their secreted or membrane-bound factors, cytokines and chemokines, as well as extracellular matrix components.

The cell types that constitute niche microenvironment and support hematopoiesis include osteoblasts, osteoclasts, mesenchymal stromal cells, reticular cells, and endothelial cells. These cells interact with HSPCs through secreted factors or membrane-bound molecules. On the other hand, adipocytes act as negative regulators of niche microenvironment and inhibit hematopoiesis [12]. Several important HSC–niche interactions have recently been demonstrated, which include jagged-1/notch interaction, sca-1/c-kit interaction, and SDF-1/CXCR4 interaction. Additionally, guanine-nucleotide-binding protein stimulatory alpha subunit, membrane-anchored plasminogen activator (urokinase receptor), and N-cadherin are all crucial in HSPC homing, engraftment, and adhesion to the BM microenvironment [13–16].

In addition to proliferation and expansion of HSPCs, another important aspect of engraftment and hematopoiesis reconstitution after HCT is to maintain a portion of HSCs in a quiescent state. HSC quiescence is critical to ensure lifelong hematopoiesis, and there are several factors in the niche microenvironment that act in concert to maintain HSCs in the quiescence state. These factors include osteopontin (a highly phosphorylated sialoprotein in the HSC niche) [17], STAT5 (a mitogenic factor) [18], Grb2-associated binding adapter proteins [19], interferon regulatory factor-2 (a transcriptional suppressor of type I IFN signaling5, 6) [20], p190-B RhoGTPase activating protein [21], and thrombopoietin receptor (Mpl) [22]. Furthermore, endosteal osteoblastic niche is a hypoxic zone of the bone marrow and hypoxia, in part via hypoxia-inducible factor-1alpha, decreases proliferation and favors quiescence [23, 24]. SDF-1/CXCR4 interaction also maintains HSCs in a quiescent state (see below for more details).

Roles of SDF-1/CXCR4 Interaction in Hematopoietic Stem Cell Homing and Engraftment

The interaction between CXCR4 on HSPCs and SDF-1 in bone marrow niche microenvironment plays an indispensable role in the homing of HSPCs following HCT. Following preparatory conditioning regimen, the SDF-1 level in the marrow niche microenvironment is significantly increased, resulting in an increased SDF-1 gradient difference between the marrow niche microenvironment and the blood circulation [25]. This increased gradient of SDF-1 attracts the migration of HSPCs out of sinusoidal vessel and homing to marrow niches [26, 27]. Preconditioning regimen also activates and cleaves complement (C)-3 in the bone marrow and the cleavage fragment product, C3a, enhances HSPC responsiveness of SDF-1 [28]. SDF-1 not only acts as chemoattractant to induce migration of HSPCs, but also enhances HSPC homing by several other mechanisms. For instance, SDF-1 augments CD9 expression on $CD34^+$ HSPCs. CD9 is a member of the tetraspanin family of proteins and has specific functions in HSC homing [29]. Furthermore, the SDF-1/CXCR4 interaction enhances adhesion of VLA-4, VLA-5, and LFA-1 on HSPCs to their endothelial ligands, VCAM-1 and ICAM-1, resulting in firm, shear-resistant attachment of HSPCs to endothelial cells [27, 30]. Additionally, SDF-1/CXCR4 interaction redistributes CD44 expression pattern of HSPCs, facilitating their transendothelial migration to marrow niche microenvironment [31, 32]. SDF-1 also increases extracellular matrix MMP-2 and MMP-9 levels, leading to degradation of base membrane and transendothelial migration of HSPC. Finally, SDF-1/CXCR4 interaction per se not only keeps HSPCs in the niche, but also enhances anchorage of HSPCs by other molecules such as VLA-4/VCAM-1 and LFA-1/ICAM-1 and fibronectin. Annexin-2 in the endosteal niche was recently found to serve as an anchor for SDF-1 to help keeping HSCs to the niche [33].

SDF-1/CXCR4 interaction also plays an important role in survival and maintenance of HSPCs in the bone marrow. At low concentration, SDF-1 acts synergistically with other cytokines promoting HSPC survival and proliferation [34–36]. At high concentration, SDF-1 induces the quiescence of primitive hematopoietic stem cells and thus maintains the HSC pool [37–39]. How SDF-1 maintains the quiescence of HSCs remains to be elucidated, but recent studies suggested that the crosstalk between SDF-1 and transforming growth factor-β (TGF-β) may be important in maintaining the balance between quiescence and proliferation of HSPCs [40].

SDF-1/CXCR4 interaction plays a critical role in HSPC homing and engraftment following HCT [41], and has several biological effects on HSPCs: (1) act as a chemoattractant to induce cell migration; (2) enhance HSPC homing; (3) tether HSCs in the bone marrow niche; (4) arrest the cycling of primitive HSCs.

Strategies to Enhance Hematopoietic Stem Cell Engraftment

Enhancing HSPC homing and engraftment is directly correlated with the success and the improved outcome of HCT. There are several strategies that can be employed to enhance the homing and engraftment of HSPCs.

Strategy 1: To Increase HSPC Homing to Bone Marrow Niches

The initial step during HSPC homing to bone marrow is the binding and rolling of HSPCs to P-selectin and E-selectin expressed on endothelial cells. Human umbilical cord blood $CD34^+$ cells have defects in binding to P-selectin due to inadequate alpha 1–3 fucosylation of selectin ligands. Treatment of umbilical cord blood $CD34^+$ cells with guanosine diphosphate fucose and exogeneous alpha 1–3 fucosyltransferase leads to alpha 1–3 fucosylation of selectin ligands and enhanced HSPC homing and engraftment in bone marrow [42]. This treatment also fucosylates the Notch receptor, leading to activation of Notch signaling and enhanced HSC engraftment [43]. Alpha 1–3 fucosylation of cord $CD34^+$ cells provides a novel approach to improve umbilical cord blood engraftment and is currently under clinical trials in several medical centers [42–44].

SDF-1/CXCR4 interaction activates the phosphatidylinositol-3-kinase (PI3K) signaling pathway. In particular, protein kinase B (PKB/c-akt), the downstream effector of PI3K, regulates HSPC homing through modulation of their adhesive and migratory properties. It was recently demonstrated that transient inhibition of PKB activity enhances HSPC homing in response to SDF-1 gradient [45]. Therefore, manipulation of PKB may provide a novel strategy to improve HSPC homing and engraftment. Hyaluronic acid and thrombin upregulate membrane type 1-MMP and thrombin activates PI3K and Rac-1 signaling pathways. Pretreatment of umbilical cord blood $CD34^+$ cells with hyaluronic acid or thrombin before transplantation improved their homing and engraftment [46], and may offer a novel approach for enhanced stem cell engraftment.

CD26, a surface serine dipeptidylpeptidase IV (DPPIV), is expressed on umbilical cord blood CD34$^+$ cells. CD26 cleaves SDF-1, leading to impaired HSPC homing. Therefore, inhibition of CD26 peptidase activity has the potential to enhance HSPC homing and engraftment. Indeed, pretreatment of cord blood CD34$^+$ cells with Diprotin A, a DPPIV inhibitor, for 15 min significantly enhanced engraftment [47–49].

Dextran sulfate increases plasma SDF-1 levels. In addition, dextran sulfate upregulates a variety of homing-related genes, including those for CXCR4, LFA-1, MMP-9, VLA-4/5, and macrophage inflammatory protein-1. Preconditioning donors with dextran sulfate increases HSPC homing efficiency and offers a novel clinical approach for improving the homing and engraftment of HSCs [50].

Strategy 2: To Provide Supportive Niche Cellular Elements to Enhance Engraftment

MSCs regulate and support hematopoiesis. MSCs provide cellular elements as well as soluble factors or membrane-bound factors for the bone marrow niche microenvironment. Studies have been performed to cotransplant MSCs and HSCs to enhance HSPC engraftment [51–54]. Recently, an open-label, randomized phase II clinical study was performed to assess the outcome of MSC coinfusion (3–5 $\times$ 10^5 cells/kg) during haploidentical hematopoietic stem cell transplantation [55]. A total of 55 patients were enrolled in the study. No immediate or long-term toxic side effects related to MSC infusion were noted, and the median times of white blood cell and platelet engraftment were comparable between the two groups. However, within 100 days, the time to a platelet concentration of >50 $\times$ 10^9 cells/L was markedly faster in the treatment group compared with the control group. Interestingly, serum SDF-1α level rose more rapidly and was significantly elevated in the MSC treatment group compared with the control group. It was thought that co-infusion of MSCs likely exerts therapeutic effects through the release of soluble factors, such as cytokines [56].

Bone marrow vascular endothelial cells constitute as well an important supporting cellular element for the niche microenvironment. Endothelial cells also possess hematopoietic activity and enhance hematological recovery after sublethal or lethal irradiation. Reestablishing endothelial cell activity provides a novel strategy to improve hematopoietic recovery following transplant. In fact, half of lethally irradiated mice that received transplant of endothelial cells alone survived, compared to 0% in untreated mice. The mice that received endothelial cell infusion demonstrated increased marrow cellularity, improved regeneration of hematopoietic stem cells, and enhanced peripheral hematological recovery [57, 58]. Further study demonstrated that VEGFR2-mediated regeneration of sinusoidal endothelial cells is critical to the engraftment and reconstitution of hematopoiesis [59, 60].

Other cell types could also be explored to enhance HSPC engraftment. For instance, CD8$^+$/TCR$^-$ graft facilitating cells (FC) are a novel cell population in bone marrow that have the potential to enhance HSPC engraftment. $CD11c^+/B220^+/CD11b^-$ plasmacytoid-precursor dendritic cell FC subpopulation also facilitate HSPC engraftment using mechanisms different from $CD8^+/TCR^-$ graft (FC) cells [61]. These cells may prove to be useful in facilitating HSPC engraftment [62].

Strategy 3: To Improve HSPC Survival to Enhance Engraftment

HSPCs that do not engraft will be eliminated via apoptosis pathway. Suppressing apoptosis will prolong the pool of circulating HSPCs and increase the chance for engraftment. Indeed, treatment of allogeneic transplant receipt mice with a caspase inhibitor, ZVAD-fmk, led to augmented engraftment of donor HSPCs and greater numbers of colony-forming units of spleen at day-12 [63]. HSPC survival is also in part regulated by receptor tyrosine kinases. Sunitinib, a multityrosine kinase inhibitor that inhibits KIT, enhances HSPC engraftment in mice [64]. Inhibiting apoptosis or improving survival provides a means to enhance engraftment.

The proliferative status of HSCs also affects their "transplantability" and engraftment. Some studies suggest that dividing HSCs are more efficient than resting HSCs in engraftment [65] and in vivo proliferation of HSCs is crucial to hematological recovery following transplantation [66, 67], while others found that proliferating HSCs displayed engraftment defect when transiting $S/G_2/M$ phase [68, 69]. Glycogen synthase kinase-3β (GSK-3β) activates the wingless (Wnt) pathway and induces cell cycle progression. 6-Bromoindirubin 3′-oxime [70], an inhibitor of GSK-3β, delayed cell cycle progression by increasing cell cycle time. Recent data suggest that transient, pharmacologic inhibition of GSK-3β provides a novel approach to improve HSPC engraftment [71].

External signals originating from the niche microenvironment regulate HSC functions and self-renewal capacity. In particular, the calcium-sensing receptor (CaR) plays a crucial role in HSC lodgment and engraftment in the bone marrow endosteal niche. CaR stimulation increases HSPC migration toward SDF-1, and treatment with a CaR agonist, Cinacalcet, increased HSC homing and engraftment [72]. Parathyroid hormone (PTH), either acting directly on osteoblasts, or indirectly through calcium, increases HSC pool and engraftment. Clinical trials of PTH treatment to enhance hematological recovery are currently ongoing in several medical centers [73].

HSPCs express prostaglandin E2 (PGE2) receptors. Treatment of HSPCs with PGE2 increases CXCR4 expression, resulting in enhanced cell migration toward SDF-1. PGE2 increases survivin expression and reduces intracellular active caspase-3, leading to improved cell survival. Transient exposure of HSPCs with PGE2 resulted in increased long-term repopulating cell and competitive repopulating unit frequency in mouse transplantation models. PGE2 is currently being tested in clinical trials as a potential therapy to enhance HSC engraftment following HCT [74, 75].

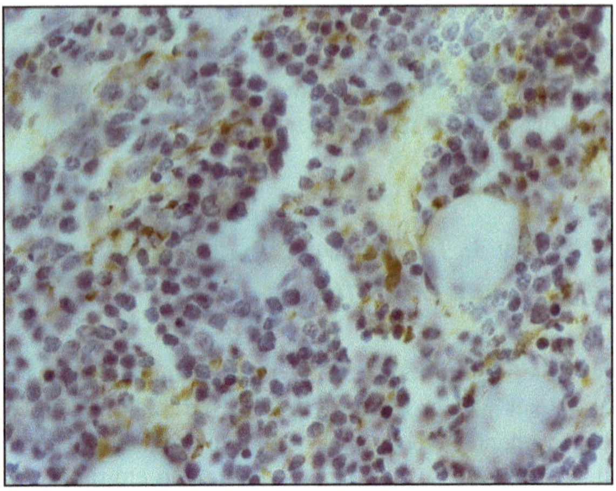

Fig. 23.1 CXCR4 expression in bone marrow. Femur bone from normal C57Bl/6 was harvested, fixed, decalcified, and labeled with CXCR4 antibody by immunohistochemical staining (40× amplification)

Strategy 4: Posttransplant Administration of CXCR4 Antagonists to Enhance HSPC Engraftment

Our laboratories have been exploring the potential of targeting CXCR4/SDF-1 interaction to enhance donor HSPC engraftment following HCT. CXCR4 is expressed on a wide variety of hematopoietic cells, including HSPCs, T cells, and dendritic cells. It was suggested that CXCR4 is also expressed on osteoblasts, endothelial cells, and other MSCs. CXCR4 expression is quite dynamic and the expression level varies with different stages of cell activation or proliferation. Binding of CXCR4 with SDF-1 not only activates several signal transduction pathways important to cell survival and migration, but also leads to downregulation of CXCR4 surface expression. The CXCR4 downregulation is mediated by arrestin binding to the C terminus of CXCR4 and subsequent phosphorylation of the cytoplasmic tail [76–78]. The re-expression of CXCR4 surface receptor is mediated by Pim (proviral insertion in murine lymphoma)-1 kinase phosphorylating Ser339 in the CXCR4 C-terminal domain [70]. At steady state, <5% of bone marrow cells express CXCR4 that are detectable by immunohistochemical staining or by flow cytometry analysis (Fig. 23.1). Further classification and determination of these CXCR4 expressing cells and investigation of the changes in bone marrow CXCR4 expression following HCT are ongoing in our laboratories.

In contrast to the dogma associated with CXCR4 antagonists, we hypothesized that posttransplant administration of a CXCR4 antagonist might actually enhance donor cell engraftment and improve hematological recovery after HCT. Our hypothesis is based upon several rationales: (1) we reasoned that even with lethal total body irradiation, there are still residual HSPCs of recipient origin that reside and occupy the niche spaces. Posttransplant administration of a CXCR4 antagonist could mobilize these cells into circulation and thus free up additional niches for donor HSPCs to engraft. (2) We reasoned that compared to recipient-origin HSPCs that have been exposed to irradiation injury during preconditioning, donor-derived HSPCs possess survival advantages and have greater chances for re-seeding in marrow niches even when they are mobilized with CXCR4 antagonists. (3) The CXCR4/SDF-1 interaction arrests the cycling of HSPCs and maintains HSCs in a quiescent state. We thus reasoned that blocking CXCR4/SDF-1 interaction with CXCR4 antagonists posttransplant would cause proliferation and expansion of engrafted HSPCs, leading to faster hematological recovery. Our last rationale for giving a CXCR4 antagonist after transplant is the possible beneficial effect of posttransplant administration of CXCR4 antagonists on thymic T cell reconstitution. With the mobilization of HSPCs comes the increased efficiency of progenitor cells seeding in thymus and an augmented immunological recovery.

To this hypothesis, we first investigated the effects of posttransplant administration of a CXCR4 antagonist on donor cell engraftment and hematological recovery using a *congeneic* mouse transplant model. We chose to use a specific and reversible CXCR4 antagonist, i.e., plerixafor (Mozobil®, Genzyme, Cambridge, MA, previously called AMD3100). Plerixafor is rapidly eliminated in vivo with an estimated distribution half-life of 0.3 h and a terminal half-life of 5.3 h [79]. Thus, giving plerixafor once every other day results in transient and pulsed blockade of SDF-1/CXCR4. Unlike genetically modified, conditioned knockout mouse models [39], using plerixafor does not permanently block CXCR4/SDF-1 interaction and thus has direct clinical application potential.

We injected sorted c-Kit^{+} Thy1^{low} Lin^{-} Sca-1^{+} hematopoietic stem cells (KTLS cells) from C57BL/Ka *CD45.1* Thy1.1 mice via tail vein into lethally irradiated C57BL/6 *CD45.2* Thy1.2 mice (250 KTLS cells/recipient mouse). Transplanted mice were then injected subcutaneously with PBS control buffer or plerixafor (5 mg/kg body weight) every Monday, Wednesday, and Friday beginning at day +2 posttransplant for a total of 56 days. In our recently published study [25], we found that posttransplant administration of plerixafor: (1) improved animal survival (Fig. 23.2a); (2) selectively enhanced donor cell engraftment (Fig. 23.2b); (3) reduced cytokine storm. We also demonstrated that this enhanced donor cell engraftment resulted from a combined effect of increased niche availability and greater cell division induced by plerixafor [25]. To investigate the effects of posttransplant administration of plerixafor on long-term repopulating HSCs, we performed secondary transplantation. We found that posttransplant administration of plerixafor preserved the long-term repopulating donor HSC pools, which is in sharp contrast to HSC exhaustion observed with conditioned SDF-1 knockout mice where CXCR4/SDF-1 interaction is permanently blocked [39].

These data support our working model as illustrated in Fig. 23.3. Blocking CXCR4/SDF-1 interaction shortly after transplant has several beneficial effects in HCT. (**a**) CXCR4 antagonist will reduce the migration of inflammatory cells and the production of pro-inflammatory cytokines and chemokines, resulting in less tissue injury, attenuated cytokine storm, and possibly reduced acute GvHD. (**b**) CXCR4 antagonist will enhance donor cell hematopoiesis through various mechanisms: (1) mobilizing residual radioresistant host HSCs, thus providing further opening of hematopoietic niches and a selective advantage for engraftment of the healthy donor

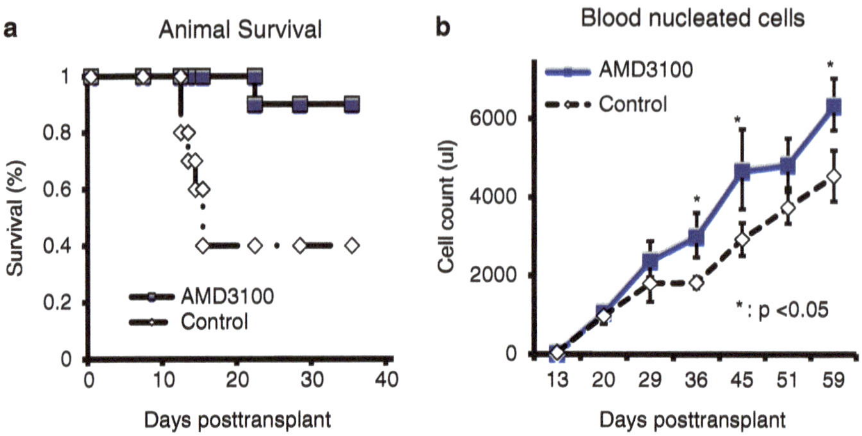

Fig. 23.2 Plerixafor improves animal survival and enhances donor cell recovery in a murine transplantation model. KTLS (c-kit^{+}Thy1.1^{low}Lin^{-}sca-1^{+}) HSC cells from C57BL/Ka *CD45.1* Thy1.1 mice were injected via tail vein into lethally irradiated C57BL/6 *CD45.2* Thy1.2 mice (250 cells/mouse). Beginning at day +2 posttransplant, the mice were injected subcutaneously with PBS control or pleirxafor at 5 mg/kg body weight every Monday, Wednesday, and Friday until day +56. The graphs are representative of three separate sets of experiments with ten mice in each group in each experiment. (**a**) Animal survival curve. (**b**) Blood nucleated cell counts (per μl) (normal range of mouse white cell counts: $1.8-10.7\times10^{3}$/μl). *$p<0.05$. Plerixafor: *blue square*. PBS control: *open diamond*

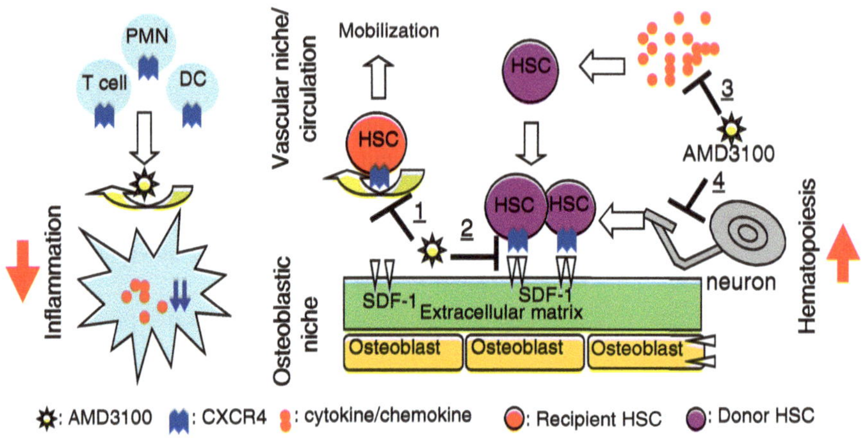

Fig. 23.3 Our rationales and working model for posttransplant administration of plerixafor to enhance donor cell reconstitution

HSCs; (2) reversing the proliferation-inhibitory effect of SDF-1, allowing for the proliferation and expansion of donor primitive HSCs; (3) modulating the levels of cytokines and chemokines in the marrow microenvironment, leading to enhanced hematopoiesis; and (4) modulating the cathecholaminergic nerve function in the

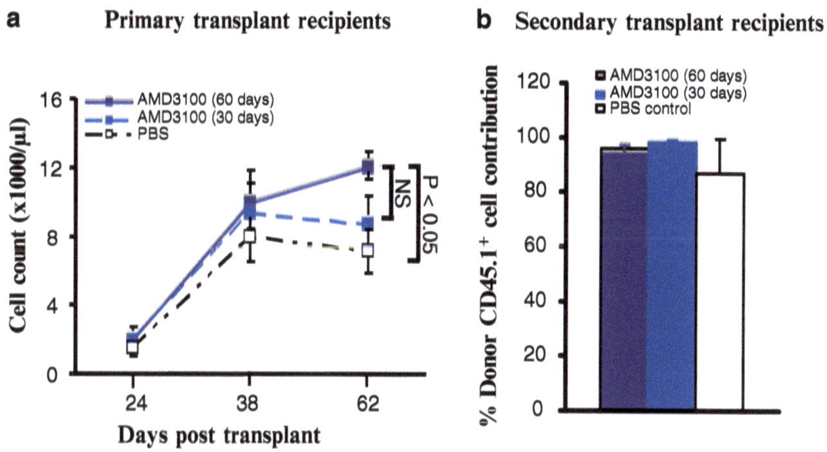

Fig. 23.4 Posttransplant administration of plerixafor enhances hematological recovery in myeloablative allogeneic mouse transplant model and maintains long-term repopulating HSC pool. Balb/C mice were lethally irradiated (8.5 Gy) and injected intravenously with whole bone marrow cells harvested from C57Bl/6 mice (5×10^6 cells/mouse). Plerixafor (5 mg/kg body weight) was administered every other day beginning at day 2 posttransplant for 30 or 60 days. Peripheral blood cell counts were performed at times as indicated (**a**). At 10 weeks after transplant, the mice were sacrificed and bone marrow cells harvested and transplanted into a second recipient mice. At 8 weeks after the second transplant, the mice were sacrificed and the donor-origin $CD45.1^+$ cells in the bone marrow were determined (**b**)

marrow, regulating the crosstalk between hematopoietic system and the marrow nervous system.

To translate our study into potential clinical application, we next investigated if posttransplant administration of plerixafor would enhance donor cell engraftment in lethally irradiated *allogeneic* mouse model. We also wished to test if shorter duration of plerixafor administration (every other day for 30 days) would have the same effect as 60 days injection. In this series of experiments, we used whole bone marrow cells instead of limited number of sorted c-Kit$^+$ Thy1^{low} Lin$^-$ Sca-1$^+$ HSCs. We injected intravenously whole bone marrow cells harvested from C57Bl/6 mice into lethally (8.5 Gy) irradiated Balb/C mice (5×10^6 cells/mouse) and administered plerixafor (5 mg/kg body weight) every other day beginning at day 2 posttransplant for 30 or 60 days. All mice including PBS-injected mice survived the transplant. Similar to congeneic mouse transplantation model, posttransplant administration of plerixafor led to enhanced hematological recovery compared to PBS-injected mice. Giving plerixafor every other day for 30 days posttransplant appears to have the same beneficial effects in enhancing donor hematopoietic recovery as those mice receiving longer treatment (i.e., 60 days) (Fig. 23.4a). Again, posttransplant administration of plerixafor did not impair long-term repopulating HSCs, as demonstrated by secondary transplantation (Fig. 23.4b).

Following our encouraging results observed with posttransplant administration of plerixafor in enhancing donor cell engraftment, one of the immediate logistic steps is

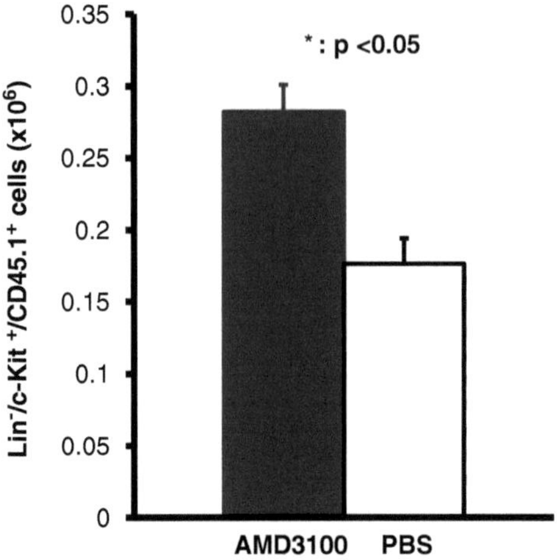

Fig. 23.5 Plerixafor given as part of conditioning regimen enhances donor cell engraftment in myeloablative allogeneic mouse transplant model. Balb/C mice were lethally irradiated (8.5 Gy) and injected intravenously with whole bone marrow cells harvested from C57Bl/6 mice (5×10^6 cells/mouse). Plerixafor (5 mg/kg body weight) was injected subcutaneously at 5 mg/kg body weight on day −1, day 0 (4 h prior to irradiation), and day +1. At 12 weeks after transplant, the mice were sacrificed and bone marrow cells harvested. $Lin^-c\text{-}Kit^+CD45.1^+$ donor-derived HSPC cells were measured and represented as cell number ($\times 10^6$) out of two tibias and one femur of each mouse

for us to test if giving plerixafor as part of conditioning regimen would enhance donor cell engraftment [80]. We hypothesized that giving plerixafor along with total body irradiation conditioning would open up more niches for donor stem cell engraftment. To test this hypothesis, we injected transplant recipient mice with plerixafor subcutaneously at 5 mg/kg body weight on day −1, day 0 (4 h prior to irradiation), and day +1. The recipient Balb/C mice were lethally irradiated with 8.5 Gy and transplanted with 5×10^6 whole bone marrow cells harvested from C57Bl/6 mice. In this particular experiment, we did not observe significant difference in peripheral blood donor cell recovery between plerixafor-conditioned recipients and PBS-injected control recipient mice. However, when we sacrificed the mice at 12 weeks posttransplantation and measured $Lin^-c^-Kit^+$ $CD45.1^+$ donor-derived hematopoietic stem/progenitor cells, we found that plerixafor-conditioned mice had significantly higher number of donor-derived $Lin^-c^-Kit^+$ HSPC cells in the marrow (Fig. 23.5). These data further support the utility of CXCR4 antagonists in enhancing donor cell engraftment.

We finally asked if plerixafor could be used as part of reduced intensity conditioning regimen to enhance donor cell engraftment while reducing cytotoxicities associated with lethal irradiation. In this series of experiments, we used a congeneic mouse transplant model and reduced the total body irradiation dose from 8.5 to 4 Gy. C57BL/6 *CD45.2* Thy1.2 mice were irradiated with 4 Gy and injected with 5×10^6 whole bone marrow cells harvested from C57BL/Ka *CD45.1* Thy1.1 mice. Plerixafor was administered to transplant recipient mice at 5 mg/kg body weight at day −1, day 0, and day +1. As shown in Fig. 23.6, giving plerixafor as part of

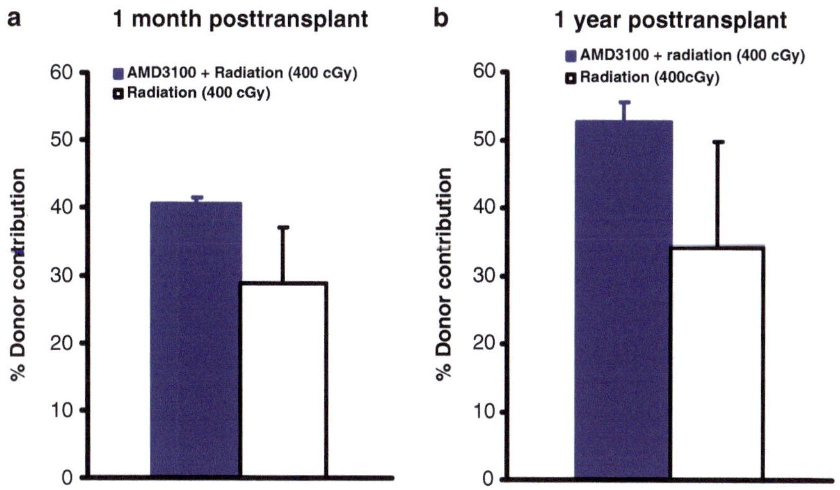

Fig. 23.6 Plerixafor given with sublethal irradiation conditioning enhanced donor cell engraftment in congeneic recipient mice. C57Bl/6 CD45.2⁺ mice were irradiated with 400 cGy and injected with bone marrow cells from C57Bl/6 CD45.1⁺ mice (5×10^6 cells/mouse). Plerixafor was given subcutaneously on day −1, day 0, and day +1. The donor contribution in blood was determined at 1 month (**a**) and 1 year (**b**) after transplantation. Plerixafor: *blue bar*. PBS control: *open bar*

reduced intensity conditioning regimen demonstrated a trend for enhanced donor cell engraftment and recovery. We are currently testing various reduced intensity conditioning regimens including fludarabine/cyclophosphomide in combination with plerixafor for enhanced donor cell engraftment.

Our studies demonstrate the therapeutic potential of CXCR4 antagonist, plerixafor, in enhancing donor cell engraftment in myeloablative and nonmyeloablative, allogeneic, and congeneic mouse transplant models. A clinical trial of posttransplant administration of plerixafor in myeloablative allogeneic transplant patients is currently planned at our two institutions. However, several questions remain to be addressed. First, it remains to be investigated if our findings could be extrapolated to other CXCR4 antagonists including CXCR4 or SDF-1 antibodies, or is only unique to plerixafor. Second, the optimal plerixafor administration schedule needs to be determined. We are currently comparing the effects of various plerixafor doses and durations on donor cell recovery. Third, the effects of posttransplant administration of plerixafor on acute and chronic graft versus host disease (GvHD) need to be investigated as plerixafor inhibits pro-inflammatory cytokine/chemokine production [25]. Finally, the effects of posttransplant administration of plerixafor on mobilization of residual leukemia cells and on graft versus leukemia activity remain to be addressed.

In summary, CXCR4/SDF-1 interaction plays a critical role in hematopoietic stem cell homing and engraftment. CXCR4 antagonists provide a novel strategy to enhance donor cell engraftment and recovery following transplantation. Additional studies are needed to further understand the molecular mechanisms and to translate these findings into clinical practice to improve the outcome and success of HCT.

References

1. Papayannopoulou T, Craddock C (1997) Homing and trafficking of hemopoietic progenitor cells. Acta Haematol 97:97–104
2. Feng Q, Chow PK, Frassoni F, Phua CM, Tan PK et al (2008) Nonhuman primate allogeneic hematopoietic stem cell transplantation by intraosseus vs intravenous injection: Engraftment, donor cell distribution, and mechanistic basis. Exp Hematol 36:1556–1566
3. Sharma M, Afrin F, Satija N, Tripathi RP, Gangenahalli GU (2011) Stromal-derived factor-1/CXCR4 signaling: indispensable role in homing and engraftment of hematopoietic stem cells in bone marrow. Stem Cells Dev 20(6):933–946
4. Li L, Xie T (2005) Stem cell niche: structure and function. Annu Rev Cell Dev Biol 21: 605–631
5. Oh IH, Kwon KR (2010) Concise review: multiple niches for hematopoietic stem cell regulations. Stem Cells 28:1243–1249
6. Xie Y, Yin T, Wiegraebe W, He XC, Miller D et al (2009) Detection of functional haematopoietic stem cell niche using real-time imaging. Nature 457:97–101
7. Mendez-Ferrer S, Michurina TV, Ferraro F, Mazloom AR, Macarthur BD et al (2010) Mesenchymal and haematopoietic stem cells form a unique bone marrow niche. Nature 466:829–834
8. Lapidot T, Dar A, Kollet O (2005) How do stem cells find their way home? Blood 106: 1901–1910
9. Mazo IB, Gutierrez-Ramos JC, Frenette PS, Hynes RO, Wagner DD et al (1998) Hematopoietic progenitor cell rolling in bone marrow microvessels: parallel contributions by endothelial selectins and vascular cell adhesion molecule 1. J Exp Med 188:465–474
10. Frenette PS, Subbarao S, Mazo IB, von Andrian UH, Wagner DD (1998) Endothelial selectins and vascular cell adhesion molecule-1 promote hematopoietic progenitor homing to bone marrow. Proc Natl Acad Sci USA 95:14423–14428
11. Ragu C, Elain G, Mylonas E, Ottolenghi C, Cagnard N et al (2010) The transcription factor Srf regulates hematopoietic stem cell adhesion. Blood 116:4464–4473
12. Naveiras O, Nardi V, Wenzel PL, Hauschka PV, Fahey F et al (2009) Bone-marrow adipocytes as negative regulators of the haematopoietic microenvironment. Nature 460:259–263
13. Adams GB, Alley IR, Chung UI, Chabner KT, Jeanson NT et al (2009) Haematopoietic stem cells depend on Galpha(s)-mediated signalling to engraft bone marrow. Nature 459:103–107
14. Tjwa M, Sidenius N, Moura R, Jansen S, Theunissen K et al (2009) Membrane-anchored uPAR regulates the proliferation, marrow pool size, engraftment, and mobilization of mouse hematopoietic stem/progenitor cells. J Clin Invest 119:1008–1018
15. Hosokawa K, Arai F, Yoshihara H, Iwasaki H, Hembree M et al (2010) Cadherin-based adhesion is a potential target for niche manipulation to protect hematopoietic stem cells in adult bone marrow. Cell Stem Cell 6:194–198
16. Hosokawa K, Arai F, Yoshihara H, Iwasaki H, Nakamura Y et al (2010) Knockdown of N-cadherin suppresses the long-term engraftment of hematopoietic stem cells. Blood 116:554–563
17. Nilsson SK, Johnston HM, Whitty GA, Williams B, Webb RJ et al (2005) Osteopontin, a key component of the hematopoietic stem cell niche and regulator of primitive hematopoietic progenitor cells. Blood 106:1232–1239
18. Wang Z, Li G, Tse W, Bunting KD (2009) Conditional deletion of STAT5 in adult mouse hematopoietic stem cells causes loss of quiescence and permits efficient nonablative stem cell replacement. Blood 113:4856–4865
19. Li G, Wang Z, Miskimen KL, Zhang Y, Tse W et al (2010) Gab2 promotes hematopoietic stem cell maintenance and self-renewal synergistically with STAT5. PLoS One 5:e9152
20. Sato T, Onai N, Yoshihara H, Arai F, Suda T et al (2009) Interferon regulatory factor-2 protects quiescent hematopoietic stem cells from type I interferon-dependent exhaustion. Nat Med 15:696–700

21. Xu H, Eleswarapu S, Geiger H, Szczur K, Daria D et al (2009) Loss of the Rho GTPase activating protein p190-B enhances hematopoietic stem cell engraftment potential. Blood 114:3557–3566
22. Yoshihara H, Arai F, Hosokawa K, Hagiwara T, Takubo K et al (2007) Thrombopoietin/MPL signaling regulates hematopoietic stem cell quiescence and interaction with the osteoblastic niche. Cell Stem Cell 1:685–697
23. Eliasson P, Rehn M, Hammar P, Larsson P, Sirenko O et al (2010) Hypoxia mediates low cell-cycle activity and increases the proportion of long-term-reconstituting hematopoietic stem cells during in vitro culture. Exp Hematol 38:301–310.e302
24. Takubo K, Goda N, Yamada W, Iriuchishima H, Ikeda E et al (2010) Regulation of the HIF-1alpha level is essential for hematopoietic stem cells. Cell Stem Cell 7:391–402
25. Kang Y, Chen BJ, Deoliveira D, Mito J, Chao NJ (2010) Selective enhancement of donor hematopoietic cell engraftment by the CXCR4 antagonist AMD3100 in a mouse transplantation model. PLoS One 5:e11316
26. Hart C, Drewel D, Mueller G, Grassinger J, Zaiss M et al (2004) Expression and function of homing-essential molecules and enhanced in vivo homing ability of human peripheral blood-derived hematopoietic progenitor cells after stimulation with stem cell factor. Stem Cells 22:580–589
27. Ponomaryov T, Peled A, Petit I, Taichman RS, Habler L et al (2000) Induction of the chemokine stromal-derived factor-1 following DNA damage improves human stem cell function. J Clin Invest 106:1331–1339
28. Wysoczynski M, Reca R, Lee H, Wu W, Ratajczak J et al (2009) Defective engraftment of C3aR–/– hematopoietic stem progenitor cells shows a novel role of the C3a-C3aR axis in bone marrow homing. Leukemia 23:1455–1461
29. Leung KT, Chan KY, Ng PC, Lau TK, Chiu WM et al (2011) The tetraspanin CD9 regulates migration, adhesion, and homing of human cord blood CD34+ hematopoietic stem and progenitor cells. Blood 117:1840–1850
30. Peled A, Kollet O, Ponomaryov T, Petit I, Franitza S et al (2000) The chemokine SDF-1 activates the integrins LFA-1, VLA-4, and VLA-5 on immature human CD34(+) cells: role in transendothelial/stromal migration and engraftment of NOD/SCID mice. Blood 95:3289–3296
31. Avigdor A, Goichberg P, Shivtiel S, Dar A, Peled A et al (2004) CD44 and hyaluronic acid cooperate with SDF-1 in the trafficking of human CD34+ stem/progenitor cells to bone marrow. Blood 103:2981–2989
32. Nilsson SK, Haylock DN, Johnston HM, Occhiodoro T, Brown TJ et al (2003) Hyaluronan is synthesized by primitive hemopoietic cells, participates in their lodgment at the endosteum following transplantation, and is involved in the regulation of their proliferation and differentiation in vitro. Blood 101:856–862
33. Jung Y, Shiozawa Y, Wang J, Patel LR, Havens AM et al (2011) Annexin-2 is a regulator of stromal cell-derived factor-1/CXCL12 function in the hematopoietic stem cell endosteal niche. Exp Hematol 39:151–166.e151
34. Porecha NK, English K, Hangoc G, Broxmeyer HE, Christopherson KW 2nd (2006) Enhanced functional response to CXCL12/SDF-1 through retroviral overexpression of CXCR4 on M07e cells: implications for hematopoietic stem cell transplantation. Stem Cells Dev 15:325–333
35. Broxmeyer HE, Cooper S, Kohli L, Hangoc G, Lee Y et al (2003) Transgenic expression of stromal cell-derived factor-1/CXC chemokine ligand 12 enhances myeloid progenitor cell survival/antiapoptosis in vitro in response to growth factor withdrawal and enhances myelopoiesis in vivo. J Immunol 170:421–429
36. Lee Y, Gotoh A, Kwon HJ, You M, Kohli L et al (2002) Enhancement of intracellular signaling associated with hematopoietic progenitor cell survival in response to SDF-1/CXCL12 in synergy with other cytokines. Blood 99:4307–4317
37. Cashman J, Clark-Lewis I, Eaves A, Eaves C (2002) Stromal-derived factor 1 inhibits the cycling of very primitive human hematopoietic cells in vitro and in NOD/SCID mice. Blood 99:792–799
38. Cashman J, Dykstra B, Clark-Lewis I, Eaves A, Eaves C (2002) Changes in the proliferative activity of human hematopoietic stem cells in NOD/SCID mice and enhancement of their transplantability after in vivo treatment with cell cycle inhibitors. J Exp Med 196:1141–1150

39. Tzeng YS, Li H, Kang YL, Chen WC, Cheng WC et al (2011) Loss of Cxcl12/Sdf-1 in adult mice decreases the quiescent state of hematopoietic stem/progenitor cells and alters the pattern of hematopoietic regeneration after myelosuppression. Blood 117:429–439
40. Chabanon A, Desterke C, Rodenburger E, Clay D, Guerton B et al (2008) A cross-talk between stromal cell-derived factor-1 and transforming growth factor-beta controls the quiescence/cycling switch of CD34(+) progenitors through FoxO3 and mammalian target of rapamycin. Stem Cells 26:3150–3161
41. Peled A, Petit I, Kollet O, Magid M, Ponomaryov T et al (1999) Dependence of human stem cell engraftment and repopulation of NOD/SCID mice on CXCR4. Science 283:845–848
42. Xia L, McDaniel JM, Yago T, Doeden A, McEver RP (2004) Surface fucosylation of human cord blood cells augments binding to P-selectin and E-selectin and enhances engraftment in bone marrow. Blood 104:3091–3096
43. Myers J, Huang Y, Wei L, Yan Q, Huang A et al (2010) Fucose-deficient hematopoietic stem cells have decreased self-renewal and aberrant marrow niche occupancy. Transfusion 50:2660–2669
44. Taupin P (2010) Ex vivo fucosylation to improve the engraftment capability and therapeutic potential of human cord blood stem cells. Drug Discov Today 15:698–699
45. Buitenhuis M, van der Linden E, Ulfman LH, Hofhuis FM, Bierings MB et al (2010) Protein kinase B (PKB/c-akt) regulates homing of hematopoietic progenitors through modulation of their adhesive and migratory properties. Blood 116:2373–2384
46. Shirvaikar N, Marquez-Curtis LA, Ratajczak MZ, Janowska-Wieczorek A (2011) Hyaluronic acid and thrombin upregulate MT1-MMP through PI3K and Rac-1 signaling and prime the homing-related responses of cord blood hematopoietic stem/progenitor cells. Stem Cells Dev 20:19–30
47. Campbell TB, Hangoc G, Liu Y, Pollok K, Broxmeyer HE (2007) Inhibition of CD26 in human cord blood CD34+ cells enhances their engraftment of nonobese diabetic/severe combined immunodeficiency mice. Stem Cells Dev 16:347–354
48. Christopherson KW 2nd, Paganessi LA, Napier S, Porecha NK (2007) CD26 inhibition on CD34+ or lineage-human umbilical cord blood donor hematopoietic stem cells/hematopoietic progenitor cells improves long-term engraftment into NOD/SCID/Beta2null immunodeficient mice. Stem Cells Dev 16:355–360
49. Peranteau WH, Endo M, Adibe OO, Merchant A, Zoltick PW et al (2006) CD26 inhibition enhances allogeneic donor-cell homing and engraftment after in utero hematopoietic-cell transplantation. Blood 108:4268–4274
50. Hayakawa J, Migita M, Ueda T, Fukazawa R, Adachi K et al (2009) Dextran sulfate and stromal cell derived factor-1 promote CXCR4 expression and improve bone marrow homing efficiency of infused hematopoietic stem cells. J Nippon Med Sch 76:198–208
51. Le Blanc K, Samuelsson H, Gustafsson B, Remberger M, Sundberg B et al (2007) Transplantation of mesenchymal stem cells to enhance engraftment of hematopoietic stem cells. Leukemia 21:1733–1738
52. Ball LM, Bernardo ME, Roelofs H, Lankester A, Cometa A et al (2007) Cotransplantation of ex vivo expanded mesenchymal stem cells accelerates lymphocyte recovery and may reduce the risk of graft failure in haploidentical hematopoietic stem-cell transplantation. Blood 110:2764–2767
53. Macmillan ML, Blazar BR, DeFor TE, Wagner JE (2009) Transplantation of ex-vivo culture-expanded parental haploidentical mesenchymal stem cells to promote engraftment in pediatric recipients of unrelated donor umbilical cord blood: results of a phase I-II clinical trial. Bone Marrow Transplant 43:447–454
54. Gonzalo-Daganzo R, Regidor C, Martin-Donaire T, Rico MA, Bautista G et al (2009) Results of a pilot study on the use of third-party donor mesenchymal stromal cells in cord blood transplantation in adults. Cytotherapy 11:278–288
55. Liu K, Chen Y, Zeng Y, Xu L, Liu D et al (2011) Coinfusion of mesenchymal stromal cells facilitates platelet recovery without increasing leukemia recurrence in haploidentical hematopoietic stem cell transplantation: a randomized, controlled clinical study. Stem Cells Dev 20(11):1679–1685

56. Horwitz EM, Prather WR (2009) Cytokines as the major mechanism of mesenchymal stem cell clinical activity: expanding the spectrum of cell therapy. Isr Med Assoc J 11:209–211
57. Chute JP, Muramoto GG, Salter AB, Meadows SK, Rickman DW et al (2007) Transplantation of vascular endothelial cells mediates the hematopoietic recovery and survival of lethally irradiated mice. Blood 109:2365–2372
58. Salter AB, Meadows SK, Muramoto GG, Himburg H, Doan P et al (2009) Endothelial progenitor cell infusion induces hematopoietic stem cell reconstitution in vivo. Blood 113:2104–2107
59. Hooper AT, Butler JM, Nolan DJ, Kranz A, Iida K et al (2009) Engraftment and reconstitution of hematopoiesis is dependent on VEGFR2-mediated regeneration of sinusoidal endothelial cells. Cell Stem Cell 4:263–274
60. Porter RL, Calvi LM (2009) Key endothelial signals required for hematopoietic recovery. Cell Stem Cell 4:187–188
61. Huang Y, Bozulic LD, Miller T, Xu H, Hussain LR et al (2011) CD8α+ plasmacytoid precursor DCs induce antigen-specific regulatory T cells that enhance HSC engraftment in vivo. Blood 117:2494–2505
62. Dominici M, Rasini V, Bussolari R, Chen X, Hofmann TJ et al (2009) Restoration and reversible expansion of the osteoblastic hematopoietic stem cell niche after marrow radioablation. Blood 114:2333–2343
63. Imai Y, Adachi Y, Shi M, Shima C, Yanai S et al (2010) Caspase inhibitor ZVAD-fmk facilitates engraftment of donor hematopoietic stem cells in intra-bone marrow-bone marrow transplantation. Stem Cells Dev 19:461–468
64. Fewkes NM, Krauss AC, Guimond M, Meadors JL, Dobre S et al (2010) Pharmacologic modulation of niche accessibility via tyrosine kinase inhibition enhances marrow and thymic engraftment after hematopoietic stem cell transplantation. Blood 115:4120–4129
65. Zhong JF, Zhan Y, Anderson WF, Zhao Y (2002) Murine hematopoietic stem cell distribution and proliferation in ablated and nonablated bone marrow transplantation. Blood 100:3521–3526
66. Verfaillie CM (2002) Optimizing hematopoietic stem cell engraftment: a novel role for thrombopoietin. J Clin Invest 110:303–304
67. Fox N, Priestley G, Papayannopoulou T, Kaushansky K (2002) Thrombopoietin expands hematopoietic stem cells after transplantation. J Clin Invest 110:389–394
68. Bowie MB, McKnight KD, Kent DG, McCaffrey L, Hoodless PA et al (2006) Hematopoietic stem cells proliferate until after birth and show a reversible phase-specific engraftment defect. J Clin Invest 116:2808–2816
69. Gothot A, van der Loo JCM, Clapp DW, Srour EF (1998) Cell cycle-related changes in repopulating capacity of human mobilized peripheral blood CD34+ cells in non-obese diabetic/severe combined immune-deficient mice. Blood 92:2641–2649
70. Grundler R, Brault L, Gasser C, Bullock AN, Dechow T et al (2009) Dissection of PIM serine/threonine kinases in FLT3-ITD-induced leukemogenesis reveals PIM1 as regulator of CXCL12-CXCR4-mediated homing and migration. J Exp Med 206:1957–1970
71. Ko KH, Holmes T, Palladinetti P, Song E, Nordon R et al (2011) GSK-3beta inhibition promotes engraftment of ex vivo-expanded hematopoietic stem cells and modulates gene expression. Stem Cells 29:108–118
72. Lam BS, Cunningham C, Adams GB (2011) Pharmacologic modulation of the calcium-sensing receptor enhances hematopoietic stem cell lodgment in the adult bone marrow. Blood 117:1167–1175
73. Rashidi N, Adams GB (2009) The influence of parathyroid hormone on the adult hematopoietic stem cell niche. Curr Osteoporos Rep 7:53–57
74. Durand EM, Zon LI (2010) Newly emerging roles for prostaglandin E2 regulation of hematopoiesis and hematopoietic stem cell engraftment. Curr Opin Hematol 17:308–312
75. Hoggatt J, Singh P, Sampath J, Pelus LM (2009) Prostaglandin E2 enhances hematopoietic stem cell homing, survival, and proliferation. Blood 113:5444–5455
76. Wong D, Korz W (2008) Translating an antagonist of chemokine receptor CXCR4: from bench to bedside. Clin Cancer Res 14:7975–7980

77. Rahimi M, George J, Tang C (2010) EGFR variant-mediated invasion by enhanced CXCR4 expression through transcriptional and post-translational mechanisms. Int J Cancer 126: 1850–1860
78. Bhandari D, Trejo J, Benovic JL, Marchese A (2007) Arrestin-2 interacts with the ubiquitin-protein isopeptide ligase atrophin-interacting protein 4 and mediates endosomal sorting of the chemokine receptor CXCR4. J Biol Chem 282:36971–36979
79. Genzyme (2009) Plerixafor injection investigator's brochure. Version 13, 27 May 2009, p 13
80. Chen J, Larochelle A, Fricker S, Bridger G, Dunbar CE et al (2006) Mobilization as a preparative regimen for hematopoietic stem cell transplantation. Blood 107:3764–3771

Chapter 24
Mobilization for Gene Therapy

Andre Larochelle and Cynthia E. Dunbar

Hematopoietic Stem Cell Gene Therapy

Hematopoietic Stem Cells as Targets for Gene Therapy

Hematopoietic stem cells (HSCs) are defined by their ability to regenerate all blood lineages, over extended periods of time, after transplantation. HSCs have the unique constellation of both self-renewal and proliferation with differentiation into multiple distinct mature cell types. Over the past five decades, analysis of these properties has led to the general view of a blood-forming system organized in a unidirectional hierarchy: rare, infrequently cycling pluripotent HSCs, a larger population of more restricted progenitor and precursor cells, and a vast pool of mature cells with defined functions (Fig. 24.1). Therefore, to achieve permanent correction of inherited or acquired disorders by gene transfer, the target cells must be the human HSCs; mature cells and committed progenitors do not have the proliferative capacity for long-term reconstitution of the entire hematopoietic system.

Approach to Gene Therapy Targeting Hematopoietic Stem Cells

At present, gene transfer to HSCs has been achieved mainly using vectors derived from wild-type, replication-competent retroviruses from which part of the genome has been removed, leaving space for insertion of a new gene. Mimicking the natural

A. Larochelle (✉) • C.E. Dunbar
Molecular Hematopoiesis Section, Hematology Branch, National Heart,
Lung and Blood Institute, National Institutes of Health, 9000 Rockville Pike,
Building 10CRC, Rm 3E-5256, Bethesda, MD 20892, USA
e-mail: larochea@nhlbi.nih.gov

S. Fruehauf et al. (eds.), *Novel Developments in Stem Cell Mobilization: Focus on CXCR4*, DOI 10.1007/978-1-4614-1960-0_24,

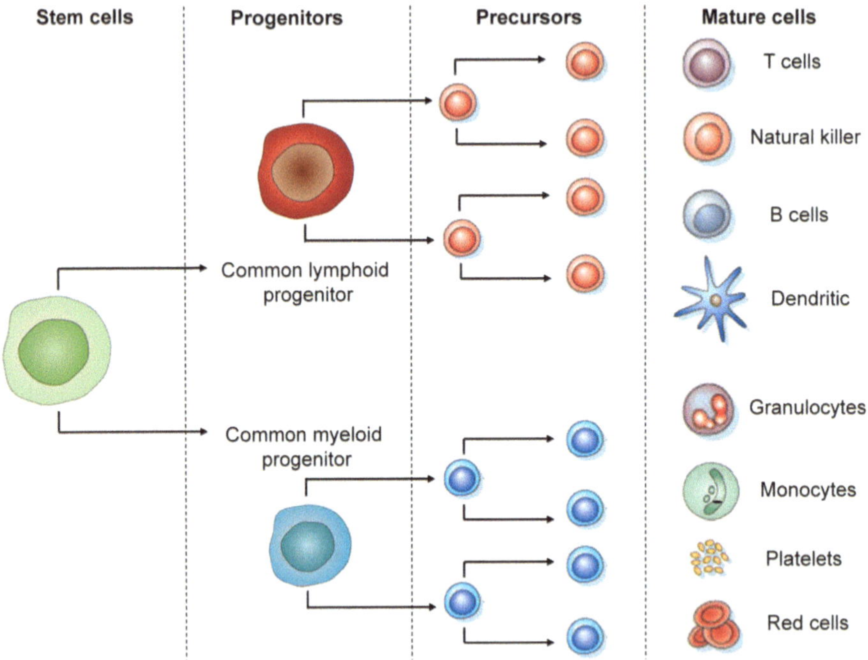

Fig. 24.1 The hematopoietic system. Hematopoietic stem cells are rare immature cells capable of self-renewal and of giving rise to all types of mature specialized cells. They are ideal targets for gene therapy applications. Progenitor and precursor cells are intermediate populations between stem cells and mature cells

life cycle of retroviruses, these vectors can stably integrate their transgene into the genomic DNA of the infected cells. All approved clinical HSC gene therapy trials to date have used modified retroviruses, namely gammaretroviruses [such as Moloney murine leukemia virus (MMLV)] and lentiviruses [such as human immunodeficiency virus type 1 (HIV-1)].

The outline of all current HSC clinical gene therapy approaches is similar (Fig. 24.2). Hematopoietic stem and progenitor cells are collected by bone marrow (BM) harvest or granulocyte-colony stimulating factor (G-CSF)-induced mobilization, and enriched for cells expressing the CD34 cell surface marker. The CD34⁺ cells are subsequently cultured with retroviral vectors expressing the desired therapeutic gene. With MMLV-based retroviral vectors, the best results occur when cells are exposed to the vectors for 72–96 h in the presence of cytokines [stem cell factor (SCF), thrombopoietin (TPO), and *fms*-like tyrosine kinase 3 ligand (Flt3-L)] [1] on a surface coated with the C-terminal fragment of fibronectin [2]. Fibronectin mimics the BM microenvironment's scaffolding, preserving the viability and engraftment potential of the HSCs, and enhancing transduction via colocalization of vectors and target cells [3]. With HIV-1-based retroviral vectors, similar conditions are used for most efficient transduction of human CD34⁺ cells, but exposure of cells to the vectors for only 24–48 h is sufficient. Transduced cells are then intravenously

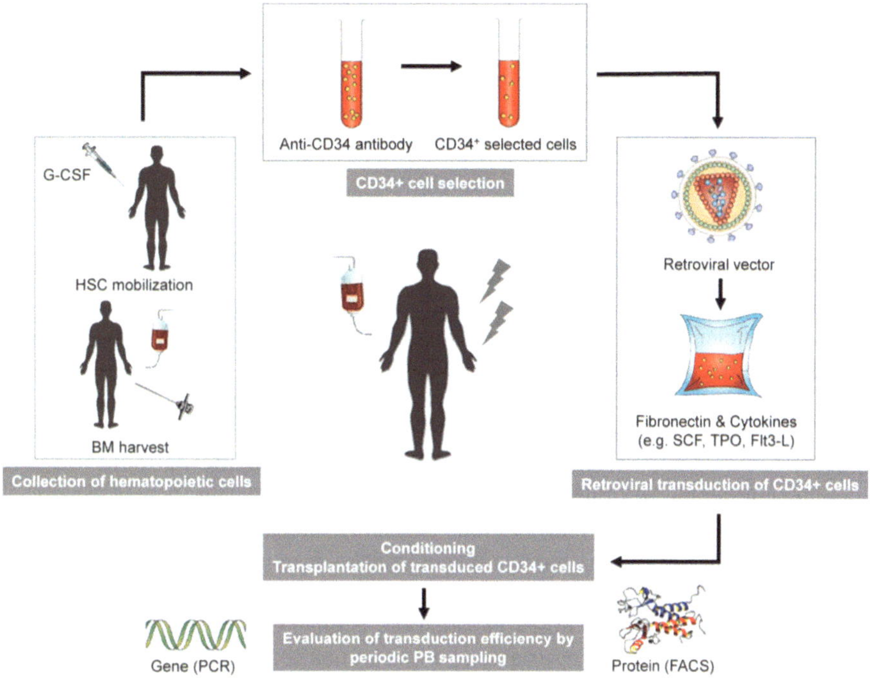

Fig. 24.2 Approach to gene therapy targeting hematopoietic stem cells (HSCs). (1) Collection of hematopoietic cells by bone marrow (BM) harvest or granulocyte-colony stimulating factor (G-CSF)-induced HSC mobilization; (2) purification of a population of hematopoietic cells enriched for HSCs, as defined by the cell surface marker CD34; (3) in vitro transduction of CD34$^+$ cells using modified retroviruses in the presence of stimulatory cytokines, including stem cell factor (SCF), thombopoietin (TPO), and fms-like tyrosine kinase 3 ligand (Flt3-L); (4) transplantation of transduced CD34$^+$ cells into a conditioned recipient; and (5) evaluation of transduction efficiency by periodic collection of peripheral blood (PB) samples

administered back into the patient, and home to the BM where they initiate hematopoiesis. For most disorders, corrected cells do not have a competitive repopulating advantage over uncorrected endogenous HSCs and their progeny. A conditioning regimen, such as radiation or chemotherapy, is thus necessary to increase the likelihood that incoming transduced cells can successfully compete for a niche in the marrow microenvironment and substantively contribute to ongoing hematopoiesis. After autologous transplantation, transduction efficiency is evaluated by periodic collection of peripheral blood (PB) samples.

Preclinical Models for Investigating Gene Transfer into HSCs

No in vitro surrogate assay capable of identifying true HSCs has yet been developed; long-term in vivo reconstitution after transplantation remains the only relevant assay.

Such in vivo reconstitution studies in the mouse have established that retroviral vectors can efficiently transfer and express new genes in primitive pluripotent HSCs capable of reconstituting all lymphoid and myeloid tissues [4–6]. Since similar experimental transplantation studies are impractical in humans, alternative preclinical transplantation models have been explored to assay for human HSC susceptibility to gene transfer.

Immunodeficient Xenogeneic Hosts

Immunodeficient hosts, namely the fetal sheep [7, 8] and the nonobese diabetic (NOD)/severe combined immunodeficiency disease (SCID) mice (known as NOD/SCID mice) [9] or NOD/SCID with IL2 receptor gamma (G) chain deficiency mice (known as NOD/SCID gamma, NSG mice) [10, 11], can be manipulated to permit human hematopoietic reconstitution. NSG mice are currently the most severely immunocompromised strain, with absence of mature T or B cells, lack of functional NK cells and deficiencies in cytokine signaling. Consequently, engraftment of human HSCs in NSG mice is more efficient than that in any other mouse strain. In the NOD/SCID and NSG models, human $CD34^+$ cells are injected into mice previously conditioned with sublethal doses of radiation. Human $CD34^+$ cells migrate to the murine BM and give rise to a sustained pool of human hematopoietic cells for weeks to months. The cells responsible for initiating human engraftment have been termed the SCID-repopulating cells (SRC) [12]. Immunodeficient mice provide an assay to estimate gene expression and gene transfer efficiency into pluripotent hematopoietic cells capable of engrafting in vivo for several weeks to months. These models have been used to validate and optimize clinical gene therapy approaches [13], including target disorders such as chronic granulomatous disease (CGD) [14, 15], adrenoleukodystrophy (ALD) [16], and lysosomal storage disease [17] (Fig. 24.3, upper panel). Follow-up of long-term human hematopoiesis is possible with NSG mice, but limited in the NOD/SCID model due to the short life span of this mutant mouse strain. Lack of cross-reactivity between murine and human cytokine and their receptors, as well as cell surface molecules important for homing and retention of cells in BM niches may limit the validity of predictions based solely on these cross-species models [18, 19].

Large Animal Models

Large animal models, including nonhuman primates (e.g. baboons and rhesus macaques), cats, and dogs, have proven invaluable in gene transfer preclinical research because of stem cell dynamics, cytokine responsiveness, and retroviral receptor properties approximating those found in humans [20, 21]. Nonhuman primates are the most widely used and the best characterized large animal models (Fig. 24.3, lower panel). Because of high purchase and husbandry cost of the animals, most experiments cannot be performed with animal numbers that allow the

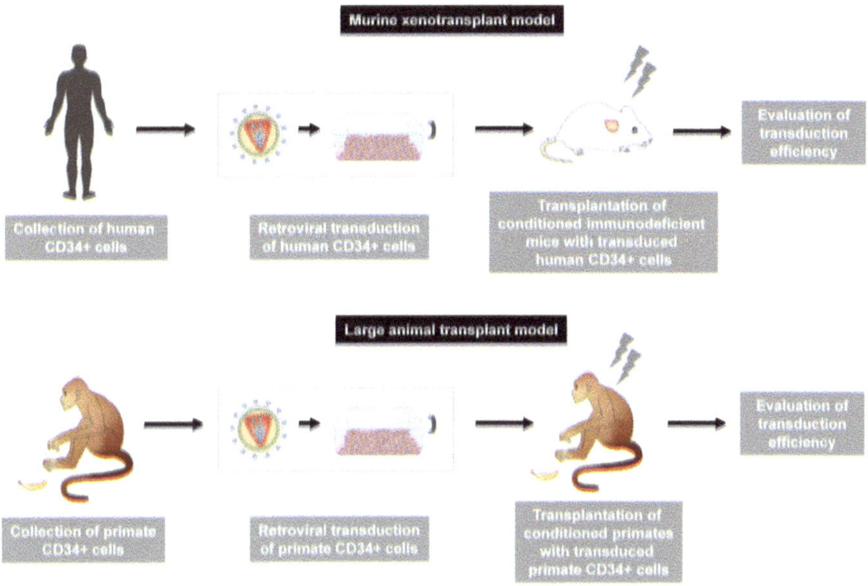

Fig. 24.3 Preclinical assays for evaluating gene transfer into hematopoietic stem cells. The mouse xenotransplant model, namely the NOD/SCID and NSG mice (*top panel*), has been validated as a practical surrogate assay system for human hematopoietic stem cells and was developed based on conventional mouse bone marrow transplantation assays for stem cell function. Large animal models, namely the nonhuman primates (*bottom panel*), have been instrumental for optimization of gene therapy strategies and results obtained using these models have been predictive of results obtained in human clinical gene therapy trials

degree of statistical power that is standard for murine models or in vitro assays. Instead, the use of internal controls, via a competitive repopulation experimental design, can yield more information with feasible animal numbers (Fig. 24.4). In this model, purified $CD34^+$ cells are split into two equal aliquots. Each aliquot is transduced under two different specific test conditions with one of two equivalent titer retroviral vectors. At the end of the culture and transduction period, the two aliquots are collected, pooled, and reinfused into the conditioned animal. After hematopoietic recovery, samples can be analyzed by PCR or flow cytometry that can distinguish the two vectors, allowing quantitation of the relative marking efficiency and contribution to hematopoiesis of cells under the two test conditions.

Conditions Influencing the Efficiency of Gene Transfer into HSCs

For more than a decade, the potential of gene transfer into human HSCs has been restricted by the inability of available methods to permit efficient gene delivery into human HSCs. Recently, improved retroviral gene transfer vectors, optimization of cytokine combination, and incorporation of a recombinant fragment of fibronectin

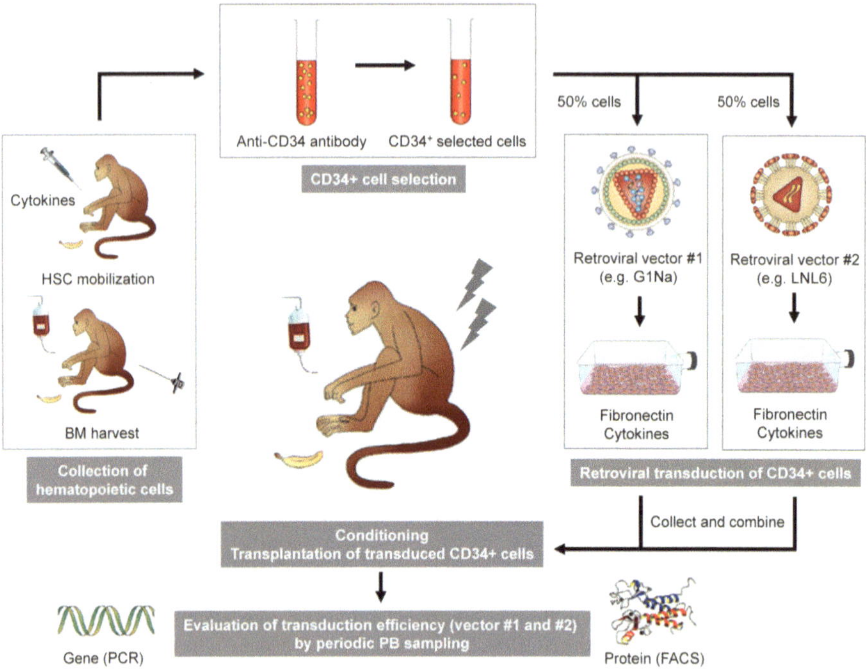

Fig. 24.4 Primate competitive repopulation assay. Rhesus macaque CD34⁺ cells purified after cytokine mobilization or bone marrow (BM) harvest are transduced under two different specific conditions with one of the two equivalent titer retroviral vectors. At the end of the transduction period, the two aliquots are pooled and reinfused into the animal after total body irradiation. After hematopoietic recovery, peripheral blood (PB) samples are collected and analyzed using assays (e.g. PCR or Southern blot) that can distinguish the two vectors, allowing quantification of the relative marking efficiency and contribution to hematopoiesis of marked BM cells and mobilized cells

during transduction have been shown to greatly improve retroviral gene transduction, with long-term in vivo gene marking levels of 10–15% or higher possible [1, 22]. These advances in the genetic manipulation of HSCs have contributed to the first successful gene therapy clinical trials in patients with SCID [23–28], CGD [29, 30], ALD [31], Wiskott-Aldrich Syndrome (WAS) [32], and β-thalassemia [33].

The efficiency of gene transfer is also influenced by the source of HSCs. Early studies transduced unfractionated or CD34⁺ steady-state BM cells. Many preclinical investigations using the NOD/SCID mouse xenotransplant model involved transduction of primitive human cord blood (CB) cells because they engraft much more efficiently in this model compared with BM. Thus, the vast majority of recently published studies on gene transfer efficiency have utilized CB target CD34⁺ cells. However, results using CB cells may not reflect the outcomes that would be obtained with more clinically relevant BM or mobilized PB HSCs. In this chapter, we discuss the considerations and experimental evidence influencing the choice of target HSC source for gene therapy applications.

Strategies for Mobilization of Hematopoietic Stem Cells for Gene Therapy

Cytokines and Chemotherapy

Mobilizing agents release HSCs from marrow to blood. As compared to HSCs collected via BM harvesting, mobilized PB HSC collections result in larger yield of $CD34^+$ cells, are obtained with less intervention and pain to donors, can be collected in even larger numbers via repeat mobilizations separated by intervals as brief as a few days to a few weeks, depending on the mobilizing agent [34], greatly shorten engraftment and immune recovery time, and result in lower overall cost [35]. Conventional stimuli used for HSC mobilization include administration of cytokines, alone or in combination with myelosuppressive chemotherapy. The cytokine G-CSF has an extensive safety profile, both as an agent for accelerating recovery from neutropenia after myelotoxic treatments (chemotherapy or radiation), and as the primary agent for PB HSC mobilization for transplantation purposes. The combination of G-CSF+SCF has proven to be a more effective mobilizing regimen compared to G-CSF alone in murine [36–38], canine [39], and nonhuman primate models [40–43]. In several randomized clinical trials, the combined use of G-CSF+SCF also led to increased median yield of $CD34^+$ cells per leukapheresis [44–48]. However, SCF has been taken off market in the United States for clinical applications because of allergic-like reactions experienced by many individuals exposed to this drug.

AMD3100

AMD3100 Is a Direct CXCR4 Antagonist

In recent years, some of the mechanisms underlying PB HSC mobilization have been elucidated, leading to the development of new mobilization strategies and a better understanding of the processes of egress and ingress of primitive hematopoietic cells from the BM microenvironment. As detailed elsewhere in this book, the interaction between CXCR4, a CXC chemokine receptor, and its ligand stromal-derived factor-1α (SDF-1α, also referred to as CXCL12) has been found to play a pivotal role in PB HSC mobilization [49]. The bicyclam molecule AMD3100 (Mozobil, Genzyme, MA, USA), shown to reversibly block the interaction between CXCR4 and SDF-1α, was initially developed for selective inhibition of CXCR4-facilitated HIV entry into cells [50–54]. Testing of AMD3100 as an anti-HIV drug was abandoned due to lack of antiviral effect and the occurrence of asymptomatic premature ventricular contractions in two patients. However, during pharmacokinetic studies with a single-dose intravenous AMD3100 administration in normal healthy volunteers, an unexpected increase in white blood cell (WBC) count was noted [55].

AMD3100 Mobilizes HSCs in Preclinical Models and in Normal Volunteers

These observations prompted studies to evaluate the effects of AMD3100 on mobilization of PB HSCs. Broxmeyer et al. [56] demonstrated rapid mobilization of murine hematopoietic progenitor cells (HPCs) and long-term repopulating cells after AMD3100 administration in various strains of mice. These studies led to the first clinical trials of AMD3100 for mobilization of $CD34^+$ cells in healthy human volunteers [57]. Maximum increase in circulating HPCs occurred in humans 6 h after intravenous injection of AMD3100. Using limiting dilution analyses in the NOD/SCID xenograft model, the frequency of SRCs per million $CD34^+$ cells in the PB of healthy donors was 4.5-fold higher than the frequency detected in comparable G-CSF-mobilized PB collections [56]. AMD3100-mobilized cells also present functional differences compared with cells mobilized with G-CSF, including a higher proportion of cells in the G1 phase of the cell cycle, a higher percentage of more primitive $CD34^+CD38^-$ cells, more cells expressing CXCR4 and VLA-4 and more B, T, and NK cells in the apheresis product [58–60]. Additional preclinical studies in the canine [61], rhesus macaque [60], and NOD/SCID [62] transplantation models demonstrated the BM repopulating capacity of AMD300-mobilized $CD34^+$ cells.

AMD3100 Acts Synergistically with G-CSF

AMD3100 has also been shown to act synergistically with G-CSF in mice [56] and healthy volunteers [56, 63]. Thus, more PB HSCs can be collected via fewer apheresis sessions, and some donors failing previous mobilization attempts with cytokines can have sufficient PB HSCs collected for transplantation following mobilization with AMD3100 or AMD3100 with G-CSF. The frequency of SRCs per kilogram in apheresis samples mobilized with G-CSF and AMD3100 was higher compared to samples mobilized with G-CSF or AMD3100 alone [56]. AMD3100, alone [64, 65] or in combination with G-CSF [59, 66–71] or G-CSF/chemotherapy [72], has been shown to be safe and effective for the rapid mobilization of $CD34^+$ cells in patients with multiple myeloma (MM) and non-Hodgkin's lymphoma (NHL) who had received prior chemotherapy. Two multicenter, double-blind placebo-controlled trials in patients with MM and NHL have shown that combination of AMD3100 and G-CSF is well tolerated and significantly more patients achieved the optimal $CD34^+$ cell target in fewer leukapheresis, compared with G-CSF alone. On the basis of the results of these two studies, AMD3100 in combination with G-CSF, was FDA-approved in December 2008 for HSC mobilization in patients with MM and NHL. A pivotal study also demonstrated safe and successful mobilization of normal donors with AMD3100 as a single agent, followed by a prompt engraftment in an allogeneic transplant setting [73].

Mobilization for Gene Therapy: Conclusions from Preclinical Transplantation Models

Transduction of G-CSF+SCF-Mobilized PB HSCs Is Superior to Steady-State BM Cells in Mouse and Rhesus Macaque Models

Mouse Transplantation Studies

In 1994, Bodine et al. [74] showed that HSCs present in mobilized PB cells collected after administration of G-CSF+SCF were transduced more efficiently with retroviral vectors compared with BM cells of mice treated with 5-fluorouracil (5-FU). Transduced murine PB HSCs mobilized with G-SCF+SCF were shown to be capable of maintaining lifelong polyclonal hematopoiesis in reconstituted mice [75]. In 1996, it was reported that BM collected 2 weeks after completion of a single 5-day mobilization course of G-CSF+SCF, referred to as "primed" marrow, had ten times the repopulating ability of baseline BM [76]. The susceptibility of these primed BM cells to gene transfer was compared with steady-state and post-5-FU marrow. All cell types were found to be equally good gene transfer targets in the murine model, but inferior to cells mobilized after G-CSF and SCF administration [77].

Rhesus Macaque Transplantation Model

Similar experiments performed in rhesus macaques indicated that day 5 G-CSF+SCF-mobilized PB and day 19 primed BM were both superior targets compared with steady-state BM, with levels of gene marking in the 1–3% or higher range in all lineages compared with <0.1% in previous studies using steady-state BM [77]. More recently, a direct competitive repopulation study (Fig. 24.4) was performed to compare the levels of genetically modified cells attainable after retroviral transduction of BM CD34$^+$ cells with CD34$^+$ cells collected from a leukapheresis product after mobilization with G-CSF+SCF. The highest marking observed was derived from G-SCF+SCF-mobilized PB in two of three animals [78].

Dog Transplantation Model

In 2003, Thomasson et al. [79] used a competitive repopulation assay in the dog to directly compare transduction efficiency of steady-state marrow, G-CSF+SCF primed BM, and G-CSF+SCF-mobilized PB. Cells from all three sources were transduced, cryopreserved, and thawed together before infusion into myeloablated dogs. While primed marrow resulted in the highest long-term marking levels, steady-state BM, in contrast to data obtained in mouse and rhesus transplantation models, was transduced at least as efficiently as G-CSF+SCF-mobilized PB in all three dogs. The discrepancy between rhesus macaque and dog studies is likely related to differences in transduction conditions, including different stimulatory cytokines and retroviral vector envelope proteins, in addition to potential species differences.

Transduction of G-CSF-Mobilized PB HSCs Is Equivalent to Steady-State BM Cells

PB HSCs mobilized with the combination of G-CSF+SCF can be transduced efficiently with retroviral vectors. However, due to serious anaphylactic reactions occurring in patients treated with SCF in combination with other agents for aplastic anemia, this cytokine is no longer available for clinical use in the United States. Instead, G-CSF-mobilized PB $CD34^+$ cells are the favored source of HSCs in clinical transplantation. However, G-CSF has been reported to precipitate severe and sometimes fatal sickle cell crisis in patients with SCD [80–84], a long-held target disorder for HSC-based gene therapy approaches. Therefore, Hematti et al. [78] conducted a study to compare the levels of genetically modified cells attainable after retroviral transduction of $CD34^+$ cells collected from a BM harvest with $CD34^+$ cells collected from a leukapheresis product after mobilization with G-CSF in the rhesus macaque autologous transplantation model. BM was equal to or better than G-CSF-mobilized PB as a source of HSCs for retroviral gene transfer and the only currently available source for patients with sickle cell disease.

Transduction of G-CSF+SCF-Mobilized PB HSCs Is Superior to PB HSCs Mobilized with Other Cytokines

Because SCF is no longer available in the United States for clinical applications, competitive repopulation experiments (Fig. 24.4) were performed in rhesus macaques to directly assess the relative gene transfer susceptibility and engraftment potential of stem cells mobilized with alternative regimens, including G-CSF alone or G-CSF combined with Flt3-L. In all animals tested, the in vivo levels of mononuclear cell (MNC) and granulocyte (Gran) marking were higher at all time points derived from target $CD34^+$ cells collected after G-CSF+SCF mobilization compared with target cells collected after G-CSF alone or G-CSF+Flt3-L mobilization [78, 85].

Transduction of AMD3100-Mobilized PB HSCs Is Comparable to G-CSF+SCF-Mobilized PB HSCs

Competitive repopulation experiments (Fig. 24.4) were also conducted in rhesus macaques to compare levels of genetically modified cells attainable after transduction of AMD3100- and G-CSF-mobilized $CD34^+$ cells with retroviral vectors containing the Neomycin resistance (Neo^R) gene [60]. Levels of in vivo MNC and Gran Neo^R

gene marking at steady-state originated predominantly from the AMD3100-mobilized fraction rather than the G-CSF-mobilized cells. In vivo gene marking levels using the AMD3100-mobilized $CD34^+$ cells were comparable to in vivo levels previously achieved in the rhesus macaque model using PB $CD34^+$ cells mobilized with a combination of G-CSF+SCF [85]. Overall, these results indicate that AMD3100-mobilized $CD34^+$ cells represent an alternative source of HSCs for genetic manipulation with integrating retroviral vectors.

Intrinsic Differences in the Target PB HSCs Mobilized with G-CSF+SCF or AMD3100 Permit More Efficient Transduction

Possible explanations have been considered for the higher marking levels achieved using the G-CSF+SCF or AMD3100-mobilized $CD34^+$ cells compared with G-CSF-mobilized $CD34^+$ cells.

Number of $CD34^+$ Cells and Repopulating HSCs

Assuming similar transduction efficiency between each mobilization regimen, it is conceivable that the larger number of $CD34^+$ cells consistently obtained after AMD3100 or G-CSF+SCF mobilization and reinfused to the animals after transduction would result in higher in vivo markings in this competitive repopulation design. However, significantly higher levels of MNC and Gran Neo^R gene marking were found to originate from the AMD3100 or the G-CSF+SCF-mobilized $CD34^+$ cells even after normalization for the number of $CD34^+$ cells infused per kilogram weight of the animal [60, 85].

Alternatively, a relative increased frequency of repopulating HSCs within the total AMD3100 or G-CSF+SCF-mobilized $CD34^+$ cells population may have accounted for the increased in vivo Neo^R gene marking. However, in vivo NOD/SCID engraftment assays do not suggest this to be the case. The frequency of SRC was found to be lower in samples mobilized with the combination G-CSF+SCF compared with G-CSF alone [86]. Similarly, the 4.5-fold increase in SRC activity noted in AMD3100-mobilized compared with G-CSF-mobilized $CD34^+$ cells [56] cannot solely account for the increase in Neo^R gene marking obtained with AMD3100-mobilized cells. Therefore, intrinsic differences in the target HSCs mobilized with G-CSF+SCF or AMD3100 likely permit more efficient transduction with retroviral vectors.

Cell Cycling Status

The increased in vivo gene marking observed in AMD3100- or G-CSF+SCF- compared with G-CSF-mobilized or steady-state BM $CD34^+$ cells may be due, in part, to a difference in cell cycling status. Gammaretroviral vectors have an absolute requirement for the target cells to enter the cell cycle in order to allow vector entry into the nucleus and the integration into the genome [87–89]. An increased proportion of AMD3100-mobilized $CD34^+$ cells was found in the G_1 phase of the cell cycle compared with G-CSF-mobilized cells, consistent with better in vivo gene marking levels [60]. AMD3100-mobilized $CD34^+$ cells will also likely be amenable to genetic manipulation with integrating lentiviral vectors, which preferentially transduce cells in the G_1 as compared with the G_0 phase of the cell cycle [90, 91].

In contrast, both G-CSF+SCF- and G-CSF-mobilized $CD34^+$ cell populations are primarily in the G_0 phase of the cell cycle [92, 93]. Using different combination of stimulatory cytokines in culture media (e.g. SCF, Flt3-L, and TPO) allows primitive hematopoietic cells to enter cell cycle. Therefore, the increased susceptibility of G-CSF+SCF-mobilized PB HSCs to retroviral transduction may be related to their ability to enter the cell cycle more frequently or rapidly than PB HSCs obtained after G-CSF administration. However, a disturbing loss of in vivo repopulating stem cell activity after prolonged culture in stimulatory cytokines has been demonstrated in murine studies [94, 95], the rhesus autologous transplantation model [93], and NOD/SCID mouse studies using human cord blood cells or mobilized peripheral blood stem cells [92, 96]. This engraftment defect has been shown to be reversible, if actively cycling cells are allowed to return to the G_0 phase of the cell cycle before transplantation. A simple culture manipulation has been identified to improve the engraftment ability of hematopoietic cells stimulated to cycle ex vivo for 4 days in stimulatory cytokines (SCF, FLT3, and TPO) by culturing these cells for an additional 2 days in non-stimulatory cytokines (SCF alone) in the presence of the CH-296 fragment of fibronectin, known to prevent apoptosis without inducing active cell cycle. Hence, this procedure may offer optimal conditions for transduction while maintaining the homing potential of the transduced cells.

Retroviral Vector Receptors

A direct correlation has been shown between retrovirus receptor expression levels in various cell types and the efficiency with which they are transduced. Orlic et al. [97] showed that the level of amphotropic receptor mRNA in HSCs from the BM of mice treated with G-CSF+SCF was 2.8- to 7.8-fold higher than in HSCs from steady-state BM. Similarly, Horwitz et al. [98] found that HSCs isolated from G-CSF-mobilized PB differ from those isolated from steady-state BM in that a significant proportion express higher levels of amphotropic receptor mRNA. Overall, these observations correlate with the increased susceptibility to amphotropic retroviral transduction of mobilized PB HSCs compared with steady-state BM. Similar studies comparing retrovirus receptor expression in G-CSF, G-CSF+SCF, and AMD3100-mobilized PB HSCs are not available.

Homing and Engraftment Potential

The differences in gene marking levels between various sources of HSCs may also be related to their variable ability to home back to the recipient BM. Human CD34⁺ cells from donors mobilized with both G-CSF and AMD3100 express higher levels of VLA-4, migrate significantly better to SDF-1, and engraft at much higher levels in NOD/SCID recipients who received transplants, compared with cells obtained from donors treated with G-CSF alone [56, 99]. Also, when healthy donors were mobilized with AMD3100 and, after 10 days of drug clearance, the same donors were mobilized with G-CSF, cells obtained after AMD3100 administration engrafted better in NOD/SCID mice compared with cells leukapheresed after G-CSF mobilization [62]. Similarly, rhesus macaque CD34⁺ cells mobilized with AMD3100 have higher VLA-4 and CXCR4 expression, SDF-1-induced migration in vitro compared with G-CSF-mobilized cells [60]. These properties of AMD3100-mobilized CD34⁺ cells more closely resemble those of steady-state BM. Thus, genetically marked AMD3100-mobilized and BM cells may engraft better after transplantation compared with G-CSF-mobilized cells, resulting in higher in vivo gene marking levels.

Mobilization with AMD3100 Can Be Used as a Conditioning Regimen Before Transplantation of Genetically Modified PB HSCs

Conditioning is a critical step before autologous transplantation of transduced HSCs in gene therapy. In the autologous setting, conditioning regimens damage (or destroy) endogenous stem cells, providing a competitive advantage to the infused transduced HSCs [100, 101]. They may also help eradicating the disease for which the transplant is being performed. Conditioning has traditionally been achieved by delivering maximally tolerated doses of chemotherapeutic agents, with or without radiation. However, these regimens are associated with significant morbidity and mortality [102]. While myeloablative regimens are justified in stem cell transplantation for malignant disorders, many of the diseases that could be targeted in gene therapy applications are chronic, indolent disorders in which the risks of myeloablative regimens outweigh the potential benefits. Also, clinically relevant engraftment of genetically modified HSCs in the absence of myeloablation remains a highly desirable goal for the therapy of genetic disorders in which the corrected cells lack a growth advantage [1, 77, 103–106].

Using a model of hematopoiesis in parabiotic mice [107], Chen et al. [108] determined that, after mobilization with AMD3100, HSCs exited marrow, transited blood, engrafted in open microenvironmental niches in partner marrow, and contributed normally to partner hematopoiesis. Thus, it was hypothesized that mobilization before HSC transplantation might vacate niches and lead to improved engraftment of donor HSCs. This hypothesis was tested in the mouse transplantation model (Fig. 24.5) [108]. When recipient mice were treated with AMD3100 2 h before transplantation of BM cells, donor cell engraftment was higher ($4.6 \pm 1.1\%$) than in

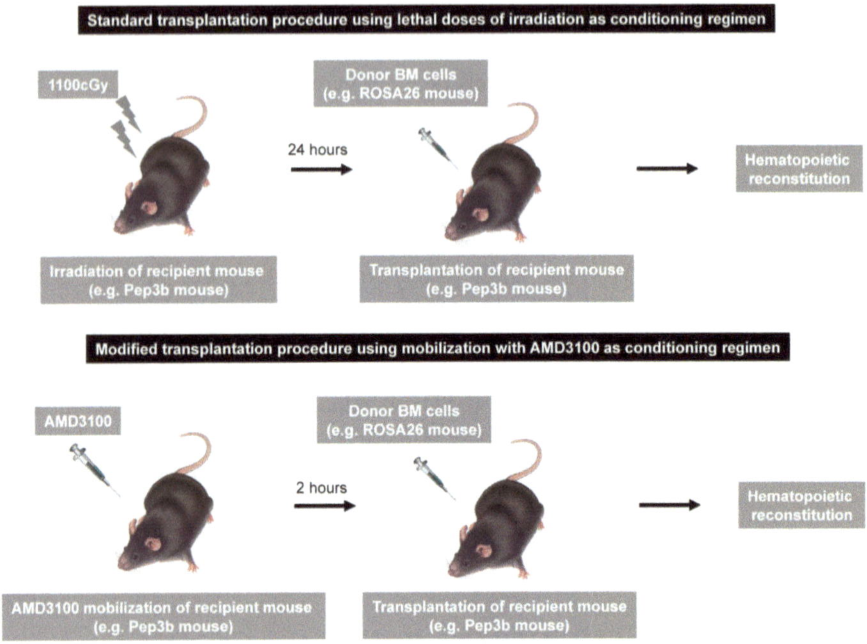

Fig. 24.5 Mobilization with AMD3100 as a conditioning regimen for hematopoietic stem cell transplantation. Standard hematopoietic stem cell (HSC) transplantation procedures use toxic myeloablative conditioning (e.g. irradiation and chemotherapy) to allow engraftment of the infused stem cells. Mobilization with AMD3100 before transplantation was shown to open microenvironmental niches and facilitate engraftment without toxic conditioning regimen in mouse models. This could provide a safer approach for HSC transplantation in clinical gene therapy applications where many of the targeted diseases are chronic, indolent disorders and the risks of myeloablative regimens outweigh their potential benefits

control animals (no AMD3100) ($1.0 \pm 0.24\%$, $p = 0.0004$). When mice received weekly injections of AMD3100 on three consecutive weeks and marrow cells were transplanted 2 h after each mobilization, donor cell engraftment further increased ($9.1 \pm 1.7\%$, $p = 0.001$). These results indicate that mobilization with AMD3100 may provide a safer conditioning regimen before HSC transplantation for gene therapy of non-malignant disorders.

Mobilization for Gene Therapy: Clinical Applications

Steady-State BM and G-CSF-Mobilized PB HSCs Are Used in Clinical HSC Gene Transfer Applications

Results derived from the preclinical transplantation models, summarized in Fig. 24.6, have contributed to the choice of target cells used for gene transfer clinical applications.

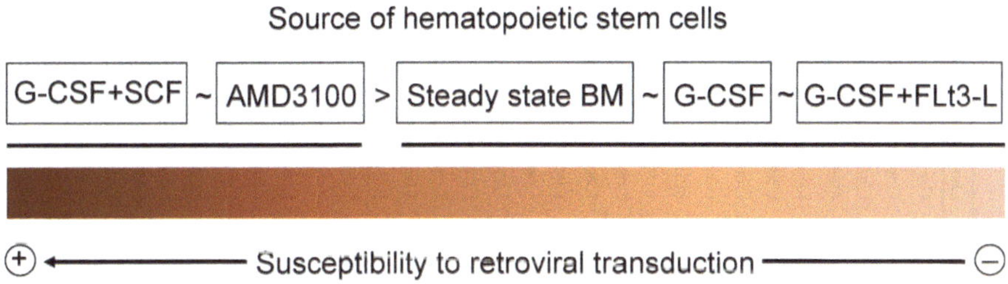

Fig. 24.6 Summary of the susceptibility of various sources of hematopoietic stem cells (HSCs) to retroviral transduction. HSCs mobilized with the combination of cytokines granulocyte-colony stimulating factor (G-CSF) and stem cell factor (SCF) have a superior susceptibility to retroviral transduction, but evidence of anaphylactic reactions in patients treated with SCF has prevented its use in clinical gene therapy trials. Gene transfer experiments in rhesus macaques have shown an efficiency of transduction in AMD3100-mobilized HSCs similar to that observed with G-CSF + SCF-mobilized HSCs, but this novel agent has not been exploited yet in clinical gene therapy applications. To date, all gene therapy trials targeting HSCs have used steady-state bone marrow or G-CSF-mobilized HSCs which offer a similar susceptibility to retroviral transduction. Mobilization with the combination of G-CSF and fms-like tyrosine kinase 3 ligand (Flt3-L) has provided no benefit for gene transfer applications

While G-CSF + SCF-mobilized PB HSCs appear a superior source of HSCs for gene therapy, this combination has not been used clinically because SCF is no longer available clinically in most of the world, secondary to concerns over anaphylactic episodes in several patients exposed to this agent. Use of alternative cytokines (e.g. G-CSF + Flt3-L) for mobilization has gained no popularity in gene therapy trials because of lack of benefit in preclinical transplantation models.

PB HSCs mobilized with AMD3100 have an equivalent susceptibility to retroviral transduction compared with G-CSF + SCF-mobilized stem cells in the rhesus macaque model. However, this agent has only recently been evaluated for its mobilization potential in healthy donors [56, 57, 63] and in patients with NHL and multiple myeloma [64, 66–72, 109, 110], but has not yet been exploited in gene therapy trials. The efficiency of transduction of cells mobilized with AMD3100, combined with the positive safety profile and the rapid mobilization kinetics of this agent will likely bring AMD3100 to the forefront as a first line mobilizing agent for future gene therapy applications. The ability to collect repeatedly with little additional toxicity and no apparent need for a rest period between collections is also attractive when cell dose is critical to achieving adequate engraftment of transduced cells in the setting of minimal myeloablation.

Preclinical models showed an equivalent susceptibility of steady-state BM cells and G-CSF-mobilized PB HSCs to retroviral gene transfer. Accordingly, success has been demonstrated in recent gene therapy trials using steady-state BM [23–25, 27, 33, 111] or G-CSF-mobilized PB HSCs [26, 29, 31, 32, 112]. Overall, for published gene therapy trials using retrovirally transduced $CD34^+$ cells for clonal gene marking or therapeutic intents, approximately half of these trials used steady-state BM as their only source of repopulating stem cells. The remainder of these trials used mobilized PB HSCs alone or in combination with steady-state BM. One study [113] transplanted newborns with transduced CB cells (Table 24.1).

Table 24.1 Gene therapy clinical trials using $CD34^+$ cells transduced with gammaretroviral or lentiviral vectors

Reference	$CD34^+$ cells	Indication	Gene	Outcome
Cavazzana-Calvo et al. [33]	Bone marrow	β-Thalassemia	β-Globin	Correction of β-thalassemia[a]
Boztug et al. [32]	G-CSF-mobilized	WAS	WAS	Correction of WAS
Cartier et al. [31]	G-CSF-mobilized	X-ALD	ABCD1	Correction of X-ALD[a]
Aiuti et al. [24]	Bone marrow	ADA-SCID	ADA	Correction of ADA-SCID
Mitsuyasu et al. [112]	G-CSF-mobilized	HIV	Anti-HIV1 ribozyme	Lower HIV-1 viral load
Chinen et al. [26]	G-CSF-mobilized	X-SCID	γ-Chain of IL2 receptor	Clinical improvement
Gaspar et al. [111]	Bone marrow	ADA-SCID	ADA	Correction of ADA-SCID
Ott et al. [29]	G-CSF-mobilized	X-CGD	$gp91^{phox}$	Correction of X-CGD
Thrasher et al. [120]	Bone marrow	X-SCID	γ-Chain of IL2 receptor	Failure to correct X-SCID
Gaspar et al. [27]	Bone marrow	X-SCID	γ-Chain of IL2 receptor	Correction of X-SCID
Amado et al. [141]	G-CSF-mobilized	HIV	Anti-HIV1 ribozyme	Low long-term gene marking
Aiuti et al. [23]	Bone marrow	ADA-SCID	ADA	Correction of ADA-SCID
Abonour et al. [142]	G-CSF-mobilized	Germ cell tumors	MDR-1	Low long-term gene marking
Cavazzana-Calvo et al. [25]	Bone marrow	X-SCID	γ-Chain of IL2 receptor	Correction of X-SCID
Liu et al. [143]	Bone marrow G-CSF-mobilized	FA	FANCC	Low long-term gene marking
Cowan et al. [144]	Bone marrow G-CSF-mobilized Cy-mobilized	Breast CA	MDR-1	Low long-term gene marking
Kohn et al. [145]	Bone marrow	HIV	RRED	Low long-term gene marking
Dunbar et al. [146]	Bone marrow G-CSF-mobilized	Gaucher	GC	Low long-term gene marking
Hesdorffer et al. [147]	Bone marrow	Breast CA ovarian CA glioblastoma	MDR-1	Low long-term gene marking
Kohn et al. [113]	Cord blood	ADA-SCID	ADA	Low long-term gene marking
Malech et al. [127]	G-CSF-mobilized	CGD	$gp91^{phox}$	Low long-term gene marking
Bordignon et al. [148]	Bone marrow	ADA-SCID	ADA	Low long-term gene marking
Dunbar et al. [104]	Bone marrow G-CSF-mobilized Cy-mobilized	Gene marking	Neo^R	Low long-term gene marking
Deisseroth et al. [149]	Bone marrow	Gene marking	MDR-1	Low long-term gene marking
Deisseroth et al. [116]	Bone marrow	Gene marking	Neo^R	Low long-term gene marking
Rill et al. [119]	Bone marrow	Gene marking	Neo^R	Low long-term gene marking
Deisseroth et al. [118]	Bone marrow	Gene marking	Neo^R	Low long-term gene marking
Brenner et al. [114]	Bone marrow	Gene marking	Neo^R	Low long-term gene marking
Brenner et al. [115]	Bone marrow	Gene marking	Neo^R	Low long-term gene marking

ADA-SCID adenosine deaminase-severe combined immunodeficiency disease, *Cy* cyclophosphamide, *FA* Fanconi anemia, *FANCC* Fanconi anemia group C, *GC* glucocerebrosidase, *HIV* human immunodeficiency virus, *Neo^R* neomycin resistance, *RRED* rev-responsive element decoy, *WAS* Wiskott-Aldrich syndrome, *X-ALD* X-linked adrenoleukodystrophy, *X-CGD* X-linked chronic granulomatous disease, *X-SCID X-linked SCID*

[a]Lentiviral vectors were used

Initial Gene Marking Clinical Trials

To gain new insights into the behavior of individual HSCs and the dynamics and origins of tumors, the first clinical trials with retroviral gene transfer targeting HSCs used retroviral vectors encoding the Neo^R gene to mark steady-state BM-derived HSCs and possible contaminating tumor cells. Although these initial trials in autologous cancer patient BM grafts proved that primitive repopulating cells could be transduced and would engraft without loss of function, the patients uniformly failed to reach and maintain therapeutically relevant levels (<0.1%) of genetically modified PB cells [114–119]. One gene marking trial in patients with multiple myeloma and breast cancer [104] directly compared contribution of BM and G-SCF- or cyclophosphamide-mobilized PB HSCs to long-term in vivo gene marking. The source of marking was both the transduced PB graft and the BM graft. However, for both fractions, the steady-state levels of marking were low, with only 1:1,000–1:10,000 cells positive. These data provided the first clinical evidence that mobilized PB HSCs can be used for gene therapy applications and that progeny of mobilized PB HSCs can contribute long-term to engraftment of multiple lineages, albeit at low levels.

Clinical Success of Gene Therapy in Treating Human Diseases

Beginning in the late 1990s, clinically relevant gene transfer levels (i.e. >5%) into long-term engrafting hematopoietic cells were finally achieved in large animals and NOD/SCID mice after optimization of the transduction conditions [1, 22]. These advances were rapidly applied in a new generation of clinical trials, with actual therapeutic intent, for immunodeficiency disorders [23–28, 111, 120] and, more recently, for other diseases, including CGD [29, 30], β-thalassemia [33], WAS [32], and ALD [31]. On the footstep of the preclinical models and the early gene marking clinical studies, both BM- and G-CSF-mobilized PB HSCs were used as a source of HSCs in these trials.

Severe Combined Immunodeficiency Disease

The first HSC gene therapy trial demonstrating unequivocal clinical benefit was led by Fischer and Cavazzana-Calvo at the Necker Hospital in France [25, 28, 121–123]. Eleven boys with X-linked SCID (X-SCID) were treated. Given the severity of this disorder, most of the children were enrolled in the first few years of life, before they were large enough to undergo apheresis. Thus, BM was the source of target $CD34^+$ cells in these boys. Each boy received autologous $CD34^+$ BM cells, transduced with a retroviral vector expressing the corrective gene (γ-chain subunit of the IL-2 receptor). The transduced cells were reinfused into these children and rapid functional B- and T-cell immune reconstitution was observed in all, but one child. The same vector insertion site could be detected in both myeloid and lymphoid cells, signifying that true HSC correction had occurred. Unfortunately, the elation after this success was short-lived; four subjects in the trial developed acute T-cell leukemia [121–123]. The gene therapy vector had inserted near the locus for *LMO2*, *BMI1*, or *CCND2* resulting in increased expression of these proto-oncogenes through the vector's enhancer activity. Chemotherapy led to sustained remission in three of the four cases of T-cell leukemia, but failed in the fourth. Patients that were successfully treated with chemotherapy continued to benefit from therapeutic gene transfer as a result of restoration of polyclonal transduced T-cell populations after chemotherapy.

BM $CD34^+$ cells were also used in a similar gene therapy trial conducted in London on ten children with X-SCID. All patients experienced substantial immunological recovery and in most patients this was accompanied by recovery of humoral immunity and withdrawal of immunoglobin supplementation [27, 124, 125]. Similar to the first clinical study of gene therapy for X-SCID, a single insertion 35 kb upstream of the transcription start site caused substantial overexpression of *LMO2* and neighboring genes in one of ten patients [124]. Leukemogenesis was thought to have been precipitated by the acquisition of other genetic abnormalities, including a gain-of-function mutation in *NOTCH1*, deletion of the tumor suppressor gene locus *CDKN2A*, and translocation of the TCR-β region to the *STIL-TAL1* locus. These data indicated that conventional murine gammaretroviral vectors (based on MMLV) present a high risk of leukemogenesis as a result of their powerful enhancer sequences in the intact long terminal repeat (LTR) regions.

While gene therapy has been effective in infants with X-SCID, minimal clinical improvement was detected in two of three pre-adolescents despite effective transduction and engraftment of G-CSF-mobilized $CD34^+$ cells [26], and complete failure of gene therapy in two adult patients was reported after transplantation of transduced BM $CD34^+$ cells [120]. Interestingly, neither the two adult X-SCID patients nor the pre-adolescent who demonstrated no clinical benefits had experienced a sustained period of normal thymic output of allogeneic T cells after a BM transplantation earlier in life. In contrast, the two pre-adolescents who showed some clinical improvement originally had full T-cell reconstitution for at least 2 years following haploidentical BM transplantation. These observations suggest that success of gene therapy in older individuals after BM transplantation may relate not only to age per se but also to prior successful T-cell production.

Bordignon's and Thrasher's groups also reported sustained engraftment of engineered HSCs and good immune reconstitution in patients with SCID resulting from adenosine deaminase (ADA) enzyme deficiency following transplantation of BM-derived transduced $CD34^+$ cells [23, 24, 111]. No cases of leukemogenesis have been reported to date in these trials consistent with the long-term analysis of integration sites revealing a polyclonal pattern along with a lack of in vivo skewing for risky insertions.

Chronic Granulomatous Disease

Individuals born with CGD have inherited phagocyte dysfunction that renders patients particularly susceptible to bacterial and fungal microorganisms. One of the most important antimicrobial systems in phagocytic cells is the NADPH phagocyte oxidase (also known as phox). CGD results from mutations in the genes encoding four essential subunits of the phagocyte oxidase [126]. The X-linked form of CGD (X-CGD) is the most common form and is related to genetic mutations in the largest subunit of the phagocyte oxidase, which is a 91-kDa glycoprotein (gp) referred to as $gp91^{phox}$.

The lack of curative options for many CGD patients and the relative genetic simplicity of its single-gene defect have made CGD a foremost candidate for somatic gene therapy applications targeted at autologous HSCs. In an attempt to genetically correct the defect in CGD patients, Manuel Grez and collaborators in Switzerland obtained G-CSF-mobilized $CD34^{+}$ cells from two CGD patients and, using a vector similar to that used in the X-SCID trials, inserted a corrective copy of one $gp91^{phox}$ gene needed to make a functional NADPH oxidase [29]. Unlike previous CGD trials [127], 3 weeks after the cells were reinfused into the patients, a surprisingly large fraction, more than 20%, of their circulating WBCs carried the corrected gene. This sustained engraftment of functionally corrected cells with therapeutically relevant levels of NADPH oxidase was unexpectedly followed by in vivo expansion of cell clones containing insertionally activated growth-promoting genes, including *MDS1-EVI1*, *PRDM16*, or *SETBP1*. These activating insertions facilitated expansion of the gene-corrected clones in both individuals, with up to 60% of their WBCs containing the corrective gene. Both patients treated on this protocol initially showed significant clinical improvement for at least 15 months and, therefore, this study represents the first demonstration of long-term clinical benefit using G-CSF-mobilized PB HSCs as a source of HSCs for gene therapy.

However, a progressive decline in blood counts was observed in both CGD patients at 15 and 28 months, respectively, after gene therapy [30, 128]. BM examination was consistent with a myelodysplastic syndrome (MDS), a group of malignant stem cell disorders characterized by dysplastic and ineffective blood cell production and a variable risk of transformation to acute leukemia. Recent evidence suggests that overexpression of EVI1 could have been an initiating event that then resulted in chromosomal instability, stimulating further chromosomal abnormalities, such as loss of chromosome 7, and progression to MDS [30, 128]. Despite the persistent high frequency of vector-corrected neutrophils, expression of NADPH oxidase dropped precipitously in both subjects over time. The silencing of NADPH oxidase occurred through progressive CpG methylation of the promoter contained in the LTR of the vector, a region important for transgene expression. These events led to a series of infections and eventual death of one patient. The second subject was referred for unrelated donor stem cell transplantation while still infection free.

Some investigators have suggested that lowering the target cell dose to the lowest amount expected to result in adequate engraftment would decrease the number of retroviral insertions the patient is exposed to and, therefore, may decrease the risk of insertional mutagenesis following gene therapy. While G-CSF-mobilized samples, as used in this trial, are more likely to provide larger cell doses per kilogram than BM samples, as used in the X-SCID trial, the demonstration of gene transfer vector-related complications following both clinical trials indicates that the source of HSC and the associated number of genetically corrected HSC infused are unlikely contributing to these adverse events. Cell dose restriction would not reduce the net insertions administered by a factor of more than 5 and patients would still receive millions of transduced cells each with the potential to transform. Moreover, infusion of smaller doses of transduced cells might confer a replicative stress to these cells, increasing the likelihood of additional genetic events, which could lead to full transformation in cooperation with vector insertion events. In a non-myeloablative setting, the therapeutic effect of lower doses of transduced cells would also be diluted by the endogenous HSC, unless the genetically corrected cells have a competitive advantage, such as in X-SCID.

Adrenoleukodystrophy

The demonstration of gene transfer vector-related complications in the X-SCID and CGD clinical trials contributed to the conclusion that the characteristics of standard gammaretroviral vectors based on MMLV preclude further application in HSC gene therapy. A new generation of clinical trials has moved forward supported by preclinical data suggesting that HIV-derived lentiviral vectors may be safer and more efficient for transduction of HSC than vectors based on gammaretroviral vectors [129–136]. The first use of a lentiviral vector was reported for the treatment of two children with X-linked ALD (X-ALD), an inherited demyelinating disorder of the central nervous system caused by mutations in *ABCD1*, a gene involved in peroxisomal import of fatty acids in the organelle [31]. In these patients, G-CSF-mobilized $CD34^+$ cells were corrected by gene transfer and reinfused to the children. Functional myelomonocytic cells derived from corrected $CD34^+$ cells migrated into the patient's central nervous system to replace diseased microglia cells. At 24 and 30 months post-transplantation, both patients had highly polyclonal reconstitution of hematopoiesis and normal levels of ALD protein, which appeared to retard the progressive cerebral demyelination process.

β-Thalassemia

Cavazzana-Calvo et al. [33] have recently provided another example of clinical success of gene therapy using lentiviral vectors by treating an 18-year-old male patient suffering from transfusion-dependent β-thalassemia. $CD34^+$ cells were isolated from the individual's BM and transduced with an HIV-derived lentiviral vector containing a functional β-globin gene. Unlike previous gene therapy trials, an intense conditioning regimen was administered to give the incoming corrected $CD34^+$ cells a competitive advantage over the endogenous diseased HSCs. The levels of genetically modified cells gradually rose up to 11% at 33 months post-transplant with concomitant increases in levels of the normal β-globin protein and improved production and quality of normal red blood cells. Remarkably, a year after treatment, the patient no longer needed red blood cell transfusions. This therapeutic benefit, however, was observed in the setting of clonal expansion resulting from integration of lentiviral vector in the HMGA2 (high mobility group AT-hook 2) gene [137]. No complication has yet been documented in this patient, but the known association between HMGA2 overexpression and benign/malignant neoplasias imposes, once more, further caution.

Wiskott-Aldrich Syndrome

WAS is an X-linked complex primary immunodeficiency disorder caused by mutations in the gene that encodes the WAS protein [138]. It is characterized by an increased susceptibility to recurrent infections associated with adaptive and innate immune deficiency, thrombocytopenia, eczema, and autoimmunity [139, 140]. Boztug et al. [32] have recently reported long-term (up to 3 years) correction of WAS in two patients through gammaretroviral infection of G-CSF-mobilized $CD34^+$ cells transfused after busulfan-induced transient myelosuppression. The frequency and severity of infections decreased in both patients after gene therapy. Within the first 12 months after treatment, both patients also experienced resolution of signs and symptoms of autoimmunity, including autoimmune hemolytic anemia, thrombocytopenia, neutropenia, and eczema. No evidence of transformation has been detected in these patients yet, but large-scale analysis of retroviral vector integration sites revealed targeting of potential oncogenes, namely CCND2 and MDS1/EVI, in active gene-corrected clones. Longer follow-up analyses will be warranted to evaluate persistence of clinical benefit without the toxic effects seen in other gammaretrovirus-based stem cell gene transfer clinical trials.

Conclusions

Preclinical animal models have been instrumental to investigate the efficiency of gene transfer into human HSCs. They have clearly established the influence of the source of HSCs on the efficiency of gene transfer. The difference in transduction efficiency of HSCs collected from different sources should be considered whenever planning clinical gene therapy trials and should preferably be tested directly in comparative studies. Steady-state BM and G-CSF-mobilized HSCs are equivalent in their susceptibility to retroviral transduction and currently the main sources of HSCs used in clinical gene therapy. No evidence suggests an increased risk of insertional mutagenesis when cells from either source are used for gene therapy applications. The newly identified mobilizing properties of the CXCR4 antagonist AMD3100 and the recent demonstration of the susceptibility of the cells mobilized with this agent to retroviral infection are likely to bring AMD3100 to the forefront for gene therapy applications.

References

1. Kiem HP, Andrews RG, Morris J et al (1998) Improved gene transfer into baboon marrow repopulating cells using recombinant human fibronectin fragment CH-296 in combination with interleukin-6, stem cell factor, FLT-3 ligand, and megakaryocyte growth and development factor. Blood 92:1878–1886
2. Moritz T, Patel VP, Williams DA (1994) Bone marrow extracellular matrix molecules improve gene transfer into human hematopoietic cells via retroviral vectors. J Clin Invest 93:1451–1457
3. Hanenberg H, Xiao XL, Dilloo D et al (1996) Colocalization of retrovirus and target cells on specific fibronectin fragments increases genetic transduction of mammalian cells. Nat Med 2:876–882
4. Dick JE, Magli MC, Huszar D, Phillips RA, Berstein A (1985) Introduction of a selectable gene into primitive stem cells capable of long-term reconstitution of the hemopoietic system of w/wv mice. Cell 42:71–79
5. Keller G, Paige C, Gilboa E, Wagner EF (1985) Expression of a foreign gene in myeloid and lymphoid cells derived from multipotent haematopoietic precursors. Nature 318:149–154
6. Lemischka IR, Raulet DH, Mulligan RC (1986) Developmental potential and dynamic behavior of hematopoietic stem cells. Cell 45:917–927
7. Porada CD, Tran ND, Almeida-Porada G et al (2002) Transduction of long-term-engrafting human hematopoietic stem cells by retroviral vectors. Hum Gene Ther 13:867–879
8. Zanjani ED, Pallavicini MG, Ascensao JL et al (1992) Engraftment and long-term expression of human fetal hemopoietic stem cells in sheep following transplantation in utero. J Clin Invest 89:1178–1188
9. Shultz LD, Schweitzer PA, Christianson SW et al (1995) Multiple defects in innate and adaptive immunologic function in NOD/LtSz-scid mice. J Immunol 154:180–191
10. Ito M, Hiramatsu H, Kobayashi K et al (2002) NOD/SCID/gamma(c)(null) mouse: an excellent recipient mouse model for engraftment of human cells. Blood 100:3175–3182
11. Shultz LD, Lyons BL, Burzenski LM et al (2005) Human lymphoid and myeloid cell development in NOD/LtSz-scid IL2R gamma null mice engrafted with mobilized human hemopoietic stem cells. J Immunol 174:6477–6489
12. Larochelle A, Vormoor J, Hanenberg H et al (1996) Identification of primitive human hematopoietic cells capable of repopulating NOD/SCID mouse bone marrow: implications for gene therapy. Nat Med 2:1329–1337
13. Schiedlmeier B, Wermann K, Kuhlcke K et al (2000) Human multidrug resistance-1 gene transfer to long-term repopulating human mobilized peripheral blood progenitor cells. Bone Marrow Transplant 25(Suppl 2):S118–S124
14. Brenner S, Whiting-Theobald NL, Linton GF et al (2003) Concentrated RD114-pseudotyped MFGS-gp91phox vector achieves high levels of functional correction of the chronic granulomatous disease oxidase defect in NOD/SCID/beta-microglobulin−/− repopulating mobilized human peripheral blood CD34+ cells. Blood 102:2789–2797
15. Roesler J, Brenner S, Bukovsky AA et al (2002) Third-generation, self-inactivating gp91(phox) lentivector corrects the oxidase defect in NOD/SCID mouse-repopulating peripheral blood-mobilized CD34+ cells from patients with X-linked chronic granulomatous disease. Blood 100:4381–4390

16. Benhamida S, Pflumio F, Dubart-Kupperschmitt A et al (2003) Transduced CD34+ cells from adrenoleukodystrophy patients with HIV-derived vector mediate long-term engraftment of NOD/SCID mice. Mol Ther 7:317–324
17. Hofling AA, Devine S, Vogler C, Sands MS (2004) Human CD34+ hematopoietic progenitor cell-directed lentiviral-mediated gene therapy in a xenotransplantation model of lysosomal storage disease. Mol Ther 9:856–865
18. Horn PA, Thomasson BM, Wood BL et al (2003) Distinct hematopoietic stem/progenitor cell populations are responsible for repopulating NOD/SCID mice versus nonhuman primates. Blood 102:4329–4335
19. Mezquita P, Beard BC, Kiem HP (2008) NOD/SCID repopulating cells contribute only to short-term repopulation in the baboon. Gene Ther 15:1460–1462
20. Abkowitz JL, Persik MT, Shelton GH et al (1995) Behavior of hematopoietic stem cells in a large animal. Proc Natl Acad Sci USA 92:2031–2035
21. Donahue RE, Dunbar CE (2001) An update on the use of non-human primate models for preclinical testing of gene therapy approaches targeting hematopoietic cells. Hum Gene Ther 12:607–617
22. Wu T, Kim HJ, Sellers SE et al (2000) Prolonged high-level detection of retrovirally-marked hematopoietic cells in non-human primates after transduction of CD34+ progenitors using clinically feasible methods. Mol Ther 1:285–293
23. Aiuti A, Slavin S, Aker M et al (2002) Correction of ADA-SCID by stem cell gene therapy combined with nonmyeloablative conditioning. Science 296:2410–2413
24. Aiuti A, Cattaneo F, Galimberti S et al (2009) Gene therapy for immunodeficiency due to adenosine deaminase deficiency. N Engl J Med 360:447–458
25. Cavazzana-Calvo M, Hacein-Bey S, de Saint Basile G et al (2000) Gene therapy of human severe combined immunodeficiency (SCID)-X1 disease. Science 288:669–672
26. Chinen J, Davis J, De Ravin SS et al (2007) Gene therapy improves immune function in preadolescents with X-linked severe combined immunodeficiency. Blood 110:67–73
27. Gaspar HB, Parsley KL, Howe S et al (2004) Gene therapy of X-linked severe combined immunodeficiency by use of a pseudotyped gammaretroviral vector. Lancet 364:2181–2187
28. Hacein-Bey-Abina S, Le Deist F, Carlier F et al (2002) Sustained correction of X-linked severe combined immunodeficiency by ex vivo gene therapy. N Engl J Med 346:1185–1193
29. Ott MG, Schmidt M, Schwarzwaelder K et al (2006) Correction of X-linked chronic granulomatous disease by gene therapy, augmented by insertional activation of MDS1-EVI1, PRDM16 or SETBP1. Nat Med 12:401–409
30. Stein S, Ott MG, Schultze-Strasser S et al (2010) Genomic instability and myelodysplasia with monosomy 7 consequent to EVI1 activation after gene therapy for chronic granulomatous disease. Nat Med 16:198–204
31. Cartier N, Hacein-Bey-Abina S, Bartholomae CC et al (2009) Hematopoietic stem cell gene therapy with a lentiviral vector in X-linked adrenoleukodystrophy. Science 326:818–823
32. Boztug K, Schmidt M, Schwarzer A et al (2010) Stem-cell gene therapy for the Wiskott-Aldrich syndrome. N Engl J Med 363:1918–1927
33. Cavazzana-Calvo M, Payen E, Negre O et al (2010) Transfusion independence and HMGA2 activation after gene therapy of human beta-thalassaemia. Nature 467:318–322
34. Shi PA, Pomper GJ, Metzger ME et al (2001) Assessment of rapid remobilization intervals with G-CSF and SCF in murine and rhesus macague models. Transfusion 41:1438–1444
35. To LB, Haylock DN, Simmons PJ, Juttner CA (1997) The biology and clinical uses of blood stem cells. Blood 89:2233–2258
36. Briddell RA, Hartley CA, Smith KA, McNiece IK (1993) Recombinant rat stem cell factor synergizes with recombinant human granulocyte colony-stimulating factor in vivo in mice to mobilize peripheral blood progenitor cells that have enhanced repopulating potential. Blood 82:1720–1723
37. Yan XQ, Briddell R, Hartley C et al (1994) Mobilization of long-term hematopoietic reconstituting cells in mice by the combination of stem cell factor plus granulocyte colony-stimulating factor. Blood 84:795–799

38. Yan XQ, Hartley C, McElroy P et al (1995) Peripheral blood progenitor cells mobilized by recombinant granulocyte colony-stimulating factor plus recombinant rat stem cell factor contain long-term engrafting cells capable of cellular proliferation for more than two years as shown by serial transplantation in mice. Blood 85:2303–2307
39. de Revel T, Appelbaum FR, Storb R et al (1994) Effects of granulocyte colony-stimulating factor and stem cell factor, alone and in combination, on the mobilization of peripheral blood cells that engraft lethally irradiated dogs. Blood 83:3795–3799
40. Andrews RG, Briddell RA, Knitter GH et al (1994) In vivo synergy between recombinant human stem cell factor and recombinant human granulocyte colony-stimulating factor in baboons enhanced circulation of progenitor cells. Blood 84:800–810
41. Andrews RG, Briddell RA, Knitter GH et al (1995) Rapid engraftment by peripheral blood progenitor cells mobilized by recombinant human stem cell factor and recombinant human granulocyte colony-stimulating factor in nonhuman primates. Blood 85:15–20
42. Andrews RG, Bensinger WI, Knitter GH et al (1992) The ligand for c-kit, stem cell factor, stimulates the circulation of cells that engraft lethally irradiated baboons. Blood 80:2715–2720
43. Donahue RE, Kirby MR, Metzger ME et al (1996) Peripheral blood CD34+ cells differ from bone marrow CD34+ cells in Thy-1 expression and cell cycle status in nonhuman primates mobilized or non mobilized with granulocyte colony-stimulating factor and/or stem cell factor. Blood 87:1644–1653
44. Facon T, Harousseau JL, Maloisel F et al (1999) Stem cell factor in combination with filgrastim after chemotherapy improves peripheral blood progenitor cell yield and reduces apheresis requirements in multiple myeloma patients: a randomized, controlled trial. Blood 94:1218–1225
45. Glaspy JA, Shpall EJ, LeMaistre CF et al (1997) Peripheral blood progenitor cell mobilization using stem cell factor in combination with filgrastim in breast cancer patients. Blood 90:2939–2951
46. Moskowitz CH, Stiff P, Gordon MS et al (1997) Recombinant methionyl human stem cell factor and filgrastim for peripheral blood progenitor cell mobilization and transplantation in non-Hodgkin's patients – results of a phase I/II trial. Blood 89:3136–3147
47. Shpall EJ, Wheeler CW, Turner SA et al (1997) A randomized phase 3 study of PBPC mobilization by stem cell factor (SCF, STEMGEN) and Filigrastim in patients with high risk breast cancer [abstract]. Blood 90:2627
48. Weaver A, Change J, Wrigley E et al (1998) Randomized comparison of progenitor-cell mobilization using chemotherapy, stem-cell factor, and filgrastim or chemotherapy plus filgrastim alone in patients with ovarian cancer. J Clin Oncol 16:2601–2602
49. Lapidot T, Petit I (2002) Current understanding of stem cell mobilization: the roles of chemokines, proteolytic enzymes, adhesion molecules, cytokines, and stromal cells. Exp Hematol 30:973–981
50. De Clercq E (2003) The bicyclam AMD3100 story. Nat Rev Drug Discov 2:581–587
51. Donzella GA, Schols D, Lin SW et al (1998) AMD3100, a small molecule inhibitor of HIV-1 entry via the CXCR4 co-receptor. Nat Med 4:72–77
52. Gerlach LO, Skerlj RT, Bridger GJ, Schwartz TW (2001) Molecular interactions of cyclam and bicyclam non-peptide antagonists with the CXCR4 chemokine receptor. J Biol Chem 276:14153–14160
53. Hatse S, Princen K, Bridger G, De Clercq E, Schols D (2002) Chemokine receptor inhibition by AMD3100 is strictly confined to CXCR4. FEBS Lett 527:255–262
54. Hatse S, Princen K, Vermeire K et al (2003) Mutations at the CXCR4 interaction sites for AMD3100 influence anti-CXCR4 antibody binding and HIV-1 entry. FEBS Lett 546:300–306
55. Hendrix CW, Flexner C, MacFarland RT et al (2000) Pharmacokinetics and safety of AMD-3100, a novel antagonist of the CXCR-4 chemokine receptor, in human volunteers. Antimicrob Agents Chemother 44:1667–1673
56. Broxmeyer HE, Orschell CM, Clapp DW et al (2005) Rapid mobilization of murine and human hematopoietic stem and progenitor cells with AMD3100, a CXCR4 antagonist. J Exp Med 201:1307–1318

57. Liles WC, Broxmeyer HE, Rodger E et al (2003) Mobilization of hematopoietic progenitor cells in healthy volunteers by AMD3100, a CXCR4 antagonist. Blood 102:2728–2730
58. Donahue RE, Jin P, Bonifacino AC et al (2009) Plerixafor (AMD3100) and granulocyte colony-stimulating factor (G-CSF) mobilize different CD34+ cell populations based on global gene and microRNA expression signatures. Blood 114:2530–2541
59. Fruehauf S, Veldwijk MR, Seeger T et al (2009) A combination of granulocyte-colony-stimulating factor (G-CSF) and plerixafor mobilizes more primitive peripheral blood progenitor cells than G-CSF alone: results of a European phase II study. Cytotherapy 11:992–1001
60. Larochelle A, Krouse A, Metzger M et al (2006) AMD3100 mobilizes hematopoietic stem cells with long-term repopulating capacity in nonhuman primates. Blood 107:3772–3778
61. Burroughs L, Mielcarek M, Little MT et al (2005) Durable engraftment of AMD3100-mobilized autologous and allogeneic peripheral-blood mononuclear cells in a canine transplantation model. Blood 106:4002–4008
62. Hess DA, Bonde J, Craft TP et al (2007) Human progenitor cells rapidly mobilized by AMD3100 repopulate NOD/SCID mice with increased frequency in comparison to cells from the same donor mobilized by granulocyte colony stimulating factor. Biol Blood Marrow Transplant 13:398–411
63. Liles WC, Rodger E, Broxmeyer HE et al (2005) Augmented mobilization and collection of CD34+ hematopoietic cells from normal human volunteers stimulated with granulocyte-colony-stimulating factor by single-dose administration of AMD3100, a CXCR4 antagonist. Transfusion 45:295–300
64. Devine SM, Flomenberg N, Vesole DH et al (2004) Rapid mobilization of CD34+ cells following administration of the CXCR4 antagonist AMD3100 to patients with multiple myeloma and non-Hodgkin's lymphoma. J Clin Oncol 22:1095–1102
65. Flomenberg N, Comenzo RL, Badel K, Calandra G (2010) Plerixafor (Mozobil) alone to mobilize hematopoietic stem cells from multiple myeloma patients for autologous transplantation. Biol Blood Marrow Transplant 16:695–700
66. Calandra G, McCarty J, McGuirk J et al (2008) AMD3100 plus G-CSF can successfully mobilize CD34+ cells from non-Hodgkin's lymphoma, Hodgkin's disease and multiple myeloma patients previously failing mobilization with chemotherapy and/or cytokine treatment: compassionate use data. Bone Marrow Transplant 41:331–338
67. Cashen A, Lopez S, Gao F et al (2008) A phase II study of plerixafor (AMD3100) plus G-CSF for autologous hematopoietic progenitor cell mobilization in patients with Hodgkin lymphoma. Biol Blood Marrow Transplant 14:1253–1261
68. Flomenberg N, Devine SM, DiPersio JF et al (2005) The use of AMD3100 plus G-CSF for autologous hematopoietic progenitor cell mobilization is superior to G-CSF alone. Blood 106:1867–1874
69. Fowler CJ, Dunn A, Hayes-Lattin B et al (2009) Rescue from failed growth factor and/or chemotherapy HSC mobilization with G-CSF and plerixafor (AMD3100): an institutional experience. Bone Marrow Transplant 43:909–917
70. Stewart DA, Smith C, MacFarland R, Calandra G (2009) Pharmacokinetics and pharmacodynamics of plerixafor in patients with non-Hodgkin lymphoma and multiple myeloma. Biol Blood Marrow Transplant 15:39–46
71. Stiff P, Micallef I, McCarthy P et al (2009) Treatment with plerixafor in non-Hodgkin's lymphoma and multiple myeloma patients to increase the number of peripheral blood stem cells when given a mobilizing regimen of G-CSF: implications for the heavily pretreated patient. Biol Blood Marrow Transplant 15:249–256
72. Dugan MJ, Maziarz RT, Bensinger WI et al (2010) Safety and preliminary efficacy of plerixafor (Mozobil) in combination with chemotherapy and G-CSF: an open-label, multicenter, exploratory trial in patients with multiple myeloma and non-Hodgkin's lymphoma undergoing stem cell mobilization. Bone Marrow Transplant 45:39–47
73. Devine SM, Vij R, Rettig M et al (2008) Rapid mobilization of functional donor hematopoietic cells without G-CSF using AMD3100, an antagonist of the CXCR4/SDF-1 interaction. Blood 112:990–998

74. Bodine DM, Seidel NE, Gale MS, Nienhuis AW, Orlic D (1994) Efficient retrovirus transduction of mouse pluripotent hematopoietic stem cells mobilized into the peripheral blood by treatment with granulocyte colony-stimulating factor and stem cell factor. Blood 84:1482–1491
75. Drize N, Chertkov J, Sadovnikova E, Tiessen S, Zander A (1997) Long-term maintenance of hematopoiesis in irradiated mice by retrovirally transduced peripheral blood stem cells. Blood 89:1811–1817
76. Bodine DM, Seidel NE, Orlic D (1996) Bone marrow collected 14 days after in vivo administration of granulocyte colony stimulating factor (G-CSF) and stem cell factor(SCF) to mice has 10 fold more repopulating ability than untreated bone marrow. Blood 88:89–97
77. Dunbar CE, Seidel NE, Doren S et al (1996) Improved retroviral gene transfer into murine and rhesus peripheral blood or bone marrow repopulating cells primed in vivo with stem cell factor and granulocyte colony-stimulating factor. Proc Natl Acad Sci USA 93:11871–11876
78. Hematti P, Tuchman S, Larochelle A et al (2004) Comparison of retroviral transduction efficiency in CD34+ cells derived from bone marrow versus G-CSF-mobilized or G-CSF plus stem cell factor-mobilized peripheral blood in nonhuman primates. Stem Cells 22:1062–1069
79. Thomasson B, Peterson L, Thompson J, Goerner M, Kiem HP (2003) Direct comparison of steady-state marrow, primed marrow, and mobilized peripheral blood for transduction of hematopoietic stem cells in dogs. Hum Gene Ther 14:1683–1686
80. Abboud M, Laver J, Blau CA (1998) Granulocytosis causing sickle-cell crisis. Lancet 351:959
81. Adler BK, Seizman DE, Carabasi MH et al (2001) Fatal sickle cell crisis after granulocyte colony-stimulating factor administration. Blood 97:3313–3314
82. Grigg AP (2001) Granulocyte colony-stimulating factor-induced sickle cell crisis and multiorgan dysfunction in a patient with compound heterozygous sickle cell/beta+ thalassemia. Blood 97:3998–3999
83. Kamble RT, Tin U, Carrum G (2006) Successful mobilization and transplantation of filgrastim mobilized hematopoietic stem cells in sickle cell-hemoglobin C disease. Bone Marrow Transplant 37:1065–1066
84. Rosenbaum C, Peace D, Rich E, Van BK (2008) Granulocyte colony-stimulating factor-based stem cell mobilization in patients with sickle cell disease. Biol Blood Marrow Transplant 14:719–723
85. Hematti P, Sellers SE, Agricola BA et al (2003) Retroviral transduction efficiency of G-CSF + SCF-mobilized peripheral blood CD34+ cells is superior to G-CSF or G-CSF + Flt3-L-mobilized cells in nonhuman primates. Blood 101:2199–2205
86. Hess DA, Levac KD, Karanu FN et al (2002) Functional analysis of human hematopoietic repopulating cells mobilized with granulocyte colony-stimulating factor alone versus granulocyte colony-stimulating factor in combination with stem cell factor. Blood 100:869–878
87. Hajihosseini M, Iavachev L, Price J (1993) Evidence that retroviruses integrate into post-replication host DNA. EMBO J 12:4969–4974
88. Miller DG, Adam MA, Miller AD (1990) Gene transfer by retrovirus vectors occurs only in cells that are actively replicating at the time of infection. Mol Cell Biol 10:4239–4242
89. Roe T-Y, Reynolds TC, Yu G, Brown PO (1993) Integration of murine leukemia virus DNA depends on mitosis. EMBO J 12:2099–2108
90. Korin YD, Zack JA (1998) Progression to the G1b phase of the cell cycle is required for completion of human immunodeficiency virus type 1 reverse transcription in T cells. J Virol 72:3161–3168
91. Sutton RE, Reitsma MJ, Uchida N, Brown PO (1999) Transduction of human progenitor hematopoietic stem cells by human immunodeficiency virus type 1-based vectors is cell cycle dependent. J Virol 73:3649–3660
92. Gothot A, van der Loo JCM, Clapp DW, Srour EF (1998) Cell cycle-related changes in repopulating capacity of human mobilized peripheral blood CD34+ cells in non-obese diabetic/severe combined immune-deficient mice. Blood 92:2641–2649
93. Takatoku M, Sellers S, Agricola BA et al (2001) Avoidance of stimulation improves engraftment of cultured and retrovirally transduced hematopoietic cells in primates. J Clin Invest 108:447–455

94. Peters SO, Kittler EL, Ramshaw HS, Quesenberry PJ (1996) Ex vivo expansion of murine marrow cells with interleukin-3 (IL-3), IL-6, IL-11, and stem cell factor leads to impaired engraftment in irradiated hosts. Blood 87:30–37
95. Peters SO, Kittler ELW, Ramshaw HS, Quesenberry PJ (1995) Murine marrow cells expanded in culture with IL-3, IL-6, IL-11, and SCF acquire an engraftment defect in normal hosts. Exp Hematol 23:461–466
96. Gan OI, Murdoch B, Larochelle A, Dick JE (1997) Differential maintenance of primitive human SCID-repopulating cells, clonogenic progenitors, and long-term culture-initiating cells after incubation on human bone marrow stromal cells. Blood 90:641–650
97. Orlic D, Girard LJ, Anderson SM et al (1998) Identification of human and mouse hematopoietic stem cell populations expressing high levels of mRNA encoding retrovirus receptors. Blood 91:3247–3254
98. Horwitz ME, Malech HL, Anderson SM et al (1999) Granulocyte colony-stimulating factor mobilized peripheral blood stem cells enter into G1 of the cell cycle and express higher levels of amphotropic retrovirus receptor mRNA. Exp Hematol 27:1160–1167
99. Srour EF, Plett PA, Dale DC et al (2003) Enhancement of G-CSF mobilization of human BM CD34+ cells with AMD3100: substantial increase in the frequency of repopulating cell through tandem administration of G-CSF and AMD3100. Blood 102:455a
100. Giri N, Kaushiva A, Wu T, Sellers SE, Tisdale JF (2001) The effects of SCF/G-CSF prestimulation on radiation sensitivity and engraftment in nonmyeloablated murine hosts. Exp Hematol 29:779–785
101. Tomita Y, Sachs DH, Sykes M (1994) Myelosuppressive conditioning is required to achieve engraftment of pluripotent stem cells contained in moderate doses of syngeneic bone marrow. Blood 83:939–948
102. Armitage JO (1996) Bone marrow transplantation. N Engl J Med 330:827–837
103. Donahue RE, Byrne ER, Thomas TE et al (1996) Transplantation and gene transfer of the human glucocerebrosidase gene into immunoselected primate CD34+ Thy-1+ cells. Blood 88:4166–4172
104. Dunbar CE, Cottler-Fox M, O'Shaughnessy J et al (1995) Retrovirally-marked CD34-enriched peripheral blood and bone marrow cells contribute to long-term engraftment after autologous transplantation. Blood 85:3048–3057
105. Emmons RV, Doren S, Zujewski J et al (1997) Retroviral gene transduction of adult peripheral blood or marrow- derived CD34+ cells for six hours without growth factors or on autologous stroma does not improve marking efficiency assessed in vivo. Blood 89:4040–4046
106. Tisdale JF, Hanazono Y, Sellers SE et al (1998) Ex vivo expansion of genetically marked rhesus peripheral blood progenitor cells results in diminished long-term repopulating ability. Blood 92:1131–1141
107. Bunster E, Meyer R (1933) Improved methods of parabiosis. Anat Rec 57:339–380
108. Chen J, Larochelle A, Fricker S et al (2006) Mobilization as a preparative regimen for hematopoietic stem cell transplantation. Blood 107:3764–3771
109. DiPersio JF, Micallef IN, Stiff PJ et al (2009) Phase III prospective randomized double-blind placebo-controlled trial of plerixafor plus granulocyte colony-stimulating factor compared with placebo plus granulocyte colony-stimulating factor for autologous stem-cell mobilization and transplantation for patients with non-Hodgkin's lymphoma. J Clin Oncol 27:4767–4773
110. DiPersio JF, Stadtmauer EA, Nademanee A et al (2009) Plerixafor and G-CSF versus placebo and G-CSF to mobilize hematopoietic stem cells for autologous stem cell transplantation in patients with multiple myeloma. Blood 113:5720–5726
111. Gaspar HB, Bjorkegren E, Parsley K et al (2006) Successful reconstitution of immunity in ADA-SCID by stem cell gene therapy following cessation of PEG-ADA and use of mild preconditioning. Mol Ther 14:505–513
112. Mitsuyasu RT, Merigan TC, Carr A et al (2009) Phase 2 gene therapy trial of an anti-HIV ribozyme in autologous CD34+ cells. Nat Med 15:285–292
113. Kohn DB, Hershfield MS, Carbonaro D et al (1998) T lymphocytes with a normal ADA gene accumulate after transplantation of transduced autologous umbilical cord blood CD34+ cells in ADA-deficient SCID neonates. Nat Med 4:775–780

114. Brenner MK, Rill DR, Moen RC et al (1993) Gene-marking to trace origin of relapse after autologous bone marrow transplantation. Lancet 341:85–86
115. Brenner MK, Rill DR, Holladay MS et al (1993) Gene marking to determine whether autologous marrow infusion restores long-term haemopoiesis in cancer patients. Lancet 342:1134–1137
116. Deisseroth AB, Zu Z, Claxton D et al (1994) Genetic marking shows that Ph+ cell present in autologous transplants of chronic myelogenous leukemia (CML) contribute to relapse after autologous bone marrow transplantation in CML. Blood 83:3068–3076
117. Deisseroth AB, Holmes F, Hortobagyi G, Champlin R (1996) Use of safety-modified retroviruses to introduce chemotherapy resistance sequences into normal hematopoietic cells for chemoprotection during the therapy of breast cancer: a pilot trial. Hum Gene Ther 7:401–416
118. Deisseroth AB, Kantarjian H, Talpaz M et al (1993) Use of two retroviral markers to test relative contribution of marrow and peripheral blood autologous cells to recovery after preparative therapy. The University of Texas M.D. Anderson Cancer Center. Division of Medicine. Hum Gene Ther 4:71–85
119. Rill DR, Santana VM, Roberts WM et al (1994) Direct demonstration that autologous bone marrow transplantation for solid tumors can return a multiplicity of tumorigenic cells. Blood 84:380–383
120. Thrasher AJ, Hacein-Bey-Abina S, Gaspar HB et al (2005) Failure of SCID-X1 gene therapy in older patients. Blood 105:4255–4257
121. Hacein-Bey-Abina S, von Kalle C, Schmidt M et al (2003) A serious adverse event after successful gene therapy for X-linked severe combined immunodeficiency. N Engl J Med 348:255–256
122. Hacein-Bey-Abina S, Garrigue A, Wang GP et al (2008) Insertional oncogenesis in 4 patients after retrovirus-mediated gene therapy of SCID-X1. J Clin Invest 118:3132–3142
123. Hacein-Bey-Abina S, von Kalle C, Schmidt M et al (2003) LMO2-associated clonal T cell proliferation in two patients after gene therapy for SCID-X1. Science 302:415–419
124. Howe SJ, Mansour MR, Schwarzwaelder K et al (2008) Insertional mutagenesis combined with acquired somatic mutations causes leukemogenesis following gene therapy of SCID-X1 patients. J Clin Invest 118:3143–3150
125. Schwarzwaelder K, Howe SJ, Schmidt M et al (2007) Gammaretrovirus-mediated correction of SCID-X1 is associated with skewed vector integration site distribution in vivo. J Clin Invest 117:2241–2249
126. Jirapongsananuruk O, Niemela JE, Malech HL, Fleisher TA (2002) CYBB mutation analysis in X-linked chronic granulomatous disease. Clin Immunol 104:73–76
127. Malech HL, Maples PB, Whiting-Theobald N et al (1997) Prolonged production of NADPH oxidase-corrected granulocytes after gene therapy of chronic granulomatous disease. Proc Natl Acad Sci USA 94:12133–12138
128. Dunbar CE, Larochelle A (2010) Gene therapy activates EVI1, destabilizes chromosomes. Nat Med 16:163–165
129. Baum C (2007) Insertional mutagenesis in gene therapy and stem cell biology. Curr Opin Hematol 14:337–342
130. Case SS, Price MA, Jordan CT et al (1999) Stable transduction of quiescent CD34+CD38– human hematopoietic cells by HIV-1-based lentiviral vectors. Proc Natl Acad Sci USA 96:2988–2993
131. Kim YJ, Kim YS, Larochelle A et al (2009) Sustained high level polyclonal hematopoietic marking and transgene expression four years following autologous transplantation of rhesus macaques with SIV lentiviral vector transduced CD34+ cells. Blood 113:5434–5443
132. Mazurier F, Gan OI, McKenzie JL, Doedens M, Dick JE (2004) Lentivector-mediated clonal tracking reveals intrinsic heterogeneity in the human hematopoietic stem cell compartment and culture-induced stem cell impairment. Blood 103:545–552
133. Miyoshi H, Smith KA, Mosier DE, Verma IM, Torbett BE (1999) Transduction of human CD34+ cells that mediate long-term engraftment of NOD/SCID mice by HIV vectors. Science 283:682–686

134. Nienhuis AW, Dunbar CE, Sorrentino BP (2006) Genotoxicity of retroviral integration in hematopoietic cells. Mol Ther 13:1031–1049
135. Trobridge GD, Beard BC, Gooch C et al (2008) Efficient transduction of pigtailed macaque hematopoietic repopulating cells with HIV-based lentiviral vectors. Blood 111:5537–5543
136. Uchida N, Sutton RE, Friera AM et al (1998) HIV, but not murine leukemia virus, vectors mediate high efficiency gene transfer into freshly isolated Go/G1 human hematopoietic stem cells. Proc Natl Acad Sci USA 95:11939–11944
137. Ikeda K, Mason PJ, Bessler M (2011) 3′UTR-truncated Hmga2 cDNA causes MPN-like hematopoiesis by conferring a clonal growth advantage at the level of HSC in mice. Blood 117:5860–5869
138. Derry JM, Ochs HD, Francke U (1994) Isolation of a novel gene mutated in Wiskott-Aldrich syndrome. Cell 78:635–644
139. Notarangelo LD, Miao CH, Ochs HD (2008) Wiskott-Aldrich syndrome. Curr Opin Hematol 15:30–36
140. Puck JM, Candotti F (2006) Lessons from the Wiskott-Aldrich syndrome. N Engl J Med 355:1759–1761
141. Amado RG, Mitsuyasu RT, Rosenblatt JD et al (2004) Anti-human immunodeficiency virus hematopoietic progenitor cell-delivered ribozyme in a phase I study: myeloid and lymphoid reconstitution in human immunodeficiency virus type-1-infected patients. Hum Gene Ther 15:251–262
142. Abonour R, Williams DA, Einhorn L et al (2000) Efficient retrovirus-mediated transfer of the multidrug resistance 1 gene into autologous human long-term repopulating hematopoietic stem cells. Nat Med 6:652–658
143. Liu JM, Kim S, Read EJ et al (1999) Engraftment of hematopoietic progenitor cells transduced with the Fanconi Anemia Group C gene (FANCC). Hum Gene Ther 10:2337–2346
144. Cowan KH, Moscow JA, Huang H et al (1999) Paclitaxel chemotherapy following autologous stem cell transplantation and engraftment of hematopoietic cells transduced with a retrovirus containing the multidrug resistance cDNA (MDR1) in metastatic breast cancer patients. Clin Cancer Res 5:1619–1628
145. Kohn DB, Bauer G, Rice CR et al (1999) A clinical trial of retroviral-mediated transfer of a rev-responsive element decoy gene into CD34(+) cells from the bone marrow of human immunodeficiency virus-1-infected children. Blood 94:368–371
146. Dunbar CE, Kohn DB, Schiffman R et al (1998) Retroviral transfer of the glucocerebrosidase gene into CD34+ cells from patients with Gaucher disease: in vivo detection of transduced cells without myeloablation. Hum Gene Ther 9:2629–2640
147. Hesdorffer C, Ayello J, Ward M et al (1998) Phase I trial of retroviral-mediated transfer of the human MDR1 gene as marrow chemoprotection in patients undergoing high-dose chemotherapy and autologous stem-cell transplantation. J Clin Oncol 16:165–172
148. Bordignon C, Notarangelo LD, Nobili N et al (1995) Gene therapy in peripheral blood lymphocytes and bone marrow for ADA-immunodeficient patients. Science 270:470–475
149. Deisseroth AB, Kavanagh J, Champlin R (1994) Use of safety-modified retroviruses to introduce chemotherapy resistance sequences into normal hematopoietic cells for chemoprotection during the therapy of ovarian cancer: a pilot trial. Hum Gene Ther 5:1507–1522

Index

S. Fruehauf et al. (eds.), *Novel Developments in Stem Cell Mobilization: Focus on CXCR4*, DOI 10.1007/978-1-4614-1960-0,

R

S

T

MIX
Papier aus verantwortungsvollen Quellen
Paper from responsible sources
FSC® C105338

If you have any concerns about our products,
you can contact us on
ProductSafety@springernature.com

In case Publisher is established outside the EU,
the EU authorized representative is:
Springer Nature Customer Service Center GmbH
Europaplatz 3, 69115 Heidelberg, Germany

Printed by Libri Plureos GmbH
in Hamburg, Germany